Psychosocial Nursing
*Care of Physically Ill Patients
and Their Families*

Psychosocial Nursing

Care of Physically Ill Patients and Their Families

THIRD EDITION

Patricia D. Barry, PhD, APRN, CS

Clinical Nurse Specialist in Consultation Liaison Psychiatry
Hartford, Connecticut

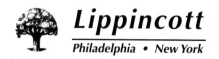

Lippincott

Philadelphia • New York

Acquisitions Editor: *Margaret Belcher*
Coordinating Editorial Assistant: *Emily Cotlier*
Project Editor: *Roberta Spivek*
Production Manager: *Helen Ewan*
Production Coordinator: *Patricia McCloskey*
Senior Design Coordinator: *Kathy Kelley-Luedtke*
Indexer: *Victoria Boyle*

Edition: Third

Library of Congress Cataloging–in–Publication Data

Barry, Patricia D.
     Psychosocial nursing: care of physically ill patients and their families /
Patricia D. Barry. -- 3rd ed.
         p.   cm.
     Rev. ed. of: Psychosocial nursing assessment and intervention /
Patricia D. Barry. 2nd ed., ©1989.
     Includes bibliographical references and index.
     ISBN 0-397-55146-0
     1. Sick--Psychology.   2. Sick--Family relationships.   3. Nursing--Psychological
aspects.   4. Nursing assessment.   I. Barry, Patricia D.   Psychosocial nursing assessment
and intervention.   II. Title.
     [DNLM: 1. Nurse-Patient Relations.   2. Adaptation, Psychological--nurses' instruction.
  3. Attitude to Health.   4. Nursing Assessment.   5. Sick Role.   WY 87 B2811p 1996]
R726.5.B36   1996
610.73--dc20

DNLM/DLC
for Library of Congress   95-40125
                                                                                  CIP

The material contained in this volume was submitted as previously unpublished material, except in the instances in which credit has been given to the source from which some of the illustrative material was derived.

Any procedure or practice described in this book should be applied by the health-care practitioner under appropriate supervision in accordance with professional standards of care used with regard to the unique circumstances that apply in each practice situation. Care has been taken to confirm the accuracy of information presented and to describe generally accepted practices. However, the authors, editors, and publisher cannot accept any responsibility for errors or omissions or for any consequences from application of the information in this book and make no warranty, express or implied, with respect to the contents of the book.

The authors and publisher have exerted every effort to ensure that drug selection and dosage set forth in this text are in accordance with current recommendations and practice at the time of publication. However, in view of ongoing research, changes in government regulations, and the constant flow of information relating to drug therapy and drug reactions, the reader is urged to check the package insert for each drug for any change in indications and dosage and for added warnings and precautions. This is particularly important when the recommended agent is a new or infrequently employed drug.

Materials appearing in this book prepared by individuals as part of their official duties as U.S. government employees are not covered by the above-mentioned copyright.

9 8 7 6 5 4 3 2

This book is dedicated to my family

and to a new life
Katherine Elizabeth Dodd
Born October 21, 1994

The inherent wisdom in her
remarkable eyes
speaks of the spirit within

and to

David Tolman Miller
who left his committed
and well-lived life on
July 21, 1993

David Miller was the editor of the first edition of this book. His support and warm encouragement were never failing. I remember fondly one telephone conversation when David and I were talking about different types of emotional states. He named several—awe, faith, joy, despair, hope, and wonder—and questioned whether they could be called emotional states. Now, several years and a Ph.D with clinical work and research in the psychophysiology of emotion later, I recognize that David was naming states of the human spirit.

David Miller was a man of spirit.
His spirit continues in the third edition of this book.
Thank you, David.

Contributors

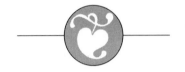

Nell Baker, M.S., R.N.
Psychiatry Clinical Nurse Specialist
Children's Medical Center of Dallas
Dallas, Texas

Marcy Bartolovic, M.S.N.
Education Specialist
Department of Education and Research
The Medical Center, Inc.
Beaver, Pennsylvania

Henrietta Bernal, R.N., Ph.D.
Associate Professor
University of Connecticut School of Nursing
Storrs, Connecticut
Center for International Community Health Studies
Department of Community Medicine
Farmington, Connecticut

Lori Clark, R.N., M.S.N.
Clinical Nurse Specialist
The Massachusetts General Hospital
Mother and Child Center of the Vincent Obstetrics Program
Boston, Massachusetts

Anne O' Rourke Cloutier, R.N., M.S.N., O.C.N.
Clinical Nurse Specialist
Department of Education
H. Lee Moffitt Cancer Center and Research Institute
Tampa, Florida

Michael Dauria
Teacher, Practitioner, and Student of Chinese Healing Practices
Farmington, Connecticut

Janet Duffey, R.N.,C., B.S.N.
Psychiatric Program Manager
Visiting Nurse Association and Hospice of Northern California
Emeryville, California

Rebecca Flannery, B.M., M.M.
Consulting Holistic Physical Therapist
Burlington, Connecticut

Sheila Ferrall, R.N., M.S., O.C.N.
Clinical Nurse Specialist
Department of Education
H. Lee Moffitt Cancer Center and Research Institute
Tampa, Florida

Miriam Hirsch, B.S., M.S.
Coordinator
American Parkinson's Disease Association
Information and Referral Service of Virginia
Department of Neurology
University of Virginia
Charlottesville, Virginia

Karen Inaba, M.S., R.N., P.M.H.N.P.
Psychiatric Mental Health Nurse Practitioner
Portland Veterans Affairs Medical Center
Portland, Oregon

Marcia Miller, R.N., M.S., C.S.
Psychiatric Program Manager
Visiting Nurse Association and Hospice of Northern California
Emeryville, California

Pamela Minarik, R.N., M.S., FAAN
Associate Professor
Yale University School of Nursing
Psychiatric Liaison Clinical Nurse Specialist
Yale-New Haven Hospital
New Haven, Connecticut

Ann Minor, R.N., C.
Holistic Nurse/Therapeutic Touch Consultant
Bristol Hospital
Bristol, Connecticut

Jane Neese, Ph.D., R.N., C.S.
Assistant Professor
School of Nursing
University of North Carolina at Charlotte
Charlotte, North Carolina

Ann Robinette, M.S.,R.N., C.S., A.R.N.P.
Psychiatric Clinical Nurse Specialist
H. Lee Moffitt Cancer Center and Research Institute
Tampa, Florida

Mary Beth Singer, R.N., M.S., C.S., O.C.N.
Adult Nurse Practitioner
New England Medical Center
Hematology/Oncology Clinical Center
Boston, Massachusetts

Dale Stover, Ph.D.
Professor
Department of Native American and Spiritual Studies
University of Nebraska
Omaha, Nebraska

Anita Thompson-Heisterman, R.N., M.S.N., C.S.
Clinical Nurse Specialist
Clinical Associate Professor of Nursing
University of Virginia
Charlottesville, Virginia

Preface

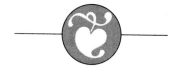

It is with pleasure that the third edition of this book is brought to press. The content is a reflection on the multiple roles of nurses in today's dynamic health care world.

The demands in today's society are occurring concurrently with sharp cutbacks in hospital admissions, lengths of stay, and outpatient services. These rapid changes have resulted in increased distress in individuals and families experiencing chronic or acute illness, who are increasingly receiving care in the home. The strong emphasis in this text on family assessment and intervention can provide a supportive foundation for nurses who are practicing in home care environments.

This edition has been written to support nurses in intensive, acute, and home care settings as they work to provide caring environments. The content in this edition is intended to provide reliable psychosocial assessment, diagnosis, planning, and intervention recommendations.

Nursing students in all clinical settings will find that this widely expanded edition provides the underlying rationale for developing workable care plans that can reduce or resolve clinical problems. Practicing nurses will find practical recommendations that can be counted on to reduce patients' and families' emotional pain and increase their potential for adaptation to illness.

New content in this edition includes a chapter on *stress and its effects on the body*. The chapter describes scientific information from the new medical science field of psychoneuroimmunology (PNI) that reviews how stress is mediated through the mind, central nervous, endocrine, and immune systems to result in systemic, biopsychosocial responses. The description of PNI in this chapter provides some basic concepts that underlie the potential contribution of stress to both physical and mental illness.

I am delighted that there are so many contributors to this edition who are experts in their fields. Their newly written chapters, described below, offer strong clinical recommendations that will provide excellent clinical resources to nurses in undergraduate and graduate school settings, as well as experienced nurses in clinical practice.

There are two newly written chapters on *ineffective coping* that address the two most common outcomes of ineffective coping: anxiety and depression. These chapters present rich new assessment and intervention recommendations that will be helpful to nurses in all settings.

The clinical specialties addressed in chapters that are new additions to this text are: oncology and hospice, pain management, home care, emergency room, maternal-child, pediatric–adolescent, general medical surgical, and older adult. These chapters were written by clinical nurse specialists (CNS's) in consultation liaison psychiatry or CNS's in the specific clinical specialties. These expert nurses bring to this text a wealth of knowledge about the specific psychosocial problems faced by patients and families in these clinical specialties.

The challenges of multicultural nursing, addressed in a *cultural assessment* chapter, are timely and pertinent for both acute and home care patients and families. A chapter on *therapeutic touch* (TT), a healing practice that is used by many nurses to reduce discomfort in patients with physical and emotional distress, focuses on a method developed by Dr. Dolores Krieger of New York University.

Because the text is based on the premise of a systemic, biopsychosocial approach to nursing care, there is a chapter on *holism and its interactive effects on health and illness.* A section in the chapter addresses different healing practices, also known as "alternative" or "complementary" therapeutic options. These alternative methods are included because it is increasingly common for individuals receiving "traditional" allopathic medical treatment to consult also with alternative health providers. Because nurses are often the confidantes of patients and families about the use of alternative treatments, it can be helpful to be familiar with these methods. The chapter also includes concepts about healing practices from the Ayurvedic, Chinese, and Native American healing traditions. These ancient practices often provide the fundamental principles for many of the current mind-body techniques practiced in many of the "new" alternative methods.

It is my sincere hope that all nurses will find their practices enhanced by the knowledge provided in this edition. The energy and impetus for the writing of this expanded third edition of *Psychosocial Nursing: Care of Physically Ill Patients and Their Families* was derived from my belief that nurses can influence the future quality of life of patients and families who might otherwise maladapt. Nurses can and do help assuage the powerful effects of acute and chronic illness in the lives of these individuals. Providing quality psychosocial care is often at the "heart" of nursing and is the source of deep satisfaction for caring nurses. This book is written for all of them.

Patricia D. Barry, Ph.D., A.P.R.N., C.S.

Contents

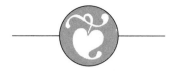

PART I

FOUNDATION CONCEPTS: PSYCHOSOCIAL ASSESSMENT IN THE PHYSICAL ILLNESS SETTING

The first part of this book includes theoretical perspectives that can form the foundations of the nursing process of assessment and diagnosis. Strategies for planning the intervention, intervening, and evaluating the intervention are developed. Part 1 includes many new concepts that generally have not been presented to nurses, as well as material perhaps already familiar from introductory courses in psychology. These concepts are integrated with recently developed theory to provide a deeper understanding of the psychosocial responses of human beings to the stress of illness.

Part 1 is designed to present the normal to abnormal range of psychosocial reactions that will be observed in patients and family members responding to physical illness. Theories about the cause, effect, and signs of psychosocial maladaptation are emphasized.

CHAPTER 1

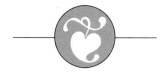

The Rationale for Psychosocial Assessment

Patricia Barry

This book will be addressing principles of psychosocial functioning. It is important for the nurse to be aware, however, that there is a crucial integration of biological processes with psychosocial dynamics. At present, research on biopsychosocial mechanisms is still in its infancy; therefore, this book is using a psychosocial perspective.

Biopsychosocial functioning can be complex to define. It involves a vast array of integrated biological, psychological, and social systems that are essential for normal human development. Biological processes are essential to the maintenance of life. Psychological functioning determines motivation, motor ability, intellectual development, perception, speech, decision-making ability, and many other characteristics that are the basis of full human functioning (Kaplan & Sadock, 1994, 1995). Social systems provide sustenance and adaptation for both the biological and psychological realms.

If a person is physically and mentally healthy, these three realms will promote well-being (Hackett et al., 1991; Kaplan & Sadock, 1994a, 1994b, 1995; Thompson, 1991). However, if a person is under physical, emotional, or social stress, then one or more of these spheres of functioning may not work properly and may cause distress for the patient, his or her family, and others in the social environment.

EVOLUTION OF CARE

THE SHIFT FROM HOSPITAL TO COMMUNITY-BASED NURSING

By the year 2000, it is anticipated that one-half of all individuals currently treated as inpatients in an acute care hospital will be cared for at home or in community-based outpatient settings. This shift, already in progress, is creating an increase in stress for patients, their families, and the nurses working in these settings.

Unknown types of experiences create challenging or threatening demands on patients and families, and can result in effective coping or ineffective coping. Effective coping can result in adaptation and new learning for all concerned (Aguilera, 1994; Carpenito, 1993).

Patricia Barry: *Psychosocial Nursing: Care of Physically Ill Patients and Their Families,* 3rd ed.
© 1996 Lippincott–Raven Publishers

When ineffective coping occurs, there will be increased stress in the physical, psychological, and social spheres of functioning (Carpenito, 1993; Charney et al., 1993; Felten et al., 1991), resulting in patients who are physically ill and also manifest psychosocial or psychiatric disturbances.

The difference between psychosocial and psychiatric disturbance is that the former is usually experienced as a temporary distress in one's psychological or social functioning. It is reversible through effective coping or well-planned psychosocial intervention. The latter, psychiatric disturbance, is often present before the physical condition occurs and may require psychiatric consultation to assist in the intervention (Hackett et al., 1991).

Correspondingly, an increase in the number of patients who are psychiatrically compromised and have a concurrent physical illness is expected. The increased number of patients with concurrent physical and mental illness being treated in inpatient, community/outpatient, and home care settings will pose new challenges for nurses practicing in these environments (Thobaben, 1990).

INCREASED INTEREST IN MIND/BODY APPROACHES

Today's health care patients and their families are increasingly knowledgeable about their health and its maintenance. One of the active health care movements occurring in Western cultures is an increasing awareness that the mind and body are one entity (Moyers, 1993). Eastern cultures have never wavered from this premise (Raheem, 1991). Increasingly, nurses are finding that their patients are asking questions about such concepts.

The orientation of nursing has traditionally been one of holism in its approach to care (Edlin & Golanty, 1992; Newberry, Jaikins-Madden, & Gerstenberger, 1991). The increased interest in mind/body health approaches provides nurses with an excellent opportunity to provide such information. Nurses' biopsychosocial orientation to health, illness, and prevention offers a unique perspective that can enhance the role of holistic nursing practice in the 21st century.

Integrating Mind and Body Concepts in a Holistic Assessment Process

Mind/body health is the term used to describe the interactions between the mind and the body (Moyers, 1993). In the fields of nursing and medicine, the professional term includes the concept of biopsychosocial interactions (Engel, 1968, 1974). This concept includes the complex interactions between psychological responses, the social environment, and the physiological effects of these three factors.

Nursing is the health profession that most frequently utilizes the biopsychosocial model in assessing human responses to stress and illness. The nurse utilizes these concepts in developing care plans to restore health and promote wellness.

The role of the nurse and nursing itself is expected to expand significantly with the health care reform movement that began in the 1990s. In order to approach the care of physically ill patients and their families in a holistic framework of assessment and intervention, it is important to understand the effects of the patient's physiological and family systems, as well as the medical caregiver system and the patient's regular social environment. These triggering effects have an ongoing impact on the response of the individual and family to illness and their motivation to return to a state of health.

THE ROLE OF CARING

Eriksson (1992) says that the foundation of the caring profession through the ages has been an inclination to help and minister to those suffering.

Eriksson (1994) believes that "true caring is based on compassion. Compassion will emerge in the meeting between suffering and love" (p. 14). She states that training in advanced skills and techniques does not necessarily result in the development of compassion, and implies that compassion is an essential quality that cannot be taught. Compassion is defined by Roach (1992) as a sensitivity to the "pain and brokenness" of the other; a way of living born out of an awareness of one's relationship with another; a quality of presence which allows one to share with and make room for the other.

Boykin and Schoenhoffer (1993) propose that the heart of nursing is caring. They built their Nursing as Caring model on the work of Mayeroff (1971), who describes the necessary ingredients of caring as:

1. *Knowing.* Explicitly and implicitly, knowing that and knowing how, knowing directly and knowing indirectly (p. 14).
2. *Alternating rhythm.* Moving back and forth between a narrower and wider framework, between action and reflection (p. 15).
3. *Patience.* Not a passive waiting, but participating with the other, giving fully of oneself (p. 17).
4. *Honesty.* Positive concept that implies openness, genuineness, and seeing truly (p. 18).
5. *Trust.* Trusting the other to grow in his or her own time and way (p. 20).
6. *Humility.* Ready and willing to learn more about other and self and what caring involves (p. 23).
7. *Hope.* An expression of the plenitude of the present, alive with a sense of the possible (p. 26).
8. *Courage.* Taking risks, going into the unknown, trusting (p. 27).

This book addresses the process of caring for the full range of human needs, using an integrated nursing model that attends to the mind, body, and spirit. This model addresses these needs within the context of the individual's social system networks of family, friends, co-workers, caregivers, and community.

The concepts contained in these pages can be applied in all settings where nurses practice: home, hospital, and community. The precepts of caring and supporting the integrity of mind, body, and spirit in the individual and family are organized into the following sections:

Part 1. Foundation Concepts: Psychosocial Assessment in the Physical Illness Setting

Part 2. The Organizing Framework of Psychosocial Assessment

Part 3. Application of the Psychosocial Component of the Nursing Process

Part 4. Psychosocial Assessment and Intervention with Ineffectively Coping Clients and Families

Part 5. Psychosocial Interventions for Specific Age Groups and Clinical Settings

Part 6. Applying Psychosocial Nursing Principles to Nurses' Self-Care

The premise of this book is that the human being is unique and complex. The effects of illness produce factors that create change in all aspects of normal human functioning: mind, body, and spirit. The caring nurse chooses to assess, diagnose, and intervene when illness results in challenge to all three domains. One of the underlying dynamics of caring is the recognition that inadequate emotional support can result in chronic maladaptation for the patient and family as a response to illness.

CARING AND HEALING PRESENCE

Another concept related to that of caring is *presence*. The healing process of *presence* as described by McKivergin and Daubenmire (1994) is the foundation of nursing practice. It includes the principles of the nursing paradigm: care, the nurse–patient relationship, the energy systems involved in the maintenance of health and wellness, self-care, and the meaning of health as expanding consciousness. The authors suggest an implied relationship between presence, healing, and consciousness—terms that are appearing frequently in publications related to the increasingly popular mind/body wellness model (Butler, 1993; Moyers, 1993). As a relational model between nurse, patient and family, *presence* is comprised of three different levels.

Levels of Therapeutic Presence

The concept of *presence* represents a comprehensive integration of the full potential of human-to-human interaction. It should be noted that the major difference between *caring* and *healing presence* (as described by Benner &

Wrubel [1989] and McKivergin & Dauben-mire [1994]) is that the term *presence* embraces the concept of spirit-to-spirit. The concepts of mind-body-spirit integration, healing, holism, and related matters will be explored in Chapter 4.

PSYCHOSOCIAL MALADAPTATION VS. FUNCTIONAL PSYCHIATRIC ILLNESS

All patients in a hospital setting experience increased physical stress. All are under increased mental stress because of concern about their well-being. However, all patients do not cope equally well with stress. People have unique personalities. With the stress of illness, certain unhealthy personality characteristics that were acquired during the patient's development may surface. These can undermine the patient's ability to adapt to the hospital environment and to the changes brought about by illness. Psychosocial maladaptation can occur and become permanent (Goldberg & Novack, 1992).

Challenged or ineffective coping that causes psychosocial maladaptation to physical illness is different from psychiatric illness. Psychosocial maladaptation is an outcome of ineffective coping with illness that can cause temporary or permanent changes in a person's normal personality functioning. These changes can undermine physical rehabilitation and affect the patient's relationships with others. They also can affect normal roles within family and social groups. Although the patient and family may experience chronic emotional stress and a decrease in the quality of normal social functioning, these changes are not severe enough to be classified as functional psychiatric illness.

A functional psychiatric disorder is one that is caused by one or more malfunctions of intrapsychic or abstract psychological processes. It is not identified as having a physical cause or etiology (Kaplan & Sadock, 1994, 1995). It is important to point out, however, that if psychosocial maladaptation is marked—if, for example, a person has a severe depres-sive reaction to a change in health status—functional psychiatric illness can result.

CONSULTATION/LIAISON PSYCHIATRY

Nurses as well as patients are becoming increasingly aware of the strong effects of psychological stress on physically ill people. A clinical science, called consultation/liaison psychiatry, has emerged that concentrates on understanding the emotional dynamics of the person who is physically ill. The word *liaison,* taken directly from the French, is defined as inter-communication for the purpose of mutual understanding (Larousse, 1955).

In the hospital, a clinician trained in this theoretical framework intervenes with the patient and all caregivers. The clinician explains the behavior of the patient and, if necessary, the family to the caregivers in order to ease the coping process for everyone. In turn, the patient and family may need assistance in understanding the hospital care system. Consultation/liaison psychiatry borrows heavily from general psychiatric theory and combines it with information gained in observing the social processes that normal persons experience in their emotional and physical adaptation to major surgery, chronic illness, or anticipated death (Hackett et al., 1991).

The Family's Response to Illness

Consultation/liaison psychiatry also examines the reactions of families when they have an ill member (McClowry, 1992). The importance of examining the responses of family members can be understood if you recall, for example, the reaction of your mother when you were a child and had a bad bruise. Most likely you received love and understanding and felt better as a result. You probably can still remember the effect her concern had on you. If you did not receive love, you can remember that also.

When a person becomes ill, the response of the patient and each of the family members will be different (McClowry, 1992). The response of one will affect the responses of the others. If a child is ill, for example, the mother will respond to her child based on what the child's illness means to her and how the child responds to the illness. The father, in turn, will respond based on his perceptions of the child's illness and his own personality and coping style. Remember, too, the child's illness introduces a whole new dynamic in the mother–father relationship, and this new stress can affect the parents' ability to support the child and each other. To complicate the picture further, the emotional responses of these three family members are never static. New dynamics enter and can cause daily changes in the way family members react to one another and to illness.

Does all this sound complex? When we begin to examine these aspects of a patient's care, it may seem so initially. Without a theoretical approach that separates and looks at the components involved in the patient and family's psychosocial functioning, these ideas may seem confusing. The ability to perform reliable psychosocial assessment is an important factor in knowing how to support the rehabilitative potential of patients and their family members.

THE NURSE AS MONITOR

Nurses may be in the best position of any member of the caregiving team to monitor and evaluate the patient's and family's psychosocial responses to illness. Nurses spend more time with patients than do any other member of the health care team. Accordingly, they have the best opportunity to observe patients' responses to illness. They also can see the patient interact with family, friends, and other members of the health care team. If psychosocial problems develop, they are most frequently observed by the nurse (O'Connor, 1991).

Nurses are usually viewed by patients as nurturing, supportive people. Patients frequently are able to talk about their feelings with their nurses if their nurses are aware of these feelings and are able to accept them. When nurses are aware of emotional disruption in their patients, they can develop a care plan that will support more adaptive responses and better outcomes. Nurses' observations and recommendations can also be communicated to other members of the health care team who

may not be aware of the difficulty the patient or family is experiencing.

It is important to discipline oneself to speak in complete sentences, avoid using slang, and state all the observed behavioral clues, rather than using one or two general adjectives to explain why a patient or family member is experiencing psychological distress. When a nurse is articulate, other caregivers listen.

The categories and defining characteristics from the North American Nursing Diagnosis Association (NANDA) are used in the majority of nursing care settings to describe psychosocial problems (Carpenito, 1993) (see Chapter 14). Nurses who use NANDA terms to describe their observations have reported informally that physicians understand and respect their opinions; they are usually open to nursing recommendations for medical assistance to reverse the ineffective coping process. The same is true for nursing recommendations given to other hospital caregivers, such as social workers and physical therapists.

A clinically observant and objective nurse who knows how to assess patients' adaptation to physical illness can promote their ability to regain their previous levels of psychic and physical functioning. Remember that living with the results of disfiguring surgery or chronic illness can seriously impair, sometimes permanently, a person's ability to enjoy life. It can also detrimentally affect the lives of family members for months and years.

Patients are often unaware of the long-term (postdischarge) consequences of illness. The effects of illness can have an impact on all aspects of functioning: physiological, intrapsychic, spiritual, interpersonal (both within the family and in the general social environment), and economic.

THE NURSE AS ADVOCATE

Because nurses often have an intuitive awareness of and a sensitivity to their patients' needs, and because patients often choose to confide in them, nurses may be in the best position of the health care team members to be the patient's advocate. Hospitals are now required to employ persons as advocates in order to safeguard patients' rights and well-being and speak out on their behalf. The advocacy role, however, continues to be unofficially carried out by nurses (Boddy, 1993; Kearney & Yeager, 1993; Schoenhofer & Boykin, 1993).

Nurses can monitor the response of the health care system to patients' needs. They can also monitor patients' responses to the health care system's interventions. Accordingly, the nurse should be able to identify those patients who seem to be coping ineffectively with their illnesses and mobilize the health care system's resources to assist them in the adaptation process. If nurses do not identify those patients who are at risk for long-term psychosocial maladaptation, who else will?

ADAPTATION AND MALADAPTATION

Adaptation is the process of adjusting to change. The term *adaptation* implies that a person has effectively coped with, accommodated, and adjusted to a changed set of internal or external conditions. However, not all adjustments are positive ones. For example, a young woman newly diagnosed with diabetes may become sullen and withdrawn. This ineffective coping response to change, if it becomes permanent, is maladaptive and can lead to ongoing maladaptation.

For ease of explanation, *adaptation* will be used here to describe positive adjustment to change; that is, after the event is over, the person's quality of life returns to normal or improves. Maladaptation, on the other hand, is the development after a major change of long-term or permanent negative characteristics that have a harmful effect on a person's physical, emotional, or social spheres (Battegay, 1991; Hagopian, 1993; Woods, Habaerman, & Packard, 1993).

The most important factor in successful adaptation is the person's ability to cope effectively. Coping is a combination of conscious and unconscious mental maneuvers used to maintain emotional stability (Weisman, 1991). Some people are emotionally stronger than others. It is the ability of an individual to cope with new situations that differentiates emotional strengths. For example, a newly admitted patient who will undergo open-heart surgery is faced with a very stressful situation. Her ability to cope with the surgery and convalescence will be largely determined by previous experiences and the way she normally copes with stress. If, in the past, she has folded easily under pressure, she will be more at risk for ineffective coping and maladaptation than someone who has coped well with a variety of difficult situations during previous years.

Roy, 1984 (Stevens Barnum, 1994; Leddy & Pepper, 1993; Parker, 1993) has identified four modes of adaptation that challenge the human being: physiological, self-concept, role function, and interdependence. If failure to adapt occurs in any or all of these modes, then the person is functioning at less than his or her former level. Adaptive functioning can be compared to a four-cylinder car that is trying to operate on three cylinders. The entire engine is working harder than normal, yet its ability and power are lessened.

In order to simplify the forms of adaptation, consider that there are two interrelated areas in which a person must adjust in order to maintain normal level of functioning: the physiological, which includes physical responses to change, and the psychosocial, which is the way the psyche reacts and the way interactions occur with other people and the environment.

THE PHYSIOLOGICAL MODE OF ADAPTATION

The physiological mode of adaptation is inseparable from the psychosocial, because the body's emotional and physical processes interact as a response to the stimulation of the sympathetic division of the autonomic nervous system (Felten et al., 1991).

This essential fact is frequently overlooked in traditional medical diagnosis and treatment. As a result, the patient's disease process is often evaluated using only physical examination data. Although there are clearly recognized cases in which psychological factors can be the presenting symptoms of an undiagnosed physical problem (as in the case of thyroid disease), the psychosocial realm is usually considered by clinicians only when the patient maladapts psychologically after illness occurs.

Instead, it may be the patient's physiological response to emotional stress that causes a physical disease process to occur (Cassem, 1991; Goldberg & Novack, 1992; Henry, 1992).

Unless a diagnostician includes in the evaluation the current intrapsychic and social stressors in the patient's life, diagnosis of the root cause of the physical problem may be overlooked (Goldberg & Novack, 1992). The implications of stress and its role in the development of physical illness will be discussed in detail in Chapter 6.

The Physiological Effects of the Stress of Illness

The physiological mode is regulated partially by the autonomic nervous system (Felten et al., 1991). The autonomic nervous system controls involuntary bodily functions, which include the following major organs: the eyes, salivary glands, blood vessels, lungs, heart, gastrointestinal tract, liver, gall bladder, pancreas, adrenal glands, sweat glands, kidneys, bladder, and internal and external genitalia.

The autonomic nervous system is subdivided into the sympathetic and parasympathetic divisions. Generally, the parasympathetic nervous system regulates automatic body processes. The sympathetic division responds to threatening or challenging events (Felten et al., 1991; Henry, 1992). Both divisions fall under the influence of the hypothalamus gland. The pituitary gland, which is called the master gland of the body, is actually controlled by the hypothalamus. The hypothalamus is a tiny anatomical structure located deep within the limbic system. The limbic system is the seat of emotions in human beings. It appears that the hypothalamus and the limbic system are the bridge between the emotional and physical domains in the human being (Murray, 1991).

How significant are the effects of the emotions on the body? Consider for a moment the body's responses when a person is almost involved in a serious accident. The heart beats rapidly, blood pressure rises, pupils dilate, the mouth feels dry, gastrointestinal activity slows down, and bronchial tubes dilate to allow more oxygen to enter the lungs. The emotion of fear causes the sympathetic nervous system to activate the various physiological responses in the body. Once the fear has subsided, the parasympathetic system takes over again and all organ systems return to their normal level of functioning (Felten et al., 1991).

Research into the relationship between stress and disease development is ongoing, with results demonstrating a far greater association between the physiological and the psychological subsystems of humans than was previously known (Kiecolt-Glaser & Glaser, 1991).

The process of adaptation involves the interaction of the mind and body. The following clinical example illustrates this process more fully:

CASE EXAMPLE

Tom, a 17-year-old high school junior, is a first-string football player and was recently named to his state's all-star football team. He has above-average intelligence. He comes from a lower-middle-class family in which there are five children. He is the oldest child. His life aspirations include attending college on a football scholarship and becoming a civil engineer. One week ago he experienced some disturbing symptoms in his left leg. After being examined by his physician, he was admitted to the hospital, where a malignant tumor of the tibia was diagnosed. In order to save his life, his leg was amputated. ☙

Tom's life, indeed, may be saved by the surgery. The surgical wound should heal rapidly because of his age. If, however, he reacts to this surgery with prolonged anger, resentment, or depression, it is possible that his physiological well-being could be affected. When a person is very angry and believes that the cause of his anger is beyond his control, his body responds the same way it does to extreme fear (Barry, 1991). Think of the detrimental effect these strong emotions could have on the vital signs of blood pressure, pulse, and respiration if they persisted for a long time. In Tom's case, his physiological integrity could be seriously undermined. It has also been discovered that a sense of loss of a valuable entity can depress the body's immunological system (Kiecolt-Glaser & Glaser, 1991), lowering its resistance to infection.

Because of the various mind–body interactions in this case, Tom could be more prone to postoperative complications if he experiences strong and prolonged negative emotion of any type (Barry, 1991). It is critical to be aware of the impact of the emotions on the autonomic nervous system in evaluating a person's adaptation in the physiological mode. Perhaps this case example can demonstrate the assessment challenge of separating the psychosocial and physiological realms.

PSYCHOSOCIAL ADAPTATION TO THE STRESS OF PHYSICAL ILLNESS

Within physical care settings, the psychosocial adaptation process may be the more complex and less understood of the two modes of adaptation. The intrapsychic aspect of this mode is abstract and can only be observed behaviorally. Intrapsychic adaptation is different in every human being; no two people ever respond emotionally in the same way to the same event. This contrasts with physiological adaptation, which is objectively observable and more predictable (Goldberg & Novack, 1992).

The complexities of personality development and the resulting intrapsychic dynamics in the human mind result in an infinite number of possible responses, whereas, on a physical level, the body reacts the same way to a given illness in the majority of persons (Kiecolt-Glaser & Glaser, 1992). For example, the physiological response to an inflamed appendix consists of the classic symptoms of appendicitis: increased white blood cell count, abdominal tenderness, and so forth (Timby & Lewis, 1992).

Psychosocial adaptation to the stress of illness imposes many new stressors on the patient and family. They usually have never experienced these stressors before; accordingly, they do not have a repertoire of coping mechanisms to relieve them. The family, which usually is a major support, is subjected to many new stressors and may temporarily be unable to meet the increased emotional needs of its loved one (McClowry, 1992).

The process of promoting psychosocial adaptation to illness involves awareness of several factors in the patient's psychosocial functioning before and during illness (Goldberg & Novack, 1992). The categories described below have been devised to provide a structure for working with the patient and helping him or her to return to a presickness level of psychosocial, as well as physical, functioning. The remaining chapters will include more specific information to help assess each of these factors.

PSYCHOSOCIAL ASSESSMENT AND THE NURSING PROCESS

Psychosocial adaptation after a major illness depends on many factors. The theory underlying these factors and the description of assessment, nursing diagnosis, care planning, intervention, and evaluation strategies will be presented in the remaining chapters in this book. The factors are:

1. *Social history.* This includes information about a patient's lifestyle and availability of people who can provide emotional support during a difficult event.
2. *Level of stress during the year before admission.* This factor assesses the patient's current life situation, including the major stressors experienced during the past year.
3. *Normal coping pattern.* People respond to difficult times in certain ways. When asked, most patients can describe what they normally do to cope when they have a serious problem or are experiencing high levels of stress.
4. *Neurovegetative changes.* Physical symptoms signal neurophysiological functioning changes from a person's normal physical patterns. They are important clinical signs of psychological stress. The normal stress response, whether caused by anxiety, depression, or some other emotional distress, alters neurotransmitter levels in the body. These neurotransmitters, such as nor-

epinephrine and serotonin, create changes in both the sympathetic and parasympathetic nervous systems (Felten et al., 1991) which affect a number of normal body functions, including sleep patterns, appetite, energy level, and sexual and bowel functioning. These physical functions and the changes in their normal patterns are called neurovegetative changes.

5. *Patient's understanding of illness.* Does the patient fully understand what is now happening and will continue to happen as a result of illness? How threatening is this illness to the patient? Think, for a moment, of Tom, described above in the case example. How long has he had to prepare psychologically for the effects his illness will have on his future? Does the patient believe that psychological stress has contributed to the cause of this illness?

6. *Mental status.* Is there any evidence of emotional, intellectual, or perceptual dysfunctioning at this time?

7. *Personality style.* This is the way a person normally interacts socially with others. Sometimes someone's personality style causes problems in the ability to adapt to hospitalization and caregivers and to the illness.

8. *Major issues of illness.* Illness can cause many types of psychosocial stresses for the patient, as well as for the family. These include disruptions in the ability to trust, maintain self-esteem, retain a sense of control, tolerate a major loss, avoid feelings of guilt, and maintain intimacy in close relationships.

Using the data collected regarding the eight psychosocial assessment factors, nurses should be able to predict with a good level of accuracy how a person will be able to cope with a sudden change in health status. If there is one or more indication of a potential problem, the nurse can observe the patient and family's responses more closely. Stronger supportive care, especially in those areas of psychosocial functioning in which warning indicators are initially observed, can be immediately planned and implemented.

The nurse cannot make the person cope. Rather, when the nurse provides external emotional support, she or he facilitates the patient's own internal coping ability to return to normal. It is common that the stress of illness causes the normal coping ability to regress to a less mature level (Hackett et al., 1991). Accordingly, during the acute phase of illness, it is unlikely that people will cope better than they do when they are well (Goldberg & Novack, 1992).

The major psychosocial issues of illness are trust, shame, self-esteem, control, loss, guilt, and intimacy. Although never formally addressed between most nurses and their patients, these issues are present in all human beings (Erikson, 1963). If the patient has a consistent relationship with a nurse, the dynamics of many of these issues will be present. Can the patient trust the caregivers and himself? How will this condition affect the patient's personal value? What if the patient can't control fear, sadness, or anger? Will life return to normal?

A sensitive nurse can listen for clues that one or more of these issues may be troubling a patient. A caring nurse who pulls up a chair next to the bed can allow the patient to examine some of these issues and begin to resolve them before they become more deeply troubling after discharge.

Immediately after a sudden illness, the adaptive mode of the psyche usually assists the patient by not being aware of the long-term implications of an illness. The immediate concerns of staying alive are all that the mind can tolerate, and it will defend itself by using unconscious defense mechanisms. (The use of defense mechanisms will be explained in Chapter 3.)

If, toward the end of the hospitalization period, a patient begins to question future functioning, questions can be answered honestly or referred to a caregiver who can answer them. This approach is preferable to reassurances that a patient or family member will recognize as untruths. Avoidance of the truth by hospital personnel only causes more feelings of anger and alienation for intelligent patients who are seeking the truth about their conditions and are struggling to regain control of their health.

CONCLUSION

The use of nursing diagnoses in the nursing process necessitates astute biopsychosocial assessment based on sound theory. This is affirmed by the fact that the majority of the nursing diagnosis categories developed by NANDA are psychosocial (Carpenito, 1993). When a psychosocial nursing diagnosis is established, good counseling techniques and knowledge of intervention theory related to ineffective coping in physical illness will be needed.

Knowledge of psychosocial assessment theory is mandatory if patients' and families' adaptations are to be supported. The first essential is to know what to look for. The second part, equally essential, is to know how to intervene when a problem is spotted.

Every day, patients and families face the crisis of physical illness, which has the potential to overwhelm them. If these crises are not averted or worked through, ineffective coping can cause a chronic or permanent deterioration in the quality of life for patients and their families. This type of psychosocial care offers great opportunities for creativity, ingenuity, and deep personal reward for all nurses.

BIBLIOGRAPHY

Aguilera, D. C. (1994). *Crisis intervention: Theory and methodology* (7th ed.) St. Louis: Mosby.

American Heritage college dictionary (3rd ed.). (1993). Boston: Houghton-Mifflin.

Barry, P. (1991). An investigation of cardiovascular, respiratory and skin temperature changes during relaxation and anger inductions. *Dissertation Abstracts International, 52-09-B,* 5012.

Battegay, R. (1991). Defense and coping in the antinomy between self-maintenance and adaptation. *Journal of the American Academy of Psychoanalysis, 19*(3), 471–483.

Benner, P., & Wrubel, J. (1989). *The primacy of caring.* Menlo Park, CA: Addison-Wesley.

Beauchamp, C. J. (1993). Qualitative approaches in nursing research. The centrality of caring: A case study. *NLN Publication, 19-2535,* 338–358.

Black, J. M., & Matassarin-Jacobs, E. (Eds.). (1993). *Luckmann and Sorensen's medical-surgical nursing: A psychophysiologic approach* (4th ed.). Philadelphia: W. B. Saunders.

Boddy, J. (1993). An ethnography of caring and control in an acute psychiatric unit. *Nursing Practice of New Zealand, 8*(1), 43.

Boykin, A., & Schoenhoffer, S. (1993). *Nursing as caring: A model for transforming practice.* New York: National League for Nursing Press.

Butler, K. (Ed.). (1993). *The heart of healing.* Atlanta: Turner Publishing.

Campbell, R. J. (1989). *Psychiatric dictionary* (6th ed.). New York: Oxford University Press.

Carpenito, L. J. (1993). *Nursing diagnosis: Application and clinical practice.* Philadelphia: J. B. Lippincott.

Cassem, N. H. (1991). Depression. In N. H. Cassem (Ed.), *Massachusetts General Hospital handbook of general hospital psychiatry* (3rd ed.) (pp. 237–268). St. Louis: Mosby Year Book.

Charney, D. S., Deutch, A. Y., Krystal, J. H., Soutwick, S. M., & Davis, M. (1993). Psychobiologic mechanisms of posttraumatic stress disorder. *Archives of General Psychiatry, 50*(4), 295–305.

Clements, S., & Cummings, S. (1991). Helplessness and powerlessness: Caring for clients in pain. *Holistic Nursing Practice, 6*(1), 76–85.

Edlin, G., & Golanty, E. (1992). *Health and wellness: A holistic approach* (4th ed.). Boston: Jones and Bartlett.

Engel, G. (1968). *Psychological development in health and disease* (3rd ed.). Philadelphia: W. B. Saunders.

Engel, G. (1974). Memorial lecture: The psychosomatic approach to individual susceptibility to disease. *Gastroenterology, 67*(6), 1085.

Erickson, E. (1963). *Childhood and society* (2nd ed.) New York: Norton.

Eriksson, K. (1994). Theories of caring as health. In D. Gaut & A. Boykin (Eds.), *Caring as healing: Renewal through hope.* New York: National League for Nursing Press.

Eriksson, K. (1992). Caring communion. In D. Gaut (Ed.), *The presence of caring in nursing.* New York: National League for Nursing Press.

Feldstein, M. A., & Rait, D. (1992). Family assessment in an oncology setting. *Cancer Nursing, 15*(3), 161–172.

Felten, D., Cohen, N., Ader, R., Felten, S., Carlson, S., & Roszman, T. (1991). Neurochemical links between the nervous and immune systems. In R. Ader, D. Felten, & N. Cohen (Eds.), *Psychoneuroimmunology* (2nd ed.). San Diego: Academic Press.

Goldberg, R. J. (1993). Depression in medical patients. *Rhode Island Medicine, 76*(8), 391–396.

Goldberg, R. J., & Novak, D. H. (1992). The psychosocial review of systems. *Social Science and Medicine, 35*(3), 261–269.

Groves, J. E., & Kurcharski, A. (1991). Brief psychotherapy. In N. H. Cassem (Ed.), *Massachusetts General Hospital handbook of general hospital psychiatry* (3rd ed.). St. Louis: Mosby Year Book.

Hagopian, G. A. (1993). Cognitive strategies used in adapting to a cancer diagnosis. *Oncology Nursing Forum, 20*(5), 759–763.

Halm, M. A., Titler, M. G., Kleiber, C., Johnson, S. K., Montgomery, L. A., Craft, M. J., Buckwalter, K., Nicholson, A., & Megivern, K. (1993). Behavioral responses of family members during critical illness. *Clinics in Nursing Research, 2*(4), 414–437.

Henry, J. P. (1992). Biological basis of stress response. *Integrating Physiology and Behavioral Science, 27*(1), 66–83.

Kaplan, H. I., & Sadock, B. J. (1995). *Comprehensive textbook of psychiatry/VI* (6th ed.). Baltimore: Williams & Wilkins.

Kearney, C., & Yeager, V. (1993). Practical applications of nursing as caring theory. *NLN Publication, 15-2548,* 93–102.

Kiecolt-Glaser, J., & Glaser, R. (1991). Stress and immune function in humans. In R. Ader, D. Felten, & N. Cohen (Eds.), *Psychoneuroimmunology* (2nd ed.). San Diego: Academic Press.

Larousse's French-English dictionary. (1955). New York: Washington Square Press.

Leddy, S., & Pepper, J. (1993). *Conceptual bases of professional nursing.* Philadelphia: J. B. Lippincott.

Levenson, J. L. (1992). Psychosocial interventions in chronic medical illness. An overview of outcome research. *General Hospital Psychiatry, 14*(6 Suppl.), 43S–49S.

Lipowski, Z. J. (1991). Consultation-liaison psychiatry 1990. *Psychotherapy and Psychosomatics, 55*(2-4), 62–68.

Mayeroff, M. (1971). *On caring.* New York: Harper & Row.

McClowry, S. G. (1992). Family functioning during a critical illness: A systems theory perspective. *Critical Care Nursing Clinics of North America, 4*(4), 559–564.

McKegney, C. P. (1993). Surviving survivors. Coping with caring for patients who have been victimized. *Primary Care, 20*(2), 481–494.

McKivergen, M. J., & Daubenmire, M. J. (1994). The healing process of presence. *Journal of Holistic Nursing, 12*(1), 65–81.

Mettlin, C. J., Bard, M., Boyd, F. J., Kushner, H. D., McKenney, S. J., Mellette, S. J., Saltzstein, S. L., Schain, W. S., Shover, L. R., & Wellisch, D. K. (1991). Patient/psychosocial issues. Patient and family education. *Cancer, 68*(5 Suppl.), 1184–1185.

Moyers, W. (1993). *Healing and the mind.* New York: Doubleday.

Murray, G. B. (1991). Limbic music. In N. H. Cassem (Ed.), *Massachusetts General Hospital handbook of general hospital psychiatry* (3rd ed.). St. Louis: Mosby Year Book.

Newberry, B. H., Jaikins-Madden, J. E., & Gerstenberger, T. J. (1991). *A holistic conceptualization of stress and disease.* New York: AMS Press.

O'Connor, S. (1991). Psychiatric liaison nursing in a changing health care system. In N. H. Cassem (Ed.), *Massachusetts General Hospital handbook of general hospital psychiatry* (3rd ed.). St. Louis: Mosby Year Book.

Parker, M. (1993). *Patterns of nursing theories in practice.* New York: National League for Nursing Press.

Raheem, A. (1991). *Soul return.* Lower Lake, CA: Aslan Publishing.

Roach, M. (1992). *The human act of caring: A blueprint for the health professions* (rev. ed.). Ottawa: Canadian Hospital Association.

Roy, C. (1984). *Introduction to nursing: An adaptation model* (2nd ed.). Englewood Cliffs, N. J.: Prentice–Hall.

Sadler, J. Z., & Hulgus, Y. F. (1992). Clinical problem solving and the biopsychosocial model. *American Journal of Psychiatry, 149*(10), 1315–1323.

Schoenhofer, S. O., & Boykin, A. (1993). Nursing as caring: An emerging general theory of nursing. *NLN Publication, 15-2548,* 83–92.

Stevens Barnum, B. (1994). *Nursing theory: Analysis, application, evaluation* (4th ed.). Philadelphia: J. B. Lippincott.

Suddarth, D. S. (Ed.). (1991). *The Lippincott manual of nursing practice* (5th ed.). Philadelphia: J. B. Lippincott.

Taylor, C. (1993). Nursing ethics: The role of caring. *AWHONNS Clinical Issues in Perinatal and Women's Health Nursing, 4*(4), 552–560.

Teasdale, K. (1993). Information and anxiety: A critical reappraisal. *Journal of Advanced Nursing, 18*(7), 1125–1132.

Thobaben, M. (1990). Depression in the medically-ill homebound patient. *Journal of Home Healthcare Nursing, 9*(4), 15–21.

Thomas, C. L. (Ed.). (1993). *Taber's cyclopedic medical dictionary* (17th ed.). Philadelphia: F. A. Davis.

Thompson, T. L. (Ed.). (1991). Research advances in consultation-liaison psychiatry. *Psychiatric Medicine, 9*(4), 503–648.

Timby, B. K., & Lewis, L. W. (1992). *Fundamental skills and concepts in patient care* (5th ed.). Philadelphia: J. B. Lippincott.

Touhy, T. (1994). The evolution of a caring-based program. In A. Boykin (Ed.), *Living a caring-based program.* New York: National League for Nursing Press.

Weisman, A.D. (1991). Coping with illness. In N. H. Cassem (Ed.), *Massachusetts General Hospital handbook of general hospital psychiatry* (3rd ed.) (pp. 309–320). St. Louis: Mosby Year Book.

Woods, N. F., Habaerman, M. R., & Packard, N. J. (1993). Demands of illness and individual, dyadic, and family adaptation in chronic illness. *Western Journal of Nursing Research, 15*(1), 10–25.

CHAPTER 2

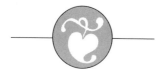

Therapeutic Communication Skills

Patricia Barry

Nurses usually have a good sense of a patient's emotional status. The ability to tune in to emotions is considered by many to be intuition. Actually, this ability develops because nurses are skilled in observing and assessing a patient's nonverbal communication: the barely perceptible cues given by eyes, voice, mood, and body posture. When exposure to patients is combined with good judgment and assessment skills, a nurse frequently is the primary force in identifying patients who need added psychosocial support in adjusting to their illnesses or to changes in lifestyle necessitated by their new body conditions.

Although many patients respond to physical illness with normal adaptive responses, many others find their coping abilities severely taxed when sudden or catastrophic illnesses occur (Aguilera, 1994; Clements & Cummings, 1991). People with immature personalities may also need additional support during their hospitalizations, although their illness itself is not considered life-threatening by hospital personnel. Entering a hospital, for whatever reason, is a severely threatening experience for many people.

At times, patients' families need extra support from hospital caregivers. If their family member is dying, chronically ill, lying in an in-tensive care unit, or waiting for a possibly frightening diagnosis, families frequently rely on nurses to provide understanding and for the opportunity to talk about their concerns. The interpersonal relationship established by a nurse with patients and family members can promote the adaptation and mature coping of all concerned.

This chapter presents a theoretical background and practical suggestions for improving a nurse's ability to alleviate some of the anxiety observed in patients and families. These skills are intended to enhance nurses' counseling skills within the professional role. With a basic knowledge of therapeutic communication theory and a warm, caring approach to patients, the nurse is in an excellent position to help patients and families. It is possible that serious emotional and physical complications may be prevented during or following hospitalizations by relieving some of the emotional stress caused by illness (Brooker & Butterworth, 1993; Burnard & Morrison, 1991; Heifner, 1993; Jones, 1992; Truant & Lohrenz, 1993).

Patricia Barry: *Psychosocial Nursing:*
Care of Physically Ill Patients and Their Families, 3rd ed.
© 1996 Lippincott–Raven Publishers

IDENTIFYING CANDIDATES FOR PSYCHOSOCIAL NURSING INTERVENTION

Any patient or family member in the general hospital, outpatient, or home care setting who demonstrates minimal to moderate levels of anxiety, depression, or any of the psychosocial diagnostic categories (see Chapters 13 and 14) is a suitable candidate for nursing intervention (Carpenito, 1993). Psychosocial nursing skills may be especially helpful with patients who have chronic conditions, such as cancer, respiratory disease, burns, orthopedic problems, and so on (O'Connor, 1991). They also can be well-used by nurses in outpatient departments or visiting nurse agencies who work with patients and families (Klebanoff & Casler, 1986).

It is essential that nurses be able to recognize whether the patient is a candidate for nursing intervention or whether psychiatric consultation is indicated. If there is any question, or if the patient's problem is moderate to severe, discuss it with a clinical supervisor. A decision can then be made about whether to approach the consultation/liaison clinical nurse specialist or the medical team about ordering a psychiatric consultation (Hackett et al., 1991; O'Connor, 1991).

With patients who need psychiatric referral, there usually are strong indications present that maladaptation to illness or hospitalization is occurring. The patient needs support in order to cope more effectively with these stresses. Other reasons for psychiatric referral in the hospital and outpatient settings are a marked change in the patient's previously observed mental status or a mental status of a patient that appears abnormal from the initial admission status (see Chapter 10). If a psychiatric consultation is ordered, talk to the consultant to obtain recommendations about the best therapeutic approaches to use with the patient.

Nurses must be cautious about using newly acquired counseling skills in their personal lives. Nurses' family members and friends often perceive them to be good listeners and advisors. However, nurses should be wary of filling the advising or counseling role with them when they have complex emotional problems.

Objectivity is difficult to maintain when people are emotionally tied to one another. Bias can sway a person from being empathetic and helpful to being overly involved and intrusive (Burnard & Morrison, 1991; Heifner, 1993; Miller, Hedrick, & Orlofsky, 1991).

When a relative or friend is in chronic or severe emotional difficulty, it is important for the nurse to recommend that the family member obtain professional counseling, rather than personally attempting it. It should be noted that psychiatric professionals routinely refer their families or friends to other psychiatric professionals when assistance is indicated.

EMPATHY VS. SYMPATHY

Empathy is an essential quality in a helping relationship. *Empathy* is differentiated from *sympathy* as follows:

> In empathy the helper borrows the patient's feelings in order to understand them fully, but is always aware of his or her own separateness. The helper realizes that the patient's feelings are not the helper's own.
>
> Sympathetic understanding, on the other hand, involves a process in which the helper loses his or her separate identity and takes on the patient's feelings and circumstances, as if the helper were in the patient's place (Barrett-Lennard, 1993; Jackson, 1992; Kelly, 1991).

The following examples may make the differences more understandable. If a person is walking near a frozen lake and sees a person fall through the ice, a helper can either:

1. Carefully walk on the ice and throw a rope or pull the person to safety with a piece of wood; or
2. Walk on the ice and, in the desire to help, get so close to the edge that the ice breaks and the helper falls in, creating the circumstance of two people who now need help.

A similar example concerns someone caught in quicksand. The helper can:

1. Find a board to slide under the trapped person's feet or hold the board so that the person can pull himself out; or

2. Get into the quicksand to help the victim out. Here the victim is not helped and the helper now needs help.

In the two examples described, the first course of action is similar to empathy in a caring relationship. The second action is comparable to sympathy, in which the desire to help a person in difficulty ultimately may cause both people to need help. A common mistake of beginning-level counselors is assuming that the person who needs help is helpless.

The process of relieving another person's psychological distress involves an empathic caring; the caring is much like the rope or board mentioned above. The person being helped is not passive. He is able to help himself. Nurses should remember that the patient, in the great majority of cases, was emotionally stable on admission. Normal coping ability has been temporarily disrupted by the multiple stressors involved in hospitalization. The objective caring of another person can lend the patient the strength to help himself. A caregiver is at risk for sympathetic overinvolvement if the caregiver needs to "jump in" to "make" the other person feel better (Barrett-Lennard, 1993; Jackson, 1992; Kelly, 1991).

There are differences between "caring for" and "caring about" that are encompassed by the term *caring*. In "caring for," the caregiver expresses concern by taking charge of another's life. This type of caregiver enjoys having an invalid or passive person to care for. The caregiver can reduce this person to an object that is predictable and controllable. "Caring about," on the other hand, describes a caregiver who meets the other as a complete person and exhibits respect for that person's abilities and decision-making capacities. In order to promote a patient or family member's normal coping abilities, it is necessary to care *about* them.

This concept can also be described in terms used in transactional analysis, a process of communication in which the communicators are described as filling the roles of adult, parent, or child (Klein, 1980). Transactional communication theory describes the parent as someone who assumes the caretaking role: one who assumes that he or she knows best, regardless of the feelings, thoughts, or abilities

of the other person. The child role describes a person who is passive and yields to the opinions and expectations of another, either willingly or in order to avoid conflict. The adult role, on the other hand, is one in which the person communicates with another by respecting the other's feelings and beliefs, but is able to state his or her own needs and expectations of the other. The ideal relationship is one in which both persons can fill the adult role, communicating honestly with respect for the feelings and reactions of the other, similar to "caring about," as described above.

Gerteis (1993), Jackson (1992), and Rogers (1976) state that the person being helped is responsible for his or her own life and has forces locked inside that will help in achieving optimal development. The helper may turn the key, but the patient must ultimately solve the problem.

INFORMAL AND FORMAL THERAPEUTIC RELATIONSHIPS

Staff nurses will usually engage in less structured types of therapeutic relationships with their patients because of time constraints. In a hospital, nurses usually find it difficult to set aside specific times to talk with patients. Instead, they frequently combine physical care with an informal counseling approach. Once the physical care has been administered, they may continue to stay and talk with the patient about the patient's concerns. Despite being called *informal counseling*, this type of relationship should not be underrated. It has the potential to be the most therapeutic emotional experience the patient has in the hospital (Gerteis, 1993; Jackson, 1992; MacKay, Hughes, & Carver, 1990; Ryden et al., 1991).

Formal counseling can be differentiated from informal counseling because it is prearranged and contacts are made on a scheduled basis. For nurses involved in a formal counseling relationship, an important component is the provision for lack of interruptions; for example, a clinician's beeper should ideally be turned off during a formal counseling interaction. Sometimes an empty room on the nursing unit can be used if privacy cannot be guaranteed elsewhere. This can be prearranged with the head nurse (Litwack, Litwack, & Ballou, 1980).

When it is not possible to find a private place on the unit and the patient has a roommate, respect your patient's need for privacy if you are engaging in a sensitive discussion about the patient's background or current illness. Always close the curtain between the two beds. One of the best ways to promote privacy under these less-than-ideal conditions is to place a chair on the side of the patient's bed that is not adjacent to the roommate's bed. The chair should be placed close to the head of the bed. This way, the conversation will be directed away from the roommate.

Whether talking with patients formally or informally, one of the most important things nurses can do to signify their interest is to sit down. The importance of this gesture to the patient cannot be overemphasized. How many times do caregivers ask, "How are things going for you?" as they stand with their hands on the door knob? The "hand-on-the-door-knob" approach is the quickest way to tell patients that the caregiver really does not have the time to find out.

The most important aspect of any therapeutic relationship is that the patient recognizes his or her need for help. A patient who is not receptive to counseling will derive little, if any, value from it. Additionally, he or she usually will become more resistant to future assistance. An important motivator for any patient in a therapeutic counseling relationship is a feeling of emotional discomfort and the desire to relieve it (Litwack, Litwack, & Ballou, 1980).

PERSONAL QUALITIES OF AN EMPATHETIC LISTENER

The most important characteristics in a helping person are:

1. A genuine feeling of warmth for the person being helped. Rogers (1976) has termed this posture one of unconditional positive regard. The helper must care about the other person and be free of judgment on what the person being helped thinks or feels. The helper accepts the other as he or she is.

2. A capacity for empathetic understanding of the patient's internal frame of reference (Rogers, 1976). This means really understanding how the patient feels. It does not mean how the helper thinks the patient feels after a quick conversation. Unbiased understanding is essential and takes time to develop. It is important to remember that total understanding of the patient's situation is never constant. The listener must always be open to changes in his or her thoughts and feelings and be able to revise his or her awareness of the patient's problems.

3. The ability to be human and real in the relationship. This quality has also been called *authenticity* (Jouard, 1971), *transparency* (Brammer & Shostrom, 1968), and *genuineness* (Cormier & Cormier, 1979). This does not mean sharing one's own opinions or personal history with the patient. It is instead a sharing of one's self. This concept has also been called *encounter* (Jouard, 1971).

A DETERRENT TO THERAPEUTIC RELATIONSHIPS: "PROFESSIONAL DISTANCING"

Because of their constant exposure to illness and death, nurses may unconsciously defend themselves psychologically in the stressful hospital environment. They may cope by pulling back their awareness of what is actually occurring emotionally in their patients and themselves. Nurses are rarely aware when this happens because it is an unconscious defensive tactic. This defense causes "professional distancing" from patients. The result is a cool, detached demeanor in which nurses give technical care and have intimate physical contact with their patients; however, they tune out their awareness of patients' emotional states.

Nurses who are professionally distanced are not capable of giving good-quality, supportive emotional care. Because of distancing and avoidance, they lack the three important personal characteristics of a counselor mentioned above. Flaskerud and colleagues (1979, p. 165) have identified five strategies that many nurses use to avoid closeness with patients:

1. Concentrating on impersonal and regimented aspects of care
2. Presenting self as impotent to change the system
3. Complaining of inadequate staffing
4. Being involved in indirect care
5. Seeking promotion and advancement

Some nurses believe that they should not show their feelings. They may also make decisions for patients rather than with them. These behaviors are the opposite of those required in an open interpersonal relationship.

THE NURSE'S ATTITUDE TOWARD THERAPEUTIC RELATIONSHIPS

Nurses must be able to analyze honestly their normal way of relating to patients if they plan to be effective in a counseling situation. If the nurse has been socialized into giving opinions and advice before patients have a chance to voice their needs, the nurse's potential for therapeutic work is diminished (Gerteis, 1993; Jackson, 1992; MacKay, Hughes, & Carver, 1990; Ryden et al., 1991).

Probably one of the most important characteristics of helpers is the attainment of healthy levels of personal growth. If helpers are immature, guarded, or professionally distanced, they will lack the ability to know themselves and be honest about their own reactions in a relationship.

The following guidelines may help nurses who are ready to move into a more active role in helping their patients cope with new or chronic health conditions:

1. There is no absolutely right way to counsel. (However, by following the guidelines you can potentially avoid the wrong ways.)
2. Know that patients have inner resources and strengths to help themselves.
3. Be nonjudgmental in listening. Let the patient or family member tell his or her story.
4. Repeat what you have heard as feedback and to ensure that you have accurately heard the story.
5. Accept patients or family members where they are.

6. Use the nursing diagnosis criteria to determine if actual or potential psychosocial problems are occurring.
7. Avoid using your own personal value system to judge the clinical appropriateness of the patient's presentation. Use a professional, clinical knowledge base in evaluating the type of intervention that would support effective coping in the patient or family member.

EMOTIONAL SUPPORT IN THERAPEUTIC RELATIONSHIPS

One of the most beneficial aspects of a good therapeutic relationship is the emotional support given to the patient. In many nursing circles, support means reassurances and words of positive encouragement; this is different from the therapeutic support demonstrated in the counseling setting. In a therapeutic relationship, the support comes from the nurse's ability to convey understanding, acceptance, and caring about the patient and the patient's problems.

Open listening is the hallmark of the supportive counselor. No matter what patients say or feel, the nurse accepts them as they are. If, for example, a diabetic man is told that his foot must be amputated, the nurse will allow him to express his feelings freely. His feelings should not be "shut off," and he should not be told that "everything will be all right." If nurses feel compelled to hold back patients' emotions, it may be due to their own anxiety (Gerteis, 1993; Jackson, 1992; MacKay, Hughes, & Carver, 1990; Ryden et al., 1991).

Such anxiety in a nurse seems to have two main sources: the nurse feels helpless in the situation and is not able to tolerate this feeling; or the nurse has experienced similar feelings as the patient and was not able to resolve them (Clements & Cummings, 1991). The patient's distress can be a reminder of the nurse's own similar anxiety. In either case, quick reassurances to the patient usually cut off the anxious feeling for the caregiver but not for the patient, whose anxiety usually increases with this approach. The patient feels even more alone and abandoned. Instead of "shutting off" patients' emotions and expressions, nurses can allow them more therapeutic ventilation of feelings and fears using techniques outlined in the remainder of this chapter.

It is also important to understand the consequences of too much support. Many nurses have a strong need to nurture and attempt to make things better for people. It is important for nurses to be aware of this tendency in themselves. Support can cause problems in a relationship if overused. If the helper helps too much, the resulting feeling in the other, if he or she is a mature person, is frequently resentment or guilt. This occurs because the helper is fostering the other's dependence on him or her. A dependent, immature person may enjoy the excessive support, but it further encourages dependency and discourages personal growth and effective coping (Aguilera, 1991).

Too much warmth from the caregiver is threatening to many people. It is especially so for those with whom a close relationship with another is difficult; it can be experienced as intrusive. Too much support by the nurse also may be interpreted by the patient or family member as shallowness or a Pollyanna attitude about a medical condition that may have inherent complications. This may sour the patient's attitude toward the caregiver. The patient may doubt the helper's honesty and pull back from the relationship. For the dependent person, too much warmth is construed as an effort on the caregiver's part to establish a relationship that will be maintained after the patient's discharge. In conclusion, too much support by a helper also risks a sympathetic rather than an empathetic relationship (remember the consequences of "falling in"?) (Barrett-Lennard, 1993; Kemper, 1992; MacKay, Hughes, & Carver, 1990).

THE "TREE" APPROACH

When nurses begin an informal or formal therapeutic relationship with a patient, their first responsibility is to assess the patient's coping ability. The theory presented in subsequent chapters can be used in assessing the patient and family's psychosocial status. The question a nurse should be able to answer af-

ter assessment is, "What treatment, by whom, is most effective for this person with this specific problem, under which set of circumstances?" This will provide the framework on which to base the intervention. As with any problem-solving process, assessment should be ongoing during the nursing process.

Two main types of approaches can be used in the psychosocial assessment process. One is rigidly structured and formal; the helper has a set format of questions and a set time in which they must be answered. The approach allows little flexibility and spontaneity. It is like an agenda that must be closely followed. If a patient presents interesting sidelights to the problem, the helper usually delays exploration of them until the established list of questions has been answered. Often they are never revisited.

The second approach is one that is informally called the "tree" approach. It is the preferred method to use in assessing psychosocial responses to illness. In this approach, the helper uses a loosely structured format and takes his or her clues about the types of questions to ask from the patient's responses to questions. The nurse asks an open-ended question; as the patient gives the answer and begins to explain a problem, the nurse tries to understand every aspect of it. The problem is explored in the same manner that a squirrel explores a tree. The squirrel usually climbs up from the trunk to a large limb, then on to the branches, then on to the twigs. It does not jump from large limb to large limb. In an assessment process that is too highly structured, the patient is asked specific questions and is told that you will "get back" to the details. In this approach the details never evolve in a natural way. Valuable information may not be obtained.

CONTENT AND PROCESS

Content and process describe what occurs in a helping relationship. *Content* is the factual recording of the conversation between the nurse and the patient or family member. *Process* is how and why the conversation occurred (Burnard & Morrison, 1991; Wachtel, 1993).

For example, a patient may say, "I am worried." The nurse may respond by saying "Oh, Mr. Jones, how can you be worried on such a nice day?" or "You are worried? Here, let me take you for a walk so that we can talk about it" or "I noticed that your wife was in earlier. Does it have something to do with her visit?" In these examples, the content includes the words in the interchange "I am worried." The process includes the underlying dynamics of what happened and why.

The dynamics of the nurse's personality respond in particular ways to the dynamics of the patient's personality and can prompt several types of responses. Similarly, the nurse's response to the patient prompts different reactions in the patient. What effect did the three different nurse responses have on you as you read them? Did one of them make you feel that you could talk freely? Did one of the responses tell you that the nurse was not "open" to the patient's feelings?

CHARACTERISTICS OF THE RELATIONSHIP

Rogers (1976, p. 407) has written, "The counseling relationship is one in which warmth of acceptance and absence of any coercion or personal pressure on the part of the counselor permits the maximum expression of feelings, attitudes, and problems by the patient." Brammer and Shostrom (1968) explain that there are various levels of the helper's impact on the one being helped:

1. *Friendship level.* The helper likes certain qualities in the patient, and the relationship is pleasurable.
2. *Encounter level.* The helper disregards qualities he or she may like or dislike in the patient and accepts the patient as he or she is.
3. *Altruistic level.* The helper loves the patient as a fellow human being.
4. *Erotic level.* The helper responds sexually to the patient, but may or may not be consciously aware of it. Effectiveness with the patient can be impaired, and objectivity can be distorted.

The ideal levels in a counseling relationship are the encounter and altruistic levels.

DYNAMICS OF THE HELPING RELATIONSHIP

There are three important dynamics present in any helping relationship. These phenomena were originally described by Freud (1933), and are called *transference, countertransference,* and *resistance.* They arise in the unconscious of the nurse and the patient; they are not part of one's normal awareness. Whenever nurses do not understand why they or their patients are reacting in particular ways, the answer may be that one or more of these dynamics are operating.

TRANSFERENCE

Kaplan and Sadock (1994, 1995) describe *transference* as an unconscious phenomenon in which the feelings, attitudes, and wishes originally linked with important figures in one's early life are projected onto others. For example, if a normally mature man, after hospitalization, begins to be very demanding and needy with a particular nurse, it is possible that there is a maternal transference. The female nurse, because of physical or personality qualities, reminds the patient of his mother. Feelings that he had long forgotten come to the surface when, because of his illness, he regresses and reverts to immature defense mechanisms or a childlike dependency.

COUNTERTRANSFERENCE

Countertransference is the conscious or unconscious emotional response of the nurse to the patient. It is determined by the nurse's inner needs, rather than by the patient's needs (Kaplan & Sadock, 1994, 1995). If, in the hospital setting, a nurse feels inexplicably drawn to, or repelled by, a particular patient, it is possible that the dynamic of countertransference is occurring; the patient may remind the caregiver of a well-loved or perhaps a disowned family member.

Take, for example, a student nurse who became heavily involved in the care of a 50-year-old man dying of cancer. She requested that he be her patient every day. When she was transferred to another unit, she continued to visit him daily. Her nursing instructor was concerned about her overinvolvement. Eventually it became known that the student's father had died of cancer, and she had never adequately resolved the loss.

When transference or countertransference issues occur in a relationship, the most important thing nurses can do is to be aware of them. It is important to remember that a patient's transference to a particular nurse and the possibly concurrent reduction in optimal emotional functioning may have two important precipitants. The first is a reduced coping level because of the stress of hospitalization (Weisman, 1991). The second is an altered mental state due to organic causes such as residual effects of anesthesia or narcotics, elevated temperature, dehydration, and so on (Goldberg & Novack, 1992). Trying to confront such a patient with the fact that he is treating you like his mother would not have any beneficial effect. Likewise, telling a patient that he reminds you of your dead father is information that is not helpful.

RESISTANCE

Resistance is the conscious or unconscious opposition to the uncovering of the unconscious. Resistance is usually linked to underlying defense mechanisms (Kaplan & Sadock, 1994, 1995). The physician has usually warned the patient that death or serious consequences will occur if her orders are not obeyed. Examples of patients who defy prohibitions are the diabetic who eats anything he wants or the individual with cardiac or respiratory disease who smokes or exercises excessively. Another patient who demonstrates the same "inability to hear" is the one recently diagnosed with terminal illness (Kumasaka & Dungan, 1993).

For each of these persons, the threat to self-image, in addition to the fear of death, causes the mind to use defense mechanisms that result in resistance. A seeming inability to hear

may be the result of the need to shut out full awareness of reality (Groves & Kucharski, 1991; Kaplan & Sadock, 1995).

The most pronounced of the defense mechanisms is denial. Others are distortion, repression, avoidance, rationalization, and suppression (see Chapter 3). For people who cope effectively, it may take only a day or two until they are able to tolerate reality. The defense may disappear and the patient is ready to accept the physician's words. For others, reality remains too threatening, and they may continue to block out the physician's diagnosis and recommendations for much longer time periods. No matter how maladaptive this resistance seems to be, it is important to remember that it protects the patient's emotional equilibrium. Without the protection of these defense mechanisms, the patient might be emotionally overwhelmed. When resistance is present, we can "test" it with gentle questions to determine its strength (Groves & Kurcharski, 1991; Kaplan & Sadock, 1995).

The following case example may clarify this approach:

CASE EXAMPLE

Ed is a 50-year-old, middle-level executive. For the past year he has become increasingly forgetful, and his working ability has deteriorated. He has poor social judgment and poor emotional control. His primary physician admitted him to the general hospital for a neurological workup and psychiatric evaluation. Diagnostic tests indicated that he was experiencing presenile dementia as a result of Alzheimer's disease. Immediately after he was told the diagnosis and prognosis, Ed continued to be very cheerful. Three days later he was very positive about the future and talked about returning to work as soon as possible. He confided to his nurse that he was hoping for a promotion to the home office in another city. ✿

This patient is behaving contrary to normal expectations of a recently diagnosed and ultimately terminal patient with a frightening illness. This should tell us that his emotional status would be very threatened if he were fully aware of the awful reality of his situation.

In working with this patient, one can ask gentle probing questions such as, "How long do you think you will be in the hospital?" or "How do you think things will go for you when you get home?" or "How does your wife feel about your illness?" The responses to these questions will be good indicators of the level of denial. He may respond that he expects to be fine when he goes home and hopes to return to work very soon. If he also tells you that his wife is hopeful and not concerned, his level of defense is very strong.

The use of such a defense is an ineffective attempt at coping. The individual is coping, but the coping is not effective and adaptive. If this ineffective coping continues on an ongoing basis, it will result in maladaptation. The maladaptation will obviously affect him; it will have profound results for his wife and family as well, as they attempt to cope with his denial of reality.

Any attempt to force reality and break through his denial may result in some type of emotional decompensation or further strengthening of his denial. As an example of the need for this defense, imagine the following situation. If you were frightened and alone in a room and someone began to threaten you on the other side of a closed door, would you open it or would you further reinforce it with a chair and anything else available? Remember that the ultimate task of the mind is to defend itself. It will do exactly what you would do in that room if you were frightened.

Frequently, the questioning approach described above will gradually help the patient to become aware of the reality of his circumstances. As he responds to the questions, the reality will slowly become apparent to him. He may become less defensive and more able to cope effectively and tolerate his new life circumstances.

Under no condition should a newly diagnosed and highly resistant patient be blatantly confronted with a statement such as, "Now, Ellen, you know you have cancer. The doctor told you you have only a year to live. Why do you keep ignoring his words?" A formal psychiatric consultation should occur whenever denial is marked and nursing intervention does not result in the desired outcome (O'Connor, 1991).

TYPES OF THERAPEUTIC RELATIONSHIPS

The many types of therapeutic relationships in which health caregivers engage with their patients include interviewing, advising, supporting, guiding, teaching, and counseling (Litwack, Litwack, & Ballou, 1980). The following descriptions of these relationships can differentiate the various roles in which nurses communicate therapeutically with their patients.

INTERVIEWING

The *interview* is primarily a question-and-answer situation in which the caregiver seeks historical data. The interviewer is usually not seeking opinions from the interviewee. *Example:* obtaining a past medical history from a newly admitted patient.

ADVISING

Advising is a helping process in which the advisor works with a person who is trying to make a decision. The advisor knows about the various options open to the advisee. Using knowledge of options and of the advisee's situation, the advisor makes a strong recommendation about the option he or she thinks is best for the advisee. The advisor essentially takes away the advisee's ability to make a decision. This role occurs less frequently due to increased awareness of the need for informed consent.

SUPPORTING

Litwack and colleagues (1980) describe a *supporting* relationship as one in which the supporter approves of the actions of the person being supported. The value system of the supporter enters strongly into the relationship.

There is a difference between *approval support* and the *acceptance support*, discussed earlier in the chapter, which is essential to a counseling relationship. In *acceptance support* the listener supports the person. In *approval sup-*

port the listener supports the person's actions and experiences.

Example: A Reach to Recovery Cancer Society volunteer visits a mastectomy patient in the hospital. She compares the patient's experiences with her own and assures the patient that her responses are within normal limits.

GUIDING

In a *guiding* relationship, the caregiver is similar to the advisor discussed above. The difference is that the caregiver knows the options open to the health care consumer and presents all of them so that the patient can make his or her own decision about the best choice in the particular circumstances (Litwack, Litwack, & Ballou, 1980).

Example: A 66-year-old man is experiencing urinary frequency. The physician diagnoses benign prostatic hypertrophy. The patient has been planning a trip to visit his daughter when she has her baby in 1 month. The physician tells the patient that he can be admitted before or after the trip for cystoscopy and a diagnostic workup. She explains the consequences if surgery is delayed until after the trip is over and then a malignancy is found. The patient ultimately makes his own decision after he has all the necessary information to do so.

TEACHING

In a *teaching* relationship, the teacher presents information about a subject he or she believes the students need to know. It is a strongly dominant–subordinate relationship. The teacher is in control of the relationship, and two-way communication is minimal (Litwack, Litwack, & Ballou, 1980). *Example:* a diabetic class on use of insulin and self-administration by syringe.

COUNSELING

In a *counseling* relationship, the counselor serves as a catalyst for self-exploration by the counselee who is striving to resolve conflicts, make decisions, and solve problems. Counsel-

ing as described in this section is very similar to psychotherapy. Both relationships contain the same elements, but the psychotherapeutic relationship also includes the use of interpretation of unconscious elements by the therapist (Litwack, Litwack, & Ballou, 1980). (Interpretation is explained later in this chapter.)

Example: A cardiac rehabilitation nurse sits with a recent myocardial infarction (MI) patient as he talks about the changes he must make in his life and his feelings about his new status. As he talks, he uncovers concerns and begins to examine ways he can learn to adjust his lifestyle.

ATTENDING BEHAVIORS IN THERAPEUTIC RELATIONSHIPS

An important aspect of a helping relationship is the way the nurse acts while with the patient. This is called *attending behavior.* Attending behavior is the manner in which a listener responds to someone. It can either encourage or discourage patients from wanting to confide (Burnard & Morrison, 1991; Davidhizar, 1992; Heifner, 1993; Jackson, 1992; Jones, 1992; McIntosh, 1991; Savage, 1991; Wachtel, 1993).

These behaviors, also called *kinesics,* include:

1. Eye contact
2. Posture
3. Gesture
4. Verbal behavior

EYE CONTACT

If the helper is an open, unthreatened person and genuinely cares for the patient, consistent eye contact communicates this.

POSTURE

In therapeutic encounters the nurse should be sitting whenever possible. The nurse should demonstrate a relaxed and attentive attitude. An erect but casual posture, rather than one in which the helper either looks ready to fall asleep or bolt out of the chair, encourages the patient to relate his or her problem.

GESTURE

The way the nurse moves his or her head, hands, arms, and legs, and shows facial expression, indicates interest or disinterest in the patient's problem. Just as a slight nod of the head signifies understanding, frequent movements of the nurse's arms and legs, arms folded across the chest, a hand held in front of the mouth, or a blank stare may indicate anxiety or an unwillingness to openly participate in the helping process.

In these attending behaviors, the emphasis is on the nonverbal messages the nurse gives the patient. In developing helping relationships, nurses should also be attentive to the nonverbal messages their patients give them. If a patient demonstrates poor eye contact or posture, or gestures with negative implications, it is possible that the patient is not motivated to be in a counseling situation. Another possibility is that anxiety, depression, or other personality conflicts may be preventing the patient from being free and open in the counseling situation. A neutral or negative response by a patient to a nurse's counseling intervention may cause the nurse to feel unfulfilled or unwanted as a caregiver.

VERBAL BEHAVIOR

The last of the attending behaviors includes the ways in which nurses usually respond to patients. These responses, if positive, will promote the relationship rather than end it prematurely. They include the three responding skills of:

1. Paraphrasing
2. Clarifying
3. Perception-checking

In *paraphrasing*, the helper feeds back only the patient's message and avoids adding ideas. In other words, the helper listens to what the patient says and repeats or rephrases it in his or her own words; the helper "mirrors it back."

Paraphrasing concentrates on the cognitive components of the patient's problem. This is also known as *reflection of content*. After paraphrasing, watch for a nod or some other sign that you have accurately understood the patient's message.

Clarifying differs from paraphrasing in that it does more than rephrase what the patient has said. Instead, the listener takes a guess about the meaning of the patient's statement. The listener asks, "Are you saying that...?" and then asks the patient if the statement is correct. It is advisable not to do this too soon. Otherwise, it is possible to misinterpret the meaning of what the patient is saying, and the patient may then feel even more alone and misunderstood. It is also possible that the patient will feel compelled to agree with the nurse's clarifying statement if he or she is intimidated by persons who represent authority.

A more perceptive paraphrasing and clarifying approach is to listen for and observe the affective or feeling component of what the patient is saying and then share the observations with the patient. If the patient's true feelings are accurately reflected, the interview can shift to a deeper and more meaningful level. The patient may respond, "Finally, someone understands."

A colostomy patient, for example, may frequently repeat that her colostomy is messy, smelly, and so on. In an informal hospital situation the nurse may respond, "Oh, Mrs. Decker, it may seem smelly to you, but I really can't smell it." Or the nurse can pull a chair up to the patient's bed and sit down and say, "Mrs. Decker, you seem worried about this colostomy."

The last of the three responding skills is *perception-checking*. It occurs after the patient has made several statements. Perceptions of the general theme of what the patient has been saying are reflected back. This statement is then followed by a request for the patient's response. For example, the nurse might say, "Mr. Paige, it sounds as if you're depressed because you don't think you'll be able to go back to work because of your respiratory disease and you wonder how you will be able to make your house payments. Is that your biggest concern at this time?"

LEADING SKILLS

Leading skills are particularly important in establishing a helping relationship. They include:

1. Indirect leading
2. Direct leading
3. Focusing
4. Questioning
   a. Open-ended
   b. Close-ended
5. Summarizing
6. Confronting
7. Interpreting
8. Advice giving

As you read about the leading skills described below, take the time to create an image of yourself in a discussion with a patient you have actually cared for. Imagine the way you would carry out each of the leading skills described in this section. If you are a student, it can be very helpful to role play these leading skills with a group of fellow students. One student can be the "patient" and can be assigned a specific diagnosis and accompanying set of psychosocial problems.

Leading types of statements invite the patient to respond. The *indirect leading* statement is deliberately vague and general, such as, "Tell me about your father." The *direct lead* asks for more specific responses, for example, "You said your father was an alcoholic?"

Focusing is best used after the patient has had the chance to discuss various topics, with the nurse using an indirect leading approach. The helper would then "zero-in" on a specific aspect of the patient's explorations. "You mentioned earlier that it was hard for you having an alcoholic father. What was it like?" The helper's focusing techniques then assist in uncovering feelings.

Questioning is a very important leading skill when open-ended questions are used. An *open-ended* question is structured to avoid a single answer from the person being questioned. It should bring forth a response from the patient that requires formulation of a more detailed answer. For example, a nurse may ask a patient, "How did you feel when your father was in the alcohol treatment center?"

A *close-ended* question is one that requires only a one-word answer. A one-word answer can bring the flow of questions to an abrupt halt. When asked "Did you ever feel angry toward your father when he was in the hospital?", the person who replies "no" may make the interviewer uncertain about how to proceed with questioning. Instead, the nurse can say, "What kind of feelings did you have when your father was in the sanitarium?"

When you are in a counseling situation with a patient, a good rule to keep in mind is that the most therapeutic outcome usually occurs when the patient's feelings are discussed. Patients, when asked about their illnesses, often will reply with cognitive statements. For example, if a patient is asked about his leg amputation scheduled for next week, he may reply, "Oh, I think it will be rough" or "I hope it will be okay." Maintain the focus on his feelings rather than on his thoughts or opinions. You can follow up with the question "How do you feel about your amputation next week?"

Often, a patient will describe physical feelings when asked how he or she feels emotionally. Remember that most caregivers are concerned with the patient's physical state. If this happens, clarify that you want to know how the patient feels emotionally. It is often a special relief for a patient to be able to talk about fears and concerns. It is highly therapeutic to release the anxiety that these fears generate.

The examples above should clarify how the process of the interview can be partially blocked or halted completely if a question is phrased poorly. The usual intellectual and affective response to an open-ended questioning approach is that the patient feels freer in the interview and experiences fewer constraints imposed by caregivers. Close-ended questions sometimes introduce the helper's judgment and bias into the interview. Another advantage of the open-ended question is that it may bring forth feelings and attitudes not previously mentioned; these responses may suggest other important and unexplored areas (Burnard & Morrison, 1991; Davidhizar, 1992; Heifner, 1993; Jackson, 1992; Jones, 1992; McIntosh, 1991; Savage, 1991; Wachtel, 1993; Brammer & Shostrom, 1968).

Summarizing is an important skill in a helping relationship. Using this skill, the helper is able to extract the essence of what a person has intellectually and affectively experienced during the discussion time. Summarizing is a statement made at the close of a discussion that describes the content and the process of the interview time. Skillfully and accurately done, it leaves the patient with a sense of affirmation about what he or she feels.

Confronting is a skill that should be used cautiously at this level of counseling. Confrontation is a direct statement made by the nurse that challenges the patient with realistic information that opposes the patient's beliefs. It can be harmful if used before adequate exploration and assessment has occurred. If, for example, a patient or family member is under exceptional stress because of hospitalization and is using denial as a way of coping with it, caregivers frequently think that the person should be confronted.

The following case is an example of how stresses other than hospitalization can have a profound effect on the patient and contribute to her need to deny the situation. In many cases, a sudden illness or hospitalization can be "the straw that breaks the camel's back."

CASE EXAMPLE

Alice was a 48-year-old executive recently transferred to the Midwest from the West coast. At age 45 she had experienced a myocardial infarction (MI). Two months after the move she had a second massive MI and was not expected to live. Her caregivers were concerned and angry that her husband did not understand the seriousness of her illness and, instead, was more concerned about finding a job in the new community.

In talking with him, the psychiatric liaison nurse discovered that his father had died 6 months earlier of a heart attack and that his two teenaged sons had been doing poorly in school since the move. In addition, he had been strongly opposed to, and was very unhappy about, the move away from his family and friends on the West Coast. ❦

Alice's husband needed a chance to talk about the anger and grief he was experiencing because of the overwhelming events that had occurred in the previous 6 months. After only two half-hour discussions, his denial about his wife's terminal status disappeared. Without

understanding the serious underlying issues, a confronting caregiver could have prodded him into a severe crisis situation. An important guideline to use when strong and apparently inappropriate denial is observed is as follows: what is the denial defending the patient or family member from knowing, and why can't he or she tolerate knowing it? This involves taking the time to know what else is occurring in the patient's life.

The type of confrontation discussed in this case example is different than that used in a professional counseling situation. In a professional counseling setting, confrontation is used to give the patient information and feedback about his or her behavior. Confrontation can aid the patient in developing insight by making the patient aware of information about himself or herself that the patient was previously unaware of.

Generally speaking, direct confrontation by a nurse in any situation is not recommended. Instead, a less threatening indirect approach such as, "Is it possible that there is a connection between the severe arguments you told me you have with your husband and the beginning of your asthma symptoms?" could be made. This approach, which still would be threatening to many people, at least gives the patient the opportunity to deny it.

When the statement is phrased as a question preceded by the words "Is it possible that...?" the patient may initially respond by saying "no." Remember, however, that the nurse's comments registered in the patient's unconscious mind. Later, when the reality is less threatening (sometimes days or weeks later), the question may reenter her conscious awareness, and, in the process of answering it by herself, she will gain insight.

Interpreting is an active helping process of explaining the meaning of events to patients so that they are able to see their problems in new ways. Interpreting is a high-level skill that requires training and expertise. It is a psychotherapeutic technique used in individual and group psychotherapy (Spero, 1992). The therapist conveys to the patient the significance and meaning of his or her behavior, constructing into a more meaningful form the patient's resistances, defenses, and transferences. It is usually used in a psychotherapy setting. Unless specially trained, nurses should not attempt to interpret in this manner. If the earlier skills of paraphrasing, clarifying, perception checking, open-ended questions, and accurate reflection of content and affect are mastered, patients usually find their own answers in the counseling setting.

Advice giving, also a leading skill, is contraindicated in almost every counseling situation and in many hospital circumstances. Many of the events that occur during hospitalization include an unexpected or crisis component (Hackett et al., 1991). Occasionally, advice can be gently inserted in a discussion. For example, an adolescent may be diagnosed as diabetic and react maladaptively by ignoring his diet, doing poorly in school, and engaging in antisocial behavior. The diabetes nurse specialist can, in addition to letting him talk about how he feels about his illness, give him information about how others have dealt with the problem. This may give him some alternatives to consider, raise his level of hope, and reverse his maladaptive pattern.

Giving advice may seem to be "the easy way out" in many situations. But ineffective advice giving has negative effects. It also may disrupt patients' rights to reach their own conclusions and informed consent. Frequently, dependent types of people will ask nurses what they should do about a particular problem. Solving problems for patients in this way further encourages their dependence on the caregiving system. Patients may blame caregivers if their situations continue to deteriorate. The caregivers then may feel angry and used.

Another negative effect of advice giving is that the caregiver may react to the patient's resulting dependence by feeling pressured to come up continually with solutions to seemingly impossible problems. Eventually, the burdened caregiver "distances" from the demanding, dependent patient. The result is that the patient feels abandoned and rejected without understanding why the caregiver is avoiding him or her.

OTHER CHARACTERISTICS OF A THERAPEUTIC RELATIONSHIP

CONTRACTS

An important aspect of any relationship is that the two people involved have an understanding of what their responsibilities are, what the relationship means to each, and what each can expect from the other. In formal counseling settings, this is known as a *contract*. The two types of contracts nurses engage in with their patients are *formal* and *informal* contracts. Formal contracts occur when nurses tell patients what their care will involve and patients agree verbally to receive their care. These are verbal contracts and appear informal, but they are taken seriously by the patient. A primary nurse, for example, is someone who makes a formal contract with a patient.

One of the first issues confronting a newly hospitalized patient is trusting an alien environment. For many patients, their nurses are the second most trusted people in the hospital (their physicians usually are first). If nurses do not value themselves properly, they may overlook their importance to patients. Accordingly, they may neglect to tell a patient that they will be off for 2 days. When told this by the head nurse or nurse's substitute, the patient's confidence in the nurse and the environment erodes.

If a clinical nurse specialist promises to see a patient every other day, the patient should be told in advance if this schedule will change. If it is necessary to cancel the visit for a particular day, a call should be made to the nursing unit. A message can be relayed to the patient by a staff member about the cancellation and another time given when the clinical nurse specialist will visit the patient.

Other types of informal contracts with patients are requests for pain medication and the medication nurse's promise to be back in 5 minutes, or a promise in the operating room that the nurse will stay with the patient until the anesthesia is given. Although these may seem incidental, they form the foundation of trust for the hospital patient.

TERMINATION

Termination is the psychological term for saying good-bye. Many people have been negatively socialized about saying good-bye. As a result, they may, figuratively speaking, bury their heads in the sand, try to avoid unpleasant feelings, and assume that there will be no consequences if they do not say good-bye. Although nurses are aware that patients will be discharged from the hospital on a specific day, they may avoid discussing their feelings about the patient's leaving until the day the person is discharged; a quick "good luck" may be the only good-bye the nurse expresses. The patient may be someone to whom the nurse has become attached during a long hospitalization, or there may have been a close primary nurse–patient relationship (Burnard & Morrison, 1991; Heifner, 1993; Jones, 1992; Kelly, 1991; Ryden et al., 1991).

In close relationships where no good-bye is said, both the patient and the nurse will suffer from avoiding talking about feelings of loss. Although they are not the same as with the loss of death, they are feelings of loss nonetheless. If not expressed, they are repressed or avoided. The more adaptive behavior is to acknowledge them and allow them to be felt.

A nurse who avoids discussing feelings about a special patient's discharge may be blocking the patient from expressing similar feelings. A special time of validation of both the patient's worth to the nurse and the nurse's worth to the patient is also lost. An important responsibility nurses have to their patients is to acknowledge the leaving before the actual moment the patient is being wheeled out the door. The patient may also express some anxiety about going home and leaving the protective hospital environment, which otherwise might not be explored. All this is a healthy and normal conclusion to the nurse–patient relationship.

If a formal type of counseling relationship has been established with a patient, termination should be discussed in sessions prior to the final meeting. This gives the patient a chance to work through some feelings about leaving the relationship, and will also promote a more mature way of handling losses in the future (Burnard & Morrison, 1991; Heifner, 1993; Wachtel, 1993).

REFERRAL

In the course of working with a patient, the nurse may become aware that the patient's mental state is deteriorating or is more im-
paired than originally evident. These symptoms of changed mental status (see Chapter 10) should be discussed with the head nurse and physician. The staff nurse in the inpatient or outpatient setting is usually the first caregiver to notice such changes. If warranted, a recommendation for psychiatric consultation can be made to the head nurse. In a primary nursing setting, make the recommendation directly to the physician, taking care to be articulate about the various aspects of the patient's mental status or psychosocial functioning that concern you. The use of terminology from NANDA diagnostic categories will assist in accurately presenting this information (Carpenito, 1993; O'Connor, 1991).

The most important reason for referring a patient to another caregiver is that the helper does not possess the skills the patient requires. The decision and rationale for referral should be discussed with the patient so that the patient does not feel abandoned or hopeless about his or her outcome. The referral can be presented with positive information about the role of the consultant. Such a statement can help allay some of the patient's anxiety about the referral. Overstating the consultant's abilities could be detrimental, however. Remember to ask the consultant what types of approaches and interventions would be most helpful to the patient and family (O'Connor, 1991).

SUPPORT GROUPS

A new role for nurses in many settings is serving as a leader or co-leader of a support group for inpatients or outpatients. Some examples are groups for parents of infants in a neonatal intensive care unit, for persons coping with cancer and their family members, or for patients who have had a myocardial infarction (Grossman & Silverstein, 1993; Rutan, 1992; Schopler & Galinsky, 1993).

It is important for nurses to understand the difference between support groups and therapy groups. The purpose of a support group is to provide people who have similar types of health problems with a setting in which they can discuss their illness-related issues with others who have the same illness. By sharing their feelings, they receive mutual support and caring from others who can fully understand the problem (Grossman & Silverstein, 1993; Rutan, 1992; Schopler & Galinsky, 1993).

The recommended training for a nurse group leader is attendance in a college-level group dynamics course that has theoretical and group membership components. The new leader also should have served as an assistant or coleader with another, more experienced support group leader for one or more years before attempting to lead a group independently.

It is essential that support group leaders realize that their clinical preparation has not prepared them to conduct a therapy group. The leader of a therapy group has had graduate-level training in psychiatric and counseling skills. The purpose of a therapy group is to examine all areas and aspects of a person's intrapsychic and interpersonal functioning. The therapy group leader is an active force in the dynamics of the group and may use interpretation as an aid to group process.

The role of the support group leader is very different: to reflect back the statements of the various members. The leader's function is to assist the group members as they support one another. A common mistake of inexperienced support group leaders is to become actively involved in the group members' process. It can be more difficult to maintain an empathic, objective stance in a group than in a one-to-one relationship because of the cumulative effect of the activity and emotional level of the group. It is easy to be swept up in the feelings of the group. Objectivity is a critically important posture of the support group leader.

In a support group, a person may raise intrapsychic and interpersonal issues not relating to the illness. The person may also raise intrapsychic and interpersonal issues that relate to the illness but are emotionally very complex. In either case, the group member can be told in the presence of the other group members that discussing these types of issues is not a function of the group and that you will talk with him or her after the session about other sources of assistance available. This will prevent the further complication of having other members raise subjects that are inappropriate and not within the group leader's training and capabilities to manage therapeutically. After

the support group session is over, the leader can discuss referral possibilities with interested group members. Patients can be encouraged to remain in the group even if they become involved in individual counseling.

When support groups fail, the leaders usually are disappointed. They wonder why patients do not return after the initial sessions. Frequently, it is because of the leader's overinvolvement in the process and lack of experience in keeping the group members focused on the original purpose of the group.

STEPS IN GROUP FORMATION

The number of people in a support group should range from eight to 12. With fewer than eight people in the beginning stage, the possibility of losing a few members during ensuing weeks may be detrimental to good group dynamics. More than 12 people results in a group with multiple dynamics that can prove too complex for the group and leader. It also results in incomplete participation from all members because of the large number. Group cohesiveness thus may not occur.

Before beginning the group, it is essential to establish admission criteria. An interview with each prospective member should be conducted. If people are automatically allowed to enter, the possibility of having inappropriate members in the group, with resulting failure of the group, is greatly increased. The purpose of the interview is to rule out people with moderate to severe psychopathology. The best clue to a potential problem is that the prospective leader feels anxious in the interview. In a group setting, this person could arouse high anxiety in the other group members, as well as in the leader, and become disruptive.

Potential leaders, in their eagerness to start a group, frequently dislike having pregroup screening interviews, but they are strongly recommended. Some of the questions that could be asked are "Why do you think the group would be helpful to you?" "What do you think you will gain from the other group members?" and "How have things been going for you following your heart attack?" The answers to these questions should give the leader a general idea of how the prospective group member relates with others. If the patient seems inappropriate for the group, a referral to a private therapist or public mental health clinic should be given.

WHEN THE GROUP BEGINS

In the pregroup interview and at the start of the first session, the rules of the group should be explained. For example, the leader can say, "The function of this group is to talk about the feelings you have about cancer and the changes it has caused in your lives." It is very important to keep the group focused on the stated goal. Because feelings are difficult to talk about, group members often will try to divert to "thinking" types of statements. If the group leader does not gently pull them back into discussing the feelings, the group usually is not as effective and the group members may gradually drop out.

The most successful support groups are ones in which feelings about the effects of the illness are discussed. The discovery of mutuality in a group is very comforting to members and is one of the most important outcomes of successful and therapeutic groups. Members begin to realize that feelings they thought were too intense or extreme, and members' responses to this unexpected life change, are normal when compared with those of the other group members.

Most support groups are of limited duration, usually 6 to 8 weeks. The duration of the group and the length of each meeting should be announced before the first session. Ninety minutes is usually the most effective time period and should be strictly adhered to.

STAGES OF GROUP DEVELOPMENT

All time-limited groups have three stages of development. If the group is of 6 weeks or 1 year duration, each of the three stages will take approximately one-third of the time; however, the middle stage in the year-long group may take up somewhat more than one-third of the total time span of the group. The stages, adapted from Yalom (1985), are as follows:

1. *Opening stage.* Search for goals and structure takes place.
2. *Middle or working stage:*
   a. Various members vie for positions within the group.
   b. A cohesive group forms; teamwork is dominant.
3. *Last or termination stage.* Characterized by increased self-disclosure; group may become more subdued; discussions of death may occur.

In a support group for people affected by a serious illness, the last stage frequently also involves a strong sense of mutual understanding, caring, and support. An intimacy may develop between members that is carried into relationships that endure beyond the group. Because of the similar problems members share, they find the support they may have lacked from other people who do not have experience with the same type of condition.

The stages described above will develop only in a group that has a specific starting and end point. This is called a *time-limited group.* It usually occurs only in an outpatient setting. In contrast, some support groups in the general hospital may have open membership, with members attending for a few sessions and dropping out when discharged. This type of group, which has no definite beginning and completion time, is called an *ongoing group.* Intimacy and mutual trust may not develop as successfully in an open-ended group as in a time-limited group with closed membership.

The counseling concepts presented in this chapter can be adapted to the group setting. The concept of process is even more dynamic in the group setting than in the individual setting (Rutan, 1992; Yalom, 1985). The transference and resistance issues of members interacting with each other and with the countertransference and possible resistance issues of one or two co-leaders has numerous results, beyond the full awareness of any group leader.

For this reason, it is strongly recommended that the entire session be tape recorded so that the leader(s) and supervisor can listen to it after the session. Usually the recording introduces many new insights that the leader(s) missed during the actual session. A request for permission to record the group can occur in the first session. If the leader explains that the recording will be confidential and helpful to the leader, members usually have no objection.

Another recommendation is for the group leader to negotiate one hour of supervision time after each group session from a psychiatrist, psychologist, psychiatric nurse specialist, or psychiatric social worker who works in the same hospital and has had experience leading groups. Support groups relating to illness usually involve discussion of life's deepest issues: dying, hopelessness, conflict within the family, anger, and so on. An inexperienced group leader can begin to feel overwhelmed if he or she does not have an experienced consultant available to review the group's progress and issues. Usually a psychiatric professional within the nurse's institution will be willing to spare an hour of time to listen to the tapes, supervise the leader's work, and answer questions.

CONCLUSION

Chapter 2 has presented numerous concepts that are part of the therapeutic nurse–patient relationship process. Nurses new to the caregiving role should be reassured that the development of counseling and group dynamic skills can take psychiatric professionals many years to acquire. This chapter has presented the principles of therapeutic communication that can assist the nurse in assessing and interviewing patients and families to support effective coping and adaptation to illness or threatening physical conditions.

Utilizing these concepts within the framework of the NANDA categories of nursing diagnosis can provide an atmosphere of psychosocial support and care planning extending from the acute care to home care settings. Ideally, communication about ineffective patient or family coping responses can be relayed by the discharging nurse to the nurse in the subsequent caregiving system.

BIBLIOGRAPHY

Aguilera, D. C. (1994). *Crisis intervention: Theory and methodology* (7th ed.). St. Louis: C. V. Mosby.

American Heritage college dictionary (3rd ed.). (1993). Boston: Houghton-Mifflin.

Barrett-Lennard, G. T. (1993). The phases and focus of empathy. *British Journal of Medical Psychology, 66*(Pt. 1), 3–14.

Brammer, L., & Shostrom, E. (1968). *Therapeutic psychology: Fundamentals of actualization counseling and psychotherapy* (2nd ed.). Englewood Cliffs, N. J.: Prentice-Hall.

Brooker, C., & Butterworth, T. (1993). Training in psychosocial intervention: The impact on the role of community psychiatric nurses. *Journal of Advanced Nursing, 18*(4), 583–590.

Burnard, P., & Morrison, P. (1991). Client-centered counselling: A study of nurses' attitudes. *Nurse Educator Today, 11*(2), 104–109.

Campbell, R. J. (1989). *Psychiatric dictionary* (6th ed.). New York: Oxford University Press.

Carpenito, L. J. (1993). *Nursing diagnosis: Application and clinical practice.* Philadelphia: J. B. Lippincott.

Carroll, R. (1993). Mourning: A concern for medical-surgical nurses. *Medical Surgical Nursing, 2*(4), 301–303.

Clements, S., & Cummings, S. (1991). Helplessness and powerlessness: Caring for clients in pain. *Holistic Nursing Practice, 6*(1), 76–85.

Cormier, W., & Cormier, L. (1979). *Interviewing strategies for helpers: A guide to assessment, treatment, and evaluation.* Monterey, CA: Brooks/Cole Publishing.

Davidhizar, R. (1992). Interpersonal communication: A review of eye contact. *Infection Control and Hospital Epidemiology, 13*(4), 222–225.

Erikson, E. (1963). *Childhood and society* (2nd ed.). New York: Norton.

Erikson, E. (1968). *Identity, youth, and crisis.* New York: Norton.

Flaskerud, J., Halloran, E., & Janken, J. (1979). Avoidance and distancing: A descriptive view of nursing. *Nurse Forum, 18*(2), 158–174.

Freud, S. (1933). *New introductory lectures on psychoanalysis.* New York: Norton.

Gerteis, M., Edgman-Levitan, S., Daley, J., & Delbanco, T. L. (1993). *Through the patient's eyes: Understanding and promoting patient-centered care.* San Francisco: Jossey-Bass.

Goldberg, R. J., & Novak, D. H. (1992). The psychosocial review of systems. *Social Science and Medicine, 35*(3), 261–269.

Grossman, A. H., & Silverstein, C. (1993). Facilitating support groups for professionals working with people with AIDS. *Social Work, 38*(2), 144–151.

Groves, J. E., & Kurcharski, A. (1991). Brief psychotherapy. In N. H. Cassem (Ed.), *Massachusetts General Hospital handbook of general hospital psychiatry* (3rd ed.). St. Louis: Mosby Year Book.

Hackett, T. P., Cassem, N. H., Stern, T. A., & Murray, G. B. (1991). Beginnings: Consultation psychiatry in a general hospital. In N. H. Cassem (Ed.), *Massachusetts General Hospital handbook of general hospital psychiatry* (3rd ed.). St. Louis: Mosby Year Book.

Heifner, C. (1993). Positive connectedness in the psychiatric nurse–patient relationship. *Archives of Psychiatric Nursing, 7*(1), 11–15.

Jackson, S. W. (1992). The listening healer in the history of psychological healing. *American Journal of Psychiatry, 149*(12), 1623–1632.

Johns, C. (1991). The Burford Nursing Development Unit holistic model of nursing practice. *Journal of Advanced Nursing, 16*(9), 1090–1098.

Jones, A. (1992). Counselling: Confronting the inevitable. *Nursing Standard, 6*(46), 54–56.

Jouard, S. (1971). *The transparent self* (rev. ed.). New York: Van Nostrand Reinhold.

Kaplan, H. I., & Sadock, B. J. (1994). *Synopsis of psychiatry: Behavioral sciences, clinical psychiatry* (7th ed.). Baltimore: Williams & Wilkins.

Kaplan, H. I., & Sadock, B. J. (1995). *Comprehensive textbook of psychiatry/VI* (6th ed.). Baltimore: Williams & Wilkins.

Kelly, R. B. (1991). The art of therapeutic communication. *Journal of Family Practice, 32*(1), 13–14.

Kemper, B. J. (1992). Therapeutic listening: Developing the concept. *Journal of Psychosocial Nursing and Mental Health Services, 30*(7), 21–23.

Klebanoff, N., & Casler, B. (1986). The psychosocial clinical nurse specialist: An untapped resource for home care. *Home Healthcare Nurse, 4*(6), 36–40.

Klein, M. (1980). *Lives people live: A textbook of transactional analysis.* New York: John Wiley & Sons.

Kumasaka, L. M., & Dungan, J. M. (1993). Nursing strategy for initial emotional response to cancer diagnosis. *Cancer Nursing, 16*(4), 296–303.

MacKay, R. C., Hughes, J. R., & Carver, E. J. (Eds.). (1990). *Empathy in the helping relationship.* New York: Springer.

McClowry, S. G. (1992). Family functioning during a critical illness: A systems theory perspective. *Critical Care Nursing Clinics of North America, 4*(4), 559–564.

McIntosh, D. (1991). Supportive therapy: The other therapy. *Perspectives in Psychiatric Care, 27*(4), 26–29.

Miller, W. R., Hedrick, K. E., & Orlofsky, D. R. (1991). The Helpful Responses Questionnaire: A procedure for measuring therapeutic empathy. *Journal of Clinical Psychology, 47*(3), 444–448.

O'Connor, S. (1991). Psychiatric liaison nursing in a changing health care system. In N. H. Cassem (Ed.), *Massachusetts General Hospital handbook of general hospital psychiatry* (3rd ed.). St. Louis: Mosby Year Book.

Rogers, C. (1976). Non-directive counseling: Client-centered therapy. In W. Sahakian (Ed.), *Psychotherapy and counseling* (2nd ed.). Chicago: Rand McNally.

Rutan, J. S. (1992). Psychodynamic group psychotherapy. *International Journal of Group Psychotherapy, 42*(1), 19–35.

Ryden, M. B., McCarthy, P. R., Lewis, M. L., & Sherman, C. (1991). A behavioral comparison of the helping styles of nursing students, psychotherapists, crisis interveners, and untrained individuals. *Archives of Psychiatric Nursing, 5*(30), 185–188.

Savage, P. (1991). Patient assessment in psychiatric nursing. *Journal of Advanced Nursing, 16*(3), 311–316.

Schopler, J. H., & Galinsky, M. J. (1993). Support groups as open systems: A model for practice and research. *Health and Social Work, 18*(3), 195–207.

Spero, M. H. (1992). Psychoanalytic reflections on language distortion and empathic listening. *American Journal of Psychoanalysis, 52*(3), 227–245.

Thomas, C. L. (Ed.). (1993). *Taber's cyclopedic medical dictionary* (17th ed.). Philadelphia: F. A. Davis.

Tommasini, N. R. (1992). The impact of a staff support group on the work environment of a specialty unit. *Archives of Psychiatric Nursing, 6*(1), 40–47.

Truant, G. S., & Lohrenz, J. G. (1993). Basic principles of psychotherapy. I. Introduction, basic goals, and the therapeutic relationship. *American Journal of Psychotherapy, 47*(1), 8–18.

Wachtel, P. L. (1993). *Therapeutic communication: Principles and effective practice.* New York: Guilford Press.

Weisman, A. D. (1991). Coping with illness. In N. H. Cassem (Ed.), *Massachusetts General Hospital handbook of general hospital psychiatry* (3rd ed.). St. Louis: Mosby Year Book.

Wilting, J. (1990). *Nurses, colleagues, and patients: Achieving congenial interpersonal relationships.* Edmonton: University of Alberta Press.

Wolfelt, A. D. (1991). Toward an understanding of complicated grief. *American Journal of Hospital Palliative Care, 8*(2), 28–30.

Yalom, I. D. (1985). *The theory and practice of group psychotherapy.* New York: Basic Books.

CHAPTER 3

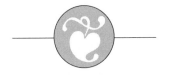

Developmental Factors in Effective Coping Responses

Patricia Barry

This chapter includes the foundation concepts regarding the development of personality factors that contribute to the outcomes of effective or ineffective coping. Coping outcomes are determined by multiple factors and multiple levels of these factors. The critical, fundamental level is determined by inborn character disposition, such as an easy-going or easily aroused and agitated physiological/neuroendocrine pattern of responses; bonding patterns; and developmental processes that contribute to personality style (Elise, 1991; Erikson, 1963; Freud, 1924; Goodyer, 1990; Kernberg, 1994; Maslow, 1970; Piaget & Inhelder, 1969; Small, 1979; Smith & Thelan, 1993). Personality style is predominantly shaped by the inborn character disposition and patterns of unconscious psychological defense mechanisms controlled by the individual's ego.

THE BUILDING BLOCKS OF EFFECTIVE COPING

The human mind is one of the most complex systems in existence. Many mental health professionals have developed theories about how the psyche develops in humans. Some of these theories may be familiar to you. Those presented in this chapter have been chosen because they are important in understanding patients' reactions to illness, in performing psychosocial assessment, and in developing interventions when ineffective coping is occurring or anticipated.

The *personality* is the combination of unique characteristics and behaviors a person acquires during development. It begins to develop at birth and is shaped by the interactions among inherited disposition, the responses of other persons in the environment, and significant external events. Every person has a unique personality that determines how others react to him or her during the person's lifetime.

DRIVE THEORY

Before attempting to absorb the various theories about personality development, it is important to examine the forces that cause the

Patricia Barry: *Psychosocial Nursing: Care of Physically Ill Patients and Their Families,* 3rd ed. © 1996 Lippincott–Raven Publishers

newborn to become aware of the environment and gradually interact with it in a unique way. These forces, which occur naturally in all humans, are the *instincts*, or *drives*. It is generally believed that people have two main drives: the drive to feel pleasure, and the aggressive drive. These drives derive from neurobiological mechanisms (Bock & Whelan, 1991; Lasky, 1993).

Drives operate in all human beings. They are essential to full human development. Without them, humans would lack the motivation to attain their needs. In some people, the drives may become dysfunctional if severe frustration occurs over a prolonged period. For example, the main drive of the infant during the first year is to feel pleasure through the mouth and to receive gratification. The infant receives this gratification by being loved by his or her mother, thus developing a sense of security in her. If, when the baby cries, the mother continually fails to respond, the baby will experience frustration in the search for the pleasure of her love. Infants can become seriously depressed if their need for love is constantly frustrated. This principle was discovered in a study of babies in orphanages. Because the infants' need for love was rarely, if ever, fulfilled, they seemed to give up. They did not cry for attention any longer. Eventually, some of them became ill and died (Spitz, 1965).

Another example of frustration of drive is a toddler who wants to be free to explore. The toddler's aggressive drive is experienced as an internal need to satisfy his or her curiosity and enabled by the new-found ability to walk. If the caregiver does not allow this active youngster some flexibility, and if, at the age of two, the toddler is still kept in a playpen most of the day with a limited number of toys, the frustration of the aggressive drive may result in an intellectually and physically inhibited child. It is the aggressive and libidinal drives that spur the child toward full emotional, intellectual, and physical development (Bullock, 1991; Lasky, 1993).

The aggressive drive is often discussed, but it is rarely spelled out that the aggressive drive is not limited to hostility. Indeed, by far the largest and most important part of the aggressive drive serves as the motor of every movement, of all activity, big and small, of motivation, survival responses and ultimately of life itself (Lasky, 1993).

In working with physically ill people in the clinical setting, many clinicians find the statement that the aggressive drive is ultimately the motor of life itself to be remarkably true. It is as if it were a life force. There are physically ill people about whom caregivers say, "I don't understand why she is going downhill so quickly." Actually, these people are demonstrating a lack of aggressive drive. They have given up, even before their bodies are ready to die. Other critically ill patients remain alive, sometimes to the wonderment of their caregivers. They cling tenaciously to life. In their cases the aggressive drive, sparked by various motivations, keeps them alive. An example is the terminal cancer patient who maintains that she will attend her son's wedding 2 weeks hence. After attending the wedding she may then slip into a coma and die by morning.

AFFECT

Affect is the overall feeling state observed in individuals. Affect is the feeling side of a thought or idea or the emotional reaction to a person or object. Affect can also be the visible sign of a drive. For example, some of the affects seen as a result of the aggressive drive are anger, rage, and hate. The term *affect* is sometimes interchanged with the term *mood*. Actually, mood should be used to describe the internal feelings experienced by a person. Affect is used when referring both to mood and to the external signs of a person's feelings.

During one's nursing career, there will be frequent requests to describe patients' affect both in nursing reports and in conversations with other caregivers. The ability to detect accurately the affect observed in patients assists the nurse in giving sensitive and understanding care. Indeed, patients often report that their nurses were the most important persons in the hospital, the ones who really understood how they were feeling and allowed them to talk about it. Box 3-1 lists many common emotions and psychospiritual states.

OBJECT RELATIONS

Another concept that is crucial in understanding patients' and families' responses to illness is object relations theory. *Object relations* are internal images of self and others and the emotional energy invested in them. Psychoanalytic theorists believe that an object can only be another person or the self (Kaplan & Sadock, 1994, 1995; Lasky, 1993). Clinicians who work with physically ill individuals and their families, however, usually consider an object to be anything to which a person is significantly emotionally attached. This can be a body part, a job, a specific role in the family, and so forth. Physical illness, especially when severe or chronic, can seriously disrupt such attachments.

The way a person interacts with others, the way he or she loves them, gets angry with them, or says good-bye to them, is part of that person's unique interpersonal style, known as object relations. Each person's style is shaped by early childhood experiences with parents and other authority figures. Children who are raised by emotionally open parents tend to develop into emotionally open adults. Similarly, children who grow up in emotionally cold, distant families are frequently cold and aloof adults (Jacobs, 1991; McClowry, 1992).

As discussed earlier, all people have drives that cause their energy to be focused on specific individuals. In order to obtain pleasure or fulfill the aggressive drive, the energy of these drives must be invested in something (Bowlby, 1973; Lasky, 1993).

One may think, for example, of the emotional reaction of a mother who never finished high school as she watches her daughter receive her college degree; years of hope and love were invested in her daughter's development and also in her own dream that someday her daughter would attend college. The son whose father is dying of chronic obstructive pulmonary disease is losing one of the most important objects in his life.

Object relations may also be seen in nurses' attachment to the patients they care for. The nurse experiences loss and grieves when her favorite patient either goes home or dies. Object relations theory applies to every patient you will ever care for. It is a simple yet profound concept, and is of great importance to people struggling with the effects of illness.

THE INTEGRATION OF MENTAL AND PHYSICAL PROCESSES

While there are several theories of personality development, there are some fundamental principles regarding personality development and functioning. One of the primary principles is related to the presence of the ego. The *ego* is an abstract structure of the mind, originally proposed by Sigmund Freud (1924). The ego begins to develop at birth, stimulated by the effects of the environment on the infant's inherited unique psychophysiological disposition. This disposition at birth is demonstrated primarily in physiological patterns of arousal—for example, whether the child is highly anxious and easily frightened or placid and relatively unperturbed by active surroundings.

BOX 3-1	Emotional States	
	Aloofness	Gullibility
	Anger	Hate
	Anxiety	Homesickness
	Bitterness	Hope
	Boredom	Jealousy
	Compassion	Joy
	Complacency	Love
	Curiosity	Masochism
	Cynicism	Mysticism
	Depression	Peace
	Despair	Petulance
	Disgust	Relief
	Disillusionment	Resignation
	Elation	Reverence
	Enthusiasm	Sadism
	Envy	Sarcasm
	Faith	Shame
	Fear	Shyness
	Fretfulness	Smugness
	Fury	Trust
	Gloating	Wistfulness
	Grief	Wonder
	Guilt	

The ego is the regulator of the personality. It watches over the instinctual energy of the id and channels it into acceptable ways of satisfying the person's drives. The ego is in touch with the world. It has conscious and unconscious components.

The ego's most important job is to adapt the psyche to reality. The ego serves as a buffer between the neurobiological drives of the id and the external judgmental environment. It consists of a large number of functions that are essential for normal human development. As you read the following list, consider the complexity of functions that the ego performs automatically (Small, 1979).

EGO FUNCTIONS

1. *Consciousness*
2. *Mastery of motor skills*
3. *Mobility.* The ability to move around in the environment.
4. *Perception.* The ability to scrutinize the environment. This is done using the senses of vision, hearing, smell, touch, and taste, all of which are controlled by the ego.
5. *Judgment.* The ability to interpret these observations.
6. *Sense of reality.* The ability to separate one's self from other people and the environment. This includes a realistic view of one's self and encompasses such concepts as self-esteem and body image.
7. *Regulation and control of emotions and impulses.* All of a person's feelings are channeled and controlled by the ego.
8. *Defense mechanisms.* These include the maneuvers the mind uses to defend itself against threatening reality. All of us have defense mechanisms that we use unconsciously. They are our greatest ally in coping with the stress of life. Defense mechanisms will be described in Chapter 6.
9. *Object relations.* Described previously. The ego controls the intensity of feelings we have about objects. It is possible for there to be too much or too little feeling about objects, depending on the undercontrol or overcontrol of the ego.
10. *Memory.* This includes long-term and recent memory. Some examples of long-term memory are the ability to file away mentally the different steps in a nursing procedure, the normal laboratory values of human blood, and what your kindergarten teacher looked like, for instance. Recent memory examples are remembering what happened this morning or a laboratory value read to you over the telephone. Whenever there is an organic impairment of the physiological functions of the brain, such as the effects of old age or a toxic reaction to an illness, the recent memory will fail before the long-term memory.
11. *Thinking.* The ability to know and learn is included in this category. Reasoning, problem solving, and all cognitive processes are controlled by this function of the ego.

It is important to be aware of the complexity of the ego because it is the nerve center of all mental function and dysfunction. Whenever a patient is confused, coping ineffectively, or has a memory disturbance, it is because one or another of the ego functions is being affected by a mental or physical disease process (Bock & Whelan, 1991; Goodyer, 1990; Noshpitz & Coddington, 1990).

THE CONSCIOUS, SUBCONSCIOUS, AND UNCONSCIOUS

The terms *conscious* and *unconscious* have already been used here. These concepts were also described by Freud (1924). He became aware of them because in his own analysis and his work with patients, he discovered that there are certain psychological processes of which a person is not aware.

THE CONSCIOUS

The *conscious* involves awareness of what is happening at a specific moment. This awareness includes what a person is thinking and feeling, that is, the internal environment, as well as awareness of his or her external environment, that is, where one is, whom one is with, and so forth.

THE SUBCONSCIOUS

The *subconscious*, also called the *preconscious*, consists of memories a person is not constantly thinking about but that can easily be recalled. This includes remembering the time and date of a dental appointment next week or a relative's telephone number.

THE UNCONSCIOUS

The *unconscious* is a psychological process that a person is not aware of and cannot control. It has been compared to a rosebud or an onion. It consists of layer upon layer of repressed memories and experiences surrounding the core of the id drives. The id itself is also part of the unconscious.

BONDING

Bonding is a concept that has gained in importance in the fields of obstetrics and neonatology (the care of the newborn infant, a subspecialty of pediatrics), as well as psychology. Bonding is an attachment process that occurs very early in the infant's life. Bonding is a two-way attachment. It is an attachment of the helpless infant to the mother and father in a manner that meets the needs of the infant's psychological and physical dependency. It also involves the bonding of the parents to their baby: their love for the baby and desire to meet their baby's needs (Klaus & Kennell, 1982). The most significant bond is formed between mother and child (Fig. 3-1).

In a critical review of studies of parent-infant bonding, it is emphasized that many variables promote positive parent-child interactions and favorable family dynamics. They include family planning, comprehensive prenatal care, postnatal infant health status, and, particularly, family supports to reduce socioenvironmental and psychological stresses.

Infants who are cared for in premature and intensive care nurseries are at special risk be-

cause of the extent to which they are deprived of contact with their parents. The mothers of infants who have spent prolonged time in such nurseries are found to lack the normal "instincts" of mothers (Koomen & Hoeksma, 1993; Symanski, 1992). Similarly, their babies frequently experience difficulties that reflect the "failure to thrive" phenomenon. In response to these findings, some hospitals have relaxed visiting hours in the intensive care and regular nurseries. Parents are encouraged to spend as much time as they want with their child.

INBORN PERSONALITY CHARACTERISTICS

In order to understand patients and their current level of personality functioning, it is important to realize that they are who they are as the result of a long continuum of development. Their psychic development actually begins when they are still fetuses and there is an awareness of the warm, dark, protective environment they are living in (Goodyer, 1990; Lasky, 1993; Schultz, 1986).

Some psychologists and obstetricians consider the process of birth to be a psychological insult to the child. They believe that the awareness of this experience remains stored in the psyche of all humans (Janov, 1970). Thus they strongly advocate natural childbirth and "quiet births" (Berezin, 1980; LeBoyer, 1975).

Formal psychiatric theorists rarely discuss the personality of the newborn. It is as if all children were born with a "blank screen" of personality characteristics, and personality was then acquired as a result of inborn biochemical drives and the impact of caregivers as they gradually mold and shape an infant's behavior.

Brazelton has demonstrated in his research that newborns enter the world with as many as 26 different behavioral characteristics and 20 reflexes that can each be observed and rated (Sepkoski et al., 1994). Brazelton's theory can be verified by observant parents, who have always been able to identify behavioral differences among their children. A parent with two, six, or ten children can report definite inborn traits, such as irritability, placidity, and alert-

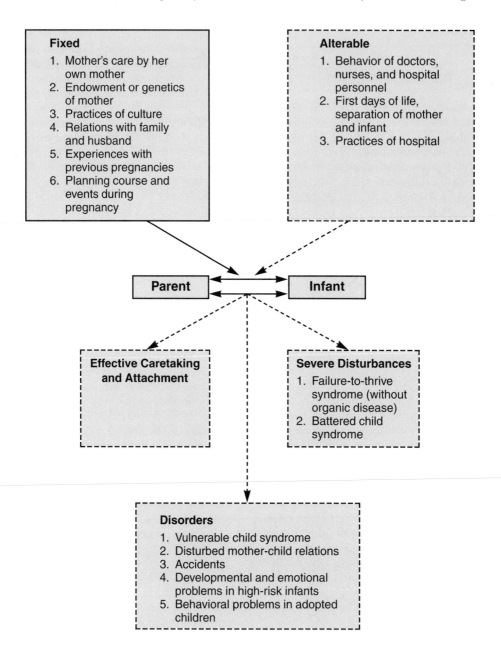

FIGURE 3-1. Influences on maternal-infant bonding. Hypothetical diagram of the major influences on maternal behavior and the resulting disturbances. Solid lines *represent unchangable determinants;* dotted lines *represent alterable determinants (Klaus, M., Kennell, J. [1976] Maternal-infant bonding. St. Louis: CV Mosby, p. 13).*

ness. Typically, their observations remain true as the child matures.

Brazelton's specific observations about newborns include the characteristics listed in Box 3-2.

Brazelton's research tells us that children are unique at birth. After birth, factors such as the child's position in the family, the way the mother and father respond to the child and to each other, and the economic circumstances that contribute to the child's risks or well-being, all shape the unique characteristics of personality.

THEORIES OF PERSONALITY DEVELOPMENT

This section presents a general overview of personality theories developed by various social scientists. These theories are helpful in understanding the emotional, cognitive, and perceptual aspects of patients' and family members' psyches. The *psyche* includes the mind and all its functions. For clarification, the emotional dimension of the psyche is called *affect*. Affect is what a person feels. The cognitive aspect of the psyche is the intellect; it controls thinking, understanding, problem solving, and other cognitive functions. Perception is the way the mind interprets all external stimuli received through the various senses. Chapter 10 will explain perceptual functions in more detail.

Four theories of personality development will be presented. They describe concepts that relate to specific periods of a person's life or are concerned with the human developmental continuum.

PIAGET: COGNITIVE STAGES OF DEVELOPMENT

Jean Piaget was a Swiss psychologist who, over several decades in the mid 1900s, studied the intellectual stages of children's development through clinical interviews, observations, and experiments. He believed that there are four stages in the intellectual development of the child.

Sensorimotor Stage (Birth to 18 Months)

The sensorimotor stage is the first level Piaget describes in a child's cognitive growth. During this stage the infant gradually learns through her senses. She is attentive to the things she sees and hears. She touches objects and explores the environment around her. She is able at times to predict the result of her actions. Thus, testing her predictions may become a game for her. For example, if the child throws her cereal bowl on the floor, she is quite certain what her mother's response will be. This type of thinking marks the beginning of simple problem solving and is the basis for all forms of higher intellectual development.

BOX 3-2	General State Observations in Infants		
	Alertness	Lability of skin color	Orientation to various auditory stimuli
	General tone	Lability of states	Defensive movements
	Cuddliness	Self-quieting activity	Compatability with intervention
	Motor maturity	Hand-to-mouth facility	
	Tremulousness	Smiles	Peak of excitement
	Activity	Response to light	Rapidity of buildup of excitement
	Irritability	Response to rattle	
	Amount of startle reflex during examination	Response to bell	Pull to sit
		Response to pinprick	
	Source: Brazelton & Lester, 1983.		

Preoperational Thought Stage
(1½ or 2 to 7 or 8 Years)

The preoperational thought stage is characterized by rigid thinking demonstrated by an inflexibility in the way the child views the environment at large. Once he has a thought or idea, it rarely changes during this stage. It is also normal for the child to be self-centered in his interactions. He is quite unable to comprehend the ideas of others if they differ from his own. This is called *egocentricity*.

Concrete Operations Stage
(8 to 11 Years)

During the stage of concrete operations, the child develops the concepts of moral judgment, numbers, and spatial relationships. The child is not yet capable of abstract reasoning. She understands things as she sees them and as they seem to be.

Formal Thought Stage
(12 Years to Adulthood)

During the stage of formal thought, the young person is able to use sequential steps in his thinking, enabling him to solve problems and form conclusions by deductive reasoning. He is able to think in an abstract manner, and is able to form and test hypotheses.

Piaget's theories provide an important theoretical foundation for assessing the responses of physically ill people and their families. One of the important roles of the nurse is to teach patients and families how to care for themselves so that rehabilitation can occur. Nurses are often called on also to correct misunderstandings about body functioning. It is important for nurses to realize that people's ability to learn such information can be affected by their cognitive states, their levels of intelligence, the amount of stress they are experiencing (which can cause regression to earlier levels of cognitive development), toxic effects of medication, and so forth.

Piaget's theories are important to nurses for many reasons. All nurses work in a pediatric setting at some time during their professional education. When patient teaching is necessary, it is important to understand the intellectual stage of cognitive development in which the child is functioning. If a nurse is preparing to teach a 9-year-old patient with diabetes about his illness, it is essential to avoid abstract concepts and those concepts that involve a level of reasoning that the child cannot perform.

These concepts are also essential in caring for adult patients, even though most adults have already progressed to Piaget's fourth stage. An important point to remember in caring for patients is that illness and hospitalization are very threatening to them. A coping device that the ego uses in threatening circumstances is regression. *Regression* is the return to an earlier level of functioning as a way of handling stress. It is an unconscious coping mechanism.

When a patient experiences high levels of stress, comprehension is impaired. He or she may regress to the concrete operations stage or even to the preoperational stage, with its inflexible thinking. We may at times think that an intelligent person is being resistant to our teaching. Instead, because of the tendency to regress, it is quite possible that the person is not capable of understanding what he or she is hearing.

Remember, too, that some patients never develop beyond the stage of concrete operations or, possibly, a lesser stage of intellectual development. When a person's IQ appears to be below normal, your teaching will be more successful if you use very basic, concrete explanations that will be more readily understood.

SKINNER: OPERANT CONDITIONING

B. F. Skinner is the psychologist who founded the field of behavioral psychology. Skinner believed that desired behavior is obtained by giving rewards when a person does what is expected of him or her. He taught that personality develops through the interaction of two variables: the intrapsychic makeup of the person (described above as id, ego, and superego) and the social environment (Kaplan & Sadock, 1994, 1995; Lasky, 1993).

Skinner's theories are important to nurses because, like Piaget's, they describe how people learn. Through them we can understand how our patients receive, process, and retain information. With this understanding, we can alter our teaching style and methods, when necessary, to ensure adequate comprehension and thus a more predictable state of well-being for patients and their families. The term *operant conditioning* refers to how a person operates in his or her environment. Operant responses are voluntary, as opposed to involuntary or reflex behavior (Kaplan & Sadock, 1994, 1995).

Positive reinforcement is similar to a reward. It increases the possibility that a person will continue the original behavior because the environment responds positively (Kuhn, 1990; Schultz, 1986).

Nurses can reshape a behavior originally adopted through positive reinforcement by ignoring or refusing to respond positively to further similar behaviors. Eventually the person will stop the behavior because of a lack of response and reinforcement from the environment. This is called *extinction* (Schultz, 1986). A nurse who tires of a patient's unnecessary extra demands may ignore the attention-seeking behavior, and the patient may respond by eventually returning to his or her normal way of interacting.

Negative reinforcement is another important concept to understand when working with patients. Negative reinforcement is the rewarding of a stoppage of an undesirable event or behavior. Frequently this concept is confused with *punishment* (Schultz, 1986). The following example may help to clarify the two.

CASE EXAMPLE

John has angina pectoris. Whenever he overexerts himself, he experiences sharp chest pain (an aversive stimulus). When he takes a nitroglycerin tablet, the pain disappears. This behavioral response causes removal of the aversive stimulus, and John feels better.

Each time a nitroglycerin tablet relieves John's chest pain, his medication-taking behavior is reinforced. Because it stops an aversive stimulus, it is called negative reinforcement. An *aversive stimulus* is any event that results in an unpleasant feeling in a person. The aversive stimulus always *precedes* the behavior. This is in contrast to punishment. With *punishment*, the aversive stimulus always *follows* the behavior. If the person is punished, he or she may choose to eliminate the behavior that results in an aversive stimulus.

Understanding and applying these concepts can make a difference in the way patients respond to nurses' teaching. Think of patients with the following conditions: cardiac disease, chronic respiratory and gastrointestinal disease, diabetes mellitus and other glandular conditions, and substance addictions (food, alcohol, drugs). In order to relieve these conditions, patients must undergo major modifications in their lifestyles. Nurses must be aware of the accompanying unpleasant feelings that new regimens produce in patients. Patients like their regular habits, and feel a loss if they must be given up. It is wise to develop a care plan that attends to the increased emotional needs that accompany the losses caused by the patient's treatment regimen.

The clinical approach called behavior modification is based on the theories of Skinner. *Behavior modification* is the restructuring of a patient's undesirable behavior using conditioning techniques designed to bring about the desired behavior. The caregiver and patient together develop a plan that is agreeable to both in order to obtain a specific goal or outcome.

ERIKSON: PSYCHOSOCIAL STAGES OF DEVELOPMENT

Erik Erikson was born in 1902 in Germany. His father abandoned his mother before he was born, and he was raised by his mother and stepfather. For many years he was unaware that his stepfather was not his real father. It is interesting that Erikson's main interests, as he developed his theories, dealt with identity and the confusion and crises that occur as people seek to understand themselves (Kaplan & Sadock, 1994, 1995).

Erikson described the psychosocial development of the human being on a continuum from birth to death. He believed that there are four major phases in life: childhood, adolescence, adulthood, and old age. He further subdivided these phases into eight psychosocial stages with specific developmental tasks.

A *developmental task* is a challenge that a person's ego must work at and resolve during sequential stages of growth. Three steps mark each stage of development: the immature phase, when the ego first becomes aware of the challenge; the critical phase, when the ego works at the challenge; and the resolution phase, which occurs if the challenge is met and the outcome is successful. The other possible outcome of the critical phase is failure to resolve the challenge of the crisis. Erikson believed that if the crisis is not worked through in the critical stage, the opportunity to resolve it will recur later (Erikson, 1963).

The stages and the developmental challenges involved are described in Table 3-1. The desired personality trait is contrasted to the trait that develops if the critical phase of that stage is not resolved.

MASLOW: HIERARCHY OF HUMAN NEEDS

Abraham Maslow was born in 1908 in New York City and died in 1970. He earned his undergraduate and graduate degrees in psychology at the University of Wisconsin, and later chaired the psychology department at Brandeis University in Waltham, Massachusetts. Maslow was one of the founders of humanistic psychology. He believed that personality develops because of a person's need for satisfaction, happiness, and growth. This is contrasted to the theories of the other main schools of psychology: behavioral, in which humans are motivated by the avoidance of punishment; and psychoanalysis, in which people develop because of the need to decrease or relieve the tension of drives (Schultz, 1986).

Maslow believed that there are five levels of needs in human beings. He called his theory the *hierarchy of human needs*. The main point of his theory is that the first level of needs must be met before one can strive for the next level, the second level must be met before one can strive for the third, and so on. The needs are organized according to their potency and primacy (Kaplan & Sadock, 1994, 1995). Compare these needs with the theories of Erikson and Skinner. Are there similarities? Differences? Consider them in relation to the adult with a major illness.

Physiological Needs

The needs for food, shelter, and sleep are physiological needs. They are essential to all human beings. If these needs are not met, death will result.

Safety Needs

All human beings, from birth through old age, need safety from harm. They need the security of a predictable social and physical environment. If safety needs are partially unfulfilled, then, depending on the severity of the deficit, serious emotional damage can occur because of the chronic effect of fear.

Love and Belonging Needs

All people need family, friends, social acceptance, and enduring intimacy. This need awakens in the older infant as he or she develops an awareness of the social environment and caregivers. The infant needs the family members. As the child matures, he or she thrives on interaction with them and with other people. The love and belonging need level is essential for full social development but is not achieved by all people. The infant will not attain this need level if the family is unable to show love. Some shy, aloof adults and adults with psychiatric disturbances are also unable to feel loved by anyone. They are frequently unable to love others or even themselves.

Esteem Needs

The need for self-worth, positive self-image, and self-acceptance is universal. It develops in the child as a result of approval received from the family. In the adult, esteem needs can be classified into two parts: a desire for a sense of one's own competence and a desire for a good reputation. The achievement of esteem depends primarily on the person's valuation of himself and his worth to his family and the community at large. Satisfaction with work is an important aspect of esteem needs. Many adults are unable to move beyond this level be-

	TABLE 3-1 Erikson's Life Stages		
Stage	**Critical Phase**	**Successfully Resolved**	**Unsuccessfully Resolved**
Early Infancy (birth to 1 year)	Trust vs. Mistrust	Trust: result of receiving affection and feeling valued Qualities acquired: drive and hope	Mistrust: result of deprivation, abuse, isolation, lack
Later Infancy (1 to 3 years)	Autonomy vs. Shame and Doubt	Autonomy: beginning of differentiation from parents (still dependent) Qualities acquired: direction and purpose	Shame and doubt: inhibition of self; poor self-confidence; afraid to develop new skills
Early Childhood (4 to 5 years)	Initiative vs. Guilt	Initiative: begins to imitate and model self after authority figures; imagination flourishes; testing behavior Qualities acquired: direction and purpose	Guilt: conscience is developing in too harsh a manner; lacking in spontaneity; evasive
Middle Childhood (6 to 11 years)	Industry vs. Inferiority	Industry: better able to set realistic goals for self; sense of accomplishment about efforts; motivated to adhere to social rules Qualities acquired: method and competence	Inferiority: feelings of inadequacy; dooms self before any new project is begun; does not assert self
Puberty and Adolescence (12 to 20 years)	Ego Identity vs. Role Confusion	Ego Identity: positive self-image and sense of identity (who am I?); idealistic; sexual preference for opposite sex; open to mentor relationships Qualities acquired: devotion and fidelity	Role confusion: self-conscious; poor value judgement; bisexual confusion; work role confusion
Early Adulthood (20 to 40 years)	Intimacy vs. Isolation	Intimacy: ability to commit self to others in meaningful relationships (developmental challenge of trust may be reawakened) Qualities acquired: affiliation and love	Isolation: aloof; overuse of avoidance or withdrawal in relationships; demeaning manner with others; promiscuous (this trait is actually denial of the basic need for a lasting, loving relationship)
Middle Adulthood (40 to 60 years)	Generativity vs. Stagnation	Generativity: productive; creative; establishing and guiding the next generation: children, younger coworkers, students Qualities acquired: productivity and ability to care for and about others	Stagnation: self-love excludes others' needs; nonproductive and noncontributing; chronic sickliness; hypochondriasis
Late Adulthood (60 years and older)	Ego Integrity vs. Despair	Ego integrity: satisfaction with self and way that life has been lived; able to let go of past; complacent about future events; sense of peace Qualities acquired: renunciation (letting go) and wisdom	Despair: fear of death; longing for past; wish to relive life and do things differently; regrets; feelings of disgust (may mask despair)

cause of a lack of self-confidence or a feeling of dissatisfaction with their role in life.

Self-Actualization Need

The need to develop to one's full potential is the self-actualization need. This need is experienced as an unspecific discontent with one's life. For example, Gail Sheehy (1974) has discussed the midlife experience of people who want to develop new skills or lifestyles. Maslow believes that a person *must* be what he or she *can* be.

It is important to remember that many people experience feelings of discontent but are restricted by their life circumstances and unable to pursue their dreams. Consider, for example, the bright young African American ghetto resident who is scorned by family and peers because of his educational and social aspirations and lacks anyone to support him emotionally or financially; the car mechanic with four children who dreams of going to college at night to become an engineer; or the woman with children in school who wants to return to her former profession, but whose husband does not support her decision.

Maslow believes that the goal of achieving full actualization is a constant drive in humans. Once survival-oriented needs are fulfilled, the human being can move on toward growth-oriented needs. The goal of achieving full actualization, or full development of one's potential, is viewed as a major life force or drive. Maslow believes it is the motivation behind all human behavior.

CHANGING DYNAMICS

These theories of personality development are important to nurses in understanding patients' responses to illness because personality dynamics are constantly changing. The forces that operated in a person as a child continue to operate in him or her as an adult. In addition, with the stress of illness, a person will normally regress to earlier levels of personality development. By being aware of these earlier levels, the nurse may be able to identify ineffective coping that can lead to maladaptive regression, or other maladaptive responses to illness.

EFFECTIVE AND INEFFECTIVE USES OF DEFENSE MECHANISMS

Whenever there is conflict in a normal person between what she wants to do and what she believes she should do, the result is an unpleasant feeling called *anxiety*. The mind attempts at all times to protect itself from unpleasant, anxiety-producing feelings and urges. This ever-watchful protectiveness results from automatic devices the mind uses to defend itself. These automatic processes are called *defense mechanisms* (Groves & Kurcharski, 1991; Kaplan & Sadock, 1994, 1995; Kernberg, 1994; Rosenbaum & Pollack, 1991; Skodol & Perry, 1993).

THE FORMATION OF DEFENSES IN THE PERSONALITY

A defense mechanism is an unconscious device used by the mind to protect itself from the feelings of conflict and anxiety that result from unacceptable impulses and drives. It is also called an *unconscious mental maneuver* or *mental mechanism*. These terms refer to the unconscious, continuous monitoring by the ego of a person's feeling state or reactions to the environment. The ego is constantly alert to events that can cause *dysphoric* (unpleasant) feelings and develops unconscious defenses to guard against them. The average person is usually unaware that he or she is using defense mechanisms. Because they are used by the ego to defend itself, the ego accepts them as natural. These are *automatic* processes.

Ego perception is like a receiving area that examines external events, sensations, or internal responses before admitting them into its conscious awareness. Anything that is compatible with the ego is allowed to enter the ego's awareness. When ideas or impulses are acceptable to the ego, they are called *ego-syntonic*. When ideas or impulses are unacceptable to the ego and could potentially cause it to feel anxiety, they are called *ego-dystonic* (Campbell, 1989). When the ego senses an ego-dystonic event, whether it is an internal impulse or external awareness, it unconsciously prepares to shut it out entirely, forget it, or distort it in some way so that it is not so unacceptable or anxiety-provoking.

Whenever the ego begins to feel anxious or threatened, it quickly reacts to protect itself. Carson (1979) has identified the various situations that cause the ego to respond with a defense mechanism:

An increase in instinctual drives at puberty.

Stimulation from without (the environment) that stirs the instinctual drives, such as a highly stimulating festive occasion or a seductive relationship.

External events that impair ego functions, such as extreme stress or the death of a loved one.

Physiological impairment of ego functions caused by such factors as alcohol, fatigue, or illness.

Less efficient ego functioning secondary to emotional stress during the formative years, the result of which is neurotic illness or personality disorder.

THE USE OF DEFENSE MECHANISMS

The ego uses defense mechanisms whenever it senses any unpleasant or potentially unpleasant feeling. The ego is determined to protect itself. The final result of a defense mechanism is that the unpleasant feeling is eliminated completely or at least minimized. If the ego is not strong enough to defend itself fully, there will be an underuse of defenses; the result will be anxiety or depression (Cassem, 1991; Rosenbaum & Pollack, 1991). When the patient's ego either overuses or underuses defense mechanisms, the possible outcome is ineffective coping (Carpenito, 1993).

Some patients never overcome the negative effects of ineffective defense mechanisms that develop during their hospitalizations. As a result of this maladaptation, they and their families may be subject to major changes in the quality of their lives. The cues that the patient is not coping or adapting well can be seen by the astute observer while the patient is still in the hospital. These cues are actually the patient's unconscious underuse or overuse of defense mechanisms, which can undermine overall coping ability.

When a patient is described as *coping ineffectively*, it may mean that his or her defense mechanisms are failing and are not being used, or that defense mechanisms are blocking out or distorting the reality of the situation. As described in Chapter 1, nurses may be the ideal clinicians to observe these cues because of the amount of time they spend with patients.

It may also be true that the patient is responding appropriately to the illness or hospitalization, but one or more family members is not. Remember that although the patient is coping well in the hospital, after discharge he or she will reenter the family system and will be detrimentally affected by ineffective coping in the family. If a wife views her husband as an invalid, for example, and develops acute anxiety or depression about his situation, it will seriously affect the man's own adjustment. Again, the nurse's observations and intervention with the family can be highly important during the hospitalization period. Sensitive observations and appropriate intervention can have a definite effect on a patient's well-being after discharge (McClowry, 1992; O'Connor, 1991).

COPING VS. DEFENSE MECHANISMS

There are no universally accepted definitions for the terms *coping* and *defense mechanism*. In this text we will use the definitions given in the *Encyclopedia and Dictionary of Medicine, Nursing, and Allied Health* (1987):

Coping. The process of contending with life difficulties in an effort to overcome or work through them (p. 295).

Defense mechanism. An unconscious mental process or coping pattern that lessens the anxiety associated with a situation or internal conflict and protects the person from mental discomfort (p. 328).

These definitions indicate that coping mechanisms are all of the mental maneuvers the mind uses to protect itself from unwanted reality in the external world or environment. *Defense mechanism* describes one type of mental maneuver the mind automatically uses to protect itself against internal reality, or what the person is feeling *inside* vs. what he or she is perceiving outside of himself or herself.

The term *coping* is used to describe the ways the mind attempts to maintain intrapsychic stability during times of increased stress. These ways include conscious stress management devices, such as talking out a problem or jogging. The other major coping strategy is the unconscious use of defense mechanisms. Because unconscious defense mechanisms can be the greatest ally of the ego in defending itself from severe anxiety or depression, they have a strong effect on a person's adaptive capacity (Cassem, 1991; Rosenbaum & Pollack, 1991). When they are maladaptive, they can result in coping failure. A broader view of coping and its components will be presented in Chapter 6.

DEVELOPMENT OF DEFENSE MECHANISMS

Defense mechanisms develop as a protective response to unacceptable drives or impulses. The mind is a creature of habit pertaining to defense mechanisms. Once it develops a certain way of dealing with either an internal or external stressor, it usually continues to defend itself in the same way.

Actually, the defense mechanisms that adults automatically use are well established by the age of six (Kernberg, 1994). These defenses form the basis of the way people respond to all types of stress and also the way they relate to others. In essence, they determine a person's personality style, the way she is viewed by others, and the way she responds to them.

LEVELS OF DEFENSE MECHANISMS

The levels of defense mechanisms include narcissistic, immature, neurotic, and mature. Table 3-2 presents these mechanisms in the order of their development in human beings.

The remainder of this chapter will present the various defenses used by normal persons as they cope with stress, in the order of their appearance during a person's psychological development. Which defense mechanisms nurses observe patients using depends on each person's previous experiences with stress and conscious ability to cope actively with illness, as well as the mind's typical use of unconscious defense mechanisms. For example, a 70-year-old man admitted to the hospital with his first exposure to major illness may find his ability to cope taxed far more than would a 30-year-old man who is chronically ill and has been hospitalized on several occasions. (These concepts will be more fully presented in Chapters 6, 12, and 16.)

It is important to remember the function of a defense mechanism; it is used whenever the mind senses danger (Lazarus, 1991). The de-

TABLE 3-2
Levels of Human Defense Mechanisms

Level and Type

Narcissistic
  Denial
  Delusional projection
  Distortion
Immature
  Acting-out behavior
  Avoidance
  Hypochondriasis
  Passive-aggressive behavior
  Projection
  Regression
Neurotic
  Displacement
  Identification
  Isolation
  Reaction formation
  Repression
Mature
  Anticipation
  Sublimation
  Humor
  Altruism
  Suppression

Adapted from Groves and Kucharski, 1991; Kaplan and Sadock, 1994, 1995; Kernberg, 1994; Vaillant, 1977.

fense mechanism's main purpose is to relieve anxiety. All types of defense mechanisms can potentially be used in an attempt to adapt to an unpleasant internal or environmental awareness. Defense mechanisms are always adaptive because they help a person cope with an otherwise difficult situation. If the defense mechanism either fails or is very rigid, however, it can result in moderate to long-lasting negative changes in the person's intrapsychic and interpersonal and physiological functioning (Aspinwall & Taylor, 1992; McClowry, 1992). At that point, the original *adaptive* mechanism becomes ineffective or *maladaptive*. It is possible for a particular defense mechanism to have either an effective (adaptive) or an ineffective (maladaptive) outcome.

NARCISSISTIC DEFENSE MECHANISMS

A person begins to use defenses very early in life. The first defenses, which occur unconsciously, begin in the child's first year. These *narcissistic defense mechanisms* are commonly used by children under age 5, then give way to a higher and more mature level of defense. They are used whenever external reality is too threatening.

The normally well-adjusted adult may regress to this early level for a brief period during very acute stress or during dreaming or periods of fantasy (Kaplan & Sadock, 1994, 1995). Narcissistic defense mechanisms, when used by persons with severe psychopathology, form the basis for psychosis.

A *psychosis* is a mental disorder in which a person loses touch with reality for varying periods. To the observer, the psychotic person appears to be in his or her own world. The intellectual, feeling, and perceptual spheres are affected. As a result, relations with other persons are impaired, and the person is dysfunctional during the psychotic episodes.

There are two main types of psychosis. Those caused by physiological disruption of the brain are called *cognitive mental disorders*. They will be described in Chapter 11. The other group of psychoses are caused by functional failure of the psyche. They include schizophrenia and manic-depressive illness. These *dysfunctional illnesses* will not be covered in this book because they are well described in most psychiatric medical and nursing textbooks.

People who routinely use narcissistic defenses have psychiatric illnesses that include active psychotic stages: schizophrenia, manic-depressive illness, acute cognitive mental disorder, and acute psychotic depression (Goff, Manschreck, & Groves, 1991; Kaplan & Sadock, 1994, 1995). The narcissistic defenses are *denial, delusional projection,* and *distortion.*

Denial

Denial is a mechanism the ego uses to shut out external reality that is too frightening or threatening to tolerate. The person sees, hears, or perceives the event through her senses but refuses to recognize it consciously. The memory of the threatening reality is stored in the unconscious, however.

Delusional Projection

Delusional projection is a mechanism by which the ego develops a false belief that is abnormal for the person's intelligence and cultural background. In delusional projection the person believes that someone is "out to get him." This mechanism has a persecutory basis. In severe psychopathology it forms the basis of paranoid psychosis.

Distortion

The ego uses the defense mechanism of *distortion* to reshape external reality to suit internal needs. The ego twists and distorts the aspects of reality that it cannot tolerate. Distortion is the basis for hallucinations and nonparanoid types of delusions.

IMMATURE DEFENSE MECHANISMS

The second level of defenses is *immature defense mechanisms.* They operate unconsciously, and occur in healthy children and adolescents between the ages of 3 and 15 or 16. They should be replaced in midadolescence by a more mature level of defense and should not be used by the adult ego unless it is under moderate to severe stress. If these mechanisms are not relinquished, but are routinely used by the adult ego, the result will be a person with major character flaws. These flaws form the basis of disabling personality disorders (see Chapter 15) and borderline states (Kernberg, 1994). The immature defenses are *acting out, avoidance, hypochondriasis, passive-aggressive behavior, projection, and regression.*

Acting-out Behavior

Acting-out behavior is the outward manifestation of an inner need that causes feelings the person cannot tolerate. The inner tension that develops is not dealt with; instead, it is acted out behaviorally in an impulsive-appearing and immature way.

Avoidance

Avoidance is a defense mechanism similar to denial. Using this mechanism, a person unconsciously shuns any situation, object, or activity that might arouse unwanted sexual or aggressive impulses. Avoidance is also unconsciously used to escape any encounter that would result in unpleasant and undesired emotional reactions. It differs from denial in that, with denial, there is an unconscious refusal to recognize a traumatic reality. With avoidance, there is an unconscious refusal to encounter a traumatic reality because it would provoke too much anxiety. The person is never aware of the reason for the change in motivation (Groves & Kurcharski, 1991; Kaplan & Sadock, 1994, 1995).

Hypochondriasis

Hypochondriasis is a defense used by the ego when it has real or imagined aggressive, critical feelings toward others and finds them unwelcome and disturbing. The critical feelings are turned back on the ego and experienced as guilt. Self-reproach may also be experienced when these feelings result from loneliness or unresolved grief. The guilt or self-reproach is then transformed into physical complaints. The unconsciously motivated development of these symptoms frequently occurs when the person experiences anger because his or her need to be cared for is not

being met. By complaining about physical ailments, the social system may respond by giving the person more care and attention.

Attention from others is unconsciously and consciously what the person has been looking for. It is called *secondary gain*. The person seeks either attention or the satisfaction of the need for love, which was never completely met during the first years of life (Campbell, 1989).

Passive-Aggressive Behavior

Passive-aggressive behavior is the outward manifestation of anger that the person is not able to express directly toward the person with whom he or she is angry. Instead, it is expressed passively in ways that are frequently self-defeating (Campbell, 1989).

Projection

Projection is a less pathological form of delusional projection, described earlier. Its basic dynamics are the same, but the ego uses it in a less disturbed way. It occurs when a person is unable to acknowledge his or her own thoughts or feelings and attributes them to others.

Regression

The ego uses *regression* when it is severely threatened by environmental stress or when there is internal psychic stress during a particular stage of personality development. As a result, the personality functioning returns to an earlier level. Regression is a normal and expectable outcome of most physical illness (Lewis & Levy, 1982).

NEUROTIC DEFENSE MECHANISMS

The next level of defenses begins to occur at approximately the same age as the immature defenses (age 3 to 15 or 16). They are distinguished from immature defenses because, although classified as *neurotic defense mechanisms*, they are used by "healthy" adults throughout their lifetimes. Seen as quirks in otherwise normally adjusted human beings, they are used to deal with stressful situations. If one or more of these defenses is heavily used and affects the person's capacity to enjoy life, it causes a neurosis (Kaplan & Sadock, 1994, 1995).

A *neurosis* differs from a psychosis in that the neurotic is not as seriously disturbed as the psychotic. In neurosis, only a part of the personality is affected and perception of reality is not grossly impaired; the quality of life is usually affected, however. In *psychosis*, most of the ego functions are disturbed and the quality of reality of the psychotic person is changed markedly.

The neurotic defenses include *displacement, identification, isolation, reaction formation*, and *repression*. They are used unconsciously by the ego. Psychiatric conditions in which the overuse of neurotic defenses occur and become crippling are *obsessive-compulsive behavior, phobias, hysteria, anxiety*, and *depressive neuroses*.

Repression

Repression (not to be confused with *regression*) is the main mechanism the ego uses to defend itself. In repression the ego unconsciously excludes awareness of thoughts, feelings, urges, fantasies, and memories that would be unacceptable or threatening if they were conscious. Anything the ego perceives as dangerous may potentially be repressed. Its concept of "dangerous" results from early childhood experiences. Events later in adulthood that seem entirely unrelated but are perceived as dangerous may result in anxiety, which causes the ego to respond by blotting out the current thought or feeling. The ego does not discriminate in a logical way when it uses repression to defend itself (Groves & Kucharski, 1991; Kaplan & Sadock, 1994, 1995; Kernberg, 1994).

The defenses of *repression* and *denial* are easily confused. The difference is that denial defends the ego against painful or unpleasant *external* reality: events occurring in the environment outside the person. Repression is used to defend against painful or unpleasant *internal* reality: feelings or thoughts occurring inside the person. In each case a reality is perceived that the ego instantly recognizes as dangerous or very unpleasant, so it shuts the awareness away into the unconscious.

In order to clarify the differences, think of a patient who hears that he has multiple sclerosis. He finds the diagnosis so threatening that he initially denies it. Denial shuts out a painful external awareness. A few days later, he is able to tolerate the diagnosis, and his denial fades.

A week after discharge, the patient may begin to experience anxiety as the full awareness of the future effects of the disease become known to him. Because his ego is unable to tolerate the anxiety, which is a distressing internal awareness, it is repressed. It is no longer in the patient's conscious awareness. As he is better able to cope with the changes the illness will cause in his life, the repression will gradually lift. He will move through the normal bereavement process as he becomes aware of the losses the illness will cause in his life. (See Chapter 9 and Chapter 24 for more information about responses to loss and the normal bereavement process.) The patient will make the necessary adjustments in his relationships and lifestyle. This is an adaptive response. If, on the other hand, the repression continues for a prolonged period and the patient develops an unresolved grief, maladaptation is the outcome.

Identification

Identification is a defense in which a person accepts the circumstances of other people as though they were actually his or her own. This acceptance can pertain to others' thoughts, attitudes, feelings, or particular experiences (Kaplan & Sadock, 1994, 1995; Kernberg, 1994).

Isolation

Isolation is a defense by which the ego separates the normal feeling associated with a particular thought or idea from that thought or idea. It then represses either the feeling or the idea so that only one of them remains. Usually, the thought content remains while the affect or feeling associated with it is repressed. Other names for this defense are *rationalization* and *intellectualization*.

Displacement

Displacement is a defense used by the ego to redirect feelings about one object to another.

Although the feelings are shifted, the instinct or motivation behind the feelings remains the same (Campbell, 1989).

Reaction Formation

Reaction formation is a defense used when an impulse or feeling is unacceptable to the ego. As a result, the ego unconsciously does a complete turnabout of the original impulse or feeling. An exact opposite impulse, feeling, thought, or behavior results. The defense of reaction formation is sometimes known as *compensation*. Anger or hostility is frequently the underlying impulse or emotion that is being guarded against.

MATURE DEFENSE MECHANISMS

The highest level of ego defenses is the category of *mature defense mechanisms*. They begin to be used around the age of 12 by well-functioning persons at all but the most stressful times. The mature defenses result from successful resolution of conflicts at earlier levels of personality development. They include *anticipation, sublimation, humor, altruism,* and *suppression*. The mature defenses are used by the ego either consciously or unconsciously (Groves & Kucharski, 1991; Kaplan & Sadock, 1994, 1995). Mature defenses are always used in an adaptive manner.

Anticipation

Anticipation is a defense by which the ego acknowledges both intellectually and emotionally an upcoming situation that is expected to provoke anxiety. By acknowledging it, some of the anxiety is worked through and resolved in advance.

Sublimation

Sublimation operates in connection with the defense of repression. In sublimation, a repressed urge or desire is expressed in a socially acceptable or useful way. As a result, the original impulse has a modified outlet, as opposed to being completely blocked.

Altruism

Altruism is a mature defense that connects the desire to satisfy one's own narcissistic needs with the desire to satisfy the needs of others. It is different from desiring to meet others' needs in order to relieve guilt feelings or meeting others' needs for other maladaptive reasons. The result of altruism is constructive and gratifying service to others.

Suppression

Suppression is a conscious or semiconscious decision to delay paying attention to an unwanted conflict or impulse until a later time. It is a commonly used coping device to postpone dealing with a normally anxiety-provoking situation until it can be dealt with properly.

CONVERSION: AN UNCLASSIFIED DEFENSE MECHANISM

Conversion is yet another defense mechanism used by the ego as a means of defending itself. It is not possible to classify it with the previous defense mechanisms because it is actually composed of elements of several mechanisms. It most frequently occurs in people who are unable to express their feelings. As a result of this inability, they react with bodily symptoms to stressors and conflicts. The inability to express feelings verbally is called *alexithymia*. The word is derived from the root derivatives *a*, meaning *without*; *lex*, from the Latin, meaning *word*; and *thymia*, from the Greek, meaning *feelings*. The words, when combined, mean "without words to describe feelings." The defense mechanisms involved are repression (of feelings) and displacement (of conflicts and feelings) into bodily symptoms. This phenomenon is sometimes called *somatization*.

In conversion, the ego changes emotional conflict related to the instinctual pleasure-seeking sexual drive or the aggressive drive into physical symptoms. The symptoms may be of short duration or may develop to cause severe physical impairment. In conversion, the person may or may not be aware of the emotional conflict that is causing the physical illness.

An important clinical dynamic frequently observed in patients with physical symptoms resulting from conversion is a history of loss or the threat of loss. Both the pleasure-seeking drive and the aggressive drive are affected when an object that was pleasurable to a person is lost. This object can be another person or an abstract entity such as one's own self-image, a job, or a role that can no longer be fulfilled. When a person's self-image is threatened, he or she will react with anxiety to this potential loss. A person's ability to work or fulfill certain roles is one of the important dynamics in a positive self-image. Both the sexual and aggressive drives motivate a person to work. The aggressive drive is also affected when there are feelings of abandonment, deep disappointment, and disillusionment regarding any object (Jacobson, 1971; Kernberg, 1994).

It is imperative that persons who are suspected of having illnesses that are psychogenic or "all in the head" have a thorough physical workup before the etiology is identified as emotional. The patient most likely to be diagnosed with psychogenic illness is one with a history of multiple illnesses, hospitalizations, and surgeries. However, people suspected of having a psychosomatic illness must not be labeled as such by caregivers. It is possible that a patient's previous illnesses may have been psychogenic but that the current illness is genuine. The patient could have a hidden tumor or some other potentially fatal condition. Information on psychosomatic illness is presented in Chapter 6.

It is important to remember that the degree of threat perceived by the ego will result in the use of differing levels of defense mechanisms. In terminal illness, one of the most threatening events a person or family can experience, there is a need for more basic and stronger levels of defense. Chapter 24 describes approaches to use in such circumstances.

CONCLUSION

Being aware of the developmental history and clinical presentation of personality dynamics in patients can assist the nurse in being more fully aware of patients' and family members' psychosocial responses to illness. In addition,

these dynamics are always operating in caregivers. A nurse who is aware of these dynamics in himself or herself will have an enhanced capacity to engage in therapeutic relationships.

The use of defense mechanisms can be both harmful and helpful to patients. The ego is a remarkable psychic structure. It usually is the best ally a person can have in making his or her way through life. Many patients who are hospitalized or treated for illness are able to cope and respond effectively because of their well-functioning egos. In many other cases, however, the ineffective defense mechanisms used by the ego to defend against threatening events are not given up after the crisis of illness is over. Instead, they are used in an ongoing manner that becomes maladaptive and can cause a deterioration in a patient's and family's quality of life.

By assessing a patient's thinking, feeling, and behavioral response to illness, it is possible to identify individuals in inpatient or outpatient settings whose egos are unconsciously using defense mechanisms either effectively or ineffectively. Assessment of psychosocial functioning and recommendations for intervention when dysfunction is observed will be discussed in subsequent chapters.

BIBLIOGRAPHY

Aguilera, D. C. (1994). *Crisis intervention: Theory and methodology*. (7th ed.). St. Louis: C .V. Mosby.

Aspinwall, L., & Taylor, S. (1992). Modeling cognitive adaptation: A longitudinal investigation of the impact of individual differences on college adjustment and performance. *Journal of Personality and Social Psychology, 63*(6), 989–1003.

Berezin, N. (1980). *The gentle birth book: A practical guide to LeBoyer family-centered delivery*. New York: Simon & Schuster.

Bertalanffy, L. von. (1968). *General system theory*. New York: Basic Books.

Bock, G. R., & Whelan, J. (1991). *The childhood environment and adult disease*. New York: Wiley.

Bowlby, J. (1973). *Attachment and loss. Volume 2: Separation*. New York: Basic Books.

Brazelton, T. B., & Lester, B. M. (Eds.). (1983). *New approaches to developmental screening of infants: Proceedings of the Fifth Johnson & Johnson Pediatric Round Table*. New York: Elsevier.

Bullock, M. (Ed.). (1991). The development of intentional action: Cognitive, motivational, and interactive processes. *Contributions to Human Development, 22*.

Campbell, R. J. (1989). *Psychiatric dictionary* (6th ed.). New York: Oxford University Press.

Carson, D. (1979). Personality development, conflict, and mechanisms of defense. In G. Usdin & J. Lewis (Eds.), *Psychiatry in general medical practice*. New York: McGraw-Hill.

Cassem, N. H. (1991). Depression. In N. H. Cassem (Ed.), *Massachusetts General Hospital handbook of general hospital psychiatry* (3rd ed.). St. Louis: Mosby Year Book.

Davis, B., & Jones, L. C. (1992). Differentiation of self and attachment among adult daughters. *Issues in Mental Health Nursing, 13*(4), 321–331.

Edlin, G., & Golanty, E. (1992). *Health and wellness: A holistic approach* (4th ed.). Boston: Jones and Bartlett.

Elise, D. (1991). An analysis of gender differences in separation–individuation. *Psychoanalytic Study of the Child, 46*, 51–67.

Encyclopedia and dictionary of medicine, nursing, and allied health (4th ed.). (1987). Philadelphia: W. B. Saunders.

Erikson, E. (1963). *Childhood and society* (2nd ed.). New York: Norton.

Freud, S. (1924). Certain neurotic mechanisms in jealousy, paranoia and homosexuality. In S. Freud, *Collected papers, Volume 22*. London: Hogarth Press.

Goff, D. C., Manschreck, T. C., & Groves, J. E. (1991). Psychotic patients. In N. H. Cassem (Ed.), *Massachusetts General Hospital handbook of general hospital psychiatry* (3rd ed.). St. Louis: Mosby Year Book.

Goodyer, I. M. (1990). *Life experiences, development, and childhood psychopathology*. New York: Wiley.

Groves, J. E., & Kurcharski, A. (1991). Brief psychotherapy. In N. H. Cassem (Ed.), *Massachusetts General Hospital handbook of general hospital psychiatry* (3rd ed.). St. Louis: Mosby Year Book.

Jacobs, E. H. (1991). Self psychology and family therapy. *American Journal of Psychotherapy, 45*(4), 483–498.

Jacobson, E. (1971). *Depression: Comparative studies of normal, neurotic, and psychotic conditions*. New York: International Universities Press.

Janov, A. (1970). *The primal scream: Primal therapy: The cure for neurosis*. New York: G. P. Putnam's Sons.

Kaplan, H. I., & Sadock, B. J. (1994). *Synopsis of psychiatry: Behavioral sciences, clinical psychiatry* (7th ed.). Baltimore: Williams & Wilkins.

Kaplan, H. I., & Sadock, B. J. (1995). *Comprehensive textbook of psychiatry/VI* (6th ed.). Baltimore: Williams & Wilkins.

Kernberg, P. F. (1994). Mechanisms of defense: Development and research perspectives. *Bulletin of the Menninger Clinic, 58*(1), 55–87.

Klaus, M., Kennell, J. (1976). *Maternal-infant bonding*. St. Louis: C. V. Mosby, p.13.

Koomen, H. M., & Hoeksma, J. B. (1993). Early hospitalization and disturbances of infant behavior and the mother–infant relationship. *Journal of Child Psychology and Psychiatry and Allied Disciplines, 34*(6), 917–934.

Kuhn, D. (Ed.). (1990). Developmental perspectives on teaching and learning thinking skills. *Contributions to Human Development, 21*.

Lasky, R. (1993). *Dynamics of development and the therapeutic process*. Northvale, N. J.: J. Aronson.

Lazarus, R. (1991). Progress on a cognitive-motivational-relational theory of emotion. *American Psychologist, 46*(8), 819–834.

LeBoyer, F. (1975). *Birth without violence*. New York: Alfred A. Knopf.

Lewis, A., & Levy, J. (1982). *Psychiatric liason nursing: The theory and clinical practice*. Reston, VA: Reston Publishing.

Mahler, M. S. (1974). Symbiosis and individuation: The psychological birth of the human infant. *Psychoanalytic Study of the Child, 29*, 89–124.

Maslow, A. (1970). *Motivation and personality* (2nd ed.). New York: Harper & Row.

Masterson, J. F., Tolpin, M., & Sifneos, P. E. (1991). *Comparing psychoanalytic psychotherapies: Developmental, self, and object relations: Self psychology, short-term dynamic*. New York: Brunner/Mazel.

McClowry, S. G. (1992). Family functioning during a critical illness: A systems theory perspective. *Critical Care Nursing Clinics of North America, 4*(4), 559–564.

Muller, M. E., & Ferketich, S. (1993). Factor analysis of the Maternal Fetal Attachment Scale. *Nursing Research, 42*(3), 144–147.

Newberry, B. H., Jaikins-Madden, J. E., & Gerstenberger, T. J. (1991). *A holistic conceptualization of stress and disease*. New York: AMS Press.

Noshpitz, J. D., & Coddington, R. D. (Eds.). (1990). *Stressors and the adjustment disorders*. New York: Wiley.

O'Connor, S. (1991). Psychiatric liaison nursing in a changing health care system. In N. H. Cassem (Ed.), *Massachusetts General Hospital handbook of general hospital psychiatry* (3rd ed.). St. Louis: Mosby Year Book.

Piaget, J., & Inhelder, B. (1969). *Psychology of the child*. New York: Basic Books.

Pine, F. (1990). *Drive, ego, object, and self: A synthesis for clinical work*. New York: Basic Books.

Rosenbaum, J. F., & Pollack, M. H. (1991). Anxiety. In N. H. Cassem (Ed.), *Massachusetts General Hospital handbook of general hospital psychiatry* (3rd ed.). St. Louis: Mosby Year Book.

Schultz, D. (1986). *Theories of personality*. Monterey, CA: Brooks/Cole Publishing.

Sepkoski, C. M., Lester, B. M., Osstheimer, G. W., & Brazelton, T. B. (1994). The effects of maternal epidural anesthesia on neonatal behavior during the first month. *Developmental Medicine and Child Neurology, 36*(1), 91–92.

Sheehy, G. (1974). *Passages*. New York: E.P. Dutton.

Skodol, A. E., & Perry, J. C. (1993). Should an axis for defense mechanisms be included in DSM-IV? *Comprehensive Psychology, 34*(2), 108–119.

Sluckin, A. (1993). My baby doesn't need me: Understanding bonding failure. *Health Visitor, 66*(11), 409–412.

Small, L. (1979). *The briefer psychotherapies*. New York: Brunner/Mazel.

Smith, L. B., & Thelen, E. (Eds.). (1993). *A Dynamic Systems approach to development*. Cambridge: MIT Press.

Spangler, G., & Grossman, K. E. (1993). Biobehavioral organization in securely and insecurely attached infants. *Child Development, 64*(5), 1439–1450.

Spitz, R. (1965). *The first year of life.* New York: International Universities Press.

Stuart, G., & Sundeen, S. (Eds.). (1987). *Principles and practice of psychiatric nursing.* (3rd ed.). St. Louis: Mosby.

Symanski, M. E. (1992). Maternal–infant bonding: Practice issues for the 1990's. *Journal of Nurse Midwifery, 37*(2 suppl.), 67S–73S.

Wykle, M. L., Kahana, E., & Kowal, J. (Eds.). (1992). *Stress and health among the elderly.* New York: Springer Publishing Company.

Vaillant, G. (1977). *Adaption to life.* Boston: Little, Brown & Co.

CHAPTER 4

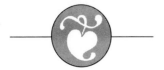

Holism: Interactive Effects of Mind, Body, and Spirit

Patricia Barry

The role of nurses as ministers to those who are suffering faces important new challenges in the future of health care. These challenges offer opportunities for nurses at all levels to enter into partnerships with patients and families who want to understand the meaning of healing and to create healing environments. The concepts of holism and healing are complex. In their depth and breadth, these concepts raise some of the most profound questions of human experience. This chapter will explore the significant philosophical issues that contribute to the creation of healing environments—in the self, the other, and the care-giving community.

WHAT IS HEALING?

In the long continuum of time, many cultures have demonstrated that the body contains the energy and mechanisms to heal many of its ills. In these cultures the unity of mind, body, and spirit within the individual is utilized to draw on these healing powers. *Healing* is the restoration to health, wholeness, or soundness. Other cultures view healing as a cure. Healing poten-

tial is enhanced in these cultures by the presence of certain belief systems: spiritual, family and community support; the ebb and flow of life and relationships; and altered states of consciousness.

In primitive cultures and in many current societies, the healing process occurs, at times, within the self, using inherent cultural beliefs about the self and healing practices. At other times, when self practices do not heal or relieve the distress, the healing presence of the shaman or medicine man may be sought. Healers in these societies serve as a medium between the visible world and the invisible spirit world (*American Heritage College Dictionary*, 1993).

Most societies in the non-Western world believe in the concepts of healing, self-healing practices, and healers who can empower the person seeking healing. Restoration to a prior level of health is the goal of healing practices. These practices occur in the cultures of Native

Patricia Barry: *Psychosocial Nursing: Care of Physically Ill Patients and Their Families*, 3rd ed.
© 1996 Lippincott–Raven Publishers

Americans, including Eskimos of North America and Siberia; Indians of the subcontinent; and Asian, South American, African, and Australian aboriginal peoples. Indeed, the number of people worldwide who engage in folk medicine and healing rituals far outnumbers those who utilize the principles of Western allopathic medicine.

It is important to note that, in these cultures, the experience of distress is holistic. Stomach pain, mental illness, or spiritual distress is experienced as whole-person distress. It is not separated systemically, as occurs in Western approaches to illness. While the healing efforts of the shaman may include elixirs that are specific to certain conditions, such as stomach, cardiac, or respiratory ailments, the mission of the healer is to restore the whole person to well-being.

CHARACTERISTICS OF THE HEALER

All persons carry within themselves the capabilities to be healing forces for themselves and others. While this capacity is present in all people, it may not be self-evident. Early psychic injuries can result in layers of protection over old traumatic hurts that can leave individuals disconnected from their own healing energies. As they work through their own early pain and shed layers of disillusionment and shame, they can discover deep intuitive wisdom, compassion and love for others, and the capacity to facilitate the healing process in self and others.

Persons who are viewed as healers possess a range of characteristics that support their healing potential. These include:

Gentleness of spirit
Compassion for the other
Respect for the dignity of the other
Respect for choices of the other
Mindfulness of the potential of the healing act to release the healing energies of the other.

There is a mutuality of purpose that is shared by the healer with the other. The healer brings to the encounter a belief that his or her actions can release healing potentials within the other (Reeder, 1994).

Brencato (1990), supporting the concept of partnership in the healing process, relates the words of an Aboriginal Australian woman:

If you have come to help me
You are wasting your time
But if you have come because
Your liberation is bound-up with mine
Then let us work together.

In traditional allopathic medical settings, the goal of the physician is to treat the diseased part of the human being. Restoration of the whole person to wellness is not the primary goal of the medical caregiver. Attending to the whole person's response to illness is and has been the goal of nursing (ANA Social Policy Statement, 1980). The nursing paradigm includes attending to all dimensions of the patient. The paradigm, when examined for the elements of holism, includes:

Person. A human being who contains integrated elements of mind, body, and spirit in dynamic balance.
Environment. Those internal or external forces that support or disrupt dynamic balance. These forces include family; community; physical, cultural, political, and economic environments; resources such as health care availability; and the value systems of health care providers.
Health. A dynamic state of mind-body-spirit balance that supports the full potential of a human being. It is a subjective state of personal well-being in contrast to a subjective state of distress.
Nursing. A process of care whose purpose is to support health.

Using the nursing paradigm as a model of health and wellness, *healing* is the process of restoring a person to health, soundness, or wholeness. The role of being a healer and participating with patients and families in this process is a choice that is open to all nurses. The remainder of the chapter will explore the physical, mental, and spiritual values that imbue the nurse with a healing presence.

QUALITIES OF A HEALING RELATIONSHIP

The foundation of a healing relationship is rooted in several guiding principles, which include:

Use of systems theory as a guiding framework

Use of change theory as a guiding framework

Application of guidelines for a therapeutic relationship

Characteristics of the caregiver relationship include:

Respect for boundaries

Awareness of the potential for over/under functioning

SYSTEMS THEORY

Systems theory is explained in Chapter 7 and the reader is referred there for fuller discussion. The fundamental concepts of systems theory are:

1. The individual is a complex, integrated system composed of interacting subsystem elements of mind, body, spirit, and social relationships. Each element consists of multiple abstract and concrete factors that have mutual feedback loops. Change or stress in any one factor has radiating effects into the subsystem; ultimately the change in the subsystem may create demand or change in the whole body/human system. Changes within the whole body system may then create challenges or threats in the family and/or other social systems, such as work, community, or health care system.

2. Responses by external systems, such as health caregivers, can create change within one or more of the human subsystem elements. Other external system factors that result in challenge or threat include an unlimited range of mental, spiritual, or physical stress factors.

3. Any type of perceived stressor can set off a cascade of responses in the whole body

system. Viewing these responses as mutually interactive in the mind-body-spirit is the focus of a healing intervention.

CHANGE THEORY

This section will address specific aspects of change theory that support the healing continuum (Jones & Bearley, 1987). They include the following conditions:

Shared vision, values, and goals. The caregiver and patient are in agreement about these three important, outcome-related criteria.

A *perceived need for change.* The patient recognizes the mind, body, spirit, or social distress that is the focus of the healing work.

A *perceived ability to change.* The patient believes that change in one or more aspects of the mind, body, spirit, or social distress is possible.

The availability of concrete options. The patient can be the subject of the healing modality, but actions and attitudes that empower the patient and the potential for healing can be taught and reviewed.

GUIDELINES FOR THERAPEUTIC RELATIONSHIPS

The foundation of a healing, therapeutic relationship is that the caregiver has a posture of respect for the autonomy, dignity, and healing potential that resides in the other.

Respect for boundaries. Boundaries are unwritten, usually unspoken rules about maintaining appropriate roles and relationships with others. Boundaries are learned in the families of origin of the caregiver and the patient.

It is particularly important that the caregiver be aware of correct, professional boundaries with patients. Because patients may place themselves in a dependent position with caregivers, they are subject to regression to earlier developmental periods. They may, for example, anticipate giving control of their healing process over to the caregiver. One of the principles of therapeutic healing relationships is that there is respect for the patient's autonomy and decision-making options. Patients may require guidance from the caregiver regarding the roles of each, so that their work together is mutually supportive of the patient's well-being.

Overinvolvement/overfunctioning vs. underinvolvement/underfunctioning. Persons who enter the healing professions have often been caregivers in their families of origin. They are frequently viewed as "givers." Indeed, one of the sources of self-esteem for most individuals is to be needed.

These characteristics can sometimes result in *overdoing* for the patient or family. When this occurs, there is a general systems effect. The patient or family does less. Overdoing on the part of the caregiver results in less control and subsequent socializing of dependent behavior in the patient or family. If the patient or family is not taught self-care principles and supported in their use, there can be erosion of the results of the healing intervention and illness behaviors are again activated.

It can be wise to begin a therapeutic relationship by reviewing the guidelines and expectations of each participant: caregiver, patient, or family member. This agreement then becomes an informal contract that sets the stage for a healing and therapeutic relationship.

WHAT IS HOLISM?

Holism is the theory that living matter or reality is made up of organic or unified wholes that are greater than the sum of their parts. *Holistic* relates to holism. As Box 4-1 indicates, the philosophy of holism "emphasizes the importance of the whole and the interdependence of its parts.... It is concerned with wholes rather than analysis or separation into parts" (*American Heritage College Dictionary,* 1993, p. 648).

Holism is the belief system that permeates all non-Western cultures and their approaches to life and all living things. Holism is an approach that was prevalent in the Western world until the advent of strong philosophical forces in the sphere of training to be medical physicians.

THE SEPARATION OF MIND AND BODY

In the 1600s, the teachers of medicine believed that it would be possible to understand the nature and cause of illness by dissecting the human body to examine its responses to disease. This intention was perceived as dangerous by authorities in the Roman Catholic Church. They held that such dissection of the body would disturb the soul. Rene Descartes, a French philosopher and mathematician who founded analytical geometry, proposed a solution that was acceptable to Church authorities. Descartes suggested that the soul is part of the mind and that the mind and body are two separate entities; emotion, intellect, and soul/spirit operate within the realm of the mind and are not part of the body (Locke & Colligan, 1986). This suggestion was well-received by Church authorities, who then determined that dissection of the human body was allowable.

The splitting of the human being into these two "separate" domains created a dualistic or Cartesian approach to the concept of health that persists to this day in Western societies and allopathic medical tradition. In the allopathic or Western medical view, the conceptualization of disease is viewed as related to matter. It must be quantifiable and able to be objectively analyzed. Without the characteristics of identifiable and quantifiable matter, an entity's reality cannot be proven (Nagel, 1993; Rossler & Rossler, 1993).

The mandate for quantifiable factors or specific measurable entities is the hallmark of the Western allopathic medical approach to disease. The difficulty in researching and "proving" the existence of entities that are valued in holistic and healing approaches is that they are difficult to quantify or measure. Such entities include mind, consciousness, spirit, suffering, transcendence, curing, self, caring, healing presence, and healing itself.

ELEMENTS OF HOLISTIC HEALTH CARE

The dimensions that support the philosophies of holism and healing are the elements at the heart of the self. These are the dimensions

BOX 4-1	**American Holistic Nurses' Association Position Statement on Social Issues**

Social Philosophy

The philosophy of the American Holistic Nurses' Association includes the belief that "health involves the harmonious balance of body, mind, and spirit in an ever-changing environment."

Thus every individual can be viewed as having three components—body, mind, and spirit—that interconnect in making the whole. Harmonious balance is achieved when conditions in an individual's life support and enhance the growth and development of each component.

Modern life presents threats and/or challenges to an individual's wholeness, whenever necessary supports for physical safety, environmental health, cognitive growth, and spiritual development are not present. AHNA supports promotion of conditions in society and in the world community that contribute to achieving universal opportunity for full development of every person. We recognize that many of these conditions are controlled by public policy and governmental decisions. For this reason, the association strives to keep its members informed of relevant social concerns and political decisions so that members may influence policy whenever possible to achieve equality and justice for all persons.

AHNA encourages socially responsible behaviors of its members regarding the nursing profession and the health care system and encourages advocacy for those groups in need of support to achieve conditions necessary for holism.

September 1992

Reprinted with permission. *Journal of Holistic Nursing, 11* (2), 1993, p. 205.

---

that exist in all human beings. They are often of a profound nature that can defy description using traditional terminology. These dimensions include:

1. Consciousness
   a. Mind
   b. Body
   c. Spirit
2. Integration or wholeness
3. Self
4. Self and other
5. Suffering
6. Hope
7. Chaos
   a. Resistance to chaos
8. Self-transcendence
9. Healing presence
   a. Centering
   b. Listening
   c. Unknowing
   d. Wisdom
10. Complementary healing methods
11. Transformation

These topics are discussed below. Although presented as specific entities, they are each integral parts of the whole human being.

CONSCIOUSNESS

Consciousness is the sum of the integrated awarenesses in the human being. These awarenesses include all elements of the mind, body, and spirit. The word *consciousness* is derived from the Latin words, *con*, meaning *together*, and *scire*, meaning *to know* (*American Heritage College Dictionary*, 1993). Consciousness encompasses the full range of self-awareness. Box 4-2 describes a compilation of definitions of consciousness.

The discussions by scientists and philosophers about the nature of consciousness continue (Harman, 1993; Nagel, 1993; Rossler & Rossler, 1993). Because of the elements that comprise the whole of consciousness, it has been impossible to arrive at a definition with clearly identifiable, discrete, and measurable components that meets the objectifiable criteria of scientific disciplines.

Burch (1994) has proposed a view of consciousness as a three-dimensional or multidimensional representation of energy in continuous movement and interaction. She describes consciousness as consisting of visible and invisible parts or entities; the invisible parts surround and permeate the visible ones. According to Burch's summary:

> Consciousness is the principle adaptive force; it is at the heart of one's ability to interact with the environment.
> Consciousness partially consists of matter and a myriad of dynamic physical processes, such as central nervous system actions, immune and endocrine effects, etc.
> Stress blocks the flow of consciousness.
> Consciousness permeates and surrounds the individual and continuously interacts with other living things and the physical environment.

Within the scope of *consciousness* are the conceptual entities of mind, body, and spirit. Using a holistic framework it is impossible to separate these entities. Employing traditional views, however, they will be described as separate entities.

Mind

Mind is viewed from many perspectives. The basic concept of mind includes all functions within the mental domains. These include cognition, perception, memory, judgment, and regulation and control of emotions and impulses.

If the reader carefully examines these mind functions, however, it becomes evident that each of them is dependent on physiological processes. For example, the neural tissue in the brain operates with remarkable physiological intricacy to support the neural processing involved with cognition—the intellectual processing of information. Perception is one's ability to use sensory processes to acquire information that is then used in cognition. The senses of vision, hearing, smell, taste, and touch are dependent on a myriad of neural networks and body systems in order for sensation and the resulting state of perception to occur.

With examination of the regulatory dimension of mind—that of mediating emotion and impulses—it is easily possible to recognize that emotion is experienced as a physiological state in the body. For example, the feelings of sadness, fear, and rage have markedly different

---

BOX 4-2	**Composite Definitions of Consciousness**

1. Joint or mutual knowledge attributed as a collective faculty to two or more people, so far as they think or feel in common.
2. A condition and concomitant of all thought, feeling, and volition.
3. The totality of the perceptions, sensations, emotions, thoughts, attitudes, desires, intentions, memories, and experience that make up a person's conscious being.
4. Sometimes limited by a qualifying epithet to a special field, such as the moral or religious consciousness.
5. Awareness, perception, or knowledge by the subject of its own acts, thoughts, feelings, or processes.
6. Inward awareness of an external object, state, or process.
7. Awareness, attention, notice, observance, realization, mindfulness, or insight with or without concern.
8. Mind or intelligence in the broadest possible sense.
9. Something in nature that is distinguished from the physical.
10. Waking life, as contrasted with sleeping, dreaming, or coma.
11. The part of mental life or psychic content in psychoanalysis that is immediately available to the ego.

SOURCE: *Collier's Encyclopedia* (1990, pp. 323–325), *Oxford English Dictionary* (1989, p. 1341), *Roget's International Thesaurus* (1977, p. 563), *Webster's Third International Dictionary* (1981, pp. 1375–1376).

subjective physical states associated with them (Barry, 1991). These states are mediated by specific psychological defenses within the mind and then by the central nervous and endocrine systems, operating through a complex neuroendocrine cascade of physiological processes. These processes infiltrate specific body systems, such as the lacrimal or tear ducts, when sadness occurs, and then loop back into cognitive and sensory processes that identify the experience as a "feeling."

Body

Body consists of the whole of all anatomical parts and physiological processes. In the dualistic view, the body is an entity that performs according to specific parameters of function. For example, cholesterol levels are ideally below a certain level so that atherosclerotic heart disease (ASHD) does not threaten physiological integrity. It is well-understood that eating foods with high fat content, particularly if there is a genetic predisposition to heart disease, will increase the risk of cardiovascular illness. These concepts fit within the view of body as matter. Physiological indicators of ASHD can be measured and quantified. Nutritional intake of fat content also can be measured and predictions about risk implied (Folkow, 1993; Johnson et al., 1992).

Mind or spirit, however, have the potential to blur the boundaries of specific body functions. When a human being is in a threatening situation, there will be an activation of the sympathetic nervous system. This activation results in multiple levels of neuroendocrine responses (see Chapter 6). When this symptho-adrenal activation occurs, one of the effects is on adipose (fat) tissue in the body. This activation releases free fatty acids and glycerol into the bloodstream (Folkow, 1993).

These fat-related substances are adaptive for the human who requires increased physical energy to fight or flee from externally occurring aggression (Cannon, 1929). When this release occurs chronically in an overweight, cardiac-illness disposed individual caught in rush hour gridlock, however, it may contribute to changes in health status (Folkow, 1993; Johnson et al., 1992). The mediating factor in the potential for release of these fatty acids will be the experience of being caught in a traffic jam and how the person responds to it. If the driver is an individual with a high level of hostility and poor coping ability accompanied by poor impulse control, his or her sympathetic nervous system will respond actively and cause a concomitant release of fatty acids (Rockstroh et al., 1992). If, on the other hand, the driver interprets the traffic tie-up as inconsequential, takes slow deep breaths, and uses the time to plan recreational activities for the weekend, the body will not receive the same ongoing symptho-adrenal activation as in the first case.

The utilization of a holistic model when assessing physiological responses to stress and their implications for health will demonstrate that the vast majority of body responses to "stress" are actually determined by the coping or "mind" response of an individual. In other words, it is the stressor's meaning to that individual that mediates the type of sympathetic nervous system activation of the full range of body systems, such as cardiovascular, gastrointestinal, muscular, skeletal, and so on. Again, it becomes virtually impossible to discern where the mind response stops and the body response begins.

Spirit

Spirit is defined as "the vital principle or animating force within living beings" and "incorporeal consciousness" (*American Heritage College Dictionary,* 1993). It is also described as "the vital center, the essence of the whole being" (Raheem, 1987, p. 19). Spirit is at the core of one's spirituality. Spirituality is described as a unifying force manifested in the self, which is expressed and experienced in the context of caring connections with oneself, others, nature, and life force or God (Burkhardt & Nagai-Jacobson, 1994). Research on spirituality has found that it is an integral aspect of well-being, life, and health (Howden, 1992). Attending to the spirit is at the core of holistic nursing approaches (Nagai-Jacobson & Burkhardt, 1989).

The North American Nursing Diagnosis Association (NANDA) has described a pattern of distress of the human spirit. The diagnosis is *Spiritual Distress*, which is defined as "the state in which the individual or group experiences or is at risk of experiencing a disturbance in the belief or value system which provides strength, hope, and meaning to life." The defining characteristic is that the individual is experiencing a disturbance in his or her belief system. Other characteristics that may be present in the individual experiencing spiritual distress include:

1. Questions credibility of belief system
2. Demonstrates discouragement or despair
3. Is unable to practice usual spiritual or religious rituals
4. Has ambivalent feelings or doubts about beliefs
5. Expresses that he has no reason for living
6. Feels a sense of spiritual emptiness
7. Shows emotional detachment from self and others
8. Expresses concern—anger, resentment, fear—over meaning of life, suffering, death
9. Requests spiritual assistance for a disturbance in belief system

The Diagnostic and Statistical Manual of Mental Disorders (DSM-IV, 1994) has, for the first time, included a spirit-related clinical problem, *Religious or Spiritual Problem*, in which "the focus of clinical attention is a religious or spiritual problem." Examples include distressing experiences that involve loss of or questioning of faith, problems associated with conversion to a new faith, or questioning of spiritual values that may not necessarily be related to an organized church or religious institution.

The NANDA and DSM-IV diagnostic categories each refer to religion and spirituality. It is important to clarify that spirituality or formal religious beliefs are subjective states that differ from person to person and within families. Some individuals have strong religious beliefs that form the primary structure through which all experience is measured. Others profess no formal religious belief system, but are imbued with the principles of spirit described earlier in this section.

The common experiences of persons with spiritual or formal religious orientation include a sense of purpose, future-orientation/hope, and connectedness with others and with an internal or external life force (Nagai-Jacobson &

Burkhardt, 1989). When these experiences of the spirit are threatened, the effects on the spirit can be profound. Fortunately, there are many resources within the individual and in the environment that work to restore spiritual balance. They include conscious coping mechanisms, unconscious defenses, dreaming (when the unconscious processes attempt to modify the underlying foundation of the distress), and the critical element of *hope* which is associated with the spirit. Environmental resources include the natural environment, as well as family, friends, and spiritual advisors. In the field of crisis intervention it is recognized that social support is one of the most important factors in averting crisis (Aguilera, 1994).

INTEGRATION OR WHOLENESS

Full comprehension of the meaning of integration may be beyond the capacities of the finite human mind. The verb *integrate* is defined as "to make a whole by bringing all parts together... to join with something else;... to make part of a larger unit" (*American Heritage College Dictionary*, 1993, p. 706). Integration can occur in human beings when the following conditions are present:

An attitude toward wholeness within the self

Awareness of defenses regarding openness within the self, with accurate insight about past psychic injuries that prevent full awareness of mind, body, and spirit connectedness

Utilization of the services of mind, body, and spiritual or healing therapists to decrease defenses that may inhibit the potential for integration within the self

What are the hallmarks that indicate a subjective sense of integration? They may include an ongoing sense of balance or knowledge to assess self equilibrium and use internal and external resources to correct imbalances. Integration may also be reflected in a subjective sense of peace, contentment, or internal harmony that may ebb and flow, but is an ongoing experience or goal of the individual. The use of a holistic model in approaching patients and families begins with caregivers who strive for the ideals of holism and integration in their own self and world views.

SELF

The concept of *self* in a holistic model can be viewed from two perspectives: the relationship of self with self, and the relationship of self with other. Before one can be fully present with another it is important that the inner life of the self is explored and viewed as an ongoing unfolding of potential.

Maslow (1970) described the self-actualized person as having fulfilled the primary needs described in his model of self-development and then moving more deeply into self-awareness in order to realize one's fullest potential. Raheem (1987) has described the experience of self-wholeness as:

> . . . one in which a person operates from a unified consciousness of body, mind, emotions, and soul. As the bonds of conditioning are shed, one begins to gain fuller awareness of a deep self-directed process that moves toward self-actualization and harmony with the cosmos. As in childhood, one becomes vulnerable again—to oneself, to other people, and to the vast mystery of life itself. . . .
>
> Where one is guided by the transcendent function of the soul and assisted by many freed parts of the personality individualized purpose can be realized. One responds to life with free thinking, open feelings, and behaviors that are congruent with the body mind. . . . The soul shines through all the layers of the personality. Such a soul-guided person is in tune with the unfolding evolutionary flow of the universe because individual purpose is part of that much bigger order in which we are all mysteriously united through spirit [pp. 16-17].

It can be helpful to realize that the work of unfolding of the self is a life-long journey; it consists of many stages, physical, psychological, and spiritual. It is a journey that is *chosen* and that requires hope, spiritual vision and connectedness with a deep life purpose. It also requires courage to delve into painful awarenesses to discover the important elements and resources of the self that lie under the layers of human distress.

SELF AND OTHER

In a holistic framework the *other* is a concept that involves the relationship of self with another living being. The fundamental approach is one of respect for the other's dignity. Another valuable dimension with respect to the other is *mindfulness,* a state of self-awareness and openness toward the self in response to the other's state. The personal qualities of the self with other may be viewed as the therapeutic self (see Chapter 2).

Another aspect of a holistic, therapeutic use of self with other is to approach the other with respect for the intrinsic wisdom and capacities that individual brings to the encounter. Such a transactional posture of caring about the other, that is, bringing an adult-adult transactional pattern to the relationship, is in contrast to a model of caretaking in which the caregiver assumes responsibility for "taking care of" the patient in a parent-child transactional style.

SUFFERING

One of the primary causes of distress of the human spirit is *suffering* (Cassell, 1992). Suffering can begin as pain in one of the human domains of the physical, psychological, spiritual, or social. When the pain is not relieved despite efforts to reduce it, there can evolve a sense of helplessness (Seligman, 1991). The experience of helplessness, if not alleviated, ultimately can lead to depression. It can be asked if, perhaps, depression and loss of hope by the spirit are the same condition.

Cassell (1992) clarifies that *suffering* is distinct from *pain*. Pain does not always lead to suffering. It is implied from Cassell's writing that spiritual resilience may safeguard the evolution of pain into suffering. He describes suffering as a "state of distress induced by the threat of loss of intactness or the disintegration of a person from whatever cause." He also adds, "Suffering is a consequence of personhood—bodies do not suffer, persons do" (p. 3). At the core of suffering, according to Cassell, is the loss of central life purpose. It is purpose, he argues, that gives guidance to life.

Suffering can occur within any dimension of the person, but it usually expands into whole-person awareness. Because the person "is a whole, thinks as a whole, and functions as a cohesive whole to the extent that something which drastically threatens a part, threatens the whole" (Cassell, 1992, p. 5), Cassell writes that when a suffering person reaches the point of loss of central purpose, he is unable to help himself and is dependent on caregivers to facilitate the restoration of meaning and purpose in life.

It has been the experience of many nurses that when a person loses a sense of central purpose and meaning, a "giving up" often occurs. This giving up is often perceived to be within the domain of the spirit. When this state becomes persistent over a period of time in a physically compromised individual, death may soon follow.

HOPE

The contrasting state to suffering and "giving up" is *hope* or optimism. Seligman (1991) describes optimistic persons as believing that a defeat is only a temporary setback. Its cause is attributed to chance or bad luck, rather than to some inherent personal flaw. When confronted with a bad situation such people view it as a challenge rather than one over which they have no control. These individuals are undaunted by defeat.

Indeed, the characteristics of hope and optimism which are the operating life principles of optimistic persons sound similar to the characteristics of the hardy personality described by Kobasa et al. (1981, 1982, 1983). These characteristics are explained in Chapter 6.

The nature of hope is more a fundamental life principle than an emotion. It is broader than a cognitive attitude. Hope is experienced at the physical level as a connected energy with the future. It is suggested that hopefulness is a life principle that resides in the spirit. This proposition includes the possibility that the home of hopefulness is in the spirit, but is inherent in the mind and body. Hopefulness within the spirit may be the fuel that supports the central purpose of an individual.

CHAOS

It is not uncommon for a time of personal change to be accompanied by a period of depression, increasing anxiety, or both states. This experience of inner change usually results in confusion and, frequently, the shift in psychological defenses results in the potentially disruptive state of *chaos*. An individual can believe that the chaotic phase cannot be survived. It is important to recognize that this subjective state of extreme distress is often the precursor to self-transcendence. The most acute aspect of the seemingly bottomless chaos stage usually lasts from 4 to 6 weeks, but may last several months. The adaptive functions of the mind, body, and spirit work at the unconscious and then conscious levels to create new patterns of physical, emotional, intellectual, and spiritual responses to the bursts of expanded consciousness.

The subjective experience of "coming to the dawn" out of the chaos occurs as swift rays of light and hope that permeate the blackness of the chaos experience. The working through, integration, and reformulation of meaning that follows the chaos period can frequently take many more months before a state of equilibrium is achieved. It is important also to recognize that "equilibrium" in the human is a state of dynamic tension, sensitive to both internal and external sensory awarenesses. Accordingly, it is not a static, fixed cognitive state of equilibrium, but rather one of fluidity and responsiveness to new awareness and experience.

Resistance to Chaos

A fleeting sense of doom can precede the experience of chaos in some individuals. Others who are strong repressors of emotion have powerful, unconscious defense mechanisms guarding against grief, anger, and the anxiety generated by conflict about the release of these emotions. It is possible that the experience of chaos can be forestalled in these persons due to the presence of strong, conscious and unconscious defenses. The psychic energy used to maintain such repression can cause a diminishment of psychic resources necessary for other developmental tasks and challenges (Aguilera, 1994). A person's life process can remain frozen at the prechaos style, sometimes for the remainder of a lifetime. Reentry into a full range of life relationships and challenges can be avoided when this frozen state persists. The person's life may be experienced as "on hold" or in decline. When this is occurring many years after the critical precipitating event, there usually is no conscious awareness of the underlying cause—unresolved grief. It is possible that a second major loss or critical event may precipitate the release of the original emotion in conjunction with that of the new loss. The accompanying grief, although repressed for many years, is experienced as freshly as if it just occurred.

SELF-TRANSCENDENCE

The emergence from chaos and the gradual return to equilibrium is described as *self-transcendence*. The characteristics of self-transcendence are:

1. Stepping back from the original traumatic experience and moving beyond what is. This characteristic is usually accompanied by a deeper awareness of self and others—a state of wisdom.
2. Extending self-boundaries. This includes reformulating one's values and sense of self to a more expanded and compassionate posture of self-acceptance and acceptance of others. This state can also include forgiveness of self and others.
3. Reaching beyond self-concern. The transcendent experience results in the desire to engage in altruism and giving to others. This characteristic is similar to the developmental stage of generativity described by Erikson (1963).

Frankl (1969) was a psychiatrist who was a prisoner in Nazi-controlled concentration camps. His stories of the inhuman treatment and terrifying experiences endured by himself and others include remarkable accounts of self-transcendence that occurred there. Frankl believes that there are three ways in which transcendence occurs:

1. Adopting an attitude of acceptance when faced with an unchangeable situation.

2. Experiencing the world through receptiveness to others and to the environment.
3. Giving to the world creatively, through family, work, or creative contributions.

Self-transcendence is the result of a healing process. It can be precipitated by either an external or internal healing catalyst or both. The result of transcendence is the movement or shift from a prior state that threatened mind/body/spirit integrity to a new set of awarenesses about which there is acceptance. While the original healing catalyst can be healer-inspired, the development and experience of transcendence can occur only within the self (Frankl, 1959; Reed, 1991b).

The original state of distress, whether initiated in the mind, body, or spirit domains, results in whole-person pain. The individual has no prior experience with such a profound event. Examples of precipitants of such distress can be the threat of terminal or life-interrupting illness; loss of a loved person through death or conflict; or loss of a job, with its resulting increase in financial anxiety, decrease in self-esteem, and loss of important work-related social relationships.

Working through the terror of terminal illness or other profound losses requires great strength and courage. Availability of support persons can be an important factor in transcending crisis events (Aguilera, 1994). The critical factor, however, is resilience within the self. The foundation of transcendence lies in the grieving process.

In each of these theories there is a period of self-doubt, high anxiety and often despair in which persons doubt that they will ever feel like "themselves" again. Self integrity or wholeness seems lost. Moods and beliefs can swing widely with no apparent order. During such a period, it can be important to work with an experienced psychotherapist who can guide the person through the "perilous waters" of chaos described by Jung (1969).

HEALING PRESENCE

The concept of *presence* has been described in many disciplines. McKivergin and Daubenmire (1994) suggest that presence as a mode of practice in nursing care may be a major thread in healing health care systems. They propose that nursing offers unique opportunities for intimacy and relationship with patients and families. By the nurse's listening and "being with" them in a centered and caring therapeutic relationship, the patient and family may be supported as they restabilize and reintegrate as a response to acute or chronic illness. Three qualities of the caring self that support the experience of healing presence for the other are centering, healing listening, and "unknowing."

Centering

Centering is a conscious act of focusing one's attention, opening one's awareness, and finding an internal reference point (Burkhardt & Nagai-Jacobson, 1994). The process of centering usually involves the steps of:

1. Attentiveness to one's breath by blowing out all of the breath as though blowing out a candle, then deeply breathing in an abdominal breath and focusing inwardly on the self and the depth of the breath within the self.
2. Awareness of connection with universal energy.
3. Intentionally choosing to be a healing presence for the other (Chiappone, 1989; Krieger, 1979).
4. Maintaining the experience of centeredness during the time of encounter with the other.

Healing Listening

"Among other things, a healer is commonly a person to whom a sufferer tells things; out of his or her listening, the healer develops the basis for therapeutic interventions," according to Jackson (1992, p. 1623). Theodore Reik (1951) describes the need for the listener to "learn how one mind speaks to another beyond words and in silence... This 'third ear' can catch what people do not say, but only feel and think"; and it can also be turned inwardly (p. 150). It can hear voices within the listener, within the self, that are usually drowned out by the listener's conscious thought processes.

This moving account by Kleinman (1988) of the experience of a medical student with a suffering child explains the meaning of healing listening.

> The...patient was a pathetic seven-year-old girl who had been badly burned over most of her body. She had to undergo a daily ordeal of a whirlpool bath during which the burnt flesh was tweezered away from her raw, open wounds. This experience was horribly painful to her. She screamed and moaned and begged the medical team, whose efforts she stubbornly fought off, not to hurt her anymore. My job as a neophyte clinical student was to hold her uninjured hand, as much to reassure and calm her as to enable the surgical resident to quickly pull away the dead, infected tissue in the pool of swirling water, which rapidly turned pinkish, then bloody red. . . . I tried to distract this little patient from her traumatic daily confrontation with terrible pain. I tried talking to her about her home, her family, her school—almost anything that might draw her vigilant attention away from her suffering. I could barely tolerate the daily horror. . . . Then one day, I made contact. . . . Uncertain what to do besides clutching the small hand, and in despair over her unrelenting anguish, I found myself asking her to tell me how she tolerated it, what the feeling was like of being so badly burned and having to experience the awful surgical ritual, day after day after day. She stopped, quite surprised, and looked at me from a face so disfigured it was difficult to read the expression; then in terms direct and simple, she told me. While she spoke, she grasped my hand harder and neither screamed nor fought off the surgeon or the nurse. Each day from then on, her trust established, she tried to give me a feeling of what she was experiencing. By the time my training took me off this rehabilitation unit, the little burned patient seemed noticeably better able to tolerate the debridement [pp. xi-xxi].

Unknowing

The example of the medical student and child described above provides the opening for an examination of adopting an *unknowing* listening posture with the other. The medical student originally approached the child believing that he "should know" the experience of the other and spoke to the child from that perspective.

Indeed, only the child knew her own pain. Healing presence or authentic person-to-person connection allows the other to feel understood. Only by asking the other to explain his or her "knowing" about the subjective experience of illness, pain, or suffering is it possible to understand the patient's own inner state.

The nursing metaparadigm of person, environment, health, and nursing (Fawcett, 1984) implies that the nurse "knows" about each of these entities of nursing practice; their meaning is clear. It is this knowing that is then brought to the patient and nursing care is "administered" by using the structure, values, and norms implicit in the particular nursing model utilized by the nurse.

Munhall (1993) presents a compelling argument that the "knowing" of these structural nursing concepts, much like the "knowing" of the medical student described above, prevents the nurse from being authentically and empathically present and fully understanding the actual experience of the patient. Munhall proposes that, in addition to the four elements of the nursing metaparadigm proposed by Fawcett, there should be a fifth pattern of knowing. Paradoxically, this level of knowing is "unknowing."

Munhall describes the state of mind of unknowing as a condition of openness. "Knowing," in contrast, leads to a form of confidence that has in it a state of closure (Munhall, 1993, p. 125). Atwood and Stolorow (1984) characterize the process of "unknowing" as a decentering from one's own organizing principles of the world.

Kurtz (1989) states that "knowledge screens the sound the third ear hears so we hear only what we know" (pp. 6–7). Kurtz also explains that "the compulsion to make sense is a resistance to unknowing." Munhall (1993) explains that "the pattern of unknowing can lead to a much deeper knowledge of another being, of different meanings and interpretations of all our various perceptions of experience" (p. 128).

Munhall describes the traditional nursing "hearing" posture of acquiring information that fits within the structure of diagnosing and prescribing to relieve patients' problems. The information obtained from the patient may be filtered through the nurse's knowledge of diagnosing and healing theories. Using this approach may then lead to premature closure without fully comprehending the cause or nature of the other's distress (1993).

Wisdom

The fourth element of healing presence to be addressed in this section is *wisdom*. Wisdom is defined as "understanding . . . what is true, right, or lasting; insight . . . common sense; good judgment (*American Heritage College Dictionary*, 1993, p. 1548).

Wisdom, sometimes also referred to as *knowing*, is a deep grounding within the self about which there is a sense of certainty. This certainty is a form of held knowledge about the self; it can also extend to others.

COMPLEMENTARY HEALING METHODS

Other therapeutic modalities can also support the healing process.

Contemporary Healing Methods

Many contemporary healing practices integrate healing traditions from a variety of sources. Table 4-1, while not all-inclusive, lists a number of contemporary complementary healing methods.

Ancient Healing Methods

Many healing methods have been utilized by ancient societies. These practices continue to be used in current cultures, including Native American, Chinese, and Ayurvedic traditions from India. Many individuals in the Western world have integrated these holistic methods in their own health regimens. They find that these practices assist in creating a sense of balance in the mind, body, and spirit. It is not uncommon that persons who are faced with life-interrupting or threatening illnesses begin to explore outside of traditional Western medicine to discover methods that support a personal healing process. Such a process involves the development of inner awareness and a search for meaning and tranquility. It is recommended that these complementary or "alternative" healing methods be used in conjunction with, rather than as a substitute for, traditional Western medical care.

Native Healing Practices*

The healing practices of the native peoples of North America are diverse, since they constitute many separate and distinct peoples. Nonetheless, their various ways of healing share common themes which are rooted in the shamanism that underlies all the world's religious and healing traditions. In shamanistic understanding, religion and healing were never separated because the natural realm and the spiritual realm were fully integrated, belonging together as the whole of things. Therefore, medicine meant the sacred power naturally present in plants and animals, in rocks and streams, in the wind and in fire, in the sun and moon and stars, and it was also the same sacred power present within the body, mind, and soul of human beings.

The use of medicine as sacred power depended upon a fundamental recognition of the kinship between human beings and all these other beings of power in the universe. Among the Lakota/Dakota people (commonly, but mistakenly called the Sioux) this vital theme of kinship is expressed in all ceremonies by the words *"mitakuye oyasin,"* which can be translated into English as "all my relations." Saying these words is a sacred way of acknowledging that you as a human being are, by your intention and your ritual acts, reaffirming a connection with all the other beings of the universe as your kin, your relatives. It is the acknowledgement of a family relationship. Indeed, animal and bird and fish peoples are referred to as nations, such as the deer nation, the eagle nation, and the salmon nation.

The kinship of all things in the universe is known by native peoples from their ancient stories, the sacred myths about how the creation of the world took place, and how the medicine, power and the kinship of all beings came to be

present in our reality, so that medicine and kinship belong to the natural order of things. These stories are taken to be true and powerful even today, because no one story rules out the truth of other stories. Any attempt to describe completely in one single tale the way all things are interconnected inevitably runs deeper and deeper into the mysteries of mind and matter where language itself is no longer adequate. The truth of these stories comes from a region beyond language, and the primary path by which the stories come into human experience is by dreams and visions, which provide us closer and deeper access to the mysteries of the universe than ordinary consciousness. Those who have mastered access to the realm of dreams and visions are the medicine men and medicine women who are the shamans of a people. Based on their knowledge of the realm of dreams and visions, they have been able to shift into non-ordinary dimensions of human consciousness through which they experience the medicine powers in our plant and animal relatives and in stone persons, thunder beings, and the winds of the four quarters of the universe, to all of which we are akin.

Since the medicine power of the universe is present both in the natural fabric of the surrounding world and within the body, mind, and soul of human beings, native healers connect together the medicine powers of the outer and inner realms by following the protocols of kinship in the sacred stories when they treat illnesses. Such connecting together takes the form of ceremony, which is a sacred way of using medicine objects, medicine songs, and the ritual acts of medicine stories to re-establish the basic reciprocities of kinship between a sick person and his or her relatives, both human and other-than-human. Typical medicine objects in native healing ceremonies today might include such items as a feather, tobacco, corn meal, and pollen. These objects are empowered with the medicine of the plants and creatures they represent. Every ceremony is apt to include medicine songs, which are sung with the assistance of a sacred drum or rattle which has the power to attune the body, mind, and soul of the sick person with the natural rhythms of the earth. By skills acquired from experience in nonordinary con-

*This section was written by Dr. Dale Stover, Professor of Native American and Spiritual Studies at the University of Nebraska.

(text continues on page 72)

TABLE 4-1
Complementary Healing Methods

Healing Method	Area Addressed	How Practitioners Work	Areas of Possible Benefit
Art Therapy	Mind, body, and spirit.	Use of creative materials and media with attention to colors and symbols. Results are then interpreted.	Insight and personal discovery, accessing the unconscious mind. Integration of the whole self.
Alexander Technique	Habitual physical alignment, coordination and functioning through lengthening the spine and freeing restrictions in the neck and head.	Teachers use verbal directions and gentle touch to engage students mentally, in movement, and in work on a table.	Back pain, slipped discs, digestion, anxiety, depression, arthritis, and rheumatism.
Acupressure, Acupuncture	A network of channels (meridians) throughout the body where life energy (chi) constantly flows.	Blocked or deficient energy is stimulated or dispersed with pressure needles at specific points on the body.	Musculoskeletal, neurological (pain), gastrological, gynecological, pediatric immunological, including allergies and asthma.
Ayurveda (Sanskrit for "science of life")	Illness is treated at the source rather than symptoms, to establish perfect balance in mind and body.	Healing and rejuvenation are achieved through a combination of meditation, herbs, diet, massage, yoga, etc.	Disorders in reproductive, digestive, circulatory, respiratory, and nervous systems.
Bach Flower Remedies	Work on the premise that disease in the body is a symptom of disturbance in the mind, heart, and spirit.	Practitioners diagnose patient's mood and mental attitude and suggest remedies which have been found to promote healing.	Various moods and attitudes, such as anxiety.
Bioenergetics	Every physical expression of the body, if fixed and habitual, has a meaning based in past experience. Limitations in motility and breathing are the result and cause of anxiety.	Special body movements and positions result in deeper contact with the body, unleashing energy bound in the musculature with a resultant improved personality function.	Self-image (body image), interpersonal relationships, quality of thinking and feeling, and enjoyment of life.
Biofeedback	EMG—A biofeedback machine gives a constant report of your body's physiological stress responses. EEG—A special form that supports deep changes in the central nervous system.	Feedback is used to guide relaxation, gain awareness and learn control of reactions underlying symptoms.	EMG—Stress-related conditions, migraines, asthma, colitis, hypertension. EEG—Addictions, learning disabilities, closed head injuries.
Body Harmony	Based on the principle that our bodies have a natural ability, inclination, and innate wisdom for healing themselves.	Practitioner helps the patient define a goal and supports the patient by following the tissue exactly. This accesses the inner wisdom of the body, enabling release of physical and emotional pain. The patient is empowered to break through old limitations.	Addresses all manner of blocks and disorders in the body.

Courtesy of Rebecca Flannery, B.M., M.M., consulting holistic movement practitioner, Burlington, CT.

TABLE 4-1 Complementary Healing Methods (Continued)			
Healing Method	**Area Addressed**	**How Practitioners Work**	**Areas of Possible Benefit**
Chiropractic	Analysis and correction of misalignments of the vertebral column to release pressure from the nerves.	The chiropractor locates spinal misalignments and adjusts them by manipulation. Various styles of chiropractic exist.	Musculoskeletal problems, back aches, headaches, neurological problems, TMJ, respiratory problems.
Core Energetics	Therapeutic work which engages the dimensions of energy and consciousness, breaking down and transforming the patient's defenses in order to reach the expressive core.	Practitioners work with patients to release emotional blocks and negative images and belief systems through work on the body to restore energy and consciousness.	Pleasure and fulfillment in life. Alleviates somatized energy.
Craniosacral Therapy	The craniosacral system consists of membranes connecting cranial and sacral bones, enclosing brain and cerebrospinal fluids.	Practitioners use hands-on techniques to rebalance this hydraulic system to its natural pulsation.	Spinal cord injuries, headaches, back pain.
The Feldenkrais Method	An educational process that retrains the mind to move the body by knowing how the body works.	In addition to giving attention to specific injury or chronic pain, the teacher guides the patient through subtle movements and teaches the patient to abandon habitual patterns and develop greater flexibility and coordination.	Improve posture and breathing, ease pain, develop efficient and flexible movement, reduce stress, move with minimum effort and maximum efficiency.
The Healing Tao	This work is a selection of Taoist/Chinese healing techniques which address the body, mind, and spirit.	Practitioners use techniques of subtle movements, i.e, Tai Chi, internal organ massage, healing sounds, the inner smile, visualization, the microcosmic orbit.	Although this widely effective work can be used for quick remedies, it is best employed over an extended period for maximum benefit and may be applied to all disease.
Homeopathy	Symptoms represent the body's effort to heal. Suppression of symptoms leads to illness. Microdoses of medicine are prescribed based on their ability to cause symptoms in the patient when taken in large doses.	Doctors diagnose the totality of symptoms and then administer minute doses of natural remedies derived from herbal, mineral, and animal substances.	Any disease or injury in which augmenting the body's defenses can provide benefit.
Hypnotherapy	Mind, body, and spirit.	Use of different methods depending on practitioner's approach, e.g., Ericson, Grove, imagery induction methods, verbal.	Whole person integration, potential release of somatic patterns associated with toxic memory or memories.

(continued)

TABLE 4-1
Complementary Healing Methods (Continued)

Healing Method	Area Addressed	How Practitioners Work	Areas of Possible Benefit
Naturopathic Medicine	Based on the healing power of nature, naturopaths aim to treat the cause rather than just the effect, do no harm, treat the whole person, see the physician as a teacher, and believe that prevention is the best cure.	Although not MDs, naturopaths are educated in conventional medical science. They use therapies from other sciences: nutrition, herbal medicine, homeopathy, hydrotherapy, counseling, etc.	All areas of family care from childbirth to geriatrics.
Polarity Therapy	Based on the premise that the balance and open flow of the energy field of the body is the foundation of good health.	The practitioner uses his or her hands to facilitate movement of energy blockages to achieve a balanced flow of energy in the body. Dietary principles, exercises, and attitudinal work	Physical and emotional distress, headaches, back ache, digestive and lymphatic system disorders.
Proprioceptive Writing	Mind, body, and spirit.	Guided writing exercises.	Insight and personal discovery, derepression of formerly unconscious memory, whole person integration.
Psychosynthesis	Combining analytic and meditative psychology to explore how the self/Self develops and expresses through personality.	Practitioner works with subpersonalities, will, guided imagery, and visualization in therapeutic sessions.	Interpersonal relationships and individual development.
Rebirthing	Use of the breath opens awareness of how past thoughts, feelings, and memories keep one from living fully in the present moment.	Practitioner guides the patient through a precisely defined circular breathing process, and provides support and anchoring for the patient.	Increased feelings of acceptance of self and others, renewal of joy in life, sense of ease and peace.
Reflexology	Based on the principle that the reflexes in the hands and feet correspond to all organs, glands, or parts of the body.	Reflexologists use thumbs and fingers to work on these reflexes, resulting in relaxation and balance.	Helps to reduce tension, improve nerve and blood supply, and normalize all major systems in the body.
Reiki	A method of activating and balancing the life-force energy in the entire body, including the organs and glands.	Practitioners gently place hands in various positions on the body to focus energy into those areas.	Used for prevention of disease and for mental, emotional, physical, and spiritual distress.

TABLE 4-1
Complementary Healing Methods (Continued)

Healing Method	Area Addressed	How Practitioners Work	Areas of Possible Benefit
Rolfing	A technique of stretching the fascial tissue (which envelopes the muscles) to lengthen and balance the body on the vertical axis. This is integrated for better functioning.	Given in a series of 10 sessions addressing surface layers and deep body tissue, which allows reorganization of the whole body. Realign and rebalance the patient's structure and teach him/her how to use his/her body well.	Structural discomfort, chronic pain; balanced, well-functioning body; integration with psychotherapy.
Rubenfeld Synergy	Connection of body, mind, and emotions. Learn how old feelings and beliefs can cause blocked energy and tension patterns. This awareness allows the possibility of change.	Patient and synergist explore physical and emotional holding patterns through use of gentle touch, verbal communication, humor, and imagination.	Increased body/mind awareness and acceptance, recovery from physical and emotional trauma, greater self-esteem and clarity.
Tai Chi	A Taoist/Chinese martial art of meditation through movement. It combines coordinated breathing with slow movements.	This form may be used for meditation, general health, or, if performed at a faster speed, for self-defense.	Supports healthy functioning of respiration, heart, digestion, glands, mind.
Therapeutic Touch	Redirecting the flow of energy towards balance and harmony of physical, emotional, and spiritual aspects.	Practitioners complete four steps: centering the self, assessing client's body energy for blockages, rebalancing patient by smoothing and redirecting, and reassessing. Work is done with hands a few inches away from the physical body.	Relief of anxiety, pain, and emotional, spiritual, or physical distress.
Yoga	Calming the mind and emotions, and toning the body through unification with Universal Spirit.	A series of stretching postures, breathing, and meditation techniques. May be done individually or in class format. Used to integrate mind and body.	Stress, feelings of separation, internal conflict, and physical stiffness.
Zero Balancing	Mind, body, and spirit.	Hands-on bodywork that balances chakras (energy vortexes) and energy.	Potential release of somatic patterns associated with toxic memory, integration of whole.

sciousness and/or by procedures in the ceremony itself, a competent medicine person will be able to discover what the root cause of the imbalance is which has manifested in the form of the illness and will be able to carry out the ceremonial forms which are appropriate for restoring wholeness.

While some ceremonies may be arranged to take place at a location which is a sacred site according to the traditions of a people, any location, even a hospital room, can be made sacred through the ceremony itself. For example, those peoples who use a sacred pipe will place a pinch of tobacco into the bowl of the pipe for the spirit powers of each of the four directions of the universe and of the sky and the earth. In this way the pipe becomes a microcosm of the whole universe, and the one who holds the pipe is standing in that moment of the ceremony at the very center of the universe. As he or she offers the filled pipe to each direction in turn, the sacred power of kinship undergirding the whole of things is brought to focus in that place and is available for healing.

Persons from nontribal backgrounds have sometimes been welcomed into ceremonies of native peoples, but not all native traditions are open to this, and being respectful of native ways means that others should not attempt to mimic or take over their practices. Nevertheless, the healing ways of tribal peoples belonged at some point in the past to everyone's traditions, and there is a widespread revival of interest in the contemporary practice of aspects of shamanic healing. The examples of native practices can assist persons who wish to enlist their dreams and visions, along with the stories, songs, places, and natural objects which become sacred to them, in order to incorporate them into the enhancement of already-existing religious ceremonies or to evolve personal forms of ceremony for individual healing. The lessons learned from native healing traditions can assist contemporary persons in understanding that the natural world is a realm of healing power and that we can access that power because we have, on the basis of kinship, a deep belonging to the whole of it and to each and every part of it.

Access to shamanic healing power is also being made available to people of modern cultures through innovative adaptations of ancient techniques to contemporary circumstances. Two forms of these which are available to people through workshops in urban centers of North America, Europe, and Australia are the "holotropic therapy" of Stanislas Grof, a psychiatrist, and the "core shamanism" of Michael Harner, an anthropologist. Both of these modern approaches make access to nonordinary states of consciousness available to ordinary people, through which the medicine powers of birds, animals, plants, and our other relatives are experienced along with the inner dimensions of body, mind, and soul.

Other Ancient Healing Practices*

Consideration of complementary healing methods involves a brief review of the basic principles underlying time-honored systems of care which evolved separately and have endured for thousands of years.

First is the concept of an all-pervasive force which surrounds and is within all things. In the early civilization of Greece it was known as *pneuma.* In ancient India it was *prana,* and in China it was *chi.* In Korea and Japan it was *ki,* in Hawaii it was *aka;* in Mexico the Maya named it *che* and the Huichol called it *kupuri,* while in the Southwestern United States the Hopi tribe named it *kuchina.* These and other traditional peoples know this force as a complementary coupling of polar energies which combine to generate the material world as well as to provide the dynamic tension for all movement, growth, healing and change. Ancient indigenous people knew this energy as the force that integrates the physical, mental, and spiritual aspects of human life with all planetary life and with the life of the universe itself.

The second concept is the perception that this force generates four or five primary components arising from essential combinations of the two polar energies within it. When these elementary units of energy are in balance, the body is in a state of health and well-being. As the strength of this force is increased in the body, it fosters greater vitality, liveliness, and the ability to regulate mind-body processes.

---

* This section was written by Michael Dauria, a teacher and practitioner of many healing modalities.

Healing methods of traditional systems include actions to remedy imbalances in components of the life force that powers the bioelectrical and biochemical energies regulating the thousands of reactions taking place within the human body each day. Approaches external to the body include stimulating and strengthening the body's energy streams; healing by touch; massage; manipulation, pressure, or energy transmission; healing with nature and environment—sunlight and colors, sounds and vibrations, aromas and textures, mineral baths, colored lakes and hot springs; experiences generated by sacred patterns, places, and living spaces. Internal approaches include diet and herbs; nutritional supplements and remedies; relaxation and meditative movement; deepening internal awareness of bodily sensations and responses to tones and colors of the sound-light continuum; and the caregivers empowering the cared-for with a sense of intention for self-healing and a sense of community through group therapy healing activities.

The classic Greek school of healing founded by Hippocrates, the "father of medicine," in the fifth century B.C. was the first Western system dedicated to the scientific understanding of health and the body. The *pneuma*, or life-force, was identified as the energy that flowed through the body linking each individual with the environment as well as with their emotional and spiritual life. The body was viewed as being composed of four humors or fluids, each a manifestation of the four basic elements of the universe: fire, water, air, and spirit. Each humor had different qualities and the equilibrium of these components was understood to determine the health or disease of the body as well as disposition and temperament.

In his *"Vis Medicatrix Naturae,"* Hippocrates endorsed the healing power of nature as the mechanism used to balance the humors of the body. Gentle therapies such as diet, herbal treatments, medicinal use of honey and wines, relaxation, and eurythmic exercises were encouraged. This tradition fostered internal energy systems taught in the Greek mystery schools and reached Galen, who brought it to the Roman Empire. There it spread vis-à-vis many other traditional healers. Today these principles are most closely associated with the contemporary healing system known as *naturopathy*.

Ayurveda, or wisdom of life, is the classic healing system of India which dates from the tenth century B.C., or before. It is considered the "mother of medicine," with roots in the matriarchal teachings of the tantra. A Sanskrit word meaning "web," tantra are experiences that stretch the mind to higher levels of awareness and knowing. The early Hindus identified *prana* as the animating force of life which provides endurance, vitality, and healing. *Prana* manifests in its physical form as the Five Bhutas, or great elements of the universe, bound together by the Three Doshas, or bioenergies. The Five Bhutas—Fire, Water, Earth, Air, and Ether—are seen as categories that describe functions and aspects of the constitution of the human body. These elements are balanced by the actions of the three bioenergies within: *vata*, which stimulates motion, circulation, thought, and communication; *pitta*, which governs digestion, assimilation, cell metabolism, and endurance; and *kapha*, which regulates structure, lubrication, reproduction, and groundedness. These energies affect the flow of *prana* through the body and whether or not it is excessive, deficient, or balanced in certain organs.

Ayurvedic healing includes gentle therapy programs: proper food and drink, herbs and supplements, cleansing therapies and massage, and meditation and exercises such as yoga. Maharishi Ayurveda is an updated version of the ancient art and is available at clinics in the United States, England, and Ireland. Transcendental meditation and yoga are taught along with programs for healing and rejuvenation.

The Chinese healing arts have developed from an ancient system known as "The Yellow Emperor's Classic of Internal Medicine," a compilation of healing information dating from as far back as the third century, B.C. Other documents describe healing arts that originated in a 10,000-year-old Chinese culture known as "The Children of the Golden Light," who are said to have lived long lives and experienced good health. It is written that they knew how to promote internal energy circulation with gentle rhythmic movements and deep breathing which relaxed the entire body, including the tendons and bones, strengthening the constitution.

Tao, defined as a way of life or path on the journey of life, is the 5,000-year-old natural philosophy at the root of the Chinese healing arts.

According to Chinese cosmology, a vast, primordial oneness gave rise to polar companions, *yin* and *yang,* which generated a cosmic life force called *chi. Chi* then divided to form the Five Qualities which in various combinations produced all physical reality, including life forms. The Five Qualities or Five Elements of *chi* energy are Fire, Water, Earth, Metal, and Wood.

In traditional Chinese medicine, the Five Qualities, or elemental activities of chi energy, associate respectively with the heart, kidneys, spleen, lungs, and liver to invigorate and regulate their functional systems. Chi flows through the body in well-defined channels called meridians. They can be likened to 12 streams of energy, each associated with a specific organ system, and two additional deep rivers of energy responsible for unifying and balancing the various organ systems. Chi energy is known to have substance, to contain information, and to have a measurable and variable charge in the electromagnetic spectrum. Eons ago, the Chinese seem to have had an intuitive knowledge of the ultimate unified field theories of complementary particle interaction which are explored in the high-energy physics laboratories of today.

Chi kung (or *qigong*) may be the earliest ancestor to all active healing therapies. Translated as "energy work" or "energy exercises," it involves standing postures, gentle rhythmic movements, and slow, deep breathing done in a calm, relaxed manner with inner-directed attention to promote the flow of chi energy throughout the body. Regular practice of chi kung exercises leads to deep inner feeling states in which sensations of accumulation and flow of internal energy are actively experienced. Meditative movement combined with mindfulness of nourishing colors, tones, vibrations, and patterns enables one to modulate the charge of inner chi energy and to rearrange its qualities. *Meridian massage* and *acupressure* are gentle methods of opening up energy blockages, removing tension and smoothing out the chi flow through its circulation systems.

Acupuncture involves the introduction of fine needles into specific points on the energy streams, as well as the use of magnets and heat to stimulate or regulate the flow of chi. Traditional Chinese medicine considers this to be a passive and more invasive therapy than the chi kung exercises, meridian massage, or acupressure therapies which form the basis of an active self-care process.

Tai chi (or *tai ji*), a meditation in motion, is a set of chi kung postures connected by flowing movements in a specific sequence. Ancient Chinese family lineages formulated their own styles which are known as particular tai chi forms. Translated as "Supreme Ultimate Source," tai chi energy exercise enhances the feelings and flow of the vital inner force of the body so that it streams in abundance, linking the essence of self with nature and cosmos to improve health and enliven the spirit.

Chinese healing arts also include Five Element nutritional therapies, extensive use of herbal formulations and treatments; *chi nei tsang*—a direct internal organ visceral manipulation procedure; external chi transmission by chi kung healers; tendon-changing and bone-marrow-washing *nei kung* exercises; Fusion Meditations to balance emotional energies; internal alchemy rejuvenation techniques; and many others which stem from a unique blend of physical, mental, and spiritual cultivation regimens.

The Yellow Emperor's Classic serves as the foundation of most of the Asian medicine, including systems adopted by Korea and Japan, and virtually all of the Oriental health systems available in the West today.

The concepts underlying the systems described above provide a foundation for and lend substance to contemporary healing arts such as Therapeutic Touch, which is similar to chi transmission healing and to the evolving field of energy medicine which encompasses the use of electromagnetic forces for established procedures such as healing bone fractures and for revolutionary therapies involving supplementation of the body's own energetic systems.

The healing methods described can be used for the most part to augment and reinforce a course of conventional medical treatment. Gentle, natural healing therapies combined with self-care and small group relaxation practices provide feelings of involvement, participation, and community, adding valuable dimensions to the healing process.

TRANSFORMATION

The human being is in a state of constant change and growth. The emotional blockages from early psychic or physical injuries result in physiologic patterns that underlie a variety of emotional states such as helplessness, helpless and frozen anger, rage, fear, grief, anxiety, depression, hopelessness, and so on. It is hypothesized that the effects of these "caught," conditioned patterns of emotional response can lead to pathophysiologic mechanisms that, over time, may result in physical or mental disorders.

Transformation is the process of "working through" or transforming the original body responses to these toxic emotional states. As described in the sections on chaos, resistance to chaos, and self-transcendence, this is usually a challenging and powerful, and sometimes frightening, endeavor. It can involve great courage. The result of transformation, which may be a years-long or lifetime process, is a dynamic state that includes being "present in the moment," and being open to the self and others. Transformation is an evolutionary process that results in resilience as a response to life events. If disruptions occur, there is an inner wisdom that is able to adapt with flexibility, find meaning in the event, and gradually return the person to a state of mind/body/spirit balance.

CONCLUSION

The concepts of holism and healing are postures associated with being "with" oneself and others. The awareness of general systems effects within the human being utilizes general systems theory to understand the rich connectedness and dynamic interactions between the mind, body, spirit and social and environmental experiences.

BIBLIOGRAPHY

Achterberg, J. (1985). *Imagery in healing: Shamanism and modern medicine.* Boston: Shambhala Publications.

Achterberg, J. (1992). Ritual: The foundation for transpersonal medicine. *Revision, 14*(3), 158–164.

Aguilera, D. C. (1994). *Crisis intervention: Theory and methodology* (7th ed.). St. Louis: Mosby.

Aldridge, D. (1991). Spirituality, healing and medicine. *British Journal of General Practice, 41*(351), 425–427.

American Heritage college dictionary (3rd ed.). (1993). Boston: Houghton-Mifflin.

American Nurses Association. (1980). *Nursing: A Social Policy Statement.* Washington, D.C.: American Nurses Publishing.

Atwood, D., & Stolorow, R. (1984). *Structures of subjectivity.* Hillsdale, New Jersey: Lawrence Erlbaum Associates.

Barnsteiner, J., Gillis-Donovan, J., Knox-Fischer, C., & McKlindon, D. (1994). Defining and implementing a standard for therapeutic relationships. *Journal of Holistic Nursing, 12*(1), 35–49.

Barry, P. (1991). An investigation of cardiovascular, respiratory, and skin temperature changes during relaxation and anger inductions. *Dissertation Abstracts International,* 52–09–B, 5012.

Beck, P. V., & Walters, A. L. (1990). *The sacred: Ways of knowledge, sources of life.* Flagstaff, AZ: Navajo College Press.

Becket, N. (1991). Clinical nurses' characterizations of patient coping problems. *Nursing Diagnosis, 2*(2), 72–78.

Brencato, H. (1990). *Women and Peacemaking* (Calendar). Erie, PA: Pax Christi, U.S.A.

Burch, S. (1994). Consciousness: How does it relate to health? *Journal of Holistic Nursing, 12*(1), 101–116.

Burkett, G. L. (1991). Culture, illness, and the biopsychosocial model. *Family Medicine, 23*(4), 287–291.

Burkhardt, M. A., & Nagai-Jacobson, M. G. (1994). Reawakening spirit in clinical practice. *Journal of Holistic Nursing, 12*(1), 9–21.

Butz, M. (1992). Chaos, an omen of transcendence in the psychotherapeutic process. *Psychological Reports, 71,* 827–843.

Campbell, R. J. (1989). *Psychiatric dictionary* (6th ed.). New York: Oxford University Press.

Cannon, W. (1929). *Bodily changes in pain, hunger, fear, and rage* (2nd ed.). New York: D. Appleton Co.

Carpenito, L. J. (Ed.) (1993). *Nursing Diagnosis: Application to clinical practice* (5th ed.). Philadelphia: J.B. Lippincott.

Carson, V. B., & Green, A. (1992). Spiritual well-being: A predictor of hardiness in patients with Acquired Immunodeficiency Syndrome. *Journal of Professional Nursing, 8*(4), 209–220.

Chang, S. T. (1986). *The complete system of self-healing.* San Francisco: Tao Publishing.

Chia, M. (1993). *Awaken healing light of the tao.* Huntington, NY: Healing Tao Books.

Chiappone, J. (1989). *The light touch.* Centerville, VA: Holistic Reflections.

Coward, D. (1991). Self-transcendence and emotional well-being in women with advanced breast cancer. *Oncology Nursing Forum, 18*(5), 857–863.

Coward, D., & Lewis, F. (1993). The lived experience of self- transcendence in gay men with AIDS. *Oncology Nursing Forum, 20*(9), 1363–1368.

Dewsbury, D. A. (1991). Psychobiology. *American Psychologist, 46*(3), 198–205.

Diagnostic and statistical manual of mental disorders (4th ed.). (1994). Washington, D. C.: American Psychiatric Association.

Doore, G. (Ed.). (1988). *Shaman's path: Healing, personal growth, and empowerment*. Boston: Shambhala Publications.

Dossey, B. M., Guzzetta, C. E., & Kenner, C. V. (1992). *Critical care nursing: Body-mind-spirit* (3rd ed.). Philadelphia: J. B. Lippincott.

Duff, V. (1994). Spiritual distress: Deciding to care. *Journal of Christian Nursing, 11*(1), 29–31.

Edlin, G., & Golanty, E. (1992). *Health and wellness: A holistic approach* (4th ed.). Boston: Jones and Bartlett.

Emblen, J. D., & Halstead, L. (1993). Spiritual needs and interventions: Comparing the views of patients, nurses, and chaplains. *Clinical Nurse Specialist, 7*(4), 175–182.

Erikson, E. (1963). *Childhood and society* (2nd ed.). New York: Norton.

Fawcett, J. (1984). The metaparadigm of nursing: Present status and future refinements. *Image: The Journal of Nursing Scholarship, 16*(3), 84.

Folkow, B. (1993). Physiological organization of neurohormonal responses to psychosocial stimuli: Implications for health and disease. *Annals of Behavioral Medicine, 15*(4), 236–244.

Frankl, V. (1959). *Man's search for meaning*. New York: Washington Square Press.

Frankl, V. (1969). *The will to meaning*. New York: New American Library.

Gaut, D.A. (Ed.) (1993). *A global agenda for caring*. New York: National League for Nursing Press.

Gerteis, M., Edgman-Levitan, S., Daley, J., & Delbanco, T. L. (1993). *Through the patient's eyes: Understanding and promoting client-centered care*. San Francisco: Jossey-Bass.

Goleman, D., & Gurin, J. (1993). *Mind-body medicine*. Yonkers, NY: Consumer Reports Books.

Grof, S. (1988). *The adventure of self-discovery*. Albany, NY: State University of New York Press.

Halifax, J. (1982). *Shaman: The wounded healer*. London: Crossroad.

Harner, M. (1980). *The way of the shaman*. New York: Harper.

Haase, J., Britt, T., Coward, D., Leidy, N. K., & Penn, P. E. (1992). Simultaneous concept analysis of spiritual perspective, hope, acceptance, and self-transcendence. *Image: The Journal of Nursing Scholarship, 24*(2), 141–147.

Harman, W. W. (1993). Mind and healing: Removing obstacles which have inhibited enquiry. *South African Medical Journal, 83*(5), 312–313.

Hartman, D., & Knudson, J. (1991). A nursing data base for initial patient assessment. *Oncology Nursing Forum, 18*(1), 125–130.

Heliker, D. (1992). Reevaluation of a nursing diagnosis: Spiritual distress. *Nursing Forum, 27*(4), 15–20.

Howden, J. W. (1992). *Development and psychometric characteristics of the Spirituality Assessment Scale*. Unpublished doctoral dissertation, Texas Women's University, Denton, TX.

Hudak, C. M., Gallo, B. M., & Benz, J. J. (Eds.). *Critical care nursing: A holistic approach* (5th ed.). Philadelphia: J. B. Lippincott.

Huxley, J. H. (1982). *Spice, time and medicine*. Boulder, CO: Shambhala.

Inagaki, K., & Hatano, G. (1993). Young children's understanding of the mind-body distinction. *Child Development, 64*(5), 1534–1549.

Institute of Noetic Sciences. (1993). *The heart of healing*. Atlanta: Turner Publishing, Inc.

Jackson, S. W. (1992). The listening healer in the history of psychological healing. *American Journal of Psychiatry, 149*(12), 1623–1632.

Jennings, J. R. (1992). Is it important that the mind is in a body? Inhibition and the heart. *Psychophysiology, 29*(4), 369–383.

Joffrion, L., & Douglas, D. (1994). Grief resolution: Facilitating self-transcendence in the bereaved. *Journal of Psychosocial Nursing, 32*(3), 13–19.

Johnson, E., Kamilaris, T., Chorous, B., & Gold, P. (1992). Mechanisms of stress: A dynamic overview of hormonal and behavioral homeostasis. *Neuroscience and Biobehavioral Reviews, 16*(2), 115–130.

Jones, J., & Bearley, W. (1987). *Managing change assertively*. Bryn Mawr, PA: Organizational Design and Development.

Jung, C. (1969). The archetypes and the collective unconscious. In *Collected Works of C. J. Jung. Vol. 9i*. Princeton, NJ: Princeton University Press.

Kaplan, H. I., & Sadock, B. J. (1994). *Synopsis of psychiatry: Behavioral sciences, clinical psychiatry* (7th ed.). Baltimore: Williams & Wilkins.

Kaplan, H. I., & Sadock, B. J. (1995). *Comprehensive textbook of psychiatry* (6th ed.). Baltimore: Williams & Wilkins.

Kleinman, A. (1988). *The illness narrative: Suffering, healing, and the human condition*. New York: Basic Books.

Kobasa, S., Maddi, S., & Courington, S. (1981). Personality and constitution as mediators in the stress-illness relationship. *Journal of Health and Social Behavior, 22*(4), 368–378.

Kobasa, S., Maddi, S., & Conn, S. (1982). Hardiness and health: A prospective study. *Journal of Personality and Social Psychology, 42*(1), 168–177.

Kobasa, S., & Puscetti, M. (1983). Personality and social resources in stress resistance. *Journal of Personality and Social Psychology, 45*(4), 839–850.

Krieger, D. (1979). *The therapeutic touch*. Englewood Cliffs, NJ: Prentice-Hall.

Kurtz, S. (1989). *The art of unknowing*. Northvale, New Jersey: Aronson, Inc.

Locke, S., & Colligan, D. (1986). *The healer within: The new medicine of mind and body*. New York: New American Library.

Mansen, T. J. (1993). The spiritual dimension of individuals: Conceptual development. *Nursing Diagnosis, 4*(4), 140–147.

Maslow, A. (1970). *Motivation and personality* (2nd ed.). New York: Harper & Row.

Mayer, G. G., Madden, M. J., & Lawrenz, E. (Eds.). (1990). *Patient care delivery models*. Rockville, MD: Aspen Publishers.

McHaffie, H. E. (1992). The assessment of coping. *Clinics in Nursing Research, 1*(1), 67–79.

McKivergin, M. J., & Daubenmire, M. J. (1994). The healing process of presence. *Journal of Holistic Nursing, 12*(1), 65–81.

Montgomery, C. L. (1992). The spiritual connection: Nurses' perceptions of the experience of caring. *NLN Publication, 15- 2465,* 39–52.

Moyers, W. (1993). *Healing and the mind.* New York: Doubleday.

Munhall, P. L. (1993). Unknowing: Toward another pattern of knowing in nursing. *Nursing Outlook, 41*(3), 125–128.

Nagai-Jacobson, M. G., & Burkhardt, M. A. (1989). Spirituality: Cornerstone of holistic nursing practice. *Holistic Nursing Practice, 3*(3), 18–26.

Nagel, T. (1993). What is the mind-body problem? *Ciba Foundation Symposium, 174,* 1–7.

Newberry, B. H., Jaikins-Madden, J. E., & Gerstenberger, T. J. (1991). *A holistic conceptualization of stress and disease.* New York: AMS Press.

O'Brien, M. E., & Pheifer, W. G. (1993). Physical and psychosocial nursing care for patients with HIV infection. *Nursing Clinics of North America, 28*(2), 303–316.

Omer, H., & London, P. (1988). Metamorphosis in psychotherapy: End of the systems era. *Psychotherapy, 25*(2), 171–180.

Raheem, R. (1987). *Soul return.* Lower Lake, CA: Aslan.

Reed, P. (1991a). Self-transcendence and mental health in oldest-old adults. *Nursing Research, 40*(1), 5–19.

Reed, P. (1991b). Toward a nursing theory of self-transcendence: Deductive reformulation using developmental theories. *Advances in Nursing Science, 13*(4), 64–77.

Reeder, F. (1994). Rituals of healing: Ever ancient, ever new. In D. Gaut & A. Boykin (Eds.), *Caring as healing: Renewal through hope.* New York: National League for Nursing Press.

Reik, T. (1951). *Listening with the third ear: The inner experience of a psychoanalyst.* Garden City, NY: Garden City Books.

Rhyner, H. H. (1994). *Ayurveda.* New York: Sterling Publishing Co.

Robinson, A. (1994). Spirituality and risk: Toward an understanding. *Holistic Nursing Practice, 8*(2), 1–7.

Rockstroh, J. K., Schmieder, R. E., Schachinger, H., & Messerli, F. H. (1992). Stress response pattern in obesity and systemic hypertension. *American Journal of Cardiology, 70*(11), 1035–1039.

Rossler, O. E., & Rossler, R. (1993). Is the mind-body interface microscopic? *Theoretical Medicine, 14*(2), 153–165.

Sabatino, F. (1993). Mind & body medicine. A new paradigm? *Hospitals, 67*(4), 66, 68, 70–72.

Savage, P. (1991). Patient assessment in psychiatric nursing. *Journal of Advanced Nursing, 16*(3), 311–316.

Seligman, M. (1991). *Learned optimism.* New York: Alfred A. Knopf.

Shih, T. K. (1994). *Qi Gong Therapy.* Barrytown, NY: Station Hill Press.

Smolan, R., Moffitt, P., & Naythons, M. (1990). *The power to heal.* New York: Prentice Hall Press.

Thomas, C. L. (Ed.). (1993). *Taber's cyclopedic medical dictionary* (17th ed.). Philadelphia: F. A. Davis.

Vessey, J. A., & Richardson, B. L. (1993). A holistic approach to symptom assessment and intervention. *Holistic Nursing Practice, 7*(2), 13–21.

Wanning, T. (1993). Healing and the mind/body arts: Massage, acupuncture, yoga, t'ai chi, and Feldenkrais. *AAOHN Journal, 41*(7), 349–351.

CHAPTER 5

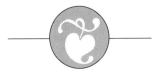

Delivering Culturally Competent Care

Henrietta Bernal

Illness and health never occur in isolation. Determining what factors within a person's cultural background influence a particular episode of illness and developing plans of care that are sensitive to these factors require specialized knowledge and skill. This chapter will present information to assist health care personnel to deliver culturally relevant care to patients who are coping with physical illness.

SOCIETAL AND PROFESSIONAL TRENDS

Delivering culturally relevant care is increasingly becoming a priority in the United States due to a number of trends in the society at large, and in the health care system in particular. These include (1) demographic shifts, (2) the push toward community-based care, (3) the concept of the "global village," (4) increasing concern for the delivery of quality care, and (5) the national dialogue among nursing leaders on the delivery of culturally competent care.

CHANGING DEMOGRAPHICS

The United States is experiencing a dramatic shift in its population profile. Culturally diverse groups that now comprise so-called minority groups are predicted to become the majority in the next century (ANA, 1991). One group in particular, Hispanics, is growing at a pace that will make it the largest minority group in the country by the year 2005, outpacing the African American population (Parker, 1990). In 1990 there were 31 million African Americans in the United States and 22 million Hispanics; by 2005 it is projected that there will be 41 million African Americans and 43 million Hispanics. Another fast-growing minority group in the United States is the Asian and Pacific Islander population. The total Asian and Pacific Islander population of the United States in 1990 was 7,272,662—a figure representing 2.9% of the total U.S. population.

Patricia Barry: *Psychosocial Nursing:*
Care of Physically Ill Patients and Their Families, 3rd ed.
© 1996 Lippincott–Raven Publishers

This population grew 95.2% during the period between 1980 and 1990 (Davis & Voegtle, 1994, p. 45).

This growth in minority populations means that there will be increased interaction between these groups and the health care system. The health care system will need to respond by increasing its ability to interact with these diverse populations and deliver care that is congruent with their lifestyles.

COMMUNITY-BASED CARE

The push toward care in the community that is discussed in Chapter 1 will pose additional challenges for health care providers because health care providers will, of necessity, have to enter the patient's world in order to deliver care. This shift from hospital to community requires a new health care delivery paradigm, one which places the patients in greater control of their care. The health care provider will confront unfamiliar territory, such as homes and communities with a larger number of culturally diverse patients. Thus, health care providers will need to understand these communities to a far greater degree than they do today.

THE "GLOBAL VILLAGE"

It is evident that no nation today can live in isolation from the rest of the world. Our lives are interdependent with other nations in ways that we do not imagine. It is not just that we as a nation provide goods and services to others; we are also dependent on other nations for our own well-being. From an economic point of view our lives are intricately linked to what happens to the Japanese yen and the European currencies. The clothes we wear, the cars we drive, the food we eat, the flowers we buy, and the conflicts we fight have a "foreign" label. We are as much part of the solution as part of the problem. Understanding other cultures and world views is a prerequisite for any professional who wants to be part of today's world. It is no longer feasible or in our best interest to have our heads in the sand. Because of our technical superiority in health care delivery,

we will increasingly be asked to provide technical consultation to other nations. Our understanding of other nations' health care systems and the cultural context of those systems will make it easier for us to be effective. On the other hand, we can learn and benefit from observing other health care systems and delivery models that have succeeded, for example, in establishing greater involvement of the family in care, in increased community participation, and in better delivery of primary care services.

DELIVERING QUALITY CARE

Increased competition among health care providers has resulted in added concern over the quality of care delivered. The assumption is that individuals will make choices based on the quality of care delivered in a particular institution. Institutions are also concerned about cost–benefit ratios. The moves toward "total quality care" and benchmarking are approaches that seek to make the institutions more responsive and effective. These models of care are generally based on the experience that institutions have had with their current patient populations. Increasingly, however, these patients come from culturally diverse groups, and their needs for "quality care" have to be considered. These patients may have unique features such as differences in language, health beliefs, family composition, traditional health care practices, and social class membership that will have to be taken into account in the delivery of quality care.

ANA POSITION STATEMENT

The American Nurses Association Position Statement on Cultural Diversity in Nursing Practice affirms the need for all nurses to have knowledge and skill in cultural diversity:

> Knowledge of cultural diversity is vital at all levels of nursing practice. Ethnocentric approaches to nursing practice are ineffective in meeting health and nursing needs of diverse cultural groups of patients. Knowledge about cultures and their impact on interactions with health care is essential for nurses, whether they are practicing in clinical settings, education, research, or administration [ANA, 1991, p.1].

Other groups, such as the American Academy of Nursing (AAN) Expert Panel on Cultural Diversity (American Academy Expert Panel, 1992), have also called for greater attention to the delivery of culturally competent care. The Expert Panel Report gives recommendations for improving the education, practice, and research in what they term "cross-cultural nursing."

KEY CONCEPTS

As in many other disciplines, there is confusion and disagreement about the meaning and use of many transcultural nursing terms that are derived from the discipline of anthropology. Some of these differences are meaningless; others, however, can lead to heated arguments about their meaning. Due to limited space only the most critical concepts needed for this chapter will be defined and discussed.

CULTURE/ETHNICITY

While definitions of culture abound, there is no agreement on a single meaning. One of the more clear definitions has been given by Schensul (1993) and will be used here for purposes of illustrating the general concept. Culture is "the patterned values, attitudes, beliefs, and social, political, economic, educational and other behaviors that emerge and are *shared* in a defined (or self-defined) group over time" (p.1).

The key aspects of this, or any other definition of culture, are the terms *patterned* and *shared*. It is these unique and distinct patterns that are shared among a particular ethnic or racial group that allow us to distinguish *between* cultural groups. For example, a shared language such as Spanish distinguishes a Mexican from a Chinese. What is not as easily understood is that elements of the culture may not be shared by all members of the group. These *within-group* differences occur as frequently as between-group differences. Factors such as economic status, education level, and patterns of family organization differentiate subgroups within the larger cultural group. Poor, African-American, inner-city dwellers may differ more in values, beliefs, and practices from their better-educated, higher-income counterparts than middle-class, professional, African Americans differ from their white, middle-class neighbors. These *intra*group variations need to be kept in mind in order to avoid the problem of stereotyping.

The three major ethnic/racial minority groups (Hispanic/Latino; African American/black; Asian/Pacific Islanders) are composed of culturally different subgroups, which adds complexity to the mosaic of cultural diversity in the United States. The African American/black population of the United States, for example, includes several groups that may have very different cultural backgrounds. These groups include descendants of slaves; recent immigrants from African countries; recent immigrants from the West Indies such as Jamaicans and Haitians; and others who may come from many different countries and identify themselves as black.

The same type of subgroupings exist both within the Asian/Pacific Islander population, and the Hispanic/Latino populations. Asian Americans include individuals from such diverse cultures as Chinese, Filipino, Japanese, Korean, Vietnamese, Cambodian, and Laotian. The United States census reports that there are 28 subgroups of Asians and 18 subgroups of Pacific Islanders living in the United States (Davis & Voegtle, 1994, p. 45). Similarly, Hispanics are represented by three large groups in the United States: Mexican Americans, Puerto Ricans, and Cubans. However, representatives of most of the Latin American countries, such as El Salvador, Guatemala, Nicaragua, Colombia, and Venezuela, can be found in most of the major urban centers of the United States.

Ethnicity and culture are often used synonymously. However, there are distinctions in the meaning of these terms that are worth noting. Culture is a general concept that applies to all members of a given group (i.e., the "American culture"). This is such a broad category, however, that it is almost meaningless. As seen in the above discussion, multiple subdivisions occur within the large cultural groupings and, most importantly, within each subgroup. One could argue that there are overarching "ideally held" views of what constitutes the "American culture": the puritan work ethic, the value of individual freedom, or the American ideal of self-determination. For practical purposes, however, these cultural categories are too broad and lead to generalizations and stereotyping. Understanding the shared patterns within smaller units such as ethnic groups yields more useful results.

Ethnicity refers to the identification which subgroups in a larger society use to distinguish themselves from each other. These differences are generally based on national origin, language, and religion. Often this identification serves as a cohesive force to help a group cope with the identity crisis and the discrimination that may result from interaction with the dominant culture (Schensul, 1993, p. 6). Each ethnic group may occupy a particular niche within the larger society that sets it apart from the rest of the culture. No doubt, too much encapsulation of an ethnic group within the larger culture can create difficulties, leading to strife between ethnic groups and competition for scarce resources. Nevertheless, U.S. society, rather than being viewed as a homogenous "melting pot," is really a mosaic of many subgroups that continue to create culture and add to its contextual richness.

BELIEFS, VALUES, NORMS

These three terms are related and can cause confusion in their interpretation. They nevertheless are important concepts to understand because they help describe the fabric of a group's identity and systems of social control. *Beliefs* are tenets having a shared meaning among members of a group and held by the group to be true, such as the belief in the existence of evil and benevolent spirits. *Values* are those aspects of culture that are held in high regard by the group and are felt to be desirable and worthy of emulation. Examples of values often attributed to the general American society are the importance of the work ethic, of a college education, and of being young and physically attractive. *Norms* refer to principles of right and wrong action binding a group and serving to guide and control the members of the group. Norms also refer to the rules of ac-

ceptable and unacceptable behavior. Sanctions, either informal or formal, such as laws, serve as deterrents for breaking these rules. For example, going topless on most beaches in the United States would be seen as breaking the social norm. In some cases this could lead to legal sanctions.

These three terms are highly interrelated and move from the abstract to the more concrete level. Beliefs are the least visible in human behavior and need to be elicited through careful interviewing. They may be inferred from observing behavior, but they are less tangible than values and norms. Values, while less abstract than beliefs, may be very much related to a group's belief system. For example, the value of religion in the everyday life of a small village in Spain is based on the existence of a strong belief system in the Catholic religion held by that group. The value of that religion for this group, however, is demonstrated through such behaviors as the contribution of time and money to the restoration of the church, or for special holiday celebrations.

Norms are the most observable of all three concepts because they influence behavior most directly. Breaking the norm or rule has consequences. One can more easily observe the norms that govern the group's behavior by observing the formal and informal sanctions imposed by groups on those who break the norms. Continuing with the village example given above, if the norm is for the members of the village to participate in the religious procession and some members choose not to participate, sanctions may occur in the form of gossip or ostracism for those members who do not participate.

Health care workers need to adapt a flexible approach in evaluating people's beliefs, values, and norms. The topless bather who would be sanctioned on U.S. beaches would be totally acceptable on many beaches around the world. Who is right and who is wrong? No one. The behavior needs to be understood in relative terms. This is not to say that there are no universal rights and wrongs. Who would approve of slavery, or torture? However, most beliefs, values, and norms are best understood from the point of view of the people who hold them.

STEREOTYPING

Stereotyping refers to the application of a particular label (positive or negative) to an individual or group, for example, "Mexican Americans are *mañana* people," or "Chinese have high IQs." Stereotyping creates a barrier between the individual doing the stereotyping and the group being stereotyped because it prevents a realistic understanding of the group's intracultural variations. Of course, some Chinese have high IQs, but many do not. To operate under this assumption in a school environment, for example, might cause other Chinese children in school who are not gifted to be pushed beyond their natural capabilities, resulting in anxiety and stress for those children. Stereotyping occurs because individuals are influenced by the views and opinions held about a group by the community at large. Nurses, as citizens of a larger community, are influenced by the larger group's views and are socialized to stereotype individuals and groups who differ from themselves. In a study of community health nurses in the Midwest, Erkel (1985) found that these nurses held the same stereotypical views of the groups they served (Mexican Americans and African Americans) as the larger community. Part of this view was that Mexican Americans were *mañana* people.

The antidote for these stereotypical views of a group that differs from ourselves is *knowledge*—not a superficial, casual awareness, but a thorough understanding of a group's shared patterns of values, beliefs, norms, and behavior.

ETHNOCENTRISM

Ethnocentrism refers to a view of the world that is generally based on the socialization experienced by individuals within their own particular culture. This point of view can be compared to the wearing of a particular set of sunglasses that only allow certain images to be seen. In this limited experience, individuals only see the world from a particular dimension. Other images and experiences are filtered out. Individuals make the assumption that the rest of the world sees the same picture, or that the picture they see is the "right"

one and others are wrong. Ethnocentrism is part of the human experience because we are all socialized to see the world in a particular way. Some individuals, however, through a series of planned or chance experiences, learn to take the culturally biased glasses off and understand and appreciate many world views.

In order to deliver culturally competent care, health care professionals have to broaden their views and open their minds to other ways of experiencing the world. One of the worst by-products of ethnocentrism is the impulse to impose our beliefs, values, and norms on others. Cultural imposition tends to create resentment and to close communication and negotiation between people. As health workers enter the patient's world in the home and community, great caution must be exercised in imposing "our ways."

THE INFLUENCE OF CULTURE ON HEALTH AND ILLNESS BEHAVIOR

While the above discussion may be interesting, it does not explain how culture influences health and illness, or what health care providers can do about its influences.

Allen Harwood (1981) developed a framework that can provide the structure to answer the first part of the question. According to Harwood, ethnicity influences four areas of interest to health care providers: rates of disease, health maintenance and home treatments, illness behavior, and utilization of health care services.

RATES OF DISEASE

Ethnic groups may share an ecological niche, a set of behaviors, and a genetic pool that can influence the incidence and prevalence of particular diseases. For example, while having higher rates of diabetes, Hispanics have lower rates of heart disease and cancer. However, homicide, AIDS and poor perinatal outcomes are among the top ten killers in this group (Torres, 1994). Some of these conditions, such as diabetes, have a genetic marker; most are directly linked to the social and environmental conditions shared by this group. Diseases that have a genetic predisposition may be influenced by the patterns of intermarriage that occur within and between groups. It stands to reason that the greater the isolation of a group, the greater is the likelihood that a particular gene will continue to be expressed in that population through intermarriage. The Pima Indians, who have been reported to have a 40% rate of diabetes, no doubt fit this pattern (Bernal, Perez-Stable, 1994).

Traditional eating habits may also play a role in the development of disease or the maintenance of health. Diets that promote high consumption of sources of complex carbohydrates, such as grains, vegetables, and fruits (e.g., Mediterranean diets) have been shown to be more healthful than those with high consumptions of animal fats.

Environmental factors such as crowding, exposure to lead-based paint, and air and water pollution all may target a particular group and result in differential rates of disease. An increasing concern has been the exposure of certain groups, usually economically disadvantaged, to nuclear and other toxic materials because of waste dumping that has occurred near their homes. They are now unable to sell their homes because of this exposure; they are unable to leave because of economic reasons.

Responses to medications have also been found to vary based on the existence of certain physiological factors that are more prevalent in a particular ethnic group. For example, differential effects for the four drug classes recommended for the initial treatment of hypertension have been reported among ethnic groups in the United States: "Possibly because hypertensive blacks tend to have low plasma renin levels, β-blockers, and ACE inhibitors are not nearly as effective as diuretics when used in monotherapy" (Caralis, 1991, p. 55).

While biological factors that may play a role in the development and treatment of disease are important to note, they play a much more limited role in disease prevalence than environmental factors. The biological hypothesis is also dangerous when it is misused and misinterpreted because it leads to the "blaming the victim" syndrome. It provides a convenient excuse for not intervening at the greater societal and environmental levels. African Americans are particularly sensitive to this issue because they have been the target of this type of discrimination.

> Early medical research often had descriptions of racial differences that had no basis in biology but were grounded in societal attitudes of the times. For example, African Americans were reported in medical journals to differ from whites in bodily secretions and fluids, brain organization, temperament, sexual appetite, and propensity for violence and crime. Socioeconomic explanations were discounted and medical treatment was thought to be ineffective in altering these basic biologic predispositions (Davis & Voegtle, 1994, p.36).

HEALTH MAINTENANCE AND HOME TREATMENTS

Culture can influence the continuum of health and illness from the general to the specific. From the general perspective, cultural habits practiced for other than specific health reasons, such as religious rituals or societal norms, may have an indirect impact on health. The practice of nightly bathing in Sri Lanka (personal communication, S. Schensul) is more of a societal norm than conscious health behavior, yet one could attribute healthful results from this practice. The *despojo* or ritual cleansing of the home with strong household detergents by Puerto Ricans who practice *Espiritismo* can also be viewed as a healthful hygienic behavior. Yet its intent is to rid the home of evil forces and as a sign of respect for certain days of the week that are deemed "special" within that belief system.

EXPLANATORY MODELS OF ILLNESS

When people experience symptoms they label them in ways that make sense within their world view (Wenger, 1993) or explanatory model of illness. A view that is rooted in the spirit or magical world, or in the ability to achieve an equilibrium of forces (e.g., hot or cold, good or bad air) will, of necessity, lead to a label or diagnosis that has to do with bad and good spirits, or the disequilibrium of forces. In a study of belief systems related to chest pain among Mexican Americans, nurse practitioners, and a lay control group, Kosko and Flaskerud (1987) found that Mexican Americans held to a more traditional, nonscientific explanatory model of causation than the other two groups. Mexican Americans were more likely to believe that chest pain was a punishment from God, that good health was a matter of good luck, and that chest pain should be treated with hot liquids. The authors conclude that Mexican Americans' beliefs about disease etiology are guided by a hot-cold theory of disease (balance of forces) and a desire for normal balance in the body. In a study of self-care behavior among 30 Vietnamese subjects suffering from respiratory illnesses, Hautman (1987) found that while supernatural causes of illness were expected, respondents gave more naturalistic causes for their illness such as weather change, cold air, and pollution.

Individuals will make decisions about care based on a number of factors, one of which may be the belief systems that are operating within their lives at a given moment in time. However, it must be kept in mind that individuals and groups change their ways of doing things, and belief systems may also change in the presence of alternative models. Therefore, health care providers must engage in a continuous process of assessment. False assumptions about a patient's belief system can create problems and even cause a chuckle or two. A Puerto Rican psychiatric patient whom the author had been visiting at home related the following story:

> Mr. O had been seen by a non-Hispanic, well-intentioned psychiatrist for several months. The patient needed to go back to Puerto Rico for a family matter, and told the therapist. The doctor then instructed him to go see an *Espiritista* (folk healer) while in Puerto Rico. When the visiting nurse asked him if he had followed up on the recommendation, he laughed and said, " I don't believe in any of that stuff!"

One can only think that the therapist had made the assumption that all Puerto Ricans practice *Espiritismo*. Research has shown that to be false. There are wide variations in the percent of Puerto Ricans who first say they believe in the system; who have used it in the

past; and who are now using it. While one may have knowledge about a particular group's folk beliefs and practices, one should operate within a system of probabilities. Yes, it is more likely that a Puerto Rican may visit an *Espiritista* for a health problem than some other person, and yes, certain characteristics may indicate a higher probability for a given individual. However, that hunch or hypothesis needs to be tested or validated with the patient by conducting a culturally competent interview. The general knowledge about a group gives one the range of options open to the patient; the interview gives specific knowledge about that particular patient's or family's approach to illness during a given illness episode.

Certain categories of illness may not be considered valid or acceptable within a cultural group. The acceptance of certain problems such as depression and/or psychosis as worthy of the sickness label requiring help and assistance is based on beliefs about the meaning of the illness. It is also based on group expectations about what constitutes an illness. Within Chinese communities, mental illness may be considered a stigma by many of the group (Louie, 1985). Seeking help for this type of illness is taboo. As a result, patients may express their psychosocial distress in other ways (i.e., somatization of the problem) and seek medical care rather than psychiatric help, or families may try to cope as best they can by denying the problem. If the problem persists, the family and patient may seek treatment with their own traditional healers, or may continue to seek help from a variety of medical providers who will continue to find nothing physiologically wrong, thus frustrating the patient. The following case illustrates this point.

CASE EXAMPLE

A 17-year-old Chinese girl was seen in the drop-in clinic for a several-week history of weakness, malaise, dizziness, palpitations, and an inability to concentrate; she had been unable to attend school. Both she and her Chinese herbalist father spoke excellent English. They were concerned that her condition was due to a previously diagnosed congenital heart condition which had already been resolved in China. Tests and exams were normal and they were told to seek psychiatric care since there was nothing physically wrong with her. The girl and her father were upset with this recommendation because they felt that she had been labeled "crazy," and sought another option. A more sensitive Asian pediatrician from their cultural background worked with them to identify factors such as high academic expectations that were creating stress, and they agreed to have counseling from the pediatrician.* ❧

TREATMENT OPTIONS

People also have a range of alternative treatments from which they may choose for a given episode of illness. These approaches may include folk and traditional therapies, modern medicine-prescribed treatments, or over-the-counter preparations obtained through pharmacies, family, and friends. Individuals may select among these options in a variety of sequential or simultaneous patterns.

In a recent study in a large metropolitan hospital, Pachter (1994) found that Hispanic parents believed in a folk illness called *Empacho*, which tends to affect children and cause a variety of GI symptoms, usually of a limited nature. Sixty-four percent of a sample of 67 parents responded that one of their children had been ill with this problem. One-third of the parents had tried to treat the illness with home-based interventions, one-third took their child to a folk therapist, and one-third took the child to a physician. In most cases the problem was resolved without physician intervention. In this study, some families chose to go to the folk practitioner first and never bothered with another treatment because the child got better. Other parents tried home treatments, then the folk practitioner, and finally the doctor. While not clear from this study, other parents could have used all three options concurrently. In the Hautman study, for example, Vietnamese patients tended to use cosmopolitan (modern) medical care and traditional therapies such as

*Adapted from Davis, B. J., & Voegtle, K. H. (1994). *Culturally competent care for adolescents.* Chicago: American Medical Association, p.7.

coin rubbing (used to get the bad air out) in combination (Hautman, 1987, 231).

Bushy (1992) describes three categories of illnesses people residing in the Northern Plain states of the United States treat with a combination of folk home remedies and over-the-counter medications. These are (1) short-term conditions, (2) chronic and incurable conditions, and (3) psychosomatic conditions. The first category includes warts, cold sores, minor menstrual problems, and muscle aches. The second group includes arthritis, weight loss, asthma, and chronic back pain; and the third includes eczema, hives, headaches, seizures, neuroses, and psychoses. A variety of treatments is reported to have been used to treat these problems: to regulate blood pressure, for example, take two or three garlic tablets every day and reduce salt intake; to prevent heart attacks, take two aspirin and run a least two miles several times per week.

TREATMENT EFFICACY

Obviously the efficacy of the treatment plays a major role in how many treatments people will employ to relieve the symptoms. Hautman (1987), in his study among Vietnamese patients with respiratory problems, found that "regardless of treatment method, subjects appeared to use the criterion of efficacy to determine which treatment was used" (p. 233). Effectiveness, however, is not always dependent on the particular therapeutic effects of the treatment but on how the patient may "feel" as a result of the treatment. In many cases the patient may still have the pathology (i.e., hypertension) but may feel better psychologically, and therefore, quality of life may improve. In other cases, the illness is self-limiting and any treatment will do; thus, all treatments will work. *Empacho* is a good example of this. In other situations, the therapies, folk or otherwise, are effective in relieving symptoms or pathology. Herbal medicines and over-the-counter preparations, as well as prescribed drugs, are examples of treatments that may have a direct effect on the existing pathology.

Knowing the treatment that patients are using is important for obvious reasons. Many of the folk treatments used—e.g., coin rubbing, massage, incantations, wearing amulets—will not usually cause any harm to the individual, but accepting the patient's use of these and talking about them will create trust between therapist and patient. Other treatments, however, may have a direct physiological effect, either positive or negative. The use of mercury in some of the *Espiritista* rituals can be seen as potentially very harmful (Wendroff, 1994). On the other hand, use of certain herbs such as *nopales* (prickly pears), have been reported to have hypoglycemic effects and are sometimes used in treating diabetes among Mexican Americans. One of the key issues existing in this area is the lack of control studies to determine actual efficacy of folk and self treatment (Anderson, 1991).

ILLNESS BEHAVIOR

Culture may also be seen to play a role in how people react to illness. There is more to being sick than recognizing that something is wrong, seeking help, and choosing appropriate treatment. Deciding when one is exempt from the normal obligations of daily living; how one reacts to certain symptoms (i.e., pain); who is allowed to care for the ill patient; where the patient should be cared for (home or hospital); and how long one should expect to be indisposed are some of the areas in which culture may influence behavior.

Many cultures expect that family members will assume responsibility for the care of patients even when hospitalized. This means that members of the family will take turns being with the patient during the entire stay, bathing and assisting with care. Some health care systems are structured to allow the family to be part of the care. This practice has very good and not-so-good consequences for the patient, family, and health care system. The point is that in countries as varied as Armenia and Spain, family care in the hospital is an expected family obligation. This expectation requires that families reorganize their lives to be with the patient during the entire hospital stay, sleeping and eating at the bedside. Immigrants from various parts of the world may still hold to these practices and will have a hard time conforming to the limitations imposed on them by our health care system.

Elderly Chinese are uncomfortable with hospitalization because they are separated from families and home, and some consider the hospital a place to die (Louie, 1985, p.20). This is a common feeling among elderly patients from many cultures who have not been exposed to modern medicine. These individuals see the home as the preferred place for treatment and expect to die if they are hospitalized. The idea of the modern hospital as the center of sick care is a rather modern invention. There are still people who have not experienced a hospitalization, and see these institutions as a foreign land where no one speaks their language, people dress differently, the food is strange, and daily routines do not allow for individuals to meet their cultural habits.

How long one should be indisposed and act out the "sick role" is also influenced by group norms. Mexican American and other Hispanics have traditionally practiced the *"quarentena"* after the birth of a child. In this practice, women are expected to be "indisposed" for forty days, while others assume the household chores. While this practice may seem exaggerated and dysfunctional to some, it does serve to give the mother a network of supports that can be very useful to her in a time of an important life transition.

UTILIZATION OF HEALTH SERVICES

Seeking care is influenced by the individual's acceptance of the set of symptoms as recognizable illness categories that are worthy of help seeking. Other factors that influence the decision to go for help have been identified by a number of researchers, most notably Mechanic (1963), who identified a set of factors that contribute to the process of help seeking. Among these are the type and severity of symptoms. Obviously, acute trauma with massive hemorrhage would be ignored by almost no one, and given the availability of a modern medical facility, help would be sought immediately from that source. As we have seen, however, most symptoms that people experience are much less dramatic in nature and are subject to a variety of interpretations regarding where, when, and to whom to go for help.

In the United States, however, the major obstacles to seeking health care have more to do with economic than cultural factors. The lack of health insurance is probably the critical issue. Even with government-supported programs such as Medicaid, patients may have difficulty finding a practitioner who will see them because payment does not cover costs, or because of the large amount of paper work involved in the reimbursement process. Poor African Americans have been reported to use clinic or outpatient services, as opposed to doctor's offices, to a far greater degree than whites. This is especially true for those with incomes under $10,000 per year (*Healthcare Trends and Transition*, 1993, p. 4). This lack of private care is felt to be responsible for the lack of primary and preventive services received by this population, which is, in turn, felt to be responsible for the high rate of preventible diseases such as certain cancers and stroke among this group. Presently the life expectancy among African Americans in the United States is 5 years less than for the general population. Poverty plays the most significant role in the differential rates of disease among poor ethnic minorities. "Regardless of race or ethnic background, people with low income have death rates that are twice as high as those with incomes above the poverty level" (*Healthcare Trends and Transition*, 1993, p. 45).

Other factors that have been blamed for the failure of certain groups, namely ethnic minorities, to seek timely and appropriate health care include: distance to care, lack of transportation, access to telephone, and access to baby sitters. System barriers such as lack of bilingual and bicultural health care providers, poor translation services, and negative attitudes are also problems once these groups gain access to care.

DELIVERING CULTURALLY COMPETENT CARE

Cultural competence is a term that has replaced "culturally sensitive care" in the social and health care literature. These terms, however, have tended to mean the same thing. Their common goal is the delivery of health care with knowledge, skill, and sensitivity to cultural factors that may play a role in a patient's health/illness behavior. Davis and Voegtle (1994) identify five components of delivering culturally competent care. These are:

1. Awareness and acceptance of cultural differences
2. Self-awareness
3. Understanding of dynamic differences
4. Basic knowledge about a patient's culture
5. Adaptation skills

DEVELOPING CULTURAL SENSITIVITY

Factors one and two above can be integrated into the process of developing cultural sensitivity. Developing cultural sensitivity requires at least three conditions: an open-minded attitude about experiencing other world views ("taking the ethnocentric glasses off"); awareness about one's own biases and attitudes that create barriers to direct interaction with a group; and experiencing culture directly.

Rooda (1993), in a study about nurses' level of knowledge and attitudes toward whites, African Americans, and Hispanics, found that registered nurses had different attitudes about the three groups. Nurses had the most positive attitudes about whites and least positive about Hispanics. Rooda concludes that cultural attitudes and cultural bias are positively correlated. Therefore, in order to take our "ethnocentric" glasses off, our attitudes toward a particular group have to be addressed.

Leininger (1991) has identified a typology of health practitioners in relation to their ability to interact effectively with other cultures. These types include the genuinely interested; the isolated and noninvolved; the one who is curious about others; the one with the hopeless image; the exploiter; the escapist; and the overprotective practitioner. As described by Leininger, the most effective type of practitioner is the "genuinely interested" type. These individuals show openness to learning from others about their way of life and engage themselves directly with the group. This type accommodates and does not impose his or her value system on the group. "This practitioner blends professional knowledge of the health world with that of the cultural group's health beliefs in skilled and appropriate ways" (Leininger, 1991, p.33). Examining one's own biases and attitudes about a cultural group is aided by involving oneself with that group in ways that allow the culture of the group, in all of its dimensions, to be experienced.

A senior nursing student during a community health experience was conducting a community assessment of a Hispanic neighborhood. In interviewing a key informant (the secretary of the Catholic church that served that community), she learned that on Good Friday there would be a procession in the streets, as was the usual custom among the Hispanic parishioners. With some encouragement and preparation, she decided to go and experience this event on her own time. This proved to be quite revealing to her in many ways. One particular observation stuck in her mind. Members of a well-known "gang" were seen following the procession in a well-dressed and very respectful manner. This caught her eye because her expectation of these gang members was quite different, based on newspaper accounts and remarks heard from friends, one of whom had said that she was very brave to have gone to this event.

The student was able to experience an important dimension of this group's life that gave her a more complete view of that culture. The friend who was concerned for her safety was projecting a one-dimensional view based on newspaper accounts of certain members of the group, the gang. Members of cultural groups are very good informants about their own culture and direct interaction with them can provide the vehicle for increasing one's knowledge of the group. Health practitioners have ready access to this source of information. All it takes is interest and skill in asking questions, and seeking opportunities to interact directly with the group.

BUILDING A KNOWLEDGE BASE

Studies (Bernal & Froman, 1994; Rooda, 1993) have shown that nurses have different levels of knowledge about three of the major ethnic groups in our society—African American, Hispanics, and Vietnamese/Southeast Asians. Bernal and Froman found that public health nurses had greater confidence in their knowledge of African American patients and least confidence in their knowledge of Southeast Asians. The amount of confidence was influenced by their past practice experience with these groups and the amount of continuing education they had attended in the area of cross-cultural nursing. Rooda found that registered nurses also varied in the amount of knowledge they had about a group depending on their educational background.

It has already been established that people from a particular target group have knowledge about themselves that they are willing to share with others. The cross-cultural literature is another source of information. While the earlier nursing cross-cultural literature tended to be unidimensional in its presentation of a particular group, more recently, data from research studies is adding a richer understanding of various cultural groups. Universities are increasing their curriculum content on cultural diversity, and continuing education programs are a useful way of increasing the knowledge base about cultural diversity. Culture, however, needs to be experienced, and so opportunities for interacting with people from the target group in their markets, eating places, social clubs, and neighborhoods need to be sought out.

Nurses have shown an ability to develop special skills and knowledge in caring for Puerto Rican patients when offered the opportunity to experience the culture and learn the language, and are provided with role models and supports (Bernal, Pardue, & Kramer, 1989; Bernal, 1994).

Developing cultural sensitivity and a knowledge base are important steps in the process of delivering culturally competent care. However, there is also a need to develop or augment specific skills that are crucial in the delivery of care to culturally diverse patients as well as others. Skills that have been identified as important include: developing language skills/using an interpreter; entering an ethnically distinct community; performing a diet review; participant observation; taking a life history; developing a genogram; and conducting a cultural assessment. Several of these will be discussed further.

DEVELOPING LANGUAGE SKILLS

Nothing is more important than direct communication with the patient. Developing the skill to speak in the patient's language is crucial. Nurses have shown the ability to learn to speak Spanish fluently through intense language immersion programs with appropriate follow-up and daily use and practice of the language (Bernal, Pardue, & Kramer, 1989). Immersion language programs are available through university modern language programs, but the follow-up phase is just as critical. This phase needs to include:

1. Vocabulary building through role playing (how to teach giving an injection of insulin).
2. Listening to the popular media (radio, television) in the target language.
3. Translating medical vocabulary and using key informant to validate accuracy or local colloquialism.
4. Grammatical drills.
5. Taping conversations in the target language and reviewing with key informant.
6. Practicing the language with patients on a daily basis.

COMMUNICATING THROUGH AN INTERPRETER

Volumes could be written about the problems in communication that occur with the improper use of translators/interpreters. The effective use of a translator is crucial since not everyone has the ability, time, or interest to learn another language. Even if all nurses could learn one other language, it is very unlikely that they could learn all of the languages needed to communicate directly with the various language groups they encounter. Therefore, while acquiring a second language may be a good but not required skill, learning to use an interpreter correctly is a *must* for all health care workers.

In a study of 37 interpreted interviews, Hatton and Webb (1993), found three types of roles played by interpreters: the voice box, the excluder, and the collaborator. This typology serves to underline some of the key issues that need to be kept in mind when using an interpreter.

In the *voice box* role, direct translation is simultaneously done and the translator tries to eliminate his or her biases and "interpretations." It is almost as though a computer were doing the translation. This approach is useful and preferred when accuracy is essential. This would include such situations as eliciting symptoms around a presenting problem, obtaining vital information regarding past medical or surgical interventions and use of prescribed or other medications, pain assessment, or cases with legal implications such as child abuse situations.

Interpreters need to be trained to be simultaneous translators; health workers using interpreters also need to have some basic skills in how to use an interpreter correctly. Box 5-1 lists some approaches that work well in a variety of settings with different types of workers.

Interpreters may find this "voice box" role limiting and in fact it may not need to be adhered to all the time. But in many cases, accurate, simultaneous translation is the only way to obtain the information you need.

The *excluder* role that Hatton and Webb describe is a role that causes frustration both for the interpreter and the health worker. In this role, the interpreter takes over most of the communication, thus absolving the nurse from his or her role, or the interpreter screens out key pieces of information as irrelevant. The control of the interview by the health care worker is lost. The nurse, for example, may ask where the patient was born, and receive an answer from the interpreter five minutes later. All other information that was exchanged in those five minutes is lost.

Hatton and Webb describe the role of the interpreter as *collaborator* in the following manner:

> The third type of interaction synthesized aspects of both the voice box and excluder. In these encounters, the nurse and interpreter were colleagues. They had worked together

BOX 5-1	Guidelines for Using a Translator

1. Slow down the communication process.
2. Give one or two sentences at a time to be translated unless the translator has been trained (i.e., U.N. translators) to do simultaneous translation.
3. Orient the patient to the process. Ask him or her to slow down communication. It may be necessary to repeat this request often.
4. Never stand during an interview; situate yourself next to the patient so that you are directly in the line of communication. Communicating with body language and eye contact is also important. This can be controlled by sitting next to the patient. Do not sit with the translator in the middle or the result will be a tennis-match style of communication.
5. Orient the translator about the topics to be covered and why it is important that accuracy be maintained.
6. Allow the translator to let you know when something is difficult to translate so that you can reword it and not be misinterpreted. Sometimes with sensitive topics translators may need coaching to ask the questions, or the translator will have to be changed. For example, a male translating questions about a sexual history may have difficulties with a female patient.
7. Do not have translators ask questions that you would not feel comfortable asking yourself. Also, do not give them the question in an angry or upset manner because they will find it difficult to translate or will want to protect the patient from your anger.
8. To avoid errors, limit the use of medical jargon in your interview. Otherwise you will force more errors as the translator goes from English medical terminology, to English lay language, to the target language. For example, if you use the term renal calculi, the translator has to translate the medical to the lay English, kidney stones; to the Spanish lay, "piedras en los riñones." The more coding and decoding the translator does the greater the chances for error.
9. Give positive praise to the translators and acknowledge their contribution. Review the positive aspects of the translation, and also those that need improvement both form the translator's and the health care provider's perspective.

for a period of time and knew each other's working styles. Viewing one another as allies, they freely discussed cases before and after dealing with patients. As collaborators, both the CHN (community health nurse) and interpreter used aspects of the voice box and excluder interactions within a context of teamwork and under specific circumstances they deemed appropriate [1993, p. 142].

ENTERING AN ETHNICALLY DISTINCT COMMUNITY AND USING KEY INFORMANTS

Individuals from the target culture can be discovered who are willing to share their knowledge and enter into a collaborative relationship with health care providers in order to serve their community better. Most communities have identifiable neighborhoods with eth-

nic organizations or other community-based organizations that seek to serve those communities. Churches that serve ethnic communities are a very important resource and can be a good starting place to obtain information about the group they serve. The example of the student nurse above demonstrates a good use of a key informant. In this case, the secretary of the rectory was Puerto Rican, and provided a wealth of information about the congregation and the community as a whole. This information served as a springboard for reaching other key groups in that community.

Health care workers have access to people from the community from all walks of life, coworkers from the target group, interpreters, members of the clergy, and patients and families. In addition, health workers can seek out organizations that need volunteers or technical expertise to serve on their boards or committees, or to volunteer their skills. This is a useful way of entering and understanding an ethnic community. A reciprocity is built in which both parties give and take from each other, thus establishing a useful and productive relationship.

Certain cautionary remarks about key informants need to be made. First, no one individual in a given community holds the full view of the community, nor the "right" view. Multiple views need to be obtained by asking people in the "know" to identify the key informants with knowledge about a particular community. Second, key informants may have axes to grind, or views about their group which they may want to promote. Third, key informants may withhold information because they do not trust the interviewer or are afraid that the information may be misused.

CONDUCTING
A CULTURAL ASSESSMENT

No step in the process of providing care is more important than the assessment phase. The failure to obtain accurate and complete data (within reason) leads to false assumptions about the patient, including errors in diagnosis. The so-called "premature closure" of a problem or jumping the gun to arrive at a diagnosis is one of the most potentially serious problems that can occur in a health care encounter. How much to assess and what to assess are important questions that will be addressed in this section.

Conducting a cultural assessment is time-consuming and requires thoughtful preparation. It is necessary to reserve this type of interview for patient situations that truly need it. The first step in this process, therefore, is to determine the need for such an interview. Keeping the discussion on intracultural diversity in mind, a health care worker cannot assume that a patient who simply looks "ethnic" or who has a last name that might indicate certain ethnic membership will behave according to the beliefs, values, and norms of his/her respective group. It is important to have "screening criteria" that help determine what patients might have the greatest probability of being influenced by their ethnic group membership.

The concept of *heritage consistency* (Spector, 1991) is one way of conducting this type of screening. Heritage consistency refers to how closely a particular person's lifestyle reflects that of his or her ethnic group. The closer an individual matches his or her ethnic group's views and lifestyle, the greater will be the groups' influence on the person's system of health care beliefs and practices. Box 5-2 presents factors identified by Spector (1991) that need to be assessed in order to determine the degree of heritage consistency. Box 5-3 presents another approach, using an Ethnic Affiliation Rating scale for a Puerto Rican patient.

Having established that a patient has a high degree of ethnic affiliation or heritage consistency, a health care worker needs to proceed to the next step in the assessment process. This step involves determining to what extent the patient's health or illness behavior is being influenced by cultural background. One approach is to assess the person's explanatory model of illness. This idea was first presented by Kleinman (1978) as a means of understanding patients' perceptions of their presenting problem and treatment. The idea is that health practitioners need to know the belief system under which patients are operating, as well as their expectations for treatment, to avoid operating at cross purposes. The patient, for example, may be expecting a cure for diabetes when medical science can only provide long-term treatment. Problems with nonadherence to the plan of care and dissatisfaction with treatment may be traced in part to a discrepancy between the practitioner's and the patient's explanatory model. Box 5-4 provides a set of questions to elicit a patient's explanatory model.

In a study by Erickson-D'Avanzo, Frye, and Froman (1994, p. 103), Cambodian respondents expressed their levels of stress through somatic manifestations. For these respondents the culturally appropriate model for describing their stress differs from the Western model. Non–Vietnamese Americans would more likely use psychological terms to express their stress, including such terms as "I'm stressed out," or "I'm anxious," or "I'm nervous." The Vietnamese respondents reported having headaches, being sick, or sleeping a

BOX 5-2	Factors Indicating Heritage Consistency

1. Childhood development occurred in the person's country of origin or in an immigrant neighborhood in the United States of like ethnic group.
2. Extended family members encourage participation in traditional religious or cultural activities.
3. Individual engages in frequent visits to country of origin or to the "old neighborhood" in the United States.
4. Family homes are within the ethnic community.
5. Individual participates in ethnic cultural events, such as religious festivals or national holidays, sometimes with singing, dancing, and costumes.
6. Individual was raised in an extended family setting.
7. Individual maintains regular contact with the extended family.
8. Individual's name has not been Americanized.
9. Individual was educated in a parochial (nonpublic) school with a religious or ethnic philosophy similar to the family's background.
10. Individual engages in social activities primarily with others of the same ethnic background.
11. Individual has knowledge of the culture and language of origin.
12. Individual possesses elements of personal pride about his or her heritage.

Reprinted with permission from Spector, R.E. (1991). *Cultural diversity in health and illness.* Norwalk, CT: Appleton and Lange, p. 55.

lot. Using this research as an example of differences in explanatory models, we can see that in a clinical situation a given Vietnamese patient experiencing stress would want relief from the headache, and might have very concrete expectations about how it should be treated. The practitioners with a different model, on the other hand, would want to get to the root of problems causing the stress, and might not deal with the patient's felt need. Both patient and health care worker could become frustrated and be at cross purposes. Asking the questions outlined in Box 5-4 can help to eliminate this type of problem.

There are a variety of guides to conducting comprehensive cultural assessments. These can be found in the work of Leininger (1991, 1984) and Tripp-Reimer (1984, 1985). Box 5-5 can serve as another example for conducting such an assessment, by generalizing the questions to the specific ethnic group of which a patient is a member.

NEGOTIATING A PLAN OF CARE

Much has been written about patient noncompliance or nonadherence to plans of care.

For example, it is estimated that half of the people who are diagnosed with hypertension are not under treatment (Caralis, 1991, p. 51). It is, therefore, imperative that we take our heads out of the sand and be more realistic about how we go about establishing plans of care *with* and not *for* patients and families. This requires negotiation between provider and patient about how best to achieve the goals of treatment. This process is assisted by understanding the patient's model and system of beliefs about the particular illness, as well as the patient's lifestyle and life patterns. The whole process of assessment has focused on the need to understand the illness from the patient's perspective, or what anthropologists call the *emic* view (as opposed to the *etic* view, which refers to the outsider's perspective of the culture). In the nursing literature this *emic* view is represented in the literature as the patient's "lived experience." Not all treatment options can be negotiated, and so patients may need to restructure the way they do things. This, however, places a great burden of responsibility on the part of the provider to conduct effective assessment and health teaching.

The following case will illustrate this point.

BOX 5-3	Degree of Ethnic Affiliation:- Screening Rating Scale for Puerto Rican Patients

1 2 3 4 5
Low   High*

1. Speaks Spanish fluently.
2. Years lived in Puerto Rico.
3. Lives in Puerto Rican neighborhood.
4. Listens to Spanish-language radio and TV programs.
5. Attends Spanish-language church services.
6. Attends Puerto Rican social clubs.
7. Reads Spanish-language newspapers and magazines.
8. Visits family and friends in Puerto Rico.
9. Attends Puerto Rican Day parade and other Puerto Rican street festivals.
10. Eats in Puerto Rican restaurants.
11. Eats Puerto Rican foods.
12. Identifies self as Puerto Rican.

*Higher scores represent higher degree of ethnic affiliation.

CASE EXAMPLE

A Hispanic child was brought to a local emergency room (ER) with what turned out to be a strep throat infection. Antibiotics were ordered and the mother and child were sent home. Less than a week later the child was brought again with the same problem. This was repeated a third time until the visiting nurse who spoke Spanish was asked to visit. A home assessment revealed that the mother had several bottles of unfinished medications in the home that had been ordered for the infection. Further interviewing revealed that the mother had not understood the directions on how to give the medication to the child. She had been giving the antibiotic medications as cough medicine. They were not given on a regular schedule, but as needed for the cough.

Frequently, the reasons given for not providing adequate health teaching are time and cost constraints. However, if we would calculate the cost in this example of three emergency room visits, plus the unused antibiotic medications, we would see that it was more costly not to have taken the time needed at the first visit to help the mother understand how to give the medication and help her plan a time schedule.

Leininger (1991) has proposed three models of clinical decision making to be used when negotiating care with culturally diverse groups. These include:

1. Culture care preservation and maintenance.
2. Culture care accommodation and negotiation.
3. Culture care patterning and restructuring.

Using this model, the health practitioner should try to support those cultural practices that are helpful or nonproblematic in a given illness episode. For example, encouraging Puerto Rican diabetics to continue to eat

BOX 5-4	Questions for Eliciting Patients' Explanatory Models of Illness

What do you call your problem? What name does it have?
What do you think has caused your problem?
Why do you think it started when it did?
What does your sickness do to you? How does it work?
How severe is it?
Will it have a short or long course?
What do you fear most about your sickness?
What are the chief problems your sickness has caused you?
What kind of treatment do you think you should receive?
What are the most important results you hope to receive from the treatment?

Adapted from Kleinman, A., Eisenberg, L., & Good, B. (1978). Culture, illness and care: Clinical lessons from anthropologic and cross-cultural research. *Annals of Internal Medicine, 88*(2), 251–258.

beans because of their high fiber content would preserve a cultural dietary habit. Providing flexible alternatives to the patient's plan of care such as establishing a glucose testing schedule and meal plan that fits within the patient's activities of daily living would be an example of culture accommodation and maintenance. When these two alternatives are not possible, then the patient needs to be helped to incorporate new lifestyle changes. An example of patterning and restructuring would be helping a male patient with asthma to stop smoking even when smoking is the "male thing" to do within his reference group. Accomplishing this may require reaching into the community to find credible role models that could support the patient in his effort.

Health care workers must keep in mind that in the home and in the community, patients are in control. They may, in fact, make choices about their lives that seem contradictory to the best recommendations of the health care worker. The health professional's responsibility is to present the options available in a respectful manner. The patient then has the right to make his or her informed choice about those treatment options.

CASE EXAMPLE: TEACHING THE HISPANIC DIABETIC

Diabetes is a chronic disease that requires life changes that may interfere with a patient's usual style of living. As a problem with a higher prevalence among Hispanic populations, especially Mexican Americans and Puerto Ricans, it is one that many nurses who care for Hispanic populations will encounter. The chronic nature of this disease makes it necessary for patients to self-manage their illness. This requires a great deal of skill and knowledge about the disease, its complications, and treatment. Research among low-income Puerto Rican diabetics (Bernal, 1984; Bernal & Froman, 1994) reveals that many (close to 50%) do not follow one or more of their care plan recommendations. The following case will illustrate some of the issues involved.

Mrs. R is a middle-aged, Puerto Rican diabetic (Type II) woman who lives in an inner-city apartment with her two daughters, one of whom is still in school. She was born in Puerto Rico and speaks very little English. She lives in a mostly Hispanic neighborhood and all of her friends and relatives are Puerto Ricans. She attends the local Pentecostal church and her minister is also Puerto Rican. The home is very well kept; she usually has the radio turned on to the Spanish-speaking radio program. The nurse receives a referral because Mrs. R's sugar is not well controlled. The referral also states that she is on a single morning dose of long-term acting insulin, and a 1200-calorie ADA diet. At the first interview with the nurse, she describes her experience with her illness as follows:

I began to feel very tired and dizzy at first and also experienced terrible thirst and blurry vision, so I went to the doctor in Puerto Rico and he examined me; he did some blood and urine tests and told me that I had diabetes. He gave a prescription for some pills—I think they were diabenase—and told to me lose weight. This was in 1974, and I had pretty good

BOX 5-5	Outline for Conducting a General Cultural Assessment
	1. Family organization
	2. Role differentiation
	3. Child care practices
	4. Utilization of health care system
	5. Types of social supports
	6. Utilization of traditional folk health practices
	7. Nutritional patterns
	8. Economic style of living
	9. Migration patterns
	10. Class structure
	11. Employment patterns
	12. Patterns of disease and illness
	13. Beliefs about health and illness
	14. Beliefs toward respect and authority
	15. Religious beliefs and patterns

Adapted from Bernal, H., Froman, R. (1987). The confidence of community health nurses in caring for ethnically diverse populations. *Image, 19* (4), p. 203.

results with the pills, but then I came to Hartford in 1978. I was feeling pretty good and stopped taking the pills. After a while, I began to have the same problems that I had in Puerto Rico and I realized that I had high blood sugar again. This time I went to the clinic and the doctor also gave me the pills to take, two every morning. Then the pills began to bother my stomach so they changed them to another kind. After a short time, I got tired of taking the pills every day and I stopped again. But then I had begun to have problems with vaginal bleeding and was told that I needed an operation to take out my womb.

The doctors wanted me to take insulin to control the sugar levels but I did not want to get used to the insulin. When I had the surgery they had to give me insulin and I have been taking it since then (1981). I have two brothers and two sisters with diabetes and one of them died after they took off his leg. That is why I was sad when they told me that I had diabetes. My other sister has had a toe taken off, but she does not take care of herself at all, she eats whatever she wants. I watch what I eat. I know that when I eat rice the night before, my test results are always bad. Also, I've been trying to lose weight because the doctor told me that it would be good for me. Sometimes, I get tired of the injections and if the test is OK I don't take the insulin, or sometimes I rush off to take my girl to school and I forget to take it or take it later in the morning. The worst thing about taking the insulin is that it makes me very hungry and if I don't eat I get very dizzy. But since I'm trying to lose weight, I don't want to eat too much. I only take some fruit to work. ❧

Answer the following questions as you analyze the case:

1. How would you rate this woman on her degree of ethnic affiliation?
2. What additional information would you need to gather about her cultural background that could have a bearing on the management of her illness?
3. What lifestyle issues need to be kept in mind when establishing a plan of care with her?
4. What problems is the present plan of care creating for her?
5. What are her knowledge and skill needs?
6. What goals would you want to negotiate with her? What accommodations can be made? What patterns will need to change? How will you go about it?

THE PAIN EXPERIENCE

We have seen in the previous discussion of symptom labeling that symptoms have cultural meaning. When individuals experience pain they react to that symptom in ways that fit what they have learned in their social network. Individuals may not experience pain only in physical terms. Pain may be perceived based on psychological dimensions such as grief, anxiety, and stress without pathophysiological manifestations. Also, what is perceived as a legitimate complaint of pain in one culture may be not reportable in another. The expression of pain or how one verbally reacts to pain and behaves also has roots within the patient's social network.

Health professionals also have perceptions about pain that are based on their own experiences and the Western scientific model of illness. These perceptions do not always match the patient's perceived reality. These incongruencies have been studied by Ruiz-Calvillo and Flaskerud (1993). They compared the perceptions of Mexican American and Anglo American women to cholecystectomy pain with nurses' attribution of pain to each of the two groups. While no significant difference was found between the two groups of women in the measures of pain, nurses assigned more pain to Anglo Americans. Also, nurses evaluated both groups as having less pain than the patients themselves indicated.

Reasons for the differential evaluation by nurses of the pain experienced by the two groups may be due to ways in which Mexican American women have been reported to express pain by moaning. Within the Mexican American culture, this expression of pain is acceptable and learned from childhood. Thus, crying out does not necessarily signify a low tolerance for pain; it may rather be seen as a coping mechanism to withstand the pain. In another study by Lipton and Marbach (Perez-Stable, 1987) of a diverse group of patients (Hispanic, African American, Jewish, and white Catholics and Protestants), the investigators found that the emotional expression of pain was similar among all of the groups, but Hispanics were *less* likely to admit to loss of control and to use the term "unbearable" when describing the pain. In the Ruiz-Calvillo and Flaskerud study (1993), both groups (Mexican Americans and Anglos) responded to pain in a stoic manner (p. 457). Nevertheless, the belief persists among health care professionals that Hispanics have a low tolerance for pain.

Stoicism is not necessarily a response that should be rewarded. Consider a white, male, middle-aged patient who experiences chest pain while shoveling snow in the early morning, but does not report it to anyone for over 2 hours because he has been taught to "grin and bear it." This delay could cost him his life. A healthier adaptation would be to complain and bring attention to the pain so that help could be sought.

The following case gives some insight as to the contextual nature of pain and the differences in pain perceptions between the individual experiencing the pain and the medical providers of care:*

CASE EXAMPLE

RJA, a 53-year-old widow with two adult sons, emigrated from Kiev to a large midwestern city in the United States. Her husband had died suddenly following a "heart attack" 4 years prior to her emigration. She was an English teacher, had a good job and friends, and did not want to leave Kiev, but did so because she "would have lost her sons" when they decided to emigrate to the United States. She was here only 2 weeks when she was hospitalized because of stomach pains. She described the onset of "liver pains" when she was 25 years old and the addition of "pancreas pain," which began after her husband died. The pain then moved to the left inter-

costal region below the heart. Now in the United States, the pains "explode all of the sudden like a bomb," including pain, nausea, and, sometimes, vomiting and diarrhea.

The metaphor of pain exploding like a bomb was important because in her view the pains had historical significance. RJA related the stomach problems to World War II, in that she and others in her age cohort often have recurring abdominal and other symptoms. During the war, food was scarce and of poor quality. In addition, she believed Russians were more "nervous" than Americans. Russians, she contended, do not know when they may be at the mercy of the government's imposition on their personal lives. Although jobs, housing, and health care were relatively secure at that time, Jews especially believed that the possibility of sociopolitical discrimination was always imminent. This belief promoted a general state of "nervousness," which she believes Americans did not experience. She repeated on several occasions that she was "a sick woman." She wondered if signs of her sickness were visible. When I related the positive signs of health I observed in her, she responded, "of course, I am talking; I am laughing. But inside here you cannot see, I am sick."

Although she appreciated the American physicians and nurses and the technology that was used to diagnose and treat her symptoms, she said that because Americans did not experience the war and do not have the "nervousness" brought on by the sociopolitical system, the health care system was not prepared to understand and treat her symptoms. "Surgeons and surgery are excellent in the United States, but not therapy," she said. She kept a large plastic bag of medication and herbs in the refrigerator, which she brought from the Soviet Union. She was not using them only because an American physician told her she must only take medications from the United States. This advice was troublesome for her, because she believed Americans had little experience with "stomach pains" that have, in part, been caused by war and "nervousness" related to political vulnerability.

She also felt deprived because she could not continue self-care as she had done in the Ukraine. There she had regularly gone to a

*Reprinted with permission of Wenger, A. F. (1993). Cultural meaning of symptoms. *Holistic Nursing Practice*, 7(2), 22–35.

health spa or "sanatorium" where she would stay a few days. There, she drank special water, ate a special diet, and rested. Her voice cooed as she said, "And I felt better." She would then feel better for 6 months, and she would look forward to another such respite. Here, she has nothing like that to look forward to. She uses the prescriptions that the physician gives her. They help somewhat to relieve the pain. ☙

Answer the following questions as you analyze the case:

1. How would you rate this woman on her degree of ethnic affiliation?
2. What additional information would you need to gather about her cultural background that could have a bearing on the management of her illness?
3. What factors in her life history are influencing the perception of her pain?
4. What problems is the present plan of care creating for her?
5. What are her knowledge and skill needs?
6. What goals would you want to negotiate with her? What accommodations can be made to incorporate her own beliefs and practices about health?

"COMPLIANCE" WITH DIETARY REGIMES

The term *compliance* has some very negative connotations. The term implies acquiescence with medical or nursing "orders" which are deemed to be "good" for the patient. In delivering care that is not culturally relevant, assumptions are made by health professionals about an individual's lifestyles and behaviors that are based on common stereotypes held about a given group. The health caregiver also assumes that a scientific knowledge base gives him or her the authority to make the right decisions for patients who do not understand the intricacies of their disease. It is important, however, to keep in mind that there are many gaps in the medical knowledge base about etiologies and treatments of the most common conditions. For example, what was thought to be appropriate dietary management for diabetes 20 years ago is no longer relevant today.

Therefore, given the imperfect knowledge base that exists, noncompliance may sometimes be a better alternative than compliance. Many times, the value judgment is made that a patient is noncompliant because he or she *won't* follow the given instructions: he won't stop smoking, won't cut down on salt intake, won't exercise three times a week, won't take his medications as prescribed. The assumption is that the patient has a choice and chooses not to do what is best for him. The following case illustrates some of these points.

CASE EXAMPLE

An elderly African American woman living in a changing black neighborhood in a middle-sized urban community is seen at the local hospital clinic with hypertension and COPD. She has pitting edema of her lower extremities, requires oxygen intermittently, and is primarily home bound. She lives alone but a son who lives in the same town comes in to check on her and provides some assistance with grocery shopping. The woman does not like to bother her son, who is married, works two jobs, and has three children. She is a deeply religious woman who enjoys reading the Bible and has visitors from her church on a weekly basis. She was born in South Carolina and had eight children delivered by a local midwife. She has enjoyed cooking all of her life and was used to preparing traditional meals for family picnics, church gatherings, and holidays. She moved north to live closer to her youngest son 10 years ago. The physician from the clinic refers the patient to the local VNA and states in the referral that she is "noncompliant with her low salt diet, despite dietary instructions, and does not have anyone to help her." The nurse makes a home visit and finds that the woman is indeed short of breath, and has moderate levels of pitting edema in her lower extremities. On this first visit the nurse asks the patient if she understands her low salt diet and the patient replies that she does. On further assessment the nurse finds that she is eating mostly frozen dinners and prepared foods because she is unable to prepare her own meals due to shortness of breath and fatigue. On further assessment, the nurse is able to find out that while the patient knows not to add salt to foods, she has no idea about the hidden salt in the frozen dinners and in the other prepared foods that she is eating. 🍎

Answer the following questions as you analyze the case:

1. How would you rate this woman on her degree of ethnic affiliation?
2. What additional information would you need to gather about her cultural background that could have a bearing on the management of her illness?
3. What assumptions had been made about her by the clinic?
4. What are the important contextual issues affecting her behavior?
5. What are her knowledge and skill needs?
6. What goals would you want to negotiate with her? What accommodations can be made to improve her intake of low salt foods?
7. How could her support network help? What additional services might be needed?

CONCLUSIONS

Health institutions will need to be more responsive to the population trends that are occurring in this country, as well as the push to deliver care in the homes and communities where patients of various ethnic, religious, and racial backgrounds live. Delivering culturally competent care is becoming a must for any health professional interested in quality care.

Delivering culturally competent care requires the acquisition of knowledge and skills as well as a willingness to become open to other world views. There are useful ways that one can go about acquiring knowledge and skill about other cultures, including self-study, continuing education, and, most importantly, experiencing other cultures directly.

The delivery of culturally competent care is based on conducting a cultural assessment once it is determined that the patient has a strong ethnic affiliation or heritage consistency. Care can then be planned through a process of negotiation, accommodation, and adaptation. Patients must be allowed to make

informed choices about their lives and health care workers must be open to offering as many options and supports as possible so that a fit between the patient's and the health care worker's model of illness can be achieved.

BIBLIOGRAPHY

American Academy Expert Panel. (1992). Report on culturally competent health care. *Nursing Outlook, 40*(6), 277–283.

American Nurses Association. (1991). *Position statement on cultural diversity in nursing care.* Washington, D.C.

Anderson, R. (1991). The efficacy of ethnomedicine: Research methods in trouble. *Medical Anthropology, 13,* 1–17.

Bernal, H., & Froman, R. (1987). The confidence of community health nurses in caring for ethnically diverse populations. *Image: The Journal of Nursing Scholarship, 19* (4), 201–203.

Bernal, H., & Froman, R. (1994). Influences on the cultural self-efficacy of community health nurses. *Journal of Transcultural Nursing, 4*(2), 24–31.

Bernal, H., Pardue, K., & Kramer, M. O. (1990). Rewards and frustrations of working with an ethnic minority population: An Hispanic unit experience. *Home Healthcare Nurse, 8*(3), 19–23.

Bernal, H., Perez-Stable, E., (1994). Diabetes in the Latino community. In C. Molina, P. Lecca, and M. Aguirre-Molina (Eds.), *Latino health: America's growing challenge.* Washington, DC.: American Public Health Association, 270–312.

Buchwald, D., Caralis, P. V., Gany, F., Hardt, E. J., Muecke, M. A., & Putsch, R. W. (1993). The medical interview across cultures. *Patient Care, 27*(7), 141–166.

Bushy, A. (1992). Cultural considerations for primary health care: Where do self-care and folk medicine fit? *Holistic Nursing Practice, 6*(3) 10–18.

Caralis, P. V. (1991). Hypertension in the Hispanic-American population. *American Journal of Medicine, 88*(3B), 95–165.

Davis, B. J., & Voegtle, K. H. (1994). *Culturally competent health care for adolescents.* Chicago: American Medical Association.

Erickson-D'Avanzo, C., Frye, B., & Froman, R. (1994). Stress in Cambodian families. *Image, 26*(2), 101–104.

Erkel, E. (1985). Conception of community health nurses regarding low-income black and Mexican/Americans and white families. Parts I and II. *Journal of Community Health Nursing, 2,*(2), 109–118.

Harwood, A. (1981). *Ethnicity and medical care.* Cambridge, MA: Harvard University Press.

Hatton, D. C., & Webb, T. (1993). Information transmission in bilingual, bicultural contexts: A field study of community health nurses and interpreters. *Journal of Community Health Nursing, 10*(3), 137–147.

Hautman, M. (1987). Self-care responses to respiratory illnesses among Vietnamese. *Western Journal of Nursing Research, 9*(2), 223–243.

Healthcare trends and transition. (1993). Eden, MD: Nex, Inc., 5(2).

Kem, B. L. (1985). Providing health care to Chinese clients. *TCN, 7*(3), 18–25.

Kleinman, A., Eisenberg, L., & Good, B. (1978). Culture, medicine, and psychiatry. *Annals of Internal Medicine, 88*(2), 251–258.

Kleinman, A., Eisenberg, L., & Good, B. (1978). Culture, illness and care: Clinical lessons from anthropologic and cross-cultural research. *Annals of Internal Medicine, 88*(2), 251–258.

Kosko, A., & Flaskerud, J. H. (1987). Mexican Americans, lay practitioner, and lay control group beliefs about cause and treatment of chest pain. *Nursing Research, 36*(4), 226–230.

Leininger, M. (1984). *Care: the essence of nursing and health.* Thorofare, NJ: Slack Incorporated.

Leininger, M. (1991). *Culture care diversity and university: A theory of nursing.* New York: National League for Nursing.

Louie, K. (1985). Providing health care to Chinese clients. *Transcultural Nursing, 7*(3), 18–25.

Mechanic, D. (1972). Social psychologic factors affecting the presentation of bodily complaints. *New England Journal of Medicine, 286*(21), 1132–1139.

Pachter, L. M. (1994). Cultural and clinical care. *JAMA, 271*(9), 690–694.

Parker, S. (1990). Hispanics in the USA. *America Today,* Sept. 14, 1990, p.1A.

Perez-Stable, E. J. (1987). Issues in Latino healthcare. *Western Journal of Medicine, 146*(2), 213–218.

Rooda, L. A. (1993). Knowledge and attitudes of nurses toward culturally different patients: Implications for nursing education. *Journal of Nursing Education, 32*(5), 209–213.

Ruiz-Calvillo, E., & Flaskerud, J. H. (1993). Evaluation of the pain response by Mexican American and Anglo American women and their nurses. *Journal of Advanced Nursing, 18*(3), 451–459.

Schensul, J. (1993). *Comments on ethnicity, culture, and cultural "competence."* Essay prepared for the Child Council Communications Retreat. Hartford, CT: Institute for Community Research.

Spector, R. E. (1991). *Cultural diversity in health and illness.* Norwalk, CT: Appleton and Lange.

Torres, S. (1994). A challenge to nursing education: Meeting the health care needs of the Hispanic community. *Deans Notes, 15*(5), 1.

Tripp-Reimer, T. (1984). Cultural assessment. In J.P. Bellack & P.A. Bumfoul (Eds.), *Nursing assessment.* Monterey, CA: Wadsworth Health Sciences Division.

Tripp-Reimer, T., & Brink, P. (1985). Culture brokerage. In G. Bulecheck & J. McCloskey (Eds.), *Nursing interventions: Treatments for nursing diagnoses.* Philadelphia: W. B. Saunders.

United States Bureau of the Census. (1990). *Current population reports.* Washington, DC: U. S. Government Printing Office.

Wendroff, A. P. (1994). More on the EPA mercury warning. *Nation's Health,* July, 2.

Wenger, A. F. (1993). Cultural meaning of symptoms. *Holistic Nursing Practice, 7*(2), 22–35.

PART II

THE ORGANIZING FRAMEWORK OF PSYCHOSOCIAL ASSESSMENT

This section presents a continuation of foundation theory for psychosocial assessment. A core concept that provides the foundation for building comprehensive assessment skills is *systems theory*—the effects of stress on the etiology and course of physical illness, and the coping ability of patients and families. The Barry Holistic Systems Model integrates systems theory concepts into the nursing paradigm of person, health, nursing, and environment, providing a model for evaluating the effects of these interacting systems on the health–illness continuum.

Major psychosocial developments are integrated with the holistic systems conceptual model to provide a framework for exploring potential causes of ineffective coping. The final chapters of this section address mental status changes and their physiological causes.

CHAPTER 6

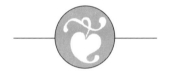

Effects of Stress When Coping With Physical Illness

Patricia Barry

This chapter will present several theories about stress. They will be discussed in three sections. The first section presents stress theories that evolve from a specific subsystem approach to stress: physiological, psychological, or social. The second section presents theories about the way stress is mediated by psychosocial functioning. The third section presents a biopsychosocial model compatible with holistic nursing concepts.

The word *stress,* when pronounced, has a dragged-out sound; it lingers. This characteristic of the word itself fits the way most people view the phenomenon of stress. In this age of increasing technology and related social pressures, the concept of stress has captured attention in most cultures. As this chapter progresses, the difficulty of separating the effects of stress into the specific realms of physical, emotional, and intellectual functioning will become obvious.

A *stressor* is a stimulus that disrupts homeostasis. The stressor may be perceived initially by either the physical or psychological domains, but ultimately, because of a general systems effect, all systems become involved in the manifestation of a stress response (Kiecolt-

Glaser & Glaser, 1992; Krueger & Krueger, 1991). The *Le Chatelier principle* from the science of physics can be applied to the effects of stress on a human being:

> If stress is applied to a system, the system will readjust to reduce the stress [Bertalanffy, 1968].

HOMEOSTASIS

Homeostasis is defined as "the ability or tendency of an organism or a cell to maintain internal equilibrium by adjusting its physiological processes (*American Heritage College Dictionary,* 1993, p. 650). The concept of homeostasis was described by a Greek philosopher, Empedocles, who applied the term to all matter. Hippocrates then used the term to describe the dynamics of health. Disturbing forces cause disease; there are inherent healing abilities within living things that restore

Patricia Barry: *Psychosocial Nursing:
Care of Physically Ill Patients and Their Families,* 3rd ed.
© 1996 Lippincott-Raven Publishers

them to health (Johnson et al., 1992). Table 6-1 shows the historical development of concepts associated with stress. Table 6-2 demonstrates the factors that contribute to homeostasis.

Usually when stress is described there are two different but associated concepts that can be identified: one, an external factor called a stressor that is perceived as challenging or threatening, results in the second, the internal distress that most people describe as "stress" (Battegay, 1991; Hagopian, 1993). An external environmental event such as taking a final examination, touching a hot iron, being in an automobile accident, getting married, or winning the grand prize in a lottery is called a stressor. A stressor is any external or internal sensory or cognitive awareness that results in demand on the person. Stress is the response to the demands of that stressor. It is a physical and psychological uneasiness that unbalances and upsets homeostatic equilibrium.

The subject of stress theory is complex. Knowledge about stress and its effects has evolved from decades of study by psychologists, sociologists, neuroscientists, and scientists in behavioral medicine and many other fields. The evolving knowledge about stress involves concepts resulting specifically from research into the physiological, psychological, social, or multisystem spheres. The resulting theories are becoming more and more intricate (Davey, Tallis, & Hodgson, 1993; Everly, 1993; Gage, 1992; Malt & Olafsen, 1992). As the body responds to a stressor it sets off a cascade of poorly understood mechanisms inherent in the mind-body complex, whose purpose is to restore homeostasis.

An important development during the last two decades, however, has been a growing awareness that it is impossible to separate the mind, body, and spirit domains of a person involved in stress responses (Krueger & Krueger, 1991; van der Kolk & Fisher, 1993). Researchers and theorists believe that the human being must be viewed holistically in its response to stress.

Accordingly, the implications of the effects of stress will be explored as they affect a person physically, emotionally, intellectually, spiritually, and socially.

PSYCHOSOCIAL MEDIATION OF STRESS

ADAPTATION TO A MAJOR LIFE EVENT

Once a stressful life event has occurred, most persons work through and adapt. The adapta-

---

TABLE 6-1
History of the Concept of Stress

Theorist	Concept
Empedocles (500–430 B.C.)	First written reference to homeostasis
Hippocrates (460–375 B.C.)	Health is the state of the harmonious balance of the elements. Disease is the state of dysharmony. Nature heals disease
Epicurus (341–270 B.C.)	Coping with emotional stressors improves the quality of life
Claude Bernard (1813–1878)	"Milieu interieur"
Walter Cannon (1871–1945)	"Fight or flight" reaction; homeostasis
Hans Selye (1907–1982)	The "General Adaptation Syndrome"

Reprinted with permission. Johnson, E., Kamilaris, T., Chorous, B., & Gold, P. (1992). Mechanisms of stress: A dynamic overview of hormonal and behavioral homeostasis. *Neuroscience and Biobehavioral Reviews, 16*(2), 116.

TABLE 6-2
The Dynamics of Homeostasis: Effects of Stress on Mind and Body

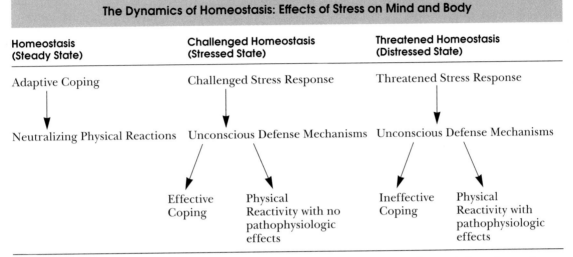

Homeostasis (Steady State)	Challenged Homeostasis (Stressed State)	Threatened Homeostasis (Distressed State)
Adaptive Coping	Challenged Stress Response	Threatened Stress Response
↓	↓	↓
Neutralizing Physical Reactions	Unconscious Defense Mechanisms	Unconscious Defense Mechanisms
	Effective Coping / Physical Reactivity with no pathophysiologic effects	Ineffective Coping / Physical Reactivity with pathophysiologic effects

Adapted from Johnson, E., Kamilaris, T., Chorous, B., & Gold, P. (1992). Mechanisms of stress: A dynamic overview of hormonal and behavioral homeostasis. *Neuroscience and Biobehavioral Reviews, 16* (2), 116.

tion process contains both conscious and unconscious elements. The common themes of this process are described by Horowitz (1976):

1. Fear of repetition of the event in real life as well as in memory.
2. Shame over helplessness or emptiness. There is a sense of loss of control because the outcome of the event was not controllable.
3. Rage or anger at the source. Although the anger may be irrational, a person needs to blame someone or something for the event.
4. Guilt or shame over aggressive impulses. The anger described above usually collides with a person's conscience and can result in guilt or shame. This can include negative feelings toward a person who has died.
5. Fear of aggressiveness. A person fears that he or she will not be able to contain angry impulses and may uncontrollably act them out.
6. Survivor guilt. If the event involves injury or death to others, the survivor, who may have had no power over the situation, often feels guilty that he or she was spared

or was less seriously injured. Awareness of this phenomenon in survivors of accidents or fires who are hospitalized will assist in giving more sensitive and compassionate care to these individuals. Gentle questioning may help the patient to verbalize feelings. The patient may be greatly relieved by being able to talk about feelings of guilt. Survivor guilt may also present itself in the form of posttraumatic nightmares about the event.

7. Fear of identification or merger with victims. This is a primitive response based on a human being's early perception of the self as "one being" with his or her mother (Mahler, 1974). Despite the unreality of this perception, it can operate at an unconscious level.
8. Sadness in relation to loss. Any major life change contains elements of loss that require adjustment.

Horowitz proposes that the two mechanisms commonly present in people who are working through these eight common themes are denial of the event alternating with intrusive and unwanted repetitions of thoughts, emotions, and behaviors related to the event.

He believes that maladaptation occurs in persons when there is ineffective coping as the result of the intrapsychic stress experienced. The stressful event is never completely worked through and resolved (1976).

RESPONSES TO STRESS

Most theorists agree that the physiological and psychological effects of a stressful event can be mediated by the presence of adaptive coping mechanisms. Ursin (1978) has identified the factors that determine whether a person's coping ability will be able to withstand a stressor:

1. The level of fear caused by a stressor
   a. Fear of some type of harm
   b. Fear of failure
2. The person's resources
   a. Familiarity with a preceding similar event
   b. Level of education and sophistication
   c. Availability of a support system
3. Role identification
4. Intellectual strategies
5. Defense mechanisms

An individual usually copes with stressful events in a consistent manner throughout adult life, depending on the underlying emotion and the early defense mechanisms that formed for self-protection. For example, if a person typically responds to stress with an angry outburst, this tends to be that person's "normal" response when under pressure of any kind.

These coping patterns, developed during childhood, tend to moderate during adolescence and then remain relatively constant during adulthood. Barry proposes that early emotional trauma related to severe states of helplessness or rage create conditioned patterns of sympathetic nervous system responses that recur whenever these emotional states occur over the lifespan (1991). If, for example a person's history indicates that he has coped effectively with stressful events in the past, it is likely that he will do so as a response to a current or future stressful event.

The reverse is also true when ineffective coping with stressful events is an established historical pattern. This is an essential concept to remember in caring for patients in inpatient or outpatient settings. In the early assessment period it is important to ascertain how an individual normally responds to pressure (see Chapter 2). If the response indicates that stress is not tolerated well, it is important to begin at that time to include extra supportive measures in the nursing care plan to avoid ineffective coping or long-term maladaptation.

Another clue that a patient's normal ability to cope is at risk is if a series of highly stressful events have occurred during the year before admission to the hospital. If the patient has experienced an unusual number of stressful events, the hospitalization, even if it appears routine, may be "the straw that breaks the camel's back" (Levine, 1993; Lipowski, 1991; Malt & Olafsen, 1992).

Discussion in this chapter is restricted to normal responses of people adapting to stress. The effects of ineffective coping and subsequent maladaptation and crisis will be discussed in later sections of the book. Figure 6-1 depicts the adaptive and maladaptive potentials of the stress response in patients and their families.

SPECIFIC SUBSYSTEM RESPONSES TO STRESS

PHYSIOLOGICAL ADAPTATION TO STRESS

There are many factors that mediate responses to a stressor, including:

1. Strength of the initial stressor; stressor may be physical, psychological, or a combination of each.
2. Physical and/or psychological, genetic disposition or constitution of the individual.
3. Current psychological and/or physical state.
4. Meaning of the event (e.g., threat or challenge).

Adaptation is the resulting effort of the individual to restore homeostatic balance. The adaptive effort is a complex integration of physiological, behavioral, intellectual, and emotional efforts and availability of social supports that are dependent on the available energy or dynamic forces to support the effort of restoration (Carpenito, 1993). The remainder of the chapter will address the specific components of the stress response.

CLASSIC THEORIES OF PHYSIOLOGICAL STRESS RESPONSE

The important thinking of pioneers in the field of physiological stress response theory includes theoretical constructs about the physiological responses to stress. Within the past few decades the explosion of understanding of the complexity of the stress response has required a multidisciplinary team approach in conducting research. Among others, the team includes experts in neuroscience, psychoendocrinology, immunology, psychosocial epidemiology of physical and mental illness, and clinical specialties of basic and medical science.

The theoretical approaches of Sternbach and Selye, described below, while relatively simple in comparison to those of current stress theorists, contain the elemental principles of our current understanding of stress responses.

Richard Sternbach: Three-Factor Theory

Sternbach (1966) identified a three-step process in the human response to stress. It involves the concepts of preferred stress response and homeostatic failure. According to the preferred stress response principle, if one of the body systems has a genetic weakness or vulnerability, when a person is stressed, it is the weak system that will experience the distress. For instance, the cardiac or gastrointestinal system, if it is weak, may manifest stress symptoms by dysfunctioning in some way. Homeostatic failure refers to the decline and ultimate failure of the normal physiological resources used by the body to balance the effects of stress.

Sternbach believed that if a person has "1) A preferred stress response, 2) Frequent trig-

gering of the stress response, and 3) Homeostatic failure of the stress response," the person will experience a stress-related disorder in the vulnerable body system (Suter, 1986, p. 83).

Hans Selye: General Adaptation Syndrome (GAS) Stress Response

One of the most recognized authorities in the field of stress research is Hans Selye. During his medical training in Czechoslovakia in the 1920s, he observed:

> Whether a man suffers from severe blood loss, an infection, or advanced cancer, he loses his appetite, strength, and ambition; usually he also loses weight and even his facial expression betrays his illness. I felt sure that the syndrome of "just being sick," which is essentially the same no matter what disease we have, could be analyzed and expressed scientifically [Selye, 1979, p. 12].

A few years after completing medical school, Selye returned to graduate school for a doctorate in biochemistry. During that time, while studying the effects of toxic substances on rats, he discovered that the rats were changed in three ways: (1) the adrenal cortex became enlarged, (2) the thymus, the spleen, the lymph nodes, and all other lymphatic structures shrank, and (3) deep, bleeding ulcers appeared in the stomach and upper gut.

Selye began to realize that these changes actually were the objective manifestations of stress. They became the basis for his stress concept, the General Adaptation Syndrome (GAS). These physiological responses are the foundation of the syndrome that Selye (1976) called "just being sick."

Selye identified three stages of the GAS. First is the alarm reaction, in which the body attempts, with all its defensive abilities, to fight off the effects of a noxious substance. After the initial shock of a stressor is met with a strong defensive response stimulated by hormones from the adrenal cortex, the body gradually settles into a less stimulated phase, during which it continues to maintain its defenses. This is the second stage: the stage of resistance. During this stage the body maintains its resistance until the noxious agent disappears and the body is

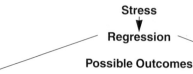

Stress

↓

Regression

Possible Outcomes

Effective Coping: **Adaptation (factors in outcome)**	**Inneffective Coping:** **Maladaptation (factors in outcome)**
Normal Mental Status	**Abnormal Mental Status**

Effective Thought Process
    Adequate memory
    Adequate problem-solving ability
    Good judgment
	Ineffective Thought Process Due to:
	    Organic mental disorder
	    Low intelligence level
	    Excessive anxiety or depression
	    Functional psychiatric disorder
	    Poor memory
	    Poor problem-solving ability
	    Poor judgment

Normal coping style
    Patient's intrapsychic defenses are adaptive
    Patient is able to use normal stress management to cope adequately with stress
    Illness is not life threatening
    Illness is not highly threatening to patient's self-esteem and body image
    Illness is not threatening to normal role functioning
	Abnormal coping style
	    Ego unconsciously underuses or overuses certain predictable defense mechanisms
	    Patient loses ability to use conscious stress management mechanisms
	    Illness is life threatening or is *perceived* as life threatening
	    Illness is threatening to self-esteem or body image
	    Illness is threatening to normal role functioning

Personality style
    Illness does not cause a major change in the way the patient normally interacts with others and environment; personality is strong enough to cope with stress
	Personality style
	    Depending on the type of illness and its particular threat to the patient, any personality style can be at risk because of the stress of major illness

Family coping style
    Family is normally able to adapt to stress
    Illness is not perceived as life threatening or causing major shifts in role of family member
    One or more family members are emotionally detached enough to allow the patient to voice concerns about self
	Family coping style
	    Family's normal response to stress may be chronically inadequate, or the family may be overwhelmed by the catastrophic illness or death of one of its members
	    Illness may cause major shift in role functioning within family
	    Patient has no family to support him or her

Other social relationships in environment
    Caregivers appropriately assess and therapeutically intervene with maladapting patient
    Patient's level of stress is responsive to caregivers' interventions
    Patient's work role is not permanently threatened
    Patient's relationships outside of the family are not permanently threatened
    Patient has friends with whom to explore concerns about illness and receive support (close friends are sometimes able to be more objective than family members)
    Physical environment supports homeostasis
	Other social relationships in environment
	    Caregivers are unable to assess and intervene with maladapting patient
	    Patient's level of stress is not responsive to caregivers' interventions
	    Patient's work role is threatened
	    Patient's role is functioning in social and work relationships is chronically or permanently threatened
	    Patient has inadequate or no social relationships for support
	    Physical environment threatens homeostasis

FIGURE 6-1. Patient and family members' responses to the stress of illness.

able to return to homeostasis. However, if the stressor is severe, such as third-degree burns or severe shock of any kind, body defenses are overwhelmed and death can result.

If the body's defensive capability is completely used up, it enters stage 3, the stage of exhaustion. If the stage of exhaustion is not reversed by removal of the toxic substance, or the body's resistance capability is not supported by medical intervention, the result is death.

PHYSIOLOGICAL STRESS RESPONSES

This section will examine the current knowledge of physiological responses to stress. There are several physiological mechanisms that contribute to biological stress response. They include:

1. Hypothalamic-Pituitary-Adrenal (HPA) Axis
2. Corticotropin-Releasing Hormone (CRH)
3. Adrenocorticotropin Hormone (ACTH)
4. Autonomic Nervous System (ANS)
    a. Sympathetic Division
    b. Parasympathetic Division

Hypothalamic-Pituitary-Adrenal (HPA) Axis

The HPA axis is the endocrine response to a stressor. The anterior lobe of the pituitary gland is stimulated by central nervous system mechanisms that initially perceive a stressor and activate corticotropin-releasing hormone (CRH).

Corticotropin-Releasing Hormone (CRH)

CRH is the principal activator of both behavioral and peripheral physiological responses to stress. CRH also stimulates the hypothalamus and pituitary glands to release peptides that result in the release of glucocorticoids.

Glucocorticoids affect cardiovascular processes, muscle function, the immune system, metabolism, and behavior. They actively regulate many body systems in an attempt to accommodate and adapt to the acute physical responses to the stressful event. It should be noted that the level of threat that is "psychologically" perceived can initiate a powerful physiological cascading effect on the physical process described above.

If the physiological or sensory perception continues to be acute or the initial physical trauma caused by the stressor is severe, the body will continue to be in a high state of arousal and the GAS effects described by Selye can result in further physiological injury, exhaustion, or death (1979).

Adrenocorticotropin Hormone (ACTH)

ACTH is released by the anterior pituitary into the systemic circulation and activates the adrenals to synthesize and secrete glucocorticoids. ACTH also sensitizes the adrenal cortex so that its response to the stressor is enhanced. It will produce an increasing amount of glucocorticoids and can continue to do so if chronic stress persists.

Autonomic Nervous System (ANS)

The autonomic nervous system has two main divisions: the sympathetic and the parasympathetic. The *sympathetic* is the reactive branch of the nervous system that responds to stressful events by stimulating various body systems. The changes in body systems were originally named the "fight or flight" syndrome by Cannon (1929). Simply stated, these physiological changes support either of two primary modes of response to a noxious or challenging stimulus—activation of the body to fight or to escape the stressful circumstances.

The sympathetic response is activated by the locus ceruleus and in turn the catecholamines epinephrine and norepinephrine are released into the systemic circulation. Enzymes are stimulated that regulate catecholamine synthesis. The catecholamine release results in arousal, vigilance, and increased anxiety. The central mechanisms of the sympathetic response also activate the adrenal medulla and sympathetic nerves in the periphery.

It should be noted that the *parasympathetic* branch of the autonomic nervous system is the "automatic" regulator of all body systems. It routinely supports the "normal," nonstressed-state body functions. When the sympathetic division is activated it overrides the routine parasympathetic actions.

If the acute stressor does not diminish, then the body response modifies from the activation described above. With chronic stress, glucocorticoids continue to be produced but the body's responsivity to them is decreased. For example, the number of glucocorticoid receptors on the various body systems and their organs will decrease when there is chronic stress. The stress arousal system may become dulled or less responsive to repeated stressful stimuli that are similar to the original stressor. In most cases, however, the introduction of a new type of stressor will result in the activation of the full stress response in all physiological systems.

PSYCHOLOGICAL STRESS AND THE COPING PROCESS

Richard Lazarus: Cognitive Appraisal

Richard Lazarus, a psychologist, is one of the leading theorists in the psychological stress field. His cognitive appraisal theory is described as follows:

> [Cognitive appraisal] is the cornerstone of his analysis of the emotions; this appraisal, from which the various emotions flow, is determined by the interplay of personality and the environmental stimulus configuration [Lazarus, 1993].

Lazarus has applied the word *transactions* to the constantly changing relationships between a person and his or her environment. These ongoing relationships involve continuous feedback loops of information between the person and the many variables in the environment. Lazarus believes that the feedback-reaction process a person has with the environment is circular, similar to the question "Which came first, the chicken or the egg?" It is not an independent cause-and-effect relationship. Lazarus' theory is rooted in a general systems framework (Lazarus, 1993).

The constant evaluation and reevaluation by humans about their life events is called cognitive appraisal. The first step in this process is primary appraisal. It involves decision-making and judgments about a person's encounters with the environment. There are three possible outcomes of primary appraisal:

1. The event is irrelevant. . . . it has no significance to the person and can be ignored (for instance, an irrelevant perceptual awareness can be the hum of the motor of an audiovisual machine during a presentation).
2. The event is benign-positive. . . . it is beneficial or desirable (for instance, eating a pleasant meal).
3. The event is stressful. . . . it involves a judgment of harm-loss, threat, or challenge:
   a. Harm-loss refers to harm or loss that has already occurred, such as a major loss of self-esteem, changes in or losses of significant relationships or role functioning, or incapacitating illness.
   b. Threat is a person's fear of the events described under harm-loss. They have not yet occurred; the fear is anticipatory.
   c. Challenge is contrasted to threat in its emotional quality. With threat, there is a negative or frightened emotional response. Challenge is a positive response to an event. It focuses on the possibility of mastery or gain (Lazarus, 1993).

Lazarus' theory of cognitive appraisal is important in conceptualizing a patient's responses to illness. For example, a person who is appraising her physical illness and hospitalization customarily will not view the event as irrelevant or benign. Rather, her appraisal will most likely fit into the third category described above; it is perceived as stressful. Figure 6-2 depicts Lazarus' conceptual model of the coping response to stress.

The next step in awareness of an environmental event is called secondary appraisal. Secondary appraisal occurs after the person answers the challenge of primary appraisal, "Am I okay or in trouble?" If she decides she is in trouble, she then asks, "What can I do about it?" During this secondary stage of cognitive appraisal, the person consciously applies coping strategies that have worked in the past.

The person continually evaluates her response to these coping efforts and makes additional coping attempts if her level of anxiety and fear is not reduced by the original efforts. Reappraisal occurs when the evaluation results in changes in her original coping attempts. This process involves continuous feedback between a person's emotional, intellectual, and physiological subsystems and the environment. Body sensations feed into the person's emotional and intellectual response.

Coping is defined as "efforts, both action-oriented and intrapsychic, to manage (that is, to master, tolerate, reduce, minimize) environmental and internal demands and conflicts which tax or exceed a person's resources." The Lazarus model divides coping into two types: problem-oriented and emotion regulation. Problem-oriented coping is an attempt to change one's own mental reaction to stress by taking conscious, intellectual actions or by changing the condition in the environment that is causing the stress. Emotion regulation refers to efforts of the psyche to maintain emotional control and reduce its own distressed feeling state (Lazarus, 1993).

The person who is physically ill or hospitalized has little control over his situation. He is not able to utilize fully the problem-oriented method of coping because the problem is within his own body. This problem did not originate in the environment and cannot be resolved by leaving or changing his surroundings. Instead, his coping must, of necessity, involve changing his own emotional reaction to the illness.

The way a person responds to illness or hospitalization depends on the following factors:

1. Change in cognition. Cognition can increase or decrease perceptual ability, thought, judgment, problem solving, motor skills, or social adaptation (Lazarus, 1993).
2. Coping responses initiated consciously in order to promote adaptation:
   a. Disturbed affect such as fear, anxiety, anger, depression, and guilt. These form the single largest category of stress responses. These emotions then trigger the unconscious defense mechanisms to assist in the coping process.
   b. Physiological change which may involve all the body systems (neurological, endocrine, cardiovascular, respiratory, gastrointestinal, and so on).
   c. Motor behavior seen most commonly as increased muscle tension (body posture, certain facial expressions, or tremor).

The sequence involved in Lazarus' theory about cognitive style, stress perception, and coping appears in Figure 6-2.

Once a person is aware of a harm-loss or threatening stressor, his or her coping ability will also determine the level of emotional and physical responses to that stressor. Two psychological factors are particularly important in understanding Lazarus' coping process: the degree of threat the person perceives and ego strength. Ego strength is the intrapsychic and primarily unconscious supply of defense mechanisms the ego uses to master the threat (Groves & Kucharski, 1991; Rosenbaum & Pollack, 1991). Lazarus scales the ego defenses in levels that range from appropriate defenses to maladaptive levels of defense (both types are discussed in Chapter 3). With coping failure, defense proceeds in a gradually deteriorating continuum from self-control to increased alertness, fantasy, displacement, panic attacks, violent loss of control, schizophrenic breaks with reality, and ultimately death.

The most mature reaction to threat occurs when the degree of threat is slight to moderate. When the degree of threat is high, even a normally well-functioning person may demonstrate a very primitive response because of the ego's inability to adapt immediately. The defense mechanisms outlined in Chapter 3 may cause the person to use denial, thereby shutting out the threat, or to reduce his or her perception of the actual degree of threat by repression or distortion.

The example of a 43-year-old woman admitted to the hospital because of bleeding of unknown etiology in her intestinal tract illustrates Lazarus' cognitive appraisal theory. According to Lazarus, a person's response to the stressor of illness or hospitalization depends on the following:

1. The individual's belief system concerning transactions with the environment.

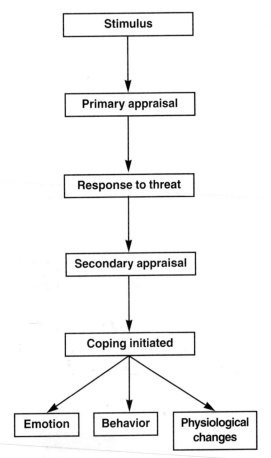

FIGURE 6-2. Lazarus stress response sequence. (Coyne, J., & Lazarus, R. [1980]. Cognitive style, stress perception and coping. In I. Kutash & L. Schlesinger [Eds.], *Handbook of Stress and Anxiety*. San Francisco; Jossey-Bass).

These include intellectual resources, education, and sophistication. The availability of these resources may make a person more or less prone to a stress reaction, depending on his or her familiarity and experience with the threat. The lack of these resources could also contribute to an incorrect threat appraisal. When a situation is believed to be threatening, whether or not it actually is so, a stress response is initiated. In the case of the patient described above, let us review her belief system. She knows that blood in the intestinal tract is abnormal. She knows it could be caused by ulcers or cancer; both are frightening diseases to her.

She remembers that her uncle had ulcers that caused him much difficulty, and she remembers that one of her neighbor's sisters died of cancer of the intestine.

2. The resources of a person to defend himself or herself from harm-losses or threats. In this case, the woman described above may have poor coping ability, and be overwhelmed by fear of the situation. She may be so threatened that denial quickly shuts out the reality; accordingly, she may delay treatment to her own detriment. She may also react with an appropriate suppression of her fears and obtain immediate treatment. If she responds by being overwhelmed or by denying her symptoms, her physical well-being is further jeopardized because of ineffective coping and maladaptive responses. If the person is in a prolonged state of panic, there is an increased rate of physiological deterioration of the body due to the GAS, in addition to the already existing disease state.

The nurse's awareness of increased psychological stress in patients is very important. If stress is undetected, no therapeutic intervention will occur that could reduce the stress level and avoid further physical demand or deterioration. In addition to the psychological stress of a threatening external stressor, unrelieved pain can produce a stress response in the body because it results in both psychological and physical distress. Care planning and interventions for people experiencing high levels of stress as the result of illness will be presented in subsequent chapters.

Psychological Hardiness

Research on the concept of *psychological hardiness* and its relatedness to mental and physical illness has identified three personality characteristics that, when present, appear to buffer the effects of moderate to high levels of life event stress (Kobasa, 1979; Kobasa, Maddi, & Conn, 1982; Kobasa, Maddi, & Courington, 1981; Kobasa & Puscetti, 1983). These personality characteristics are contrasted to those that were found to undermine adaptive stress responses.

Individuals with characteristics of hardiness who had moderate to high levels of stress reported less physical and mental illness than persons who measured low on the three characteristics. Psychosocial assessment of the factors described below, when accompanied by interventions designed to address specific coping problems associated with one or more of these factors, can result in more effective coping.

The three personality factors identified as being related to hardiness are:

Control vs. Helplessness. A person believes that he has control over what happens to him. This characteristic can be compared to the concept of internal locus of control described in Chapter 9. It is contrasted by Kobasa, Maddi, and Conn (1982) to the experience of helplessness.

Commitment vs. Alienation. A person believes that there is a purpose to her actions and she becomes actively involved in bettering her or others' situations. This concept is contrasted to alienation. Alienation is defined as "emotional isolation or dissociation. A state of estrangement between the self and the objective world or between different parts of the personality" (*American Heritage College Dictionary,* 1993, p.34).

Challenge vs. Threat. A person perceives an event as one that promotes change and an opportunity for growth. Challenge is contrasted to threat. Please see the section on Lazarus' theory of cognitive appraisal, above, for discussion of the difference in perception between challenge and threat.

Of particular clinical significance is the perception of control vs. helplessness. *Helplessness* is a psychological state that has been described by Seligman (1991). It occurs as a response to repeated unsuccessful attempts to improve a given situation. Seligman's early work with laboratory animals resulted in a phenomenon of "giving up." This phenomenon of *learned helplessness* in animals was accompanied by marked withdrawal and passivity, as well as significant changes in physiological measures. This animal model of learned helplessness has been proposed as the human model of depression (Weiss & Simon, 1985). Indeed, helplessness is the opposite experience of feeling in control. Barry describes the sense of loss of control or

helplessness as perhaps the most pervasive mental state that contributes to ineffective coping (1991). Box 6-1 depicts physiological response to the control, and reaction in the striving and helpless states.

In planning psychosocial interventions, it may be possible to assist the patient in reframing the stressful event. Reframing is the exploration of distressing issues with new perspectives. By reframing the stressful event from the original experience of helplessness, alienation, or threat to new perspectives regarding control, commitment, and challenge, it is possible that changed awarenesses in patients and families can occur.

BIOPSYCHOSOCIAL MEDIATION OF STRESSFUL EVENTS

Experts in the fields of medical science and physical pathology have previously considered the cause of physical disease to be the failure of normal organ functioning due to purely physiological causes. The premise of this book is that it is not possible to separate physical phenomena from psychologic phenomena. The physical subsystems are constantly interacting with the psychological subsystems because both are part of one body system. They both respond continuously to stressors such as social and environmental demands (Charney et al., 1993; Everly, 1993; Kiecolt-Glaser & Glaser, 1992; Puglisi-Allegra & Oliverio, 1990; van der Kolk & Fisher, 1993). During the past decade, nursing theory has developed a holistic or systems approach toward understanding the functioning of human beings and the etiology and course of illness. The systems approach includes the principles of biopsychosocial phenomena in the etiology and treatment of disease (Dossey, Guzzetta, & Kenner, 1992).

THE PSYCHOBIOLOGY OF STRESS MEDIATION: THE MIND-BODY BRIDGE

Many nursing caregivers have clinically observed a relationship between how a person feels emotionally and that person's physical state (Black & Matassarin-Jacobs, 1993; Stanhope & Lancaster, 1992). However, until recently, it was impossible to document a definite association between the two. Lack of high-level technology inhibited psychosomatic research.

A systems approach to understanding stress tells us that not only does physical illness cause emotional and social stress, but emotional and social stress may cause physical illness. There is a constant, circular relationship between these factors. When coping fails, there is increased stress on all the subsystems, and physical illness can result. Effective coping can usually reduce or stop the cycle of psychological distress (Davey, Tallis, & Hodgson, 1993; Gage, 1992; Goldstein & Niaura, 1992; Hagopian, 1993; Levine, 1993; Small & Graydon, 1992; Woods, Habaerman, & Packard, 1993).

For acute or chronic psychological stress to induce disease in an organ, the stress would have to be transmitted from the brain to that organ by the autonomic nervous system or neuroendocrine pathways. The autonomic nervous system and the neuroendocrine system are routes by which the brain can directly affect the activity of the internal organs. Both the autonomic nervous system and the neuroendocrine system are relatively autonomous, taking care of the routine business of keeping the internal environment constant. However, this ordinary reflex activity can be overridden by higher centers of the brain when they sense some change in the environment and prepare the body to meet it (Charney et al., 1993; van der Kolk & Fisher, 1993; Yehuda, Giller, & Mason, 1993).

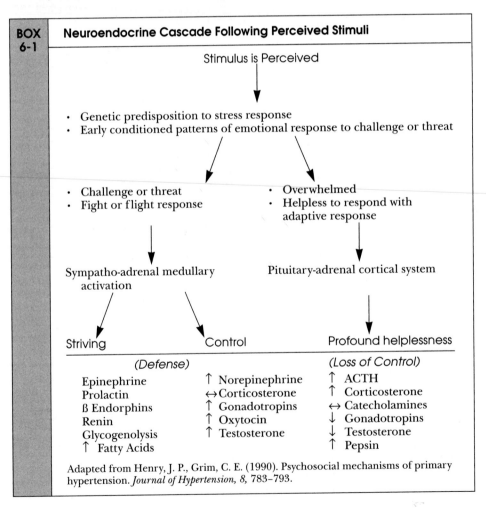

BOX 6-1

Neuroendocrine Cascade Following Perceived Stimuli

Stimulus is Perceived

- Genetic predisposition to stress response
- Early conditioned patterns of emotional response to challenge or threat

- Challenge or threat
- Fight or flight response

- Overwhelmed
- Helpless to respond with adaptive response

Sympatho-adrenal medullary activation

Pituitary-adrenal cortical system

Striving   Control   Profound helplessness

(Defense)		*(Loss of Control)*
Epinephrine	↑ Norepinephrine	↑ ACTH
Prolactin	↔ Corticosterone	↑ Corticosterone
ß Endorphins	↑ Gonadotropins	↔ Catecholamines
Renin	↑ Oxytocin	↓ Gonadotropins
Glycogenolysis	↑ Testosterone	↓ Testosterone
↑ Fatty Acids		↑ Pepsin

Adapted from Henry, J. P., Grim, C. E. (1990). Psychosocial mechanisms of primary hypertension. *Journal of Hypertension, 8,* 783–793.

Many studies have shown that the structures of the limbic system are involved with basic drive states such as fear, hunger, sexual excitement, and aggression. The limbic structures, including the locus ceruleus, are shaped like a "C," forming a ring around an even older, more basic structure called the brain stem. The brain stem contains centers which are involved in regulating basic vegetative functions. For example, the centers for temperature control, blood pressure regulation, and sleep-wake activation are located in the brain stem. The brain stem passes information to the internal organs by way of the autonomic nervous system. Thus the emotion of fear, generated in the limbic system, influences the nearby brain stem structures to alter the activity of the internal organs. Blood pressure rises, rapid breathing begins, the heart starts to pound, and muscles fill with blood (Murray, 1991; Sack, 1980).

The autonomic nervous system (ANS) has two major divisions, the sympathetic and the parasympathetic. In general, the sympathetic division of the ANS mediates the response to challenges presented by the environment. The adrenal medulla is a specialized and enlarged sympathetic ganglion. When stimulated, the adrenal gland releases epinephrine, which is also called adrenaline. The parasympathetic division of the ANS is involved during periods of physiological restoration—for example, when digesting a meal. Both divisions of the autonomic nervous system have been implicated in psychosomatic illness (Murray, 1991; Sack, 1980).

In addition to the autonomic nervous system, the other major route by which psychological stress is transmitted to the internal organs is the hypothalamic-pituitary neuroendocrine system. The hypothalamus lies at the base of the brain and receives input from most other parts of the brain. Electrical messages from other brain areas are translated to chemical messages in special hypothalamic cells; these cells secrete polypeptide hormones. These polypeptides from the hypothalamus, also known as releasing factors, travel down into the pituitary gland via a special blood vessel network.

The pituitary, sometimes called the master gland, secretes hormones into the general circulation when activated by hypothalamic polypeptide hormones. The pituitary hormones may act directly on other organ systems, or they may stimulate other endocrine glands such as the thyroid and adrenal cortex to release hormones (Murray, 1991; Sack, 1980). Table 6-4 depicts neurohormonal responses to stress in the form of psychosocial stimuli.

Thus, in addition to autonomic arousal, psychological stress can activate a chain of hormonal responses that eventually alters the activity of the internal organs (Sack, 1980).

Sack presents the rationale for the potential relationship between the etiology of physical illness and psychic stress. Sack does not address the impact of social and environmental factors, however. Perception of social or environmental stressors typically triggers a cognitive appraisal or physiological response that can result in the activation process described above. The interactive effects of stress on the mind and body cannot be isolated from the multiple social stressors, such as sitting for final examinations or being involved in an argument, or environmental stressors, such as extremes of temperature or exposure to infectious disease. Individuals are constantly exposed and responding to such stressors. Accordingly, the effects of stress must be studied within the context of general systems effects.

HISTORICAL DEVELOPMENT OF A SYSTEMS APPROACH TO STRESS

A systems approach to illness has been evolving for centuries. The Bible and Socrates' writings both evidence a relationship between hopelessness or melancholy and the development of physical illness. On occasion, similar references appeared in medical literature before the 20th century.

During the early 20th century, Cannon (1929) attempted to prove an association between mental states and the endocrine system. Because of inadequate laboratory facilities, his attempts were doomed to failure. However, his theories about a possible association between the two formed the basis of research in later decades.

Alexander was another important theorist in the field of psychosomatic medicine. Beginning in the 1930s, he and his associates spent several decades attempting to prove that people with certain personality styles were prone to specific types of illnesses. The development of illness was believed to represent certain types of intrapsychic conflict.

The diseases they studied were duodenal peptic ulcers, bronchial asthma, rheumatoid arthritis, ulcerative colitis, essential hypertension, neurodermatitis, and thyrotoxicosis. Their research focus identified factors that they believed would result in the development of one of these illnesses. The factors were predominantly intrapsychic and were believed to be related to the physiological subsystem by direct action on the end organs by the peripheral mechanisms of the autonomic nervous system (Alexander, 1987). These theories are now considered by some to be oversimplified in the light of recent advances in understanding the complexity of the mind-body interaction (Folkow, 1993; Goldstein & Niaura, 1992; Kaplan & Sadock, 1994; Reiser, 1984; Solomon, 1985; Temoshok, 1987).

The study of the effects of stress in the development of illness continues. More attention is being paid to the interactive effects of physiological and psychological genetic dispositions, the personality structure developed in response to family dynamics, the overall social system, and the environment; these factors were identified by research demonstrating their impact on the development of illness.

THE EFFECT OF STRESS ON THE DEVELOPMENT OF PHYSICAL ILLNESS

Currently, stress is implicated in the development of many physical illnesses. Many researchers and theorists propose that there is a relationship between stress, inadequate coping, and immunosuppression (Kiecolt-Glaser & Glaser, 1991; Stein, Miller, & Trestman, 1991).

The Role of Neurotransmitters

All thoughts and feelings emanate from information-processing events in the brain.

Less well appreciated is the fact that virtually all this information processing involves communications between nerve cells (which are called neurons) via chemicals known as neurotransmitters [Felten et al., 1991].

The most basic connecting link in the bridge between the mind and the body is the neurotransmitter, a chemical messenger that relays information between neurons (Snyder, 1980). A neuron is the basic unit of the nervous system. It consists of a body, an axon, and one or more dendrites. The axon sends impulses or messages away from the neuron body; the dendrites receive messages from other neurons.

Neurons do not actually touch one another in the process of sending and receiving messages. Instead, there is a slight space between them called a synapse. When the cell body initiates an impulse to its axon, the axon automatically releases a neurotransmitter substance that will carry the message across the synapse to the dendrites of hundreds or thousands of neighboring neurons.

Different parts of the brain contain specific types of neurons with particular functions. The neurotransmitters they release differ chemically from those of other neurons. There are probably hundreds of different types of neurotransmitters in the brain. Each of them has a different stimulating or inhibiting effect on neurons. All brain functioning, whether it involves thinking, feeling, or sending messages to the muscles of the limbs or organs, depends on these neurotransmitters (Snyder, 1980).

Neuroscientists are only beginning to scratch the surface in understanding the importance of these chemical substances in the body. By studying the effects of having too much or too little of these biochemicals in humans and laboratory animals, their specific roles in neuroendocrine functioning will be increasingly documented. In fact, some theorists believe that further research on these substances will show that they hold the key to whether people will become ill as a result of immune system failure or whether they will remain well (Locke & Colligan, 1986).

Neurotransmitter Effects on the Immune System

One of the most significant physiological discoveries in recent years is that the various

TABLE 6-3
A Model Depicting the Interaction of Stress and the Organism

Level	Adaptive Capacity	Stressors	Alarm Reaction	Defensive Reaction	Pathological End-State
Biological	State of physique, nutrition, vigor Natural or acquired immunities	Deprivation of biological needs Excess inputs of physical or biological agents	Arousal—hunger, thirst, pain, fatigue Changes in physiological function	GAS Physiological compensation Shifts in metabolism Changes in pain threshold	Deficiency diseases "Exhaustion" Addictions Chronic dysfunction Structural damage
Psychological	Resourcefulness, problem-solving ability Ego strength Flexibility Social skills	Perceptions and interpretations of danger, threat, loss, disappointment, frustration, or sense of failure or hopelessness Loss of self-acceptance Threat to security	Feelings of deprivation—boredom, grief, sadness Feelings of anxiety, pressure, guilt Fear of danger	Ego defenses—denial, repression, projection Defensive neuroses Perceptual defenses—wishes, fantasies, motives Planning Problem solving	Despair, apathy-Chronic personality pattern disturbances Psychoses Chronic affective disorders Meaninglessness
Interpersonal	Primary relationships including family Network of social supports	Social isolation Lack of acceptance Insults, punishments, rejections Changes in social groups, especially losses	Antagonism, conflict, suspicion Withdrawal Feelings of rejection, punishment	Defensive, rigid social relating Avoidance Assuming sick role Aggressiveness "Acting out" Enlisting social supports	Chronic exploitation Becoming an outcast Imprisonment Permanent disruption of interpersonal ties Chronic failure to fulfill roles
Sociocultural	Values Norms and practices "Therapeutic" social institutions Systems of knowledge and technology	Cultural change Role conflict Status incongruity Value conflicts with important others Forced change in life situation	Communication of concern and alarm Expressive behavior of crowds Mobilization of social structures	Culturally prescribed defenses—scapegoating, prejudice Explanatory ideologies Legal and moral systems Use of curers and institutions	Alienation, anomie Breakdown of social order Disintegration of the cultural systems of values and norms

Jenkins, D. (1979). Psychosocial modifiers of response to stress. In Barrett, J., Rose, R., Klerman, G. (Eds.), *Stress and Mental Disorder,* New York: Raven Press, p. 269.

cells in the immune system contain receptor sites for neurotransmitters, which are known to have an active role in the mediation of stress (Good, 1986). Stressors stimulate release of a number of types of neurotransmitters, such as norepinephrine and serotonin. These neurotransmitters stimulate receptors on cells in the immune system; if strong enough, they eventually suppress the normal immune response (Felten et al., 1991; Madden & Livnat, 1991; Roszman & Carlson, 1991). A more complete discussion of immune system responses to psychological stress appears below in the section on psychoneuroimmunology.

The Role of Stress in Myocardial Infarction

Stress has also been suggested as a cause of atherosclerotic heart disease. Rahe and Lind (Folkow, 1993; Johnson et al., 1992), in questioning the families of people who died from myocardial infarction (MI), discovered that the amount of life change and stress the victims experienced during the year preceding death (see the Holmes and Rahe stress scale) was significantly higher than the stress they experienced during the 2 years preceding it. The 6 months preceding death showed the highest increase of all.

One possible cause of the relationship between stress and the development of atherosclerosis is that stimulation of the sympathetic nervous system is known to cause the release of fatty acids and glycerol from the fat tissues. Carruthers (1969) has theorized that sympathetic adrenal medullary stimulation could repeatedly raise blood fatty acid levels, resulting, after several biochemical steps, in the buildup of fatty acid deposits on the walls of arteries (atherosclerosis). Accordingly, it is possible that both high blood pressure and the development of coronary heart disease are precipitated by stress (Folkow, 1993; Johnson et al., 1992; Sack, 1980).

In reviewing the types of stressful events that occurred in the lives of subsequent MI patients, Hurst and colleagues (1979) discovered that different people reported varying levels of distress about a given life event. Accordingly, they propose that it is the unique

responses to events that are personally upsetting that can undermine an individual's coronary status.

The most up-to-date theory about the relationship between stress and physical illness suggests that many factors influence the development of illness:

1. The genetic personality and physical dispositions the person inherits (see Chapter 3)
2. Effects of the environment on personality development as determined by:
   a. Family dynamics
   b. Type of defense mechanisms that develop in response to the conflict between the person's needs and those of the family system
   c. The person's overall coping ability (see Chapters 2, 3, 6–10)
3. Mutual feedback between the mind, the body, and the environment as discussed earlier and initiated by factors such as biological body rhythms, fatigue, impact of psychosocial events, and availability of a social support system.

A COMPREHENSIVE MODEL FOR EVALUATING STRESS

Integration of the concepts presented in this chapter is assisted by the model proposed by Jenkins (1979). About the traditional stress models, he wrote:

A major weakness of most stress research has been its limitation to a two-variable research design: a noxious stimulus is introduced and a response of discomfort or disease is observed . . . defined in terms of the presence of a physical or psychiatric illness [Jenkins, 1979, p. 265].

His solution to the incompleteness he found in the traditional approaches to stress was to introduce five variables:

1. The person's adaptive capacity
2. The stressor
3. The alarm reaction
4. The defensive reaction
5. The pathological reaction

Jenkins has found that a person's ability to adapt to stress also depends on his interpersonal relationships and the overall society in which he functions. Table 6-3 shows the many possible responses to stress and the potential for negative effects of stress on patients who are unable to cope with their illness or hospitalization.

THE PATIENT'S RESPONSE TO THE STRESS OF ILLNESS

Another important consideration in the care of the person with physical illness is that the illness generates an increased amount of stress for the patient and family. The new level of stress requires a higher order of coping responses. This demand on the patient-family system creates stress throughout the biopsychosocial realms of each person in the family. Their responses may be effective or ineffective. As noted earlier in Figure 6-1, the two major coping styles have very different outcomes.

Psychoneuroimmunology and the Stress Response

Early research on the role of psychological factors on physiological states focused on endocrine hormones (Besedovsky, 1977; Calvet & Gresser, 1979; Goldstein, Slader, & White, 1966; Isakovic & Jankovic, 1973; Tyrey & Nalbandov, 1972). Adrenocortical and lymphocytic relationships with stress responses were also studied by the pioneers in the medical science field of psychoneuroimmunology (Bartrop et al., 1977; Blalock, 1984; Ader & Cohen, 1982, 1985, 1991; Schleifer et al., 1983; Stein et al., 1991).

As basic medical science and clinical medicine disciplines engaged in research on the effects of "stress," it behooved researchers to develop multidisciplinary terms so that systemic stress-related factors could be comprehensively addressed. The name psychoneuroimmunology emerged because it incorporates the critical elements of the full stress response (Ader, Felten, & Cohen, 1991).

Work in this field gained impetus because of the human immunodeficiency virus (HIV) and AIDS, and the interest in examining all potential factors that could support longevity and quality of life for AIDS-infected or HIV-positive individuals. Temoshok (1987) has identified the possible role of psychosocial stressors as epidemiologic factors in cancer etiology. Research studies are probing the role of psychosocial stress and viral infections such as upper respiratory infections and herpes simplex (Cappel, Gregoire, Thiry, & Sprecher, 1978; Kiecolt-Glaser & Glaser, 1986).

These studies have demonstrated the downward modulation of immune function as a response to different types of stressors. One of the immune functions that shows stress-related immunocompetence is natural killer (NK) cell activity. The NK cell is the tumor- and virus-vigilant cell of the immune system (Kiecolt-Glaser & Glaser, 1992). The implications of significantly reduced numbers of NK cells when an individual is actively stressed speaks to the importance of developing psychosocial interventions that can support effective coping during all critical stress incidents. It should be emphasized also that due to the finding of stress-related immune system suppression, the psychosocial support of persons with newly diagnosed, life-threatening illness is an essential part of comprehensive patient care.

A psychoneuroimmunology study reported in 1993 found altered immune responses to breast cancer patients with high trait anxiety who were undergoing adjuvant chemotherapy compared to breast cancer patients with low trait anxiety. The specific differences were in monocytes, NK cells, and helper/inducer T-cells. The high-anxiety women also had increased numbers of granulocytes. In prior studies, increased granulocytes were related to higher/elevated anticipatory stress and conditioning responses (Fredrikson et al., 1993).

Other stress-related indications of decreased immune system function include decreases in mitogen response, T-cell proliferation, neuroendocrine receptors on T-cells, and platelets that are essential to a full immune response (Gatti et al., 1993; Helig et al., 1993; Kiecolt-Glaser & Glaser, 1992; Wood et al., 1993).

CONCLUSION

The effects of stress on the body are increasingly recognized by nursing and medical

TABLE 6–4 Neurohormonal Responses to Psychosocial Stimuli	
Level of Control	**Affected Body Mechanisms**
Central Nervous System	Somatomotor: behavior Visceromotor: digestive and circulatory systems Hormonal: endocrine levels, metabolism rates, electrolyte balance
Bulbar (systemic)	Neurohormonal/cardiovascular mechanisms; body fluid volume levels, flow and resistance
Local	Neurotransmission and feedback mechanisms in specific organs and tissues
Allular	Cell metabolism, antibody response
Sub-cellular	Neurochemistry and homeostasis in cellular membranes, organelles
Molecular	DNA, molecular integrity

Adapted from Läkartiningen, (1993) 90: 4339–4342.

practitioners as well as scientists in many fields. In general hospital and traditional medical care settings, however, many patients continue to be treated with a biomedical model based on diagnosis and treatment of physical pathology. There may be little attention paid to the effects of the psychological and social subsystems in the etiology and course of illness. Similarly, there may be little consideration given to the interaction of the mind, body, and spiritual states during the active treatment process.

Professional nursing has identified the significance of assessing the patient from a holistic perspective. The use of nursing diagnosis as an essential part of the nursing process has especially highlighted the nurse's importance as the monitor of the patient's biopsychosocial response to illness (Carpenito, 1993; McFarland, Wasli, & Gerety, 1992).

The information presented in this chapter further emphasizes the impact of the psychosocial spheres on both the development of illness and the patient's response to illness. The effects of stress and inadequate coping promote an ongoing illness potential in all people. When stress overcomes a person's ability to cope, the potential for maladaptation or crisis in the physical, psychological, spiritual, or social spheres increases. Crisis assessment

and intervention recommendations appear in Chapter 16.

BIBLIOGRAPHY

Ader, R., & Cohen, N. (1982). Behaviorally conditioned immunosuppression and murine systemic lupus erythematosus. *Science, 215,* 1534–1536.

Ader, R., & Cohen, N. (1985). CNS-immune system interactions: Conditioning phenomena. *Behavioral and Brain Sciences, 8,* 379–426.

Ader, R., Cohen, N., & Felten, D.L. (1987). Brain, behavior and immunity. *Brain, behavior and immunity, 1*(1), 1–6.

Ader, R., Felten, D., & Cohen, N. (Eds.). (1991). *Psychoneuroimmunology* (2nd ed.). New York: Academic Press.

American Heritage college dictionary (3rd ed.). (1993). Boston: Houghton-Mifflin.

Barry, P. (1991). An investigation of cardiovascular, respiratory, and skin temperature changes during relaxation and anger inductions. *Dissertation Abstracts International, 52-09-B,* 5012.

Bartrop, R.W., Lazarus, L., Luckherst, E., Kiloh, L.G. & Penny, R. (1977). Depressed lymphocyte function after bereavement. *Lancet, 1,* 834–836.

Battegay, R. (1991). Defense and coping in the antinomy between self-maintenance and adaptation. *Journal of the American Academy of Psychoanalysis, 19*(3), 471–483.

Bertalanffy, L. von. (1968). *General system theory.* New York: Basic Books.

Besedovsky, H., Sorkin, E., Felix, D., & Haas, H. (1977). Hypothalamic changes during the immune response. *European Journal of Immunology, 7,* 323–325.

Black, J. M., & Matassarin-Jacobs, E. (Eds.). (1993). *Luckmann and Sorensen's medical-surgical nursing: A psychophysiologic approach* (4th ed.). Philadelphia: W. B. Saunders.

Blalock, J. (1984). The immune system as a sensory organ. *Journal of Immunology, 132*, 1067–1070.

Brown, G. W., & Harris, T. O. (Eds.). (1989). *Life events and illness.* New York: Guilford Press.

Buss, D. M. (1991). Evolutionary personality psychology. *Annual Review of Psychology, 42*, 459–491.

Calvet, M., & Gressler, I. (1979). Interferon enhances the excitability of cultured neurons. *Nature* (London). 278, 558–560.

Campbell, R. J. (1989). *Psychiatric dictionary* (6th ed.). New York: Oxford University Press.

Cannon, W. (1929). *Bodily changes in pain, hunger, fear, and rage* (2nd ed.). New York: D. Appleton Co.

Cappel, R., Gregoire, F., Thiry, L., & Sprecher, S. (1978). Antibody and cell-mediated immunity to herpes simplex virus in psychotic depression. *Journal of Clinical Psychiatry*, 39 (3), 266–268.

Carruthers, M. (1969). Aggression and atheroma. *Lancet*, 2(631), 1170–1171.

Creamer, M., Burgess, P., & Pattison, P. (1992). Reaction to trauma: A cognitive processing model. *Journal of Abnormal Psychology, 101*(3), 452–459.

Dewsbury, D. A. (1991). Psychobiology. *American Psychologist, 46*(3), 198–205.

Edlin, G., & Golanty, E. (1992). *Health and wellness: A holistic approach* (4th ed.). Boston: Jones and Bartlett.

Engel, G. (1968). *Psychological development in health and disease* (2nd ed.). Philadelphia: W. B. Saunders.

Everly, G. S. (1993). Psychotraumatology: A two-factor formulation of posttraumatic stress. *Integrative Physiological and Behavioral Science, 28*(3), 270–278.

Felten, D. L., Cohen, N., Ader, R., Felten, S., Carlson, S., & Roszman, T. L. (1991). Central neural circuits involved in neural-immune interactions. In R. Ader, D. Felten, & N. Cohen (Eds.), *Psychoneuroimmunology* (2nd ed.). New York: Academic Press.

Felten, D.L., Overhage, J.M., Felten, S.Y., & Schmedtje, J.F. (1981). Noradrenergic sympathetic innervation of lymploid tissue in the rabbit appendix: Further evidence for a link between the nervous and immune systems. *Brain Research Bulletin, 7*, 595–612.

Folkow, B. (1993). Physiological organization of neurohormonal responses to psychosocial stimuli: Implications for health and disease. *Annals of Behavioral Medicine, 15*(4), 236–243.

Fredrikson, M., Furst, C., Lekander, M., Rotstein, S., & Blomgren, H. (1993). Trait anxiety and anticipatory immune reactions in women receiving adjuvant chemotherapy for breast cancer. *Brain, Behavior, and Immunity, 7*(1), 79–90.

Gage, M. (1992). The appraisal model of coping: An assessment and intervention model for occupational therapy. *American Journal of Occupational Therapy, 46*(4), 353–362.

Gatti, G., Masera, R., Pallavicini, L., Sartori, M., Staurenghi, A., Orlandi, F., & Angeli, A. (1993). Interplay in vitro between ACTH, beta-endorphin, and glucocorticoids in the modulation of spontaneous and lymphokine-inducible human natural killer (NK) cell activity. *Brain, Behavior, and Immunity, 7*(1), 16–28.

Giron, I.T., Crutcher, K.A. & Davis, J.N. (1980). Lymph nodes—a possible site for sympathetic neuronal regulation of immune responses. *Annals of Neurology, 8*, 520–525.

Goldberg, R. J., & Novack, D. H. (1992). The psychosocial review of systems. *Social Science and Medicine, 35*(3), 261–269.

Goldstein, A., Slader, F., & White, A. (1966). Preparation, assay and partial purification of a thymic lymphatocytopoietic faction (thymosin). *Proceedings of the National Academy of Sciences of the U.S.A., 56*, 1010.

Goldstein, M. G., & Niaura, R. (1992). Psychological factors affecting physical condition. Cardiovascular disease literature review. Part I: Coronary artery disease and sudden death. *Psychosomatics, 33*(2), 134–145.

Good, R. (1986). *Enkephalins and endorphins: Stress and the immune system.* New York: Plenum Press.

Goodyer, I. M. (1990). *Life experiences, development, and childhood psychopathology.* New York: Wiley.

Halm, M. A., Titler, M. G., Kleiber, C., Johnson, S. K., Montgomery, L. A., Craft, M. J., Buckwalter, K., Nicholson, A., & Megivern, K. (1993). Behavioral responses of family members during critical illness. *Clinics in Nursing Research, 2*(4), 414–437.

Helig, M., Irwin, M., Grewal, I., & Sevcarz, E. (1993). Sympathetic regulation of T-helper cell function. *Brain, Behavior, and Immunity, 7*(1), 154–163.

Henry, J. P. (1992). Biological basis of stress response. *Integrative Physiological and Behavioral Science, 27*(1), 66–83.

Horowitz, M. (1976). *Stress response syndromes.* New York: Aronson.

Hurst, M., Jenkins, C., & Rose, R. (1979). The relation of psychological stress to onset of medical illness. In C. Garfield (Ed.), *Stress and survival: The emotional realities of life-threatening illness.* St. Louis: Mosby.

Isakovic, K., & Jankovic, B. (1973). Neuro-endocrine correlates of immune response. II. Changes in the lymphatic organs of brain lesioned rats. *International Archives of Allergy and Applied Immunology, 45*, 373–384.

Jenkins, C. (1979). Psychosocial modifiers of response to stress. In J. Barrett, R. Rose, & G. Klerman (Eds.), *Stress and mental disorder.* New York: Raven Press.

Johnson, E., Kamilaris, T., Chorous, B., & Gold, P. (1992). Mechanisms of stress: A dynamic overview of hormonal and behavioral homeostasis. *Neuroscience and Biobehavioral Reviews, 16*(2), 115–130.

Kaplan, H. I., & Sadock, B. J. (1994). *Synopsis of psychiatry: Behavioral sciences, clinical psychiatry* (7th ed.). Baltimore: Williams & Wilkins.

Kaplan, H. I., & Sadock, B. J. (1995). *Comprehensive textbook of psychiatry/VI* (6th ed.). Baltimore: Williams & Wilkins.

Kawahara, G., & Osada, N. (1962). Studies on the innervation of bone marrow with special reference to the intramedullary fibers in the dog and goat. *Archivum Histologicum Japonicum, 24*, 471–487.

Kiecolt-Glaser, J.K., & Glaser, R. (1986). Psychological influences on immunity. *Psychosomatics, 27*(9), 621–624.

Kiecolt-Glaser, J. K., & Glaser, R. (1992). Psychoneuroimmunology: Can psychological interventions modulate immunity? *Journal of Consulting Clinical Psychology, 60*(4), 569–575.

Kiecolt-Glaser, J. K., Cacioppo, J. T., Malarkey, W. B., & Glaser, R. (1992). Acute psychological stressors and short-term immune changes: What, why, for whom, and to what extent? *Psychosomatic Medicine, 54*(6), 680–685.

Kobasa, S. (1979). Stressful life events, personality, and health: An inquiry into hardiness. *Journal of Personality and Social Psychology, 37*(1), 1–11.

Kobasa, S., Maddi, S., & Conn, S. (1982). Hardiness and health: A prospective study. *Journal of Personality and Social Psychology, 42*(1), 168–177.

Kobasa, S., Maddi, S., & Courington, S. (1981). Personality and constitution as mediators in the stress-illness relationship. *Journal of Health and Social Behavior, 22*(4), 368–378.

Kobasa, S., & Puscetti, M. (1983). Personality and social resources in stress resistance. *Journal of Personality and Social Psychology, 45*(4), 839–850.

Kolk, B. A. van der, & Fisher, R. E. (1993). The biologic basis of posttraumatic stress. *Primary Care, 20*(2), 417–432.

Krueger, E., & Krueger, G. R. (1991). How does the subjective experience of stress relate to the breakdown of the human immune system? *In Vivo, 5*(3), 207–215.

Lazarus, R. S. (1966). *Psychological stress and the coping process.* New York: McGraw-Hill.

Lazarus, R. S. (1970). Cognitive and personality factors underlying threat and coping. In S. Levine & N. Scotch (Eds.), *Social stress.* Chicago: Aldine.

Lazarus, R. S. (1992). Coping with the stress of illness. *WHO Regional Publication, European Series, 44,* 11–31.

Lazarus, R. S. (1993). Coping theory and research: Past, present, and future. *Psychosomatic Medicine, 55*(3), 234–247.

Locke, S., & Colligan, D. (1986). *The healer within: The new medicine of mind and body.* New York: New American Library.

Madden, K., & Livnat, S. (1991). Catecholamine action and immunologic reactivity. In R. Ader, D. L. Felten, & N. Cohen (Eds.), *Psychoneuroimmunology* (2nd ed.). New York: Academic Press.

Mahler, M.S. (1974). Symbiosis and individuation: The psychological birth of the human infant. *Psychoanalytic Study of the Child, 29,* 89–124.

McCarthy, S. M., & Gallo, A. M. (1992). A case illustration of family management style. *Journal of Pediatric Nursing, 7*(6), 395–402.

McClowry, S. G. (1992). Family functioning during a critical illness: A systems theory perspective. *Critical Care Nursing Clinics of North America, 4*(4), 559–564.

McFarland, G. K., Wasli, E. L, & Gerety, E. K. (1992). *Nursing diagnoses and process in psychiatric mental health nursing* (2nd ed.). Philadelphia: J. B. Lippincott.

McHaffie, H. E. (1992). The assessment of coping. *Clinics in Nursing Research, 1*(1), 67–79.

Miller, T. W. (Ed.). (1989). *Stressful life events.* Madison, CT: International Universities Press.

Moore, A. D., & Stambrook, M. (1992). Coping strategies and locus of control following traumatic brain injury: Relationship to long-term outcome. *Brain Injury, 6*(1), 89–94.

Murray, G. B. (1991). Limbic music. In N. H. Cassem (Ed.), *Massachusetts General Hospital handbook of general hospital psychiatry* (3rd ed.). St. Louis: Mosby Year Book.

Newberry, B. H., Jaikins-Madden, J. E., & Gerstenberger, T. J. (1991). *A holistic conceptualization of stress and disease.* New York: AMS Press.

Niaura, R., & Goldstein, M. G. (1992). Psychological factors affecting physical condition. Cardiovascular disease literature review. Part II: Coronary artery disease and sudden death and hypertension. *Psychosomatics, 33*(2), 146–155.

Noshpitz, J. D., & Coddington, R. D. (Eds.). (1990). *Stressors and the adjustment disorders.* New York: Wiley.

O'Brien, M. T. (1993). Multiple sclerosis: Stressors and coping strategies in spousal caregivers. *Journal of Community Health Nursing, 10*(3), 123–135.

Puglisi-Allegra, S., & Oliverio, A. (Eds.). (1990). *Psychobiology of stress.* Boston: Kluwer Academic Publishers.

Reilly, F.D., McCuskey, R.S., & Meineke, H.A. (1975). Studies of the hemopoietic microenvironment: VIII. Adrenergic and cholinergic innervation of the murine spleen. *Anatomical Record, 185,* 109–118.

Reiser, M. (1984). *Mind, brain, body.* New York: Basic Books.

Robinson, K. R. (1993). Denial: An adaptive response. *Dimensions of Critical Care Nursing, 12*(2), 102–106.

Rosenbaum, J. F., & Pollack, M. H. (1991). Anxiety. In N. H. Cassem (Ed.), *Massachusetts General Hospital handbook of general hospital psychiatry* (3rd ed.). St. Louis: Mosby Year Book.

Roszman, T., & Carlson, S. (1991). Neurotransmitters and molecular signaling in the immune response. In R. Ader, D. L. Felten, & N. Cohen (Eds.), *Psychoneuroimmunology* (2nd ed.). New York: Academic Press.

Sack, R. (1980). Psychosomatic disorders. In S. Snyder (Ed.), *Biological aspects of mental disorder.* New York: Oxford University Press.

Sadler, J. Z., & Hulgus, Y. F. (1992). Clinical problem solving and the biopsychosocial model. *American Journal of Psychiatry, 149*(10), 1315–1323.

Schleifer, S.J., Keller, S.E., Camerino, M., Thornton, J.C., & Stein, M. (1983). Suppression of lymphocyte stimulation following bereavement. *JAMA, the Journal of the American Medical Association, 250,* 374–377.

Seligman, M. (1991). *Learned optimism.* New York: Alfred A. Knopf.

Selye, H. (1976). *Stress in health and disease.* Boston: Butterworth & Co.

Selye, H. (1979). Stress without distress. In C. Garfield (Ed.), *Stress and survival: The emotional realities of life-threatening illness.* St. Louis: C. V. Mosby.

Sherer, M. (1992). Affective control efficacy and cognitive control efficacy: A comment. *Psychological Reports, 70*(3 Pt. 2), 1230.

Showers, C. (1992). The motivational and emotional consequences of considering positive or negative possibilities for an upcoming event. *Journal of Personality and Social Psychology, 63*(3), 474–484.

Small, S. P., & Graydon, J. E. (1992). Perceived uncertainty, physical symptoms, and negative mood in hospitalized patients with chronic obstructive pulmonary disease. *Heart and Lung, 21*(6), 568–574.

Smolan, R., Moffitt, P., & Naythons, M. (1990). *The power to heal.* New York: Prentice Hall Press.

Snyder, S. (1980). *Biological aspects of mental disorders.* New York: Oxford University Press.

Solomon, G. F. (1985). The emerging field of psychoneuroimmunology, with a special note on AIDS. *Advances, 2*(1), 6–19.

Spurrell, M. T., & McFarlane, A. C. (1993). Post-traumatic stress disorder and coping after a natural disaster. *Social Psychiatry and Psychiatric Epidemiology, 28*(4), 194–200.

Stanhope, M., & Lancaster, J. (Eds.). (1992). *Community health nursing: Process and practice for promoting health.* St. Louis: Mosby Year Book.

Stein, M., Miller, A., & Trestman, R. (1991). Depression and the immune system. In R. Ader, D. L. Felten, & N. Cohen (Eds.), *Psychoneuroimmunology* (2nd ed.). New York: Academic Press.

Sternbach, R. A. (1966). *Principles of psychophysiology.* New York: Academic Press.

Suddarth, D. S. (Ed.). (1991). *The Lippincott manual of nursing practice* (5th ed.). Philadelphia: J. B. Lippincott.

Suter, S. (1986). *Health psychophysiology: Mind-body interactions in wellness and illness.* Hillsdale, NJ: L. Erlbaum Associates.

Temoshok, L. (1987). Personality, coping style, emotion and cancer: Towards an integrative model. *Cancer Surveys, 6*(3), 545–567.

Temoshok, L., & Dreher, H. (1993). *The type-C connection: The mind-body link to cancer and your health.* New York: New American Library.

Thomas, C. L. (Ed.). (1993). *Taber's cyclopedic medical dictionary* (17th ed.). Philadelphia: F. A. Davis.

Tyrey, L., & Nalbandor, A. (1972). Influence of interior hypothalmic lesions on circulating antibody titers in the rat. *American Journal of Physiology, 222,* 179–185.

Ursin, H. (1978). Activation, coping, and psychosomatics. In H. Ursin, E. Baade, & S. Levine (Eds.), *Psychobiology of stress: A study of coping men.* New York: Academic Press.

Weiss, J. M., & Simson, P. G. (1985). Neurochemical basis of depression. *Psychopharmacology Bulletin, 21*(3), 447–457.

Witt, P. H., Greenfield, D. P., & Steinberg, J. (1993). Evaluation and treatment of post-traumatic stress disorder. *New Jersey Medicine, 90*(6), 464–467.

Wood, P., Karol, M., Kusnecov, A., & Rabin, B. (1993). Enhancement of antigen-specific humoral and cell-mediated immunity by electric footshock stress in rats. *Brain, Behavior, and Immunity, 7*(1), 121–134.

Woods, N. F., Habaerman, M. R., & Packard, N. J. (1993). Demands of illness and individual, dyadic, and family adaptation in chronic illness. *Western Journal of Nursing Research, 15*(1), 10–25.

Yehuda, R., Giller, E. L., & Mason, J. W. (1993). Psychoneuroendocrine assessment of posttraumatic stress disorder: Current progress and new directions. *Progress in Neuropsychopharmacology and Biological Psychiatry, 17*(4), 541–550.

CHAPTER 7

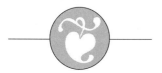

General Systems Theory Applied to Individual and Family Coping Responses

Patricia Barry

Illness is a disrupting psychological event for anyone. It presents even more challenges to the ill person when it is compounded by the family's reactions to it. For each family member, the illness has unique implications and poses a unique threat. The effect within the family of one member's illness can be compared to a hanging mobile. When you flick one of the figures with your finger, the entire mobile moves. Each figure is now in motion because it was affected by the change to just one figure. Illness creates similar change and disruption in the family. An important concept that is helpful in understanding how and why illness can have such a profound effect on the family is systems theory (Bertalanffy, 1968; Dewsbury, 1991; Dohms & Metz, 1991; Engel, 1962; Goldberg & Novack, 1992).

WHAT IS A SYSTEM?

The word *system* is defined as:
   A group of interacting, interrelated or interdependent elements forming a complex whole . . . A social, economic or political orga-

nizational form [*American Heritage College Dictionary,* 1993, p. 1378].

   The essence of systems theory is that any action, whether social or biological, causes a reaction within its own environment. The action also changes the relationship of that object to all the other objects in its environment. These changes or adjustments alter the overall system to which they belong. Using these definitions, think of some objects that can be classified as systems. Is a television set a system? It has a series of parts that operate together and cause it to be a television set. Is a family a system? It has a series of parts that cause it to be a complex unit. Is a human being a system? What kinds of parts go into a human being? Your first answer will probably be anatomical parts. Are there any other parts? What about psychological functioning, that is, the ability to think and feel? A person can function psychologically whether alone or with someone else. Another

Patricia Barry: *Psychosocial Nursing:
Care of Physically Ill Patients and Their Families,* 3rd ed.
© 1996 Lippincott–Raven Publishers

very important part of a person is social functioning. To function socially, a person must interact with others. Once a person interacts with others, he or she is open to many opportunities as well as risks.

A human being belongs to many types of systems, some of them social: a family, work force, social clubs, friendships, and so on. He or she is also a part of the ecological supersystem of the environment. The human is a vital link in the earth's biological chain, for example, inhaling oxygen produced by the photosynthesis of the earth's greenery. After the human body uses oxygen, it exhales carbon dioxide, which is essential to the same plants and trees in their production of oxygen. The human body is a large system made up of many smaller physiological subsystems, each of them essential to the functioning of the total body equilibrium. Optimally, they operate in unison to support the integrity of the entire body.

All living things and all social groups are dynamic. The word *dynamic* used in this manner means it is related to the branch of physics concerned with the production of motion due to various forces. It also deals with the effects of these forces on bodies in motion or at rest. When used as a noun, *dynamics* (within the context of psychosocial functioning) are the multiple and ever-changing forces or factors behind the actions of human beings.

Systems theory is an exciting concept that can help nurses be far more aware of the impact of multiple-factor relationships everywhere: in the body, in intrapsychic psychological functioning, in families, in the medical care system, and in all types of social relationships.

TYPES OF SYSTEMS

All systems can be generally classified by how many contributing factors or how much input has the potential to cause change within the system. Systems fall into two main categories, open and closed:

Open system. An open system is marked by its ability to be flexible and responsive to change. It has an unlimited number of ever-changing dynamics. A normal family can be called a relatively open system because all of its members are subject to change.

The openness in a system comes from the vast number of subsystems that exist within the overall system. In a family there are various members, each of whom contains intrapsychic, physical, and social subsystem components. Each component has the potential to change the dynamics in that person, as well as the dynamics of the other members, because of the constant interaction that occurs in a family. The more open a system, the less predictable is the outcome of any change in the system.

Closed system. A closed system is relatively inflexible and resistant to change. It consists of specific variables that react with a predictable outcome. These variables are usually rigid and do not respond to change with a significantly different way of functioning.

Within the body, an example of a closed system is any of the main body subsystems. None of them is ever static; they are all subject to change based on the external or internal stresses they are subjected to. The amount of change is not infinite, however. There is a normal range of variation beyond which the subsystem, and eventually the entire body system, would fail. For example, a body temperature of 94°F to 106°F will continue to sustain life. If it goes below or above this range for a prolonged period, most body systems would soon fail. Body temperature adjustment mechanisms are fairly rigid. Once exhausted, they stop working. They cannot tolerate an infinite range of temperature variation. The temperature-regulating mechanism is a moderately closed system (Dewsbury, 1991; Dohms & Metz, 1991; Kiecolt-Glaser & Glaser, 1991).

All the physiological subsystems that may initially seem distinct and separate are interdependent. One cannot live without the others. If the gastrointestinal system lost its blood supply, its tissues would die. It would also die because it would have no way of eliminating toxic wastes. All the tissues in the other body systems would fail because of lack of carbohydrates, fats, proteins, minerals, vitamins, and water, which are the end products of digestion.

Physiological subsystems are not the only subsystems influencing the human being and his or her actions. Even when a person is asleep, the intrapsychic subsystem never ceases its dynamic process. It is constantly affected by external events and its own reaction to them. It also responds continually to neurotransmitters and other biochemical substances of the physiological subsystem. The physiological and intrapsychic subsystems operate interdependently. None of them operates in isolation.

Before moving on to discuss family systems, it is helpful to develop a broader understanding of systems theory as applied to the individual.

GENERAL SYSTEMS THEORY

HISTORY

Although there are all types of systems, the formal idea of systems theory was not conceptualized until the late 1920s, when the biologist Ludwig von Bertalanffy described his organismic viewpoint, noting that all organisms are organized things. In studying the metabolism, growth, and biophysics of organisms, von Bertalanffy (1968) was struck by the interdependence of biological systems. He was the first to describe the concept that, rather than being distinct and separate systems, biological systems are actually a part of a still larger system.

As von Bertalanffy's theory emerged in the early 1930s, scholars from many disciplines discovered that the concept of general systems theory applied equally well to their own fields, such as chemistry, physics, and the social sciences. The application of general systems theory to psychiatry was helpful in conceptualizing the development of personality.

APPLICATION TO PERSONALITY DEVELOPMENT

The development of the psyche is an abstract process occurring within the human being's emotional system. It is affected by many factors. Brazelton (1973) has theorized that the infant is born with an inherited set of unique personality characteristics. The "fit" of the parents' personality characteristics with the unique characteristics of the child can subdue or cause a marked increase in the strength of those characteristics (Burr, 1991; Smith & Thelen, 1993).

Catecholamine research has demonstrated that greater or lesser amounts of biochemical neurotransmitters—substances known to be in the physiological realm—affect the emotional realm. In fact, the two major drives of human beings, pleasure-seeking and aggressive, are inseparable from the endocrine subsystem. Here we can see a multiple interaction relationship between a physiological subsystem and an abstract psychological subsystem. External influences such as infection, trauma, or natural disaster can also have a profound impact on these internal subsystems (Dewsbury, 1991; Felten et al., 1991; Felten & Felten, 1991).

The emotional stress of physical illness can result in increased stress on an already impaired physiological subsystem (Dewsbury, 1991). The increased stress the family experiences during hospitalization of one of its members also affects the ill member (Franks, Campbell, & Shields, 1992; Halm et al., 1993). In general, the more open a system, the more tolerance it has for stress and the less likely psychosocial or physiological dysfunction will occur. For example, a family may have a father who has maintained "iron" rule over his wife and children. The wife and children have always adhered to his authority. Their functioning in the family and in their roles outside of the family has always been in line with the father's expectations. This family demonstrates "closedness." There is little flexibility. If this father were to become seriously ill or die, the remaining family members would be at far more risk for dysfunction because of their own lack of development as independent beings (Donley, 1993; Franks, Campbell, & Shields, 1992; Halm et al., 1993). So too with body functioning.

Although the physiological subsystems operate within the ranges required to sustain life and can be classified as closed systems, there can be differences in the range of closedness. For example, a person who has chronic obstructive respiratory disease complicated by frequent infections has a more closed body system than a healthy person. Both the emotional and physiological stresses of illness have a greater potential to promote dysfunction in the person with a more closed body system (Dewsbury, 1991; Dohms & Metz, 1993).

Systems theory can be applied to all patients. Nurses should be aware of the complex impact that a set of circumstances can have on several aspects of a patient's life. Major illness, for example, affects not only the patient's physiological and psychological subsystems but also the familial and extrafamilial supersystems (Harrison & Cole, 1991; McClowry, 1992). The effects are similar to the ever-widening set of ripples set off by a stone tossed into a pool. When a systems approach is used in designing and implementing care plans, a more holistic, realistic, and compassionate care will be delivered than if the patient is viewed as a sick being with an acute medical disease who is temporarily isolated from all other aspects of existence.

APPLICATION TO NURSING PRACTICE

A person with any type of illness, chronic or acute, is affected by many factors, including what the illness means to him or her, its physical and emotional effects, the quality of medical care available, the quality of nursing care available, and how family and friends react to the illness. In reviewing these factors, is any one separate and distinct from the others? Is it possible for one of these factors to influence another? Is it also possible for one factor to influence all the others? A careful review should illustrate the interrelationship of factors and how one of them, depending on the degree of its impact, can cause a varying response in the others.

What the Illness Means to the Patient

Imagine that a patient has been admitted for a hemorrhoidectomy. As a nurse, this illness may be classified as nonthreatening. The way the patient perceives her illness, however, may be quite different.

The hemorrhoidectomy patient may be someone who is normally fearful in a new situation. This patient may be a woman with a very low pain tolerance who has never before been hospitalized and her coping ability during stressful periods may be known to be poor. Her physician has cautioned her that the pain from the surgery may be severe for the first few days. She has had chronic constipation for years, and the idea of moving her bowels after surgery already frightens her. In addition, her cousin died many years ago while undergoing anesthesia for a minor surgical procedure. She fears that she too could die during surgery.

In assessing this patient's perception of her illness, we find that her illness is very threatening to her. Many of her perceptions are based on accurate cognitive awarenesses. She has definite reasons why she is fearful.

Let's examine the effect of the illness's meaning to a patient on the various factors above. An asterisk will mark each instance in which one factor is capable of setting off a response and triggering a series of changes in other subsystems.

Will the Patient's High Level of Fearfulness Have a Physical Effect?

In reviewing this patient's potential postoperative response, assess the following: Will she be unusually tense and frightened?[*] Will this psychic tension and alarm trigger her sympathetic nervous system?[*] What are some of the effects of the neuroendocrine subsystem on vital signs[*] and on the musculoskeletal subsystem?[*] Will this affect all her muscles?[*] Could her vital signs be altered as a result of her high level of muscle tension?[*] Perform the following exercise:

Make a fist with your right hand. Tense the muscles in your right arm and squeeze your fist. What effect do you think this tenseness has on your pulse, blood pressure, and respirations? In this example, the patient's vital signs are already affected by the neuroendocrine response to her fear. The accompanying muscular tension heightens and aggravates the already stressed cardiovascular and pulmonary systems.

Will she perhaps need more analgesia or more frequent analgesia than a normal hemorrhoidectomy patient? Will this analgesia alter other physiological responses?* Will her first bowel movement be complicated by an unusually tight anal sphincter (gastrointestinal subsystem)?* Could there be bleeding complications as a result (cardiovascular subsystem)?* Will she ambulate well (musculoskeletal subsystem)?* If not, could venous or pulmonary complications be precipitated (cardiovascular and respiratory subsystems)* if she is inactive due to her pain and level of fearfulness (central nervous system)?

Will the Patient's Perceptions of the Seriousness of Her Illness Affect Her Emotional Functioning?

Because of her high level of anxiety, is it possible that this patient will be fully receptive to preoperative teaching (affective and cognitive-intellectual parts of intrapsychic system)?* Could her fear actually cause her to blot out the nurse's words? Her ego is prepared to protect her from hearing anything that may overload and overwhelm her (affective and ego defensive parts of intrapsychic mental system).* As a result, when she awakens in the recovery room, she may be unprepared for the experience, and her level of anxiety may be high.*

In the recovery room, she may not comply with the normal postoperative precautions of turning, coughing, and deep breathing.* Her emotional response to pain* and her level of fearfulness* about the anticipated bowel movement may even cause her to require sedative medication.* Her anxiety may also cause her to be demanding and difficult with the medical* and nursing* staff and with her family.*

Will the Patient's Perceptions of the Seriousness of Her Illness Affect the Quality of Medical Care?

The quality of medical care available to a patient can differ from institution to institution and, within one institution, from physician to physician, from nursing unit to nursing unit, and from nurse to nurse. Ideally, physicians respond with a caring and professional manner to all patients. However, they can be affected by patients' responses to their illnesses. A compliant, noncomplaining, respectful, and friendly patient will promote a more positive physician-patient relationship. A patient with an inappropriate level of fear who lacks trust in her physicians and questions them about all aspects of her care may invite a negative response.*

Nurses may complain to the physician about the patient* with comments such as, "She's asking for pain medication," or, "When she had her first bowel movement yesterday, she had to have someone stay with her the entire time. Every time the nurse would start to leave she would become nearly hysterical." These comments further reinforce the idea in the physician that his or her patient is a nuisance. He or she may be inclined to interact with the patient as briefly and superficially as possible.*

The frightened patient then perceives the physician's abruptness as impatience with her (she may be correct) and becomes even more anxious.* Unfortunately, she may have contributed to this changed impression without being aware of it.

Will the Patient's Perceptions of the Seriousness of Her Illness Affect the Quality of Nursing Care?

Nurses who care for this patient may eventually become exasperated and impatient if her "negative" behavior continues.* They may begin to withdraw from her because she is difficult to be with and because they want to avoid losing their tempers.* They may eventually respond less promptly to her requests for pain medication* if she asks for more medication than they believe is necessary for a postoperative hemorrhoidectomy patient.

Will the Patient's Perceptions of the Seriousness of Her Illness Affect the Reactions of Her Family and Friends?

The patient may react to her illness with demonstrations that she is in great pain. Accordingly, she may arouse much sympathy in her family.* They will frequently approach nurses about being more attentive to their wife's or mother's needs.* Friends also may respond with much sympathy to the patient and, by doing so, may cause a prolongation of pain behavior* because of the secondary gain the patient derives from their attention. Secondary gain includes the benefits a person obtains from illness, such as increased attention, decreased responsibilities, and so on. They eventually may become tired of her need for attention (Kaplan & Sadock, 1994, 1995).

On the other hand, the patient's pain experiences may encourage her family to defend her actions with the nurses and her physicians.* If, for example, the patient senses the rejection of caregivers because of her negative response to her hospitalization, she may cause her spouse or her children to admonish the nurses for their "poor" care*; to report the nurses to the physician*; to report nurses, house officers, or attending physicians to the hospital administration*; or to complain to contacts in the community about the "poor" care available at the hospital.* These comments, if convincing, may influence their acquaintances' attitude toward the hospital.*

This example of a patient's response to illness illustrates the many effects that just one factor can have on only five of the many factors that affect responses to physical illness. It is clear that one component of illness can trigger a whole series of responses. Each of those responses can then trigger another chain of events within the overall system, some physical, some emotional, some affecting hospital personnel, some affecting the family's emotional and social response, and some affecting the hospital and the community at large (Dewsbury, 1991; Lipowski, 1991).

All the concepts that contribute to the nursing diagnosis (which will be introduced in Chapters 12, 13, and 14) are strongly influenced by general systems effects. Understanding of general systems effects in the assessment, planning, intervention, and evaluation steps of the nursing process can assist in understanding more fully the effects of a particular illness on a specific patient and family. By using a holistic systems framework, nursing care can promote an adaptive response in the patient and family.

THE FAMILY AS A SYSTEM

Systems theory has been applied to a special type of social group that is essential to the development of all human beings: the family. The family system is ever changing and is constantly affected by the larger social order as well as by events that impact each member. The intrapsychic reaction of each family member to a specific event will determine his or her interactions with each of the other members. These reactions are based on many dynamics within the family group: the role each member fills within the family, who has the real power in the family, the unwritten rules of the family, and so on (Fisher et al., 1992; Halm et al., 1993).

Theories about family functioning have been proposed by psychiatric researchers attempting to discover the roots of psychopathology in patients with severe psychiatric disturbance. In one study, a patient's entire family was admitted to the hospital with him, and methods of communicating were closely observed (Bateson, Jackson, & Haley, 1956). During the last several decades, the many types of relationships and communication styles that exist between family members in well-functioning as well as in poorly functioning families have been described (Boszormenyi-Nagy & Framo, 1985; Green & Framo, 1981; Haley, 1984; Minuchin & Fishman, 1981; Wolman & Stricker, 1983).

Family systems theory can be generally applied to all social groups, for example, nursing units, social clubs, and school classrooms. These concepts have a strong impact on nurses in any nursing setting. They can be applied to a visiting nurse agency, a general hospital unit, a nursing faculty group, or any other working environment in which there is a group of people whose membership and leadership remains fairly stable. Family systems theory offers a better understanding of the "rules" and dynamics that affect relationships within a social system (Baum & Page, 1991; Burr, 1991; Clement, 1991; McClowry, 1992).

Nurses find family systems theory particularly helpful in understanding and caring for patients. Most patients are members of families; they have certain roles in their families that are disrupted by their illnesses and hospitalizations (Burr, 1991; Clement, 1991; Halm et al., 1993; McDaniel, Campbell, & Seaburn, 1990; Woods, Habaerman, & Packard, 1993). The loss of a person in his or her normal family role results in shifts in functioning in all other family members. For example, if a mother is admitted to the hospital, other family members usually assume some of her responsibilities. In addition, because of their concern about her illness and prognosis, they may all become more emotionally demanding. If all the members need increased support, they may be unable to satisfy these emotional needs within the immediate family, so they may turn to extended family members, friends, or professionals (Lipowski, 1991; O'Connor, 1991). A family member who is normally shy and aloof may be unable to ask for emotional support or unable to receive it, even if it is available. If the emotional stress of a family member is severe and is unrelieved for an extended period, physical or emotional illness could be the outcome (Engel, 1962).

At the same time that the family members are adapting emotionally, the ill member, who is actually precipitating the emotional stress of the others, is going through an emotional process of his or her own. Because of the different dynamics in each member, adaptation processes do not occur at the same rate. A shutdown in communication in order to protect one another may occur. Conflict is another possibility. Many families find it difficult to maintain open and empathetic communication among all members during a time of acute stress (Halm et al., 1993; McClowry, 1992).

Duvall (1977) has described six functions of a family:

1. Generating affection between husband and wife, between parents and children, and among members of the generations.
2. Providing personal security and acceptance.
3. Giving satisfaction and a sense of purpose.
4. Assuring continuity of companionship (a sense of permanence in a rapidly shifting environment).
5. Guaranteeing social placement and socialization.

6. Calculating controls and a sense of what is right.

Chronic or catastrophic illness disrupts the family in each of the functions Duvall described. The extent and nature of the changes depend on the unique characteristics of the family and individuals involved.

FAMILY SYSTEMS TERMINOLOGY

The following terms are defined here in order to clarify the ways they are used in this chapter.

Family of origin. The family of origin is the family into which a person is born. It includes the immediate family members (mother, father, siblings, and any other person who is a consistent member of the household). Any person, by living permanently in the home, influences the overall dynamics of the family.

Nuclear family. The nuclear family is a new family that is created by two partners. It consists of an individual or two partners (each of whom has a family of origin and an extended family) and their children or the children they might bring from previous relationships.

Extended family. The extended family is the family network beyond the family of origin. It includes stepparents, grandparents, aunts, uncles, cousins, nieces, nephews, and grandchildren. It is significant because of dynamics passed on from one generation to the next. For example, if a grandmother has a tendency toward multiple illnesses with much secondary gain, this pattern will often be repeated in succeeding generations in her niece, granddaughter, and so on (Kaplan & Sadock, 1994, 1995). In today's rapidly changing family environments, given the frequency of relocation away from one's place of birth and prevalence of transitional living arrangements, the role of the extended family is often relegated to friends, day care workers, professionals, and so on.

DIFFERENTIATION OF SELF

Before we can examine the family as a group, or understand the patient as he or she relates with other family members, we must first understand the functioning of the patient. A concept proposed by Murray Bowen (1976, p. 65; Papero, 1990), *differentiation of self,* is helpful toward this end. Differentiation of self is the degree to which either a person's intellect or emotions control his or her functioning. It "defines people according to the degree of fusion or differentiation between emotional and intellectual functioning."

An example of good differentiation is the response of a nurse who is told by the head nurse that she should spend less time talking with her newly admitted patient. Instead of being overwhelmed by feelings of guilt or anger toward the head nurse (emotional fusion), her intellect dominates and she says to herself, "Mrs. Ames doesn't know that this new patient is being admitted directly from attending her husband's funeral. The patient is very upset and needs to talk with me. I'll explain it to Mrs. Ames later." The nurse's intellect is well-differentiated. A distinct boundary separates a "feeling" response from a "thinking" response.

Bowen writes that this concept is so universal that all people can be categorized on a single continuum (Fig. 7-1). There are people whose emotions and intellect are so inseparable that everything they do is dominated by their emotions. They are at the fusion level of the continuum. Their life energy is devoted to avoiding feelings of displeasure, unhappiness, guilt, anger, jealousy, and so on. Their intellect is totally dominated by their feeling state. Few people are totally controlled by their feelings, but many dependent people and a number who develop chronic illness as an unconscious means of avoiding the demands of adulthood fall on the first 25% of the continuum.

Another aspect of Bowen's theory is *undifferentiated ego mass.* An undifferentiated ego mass operates in a family when one person feels anxiety and one or more other members automatically begin to feel the same anxiety. They are not able to differentiate their own feelings from those of their family member. They are not able to maintain their own feelings if they are different.

Bowen's theory explains the likelihood that like-minded emotional parents will raise their children in an environment that fosters emotionalism. When a person from such a family, who has a low level of differentiation, is admitted to the hospital, he may flounder because he has lost the highly charged emotional setting in which he is comfortable and accepted. Instead, the hospital system is cool and clinical and is unable to tolerate lack of emotional control in patients. Frequently, hospital staff members attempt to confine emotionalism by being authoritative, using an intellectual approach, and withholding their acceptance. This will increase the patient's level of anxiety and may cause an already minimal coping ability to be even more threatened. By understanding the patient's normal level of functioning, you can design a care plan that encourages stronger emotional support from caregivers. Kind and caring limit-setting can help the patient's attempts to retain a level of emotionalism that is tolerated by the staff and that will not cause them to abandon him.

WHAT IS THE SELF?

Bowen has described two ways in which people function in regard to their beliefs about themselves. The *solid self* includes the beliefs a person has about him or her self and environment resulting from life experiences since birth. The *pseudo self* is the self a person presents to the world. (*Pseudo* is derived from the Greek *pseudes,* meaning false.) It is the result of the emotional pressure applied on a person by the social system to conform to specific role expectations. For example, a woman who is a lawyer may fill many roles. She may behave somewhat differently in each one based on the expecta-

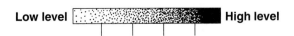

Low level **High level**

(feelings in total control)   (intellect in total control)

FIGURE 7-1. Differentiation-of-self continuum.

tions of others and her level of self-differentiation. These roles may include:

A woman
A girlfriend or wife
A mother
A daughter
A part-time college professor
A high-level professional (within her professional role she may relate differently to other lawyers in her firm who rank above or below her or other workers who are in subordinate roles)

Ideally, if the level of solid self is high, people should behave according to their own beliefs, rather than demonstrating changes in behavior based on the particular role they are filling at the time.

If the level of pseudo self is high, the person presents himself differently in each social relationship. The primary motivation for this person is to ensure acceptance by others. He is never really himself. For example, one man may be an unresponsive husband; a demanding and insensitive father; a passive, acquiescing son; a bullying foreman; a "good old boy" bowling-team member; and a "tough guy" neighbor. Actually, this man does not appear to have a "down deep" solid type of self.

The hospital system and the outpatient care system tend to encourage patients to suppress or deny their own needs and conform to the care system's expectations of appropriate patient behavior. The individualist with a strong sense of solid self may clash with physicians or nurses who have expectations regarding compliance. It is wise to remember that the main objective in caring for patients is to assist them in returning to the preillness state. Requiring them to change their normal level of interpersonal behavior to cope with the caregiving environment may be easier for the caregiver but it may be detrimental to patients and their families (Hackett et al., 1991; Lipowski, 1991; O'Connor, 1991).

THE LEVELS OF
SELF-DIFFERENTIATION

The concept of level of differentiation is important in evaluating the patient's response to

the illness and the hospital care system. It is also valuable in assessing the patient's preillness level of emotional functioning; his or her coping capacity and adaptation potential in the hospital system and when discharged into the normal family system (these settings may impose very different expectations); his or her emotional reaction to the illness; the family's emotional reaction to the illness; and his or her reaction to the family's reaction to the illness.

The factor of the patient's reaction to the family's reaction to the illness may be clarified with the example of a cancer patient who has a low level of emotional self-differentiation. On his own, in the hospital, he might be able to achieve a reasonable level of psychological adaptation. If he is discharged into a family with an undifferentiated ego mass, and they feel helpless and hopeless about his cancer, their feelings may overwhelm him and he will be unable to maintain his own feelings and beliefs (Papero, 1990).

When the stress of illness occurs, the patient may regress to a lower coping level. Viewed within the context of the stress of illness, the level of differentiation is indicated by the degree of dysfunctioning that occurs when a person or loved one is seriously ill. The level of dysfunctioning that occurs and the time it takes to regain equilibrium depend on the level of emotional differentiation in the person as well as in the family group. For example, the person or family with poor differentiation is more likely to become emotionally overwhelmed by illness (Papero, 1990).

The person and family with a moderate to high level of differentiation will be more likely to maintain control and cope adaptively. Another possibility is the family in which one or more members regress to a less effective level of coping because of the emotional stress they experience due to their loved one's illness. How would differences in coping levels affect intrafamily relationships, communications, and overall coping ability?

LOW LEVEL

At the low level of differentiation of self, the intellect and its ability to reason and analyze situations are dominated by feelings. Feelings tend to govern the intellect. People functioning at this level have a strong need to keep relationships in harmony as a way of avoiding anxiety. Accordingly, the solid self submits almost entirely to the pseudo self.

The avoidance of anxiety, guilt, and other negative feelings has a strong influence on the person's actions and the choices he or she makes in life. The person and his or her family members do not integrate easily into the world at large; they usually remain close-knit. Relationships outside of the immediate or extended family are not strongly encouraged. If a member of the family attempts to separate from the family, strong pressure is exerted by other members to conform to their expectations (Papero, 1990; Woods, Habaerman, & Packard, 1993).

When working with patients in this category, especially when planning for home care or outpatient work of any kind, it is important to include one or more family members in the process. Unless someone in the patient's family shares the experience and understands the treatment recommendations, the family's expectations of the patient after discharge may cause noncompliace with the prescribed plan. Other family members should be included in the steps of nursing process, as well.

Assessment of highly anxious family members includes identifying their specific fears. During the planning and intervention steps, it is important to spend time talking with them. In doing so, their anxiety, which is probably due to an unknown cause, may be narrowed to a definite fear. Once their fear is identified and talked about, their level of anxiety usually decreases (Carpenito, 1993).

MODERATE LEVEL

People with a moderate level of differentiation fluctuate between behavior governed by intellect and feelings. Their lives are relationship-oriented. They are more open and honest in expressing feelings than people on the lower level of the continuum. Their relationships and communication styles are largely pseudo self in expression because of their need to meet others' expectations. This type of person

usually adapts well to the hospital environment. The patient and family are able to understand the expectations of the hospital and their caregivers. They rarely have difficulty in conforming (McCarthy & Gallo, 1992; Woods, Habaerman, & Packard, 1993).

HIGH LEVEL

The person with a high level of differentiation demonstrates strong evidence of solid self. She is confident in her own value system and does not feel a strong need to meet others' expectations; she enjoys relationships and is free to be herself. She remains independent when she so chooses (Bowen, 1974, 1976, ; Papero, 1990). The highly differentiated person is fully aware of herself as a person. Bowen (1976, p. 73) writes, "They are remarkably free from the full range of human problems." Note however, that the highly differentiated person is not rigidly cold and controlled. The highly controlled person has a strong need to avoid her own affect, and many of her emotions may be repressed (Groves & Kurcharski, 1991). The person with a high level of differentiation, on the other hand, is fully aware of her feelings.

OTHER CONCEPTS OF FAMILY SYSTEMS THEORY

Other family systems concepts can help to determine a person's level of psychosocial functioning and in-hospital coping potential, as well as provide an indication of how a person will function after discharge. These concepts may also help explain the dynamics in the social systems of family, working environment, relationships with roommates or classmates, and any other social group.

BALANCE IN THE FAMILY

Boszormenyi-Nagy views families within the context of their extended family environment. He believes that families are always attempting to maintain balance and fairness within their unit. This requires giving and receiving on the part of all family members. Although there may be members within the family who appear unable to give, they are aware of their indebtedness to the family system. All members carry an unconscious awareness of the balance "ledger" (Boszormenyi-Nagy & Framo, 1985).

The development of physical illness within the family presents a dynamic that can temporarily unbalance the ledger as family roles shift. This can have a positive as well as a negative effect. For example, one family member may have been primarily on the "receiving" end in the family. If the ill member has been a giver, it is possible that the "receiving" person can temporarily move into a giving role. His view of himself and of other family members can become more positive, and the potential that he will become a contributing member within the family system is enhanced (Baum & Page, 1991; Burr, 1991; Clement, 1991).

SUBSYSTEM

A subsystem is a working unit in a larger structure called a system. Each person in a family is a subsystem who belongs to many systems. She is a subsystem within her own family, and she is a subsystem in each social group to which she belongs. These social groups include the work place, social support network, and nuclear and extended family. She may function differently in each of them depending on her role as wife, mother, daughter, niece, granddaughter, and so on.

In each of these roles she has different levels of power and different functions (Minuchin, 1974; Minuchin et al., 1978). "Subsystems can also consist of more than one individual such as a dyad of husband and wife or a dyad of mother and child" (Jones, 1980, p. 63). Subsystem dyads can also occur in other combinations, such as two persons within a family who share the same interests, are of the same gender, serve the same function (for example, two brothers-in-law), or even share the same illness (Burr, 1991; Clement, 1991; Woods, Habaerman, & Packard, 1993).

OPEN AND CLOSED FAMILY SYSTEMS

Another dynamic that can affect the adaptability of a family experiencing illness is whether the family is *open* or *closed*. In an open family the members are differentiated from one another; one member can express a view or feeling different from another or from the family at large, but continue to receive respect and caring within the family. The closed family does not tolerate dissension from its mutually experienced feelings. Responses to events are primarily rigid and fixed. There is little opportunity for members to express emotion. Similarly, they are discouraged from obtaining support beyond the immediate family. Thus there is no safe outlet for emotion. Members of the closed family repress and avoid feelings (Burr, 1991; Clement, 1991; Woods, Habaerman, & Packard, 1993). Table 7-1 describes the differences between open and closed families.

SIBLING POSITION IN FAMILY OF ORIGIN

A concept of family systems theory that is helpful in understanding why patients behave as they do is the idea that the particular role occupied by a child in his or her original family exerts an influence on interpersonal functioning in adult life. No matter where the person is or what the social situation, he or she will continue to demonstrate many of the traits that developed and were tolerated by parents and siblings (Eisenman, 1992; Elliot, 1992; Toman, 1976).

> This does not mean to imply an inescapable determinism, but recent and contemporary influences should not be overestimated in view of the early experiences that have been having their effect for much longer. . . . They appear in sentiments and attitudes, in basic wishes and interests of which the person may be partly unaware. They do affect his social behavior, and, to be sure, they often do so more strongly, the less conscious they are [Toman, 1976, p. 6].

Consider the following case example of a 61-year-old lathe operator who was admitted to the hospital because of lower extremity vascular insufficiency caused by diabetes. This example also includes the concept of systems intervention.

CASE EXAMPLE

Henry was the youngest of six children. As the youngest child his needs were met, frequently before he became aware of them, by his mother and his next three closest siblings, who were sisters 2, 3, and 5 years older than he. He enjoyed their attention to his needs, and they enjoyed taking care of him. He lived at home until he married. As he approached his mid-20s, he imagined marriage to various young women he knew. Those who seemed passive and dependent did not particularly appeal to him. Instead, a very motherly, nurturing young woman who seemed capable and self-assured became his bride. In their marriage she was the dominant partner. She enjoyed her dominant role in the home, and he found it pleasant to be taken care of.

After 2 weeks of hospitalization, Henry's surgeons decided that bilateral, below-the-knee amputations were unavoidable. After surgery the nurses who were caring for him began to encourage self-care during his bath and other activities. Henry refused to participate in his own care, claiming that it was too tiring. Each morning, shortly after the nurse left him with a wash basin and other items for morning care, his wife appeared and gave him a complete bath. The frustrated nurses soon discovered that as soon as they left him with instructions to complete as much of his care as possible, he telephoned his wife who lived near the hospital and asked her to come and help him because "the nurses were not doing their jobs." ❦

In this example, it is possible to see the effects of this man's upbringing on his choice of a mate and on his behavior during hospitalization. If nurses are to succeed in motivating such a patient to become more independent, they first have to assess the type of social system to which he is normally accustomed. This is one of the most important steps in psychosocial assessment. Supporting the patient to return to his normal level of adaptation is a more realistic nursing care goal than expecting a higher level of social functioning after a major illness.

TABLE 7–1
Characteristics of Open and Closed Family Systems

	Open System	Closed System
Communication	• Direct, clear, specific, congruent, leveling (honest), growth-producing	• Indirect, unclear, unspecific, incongruent, computing, blaming, placating, distracting, growth-impeding
Rules	• Overt, up-to-date, human rules; rules change when need arises • Full freedom to comment on anything	• Covert, out-of-date, inhuman rules; remain fixed, change needs to conform to established rules • Restrictions on commenting
Outcome	• Related to reality, appropriate, constructive • Self-worth: person grows even more confident and draws increasingly more from the self	• Accidental, chaotic, inappropriate, destructive • Self-worth: a person grows even more doubtful and leans more and more heavily on the outside for support

Adapted from Satir, V. (1972). *Peoplemaking*. Palo Alto, CA: Science and Behavior Books, pp.116, 117.

Temporary emotional and intellectual regression is normal in adaptation to illness . Henry had regressed to the point where he could not respond to the nurses' intellectual reasoning. Instead, he circumvented the nurses in order to receive the type of nurturing he needed, both emotionally and physically. The nurses had to identify this situation as a problem stemming from his social system. His nurse, acting on her own, was not going to be able to modify this patient's self-defeating behavior. Instead, his wife, his children, and the other nurses on the unit all needed to modify their behavior to him and maintain a systems approach in giving care. A systems approach is a unified approach in which all caregivers are consistent in their caregiving style.

Before rehabilitation could be promoted, it was important to ask his wife to come in to talk with the nurse. She needed to understand that her coming in to give Henry a bath, which was her usual way of responding, had negative effects. The nurse could explain the importance to both her and her husband that he gain the ability to be independent.

One of the best ways to persuade people to do something is to point out the advantages to them if they follow the recommendation. By pointing out the advantages to the person who is making the recommendation, the compliance of the patient or family may not be as complete or as long-lasting. In this case, Henry's dependence on his wife was encouraged by her constant attendance to his needs in the hospital; he could potentially become a permanent invalid requiring her constant presence and care. After he returned home, her quality of life as well as his would be affected.

In this case example, the nurse asked the wife to support the nurse's insistence that Henry do as much for himself as possible. The nurse explained to the wife that she understood that the wife wanted to help him and that withholding her help was untypical. The nurse emphasized that in this case it was more helpful to withhold assistance; if she continued coming every time he called her, there was a risk of prolonging her husband's rehabilitation. It was also a relief to the spouse not to have to be so readily available, she admitted, because she was becoming very tired.

As part of a general systems and family systems approach, the nurse asked the wife to be present when she explained to the patient the importance of his caring for himself. When the three of them were together, the nurse explained to the patient that she had talked to his wife about not coming in when he called to ask her for help. His wife told him that she would come in to visit but would no longer give him his bath or feed him. The patient's self-care program was listed in detail in the nursing care plan so that all caregivers would support his rehabilitation in the same way.

FAMILY RULES

Within a family certain rules are unwritten and may also be unspoken. These rules have been passed down from generation to generation. When a man from one family marries a woman from another family, they combine their respective rules into expectations of their own and their children's functioning. Most people instinctively choose a spouse whose inherited rule system or values are comparable to their own.

Family rules can be modified based on the effects of education and enlightenment; however, within an extended family, the majority of couples in the younger generation retain many of their families' fundamental values and expectations. Those who establish different rules are often ridiculed or encouraged in more subtle ways to conform.

When adolescent and adult children break markedly from family rules and expectations, there is often serious conflict between generations (e.g., the brothers and sisters of the older generation vs. the younger generation), and in all other sets of relationships in the family (cousin vs. cousin, aunts and uncles vs. nieces and nephews).

If the spouses' rules do not combine well, either the husband or the wife will assert himself or herself, compromises will be agreed on, active conflict will continually recur over the unresolved difference, or the problem will be repressed.

Religious beliefs are an important aspect of family rules. After the marriage, other family rules will be decided on as the need arises. For example, at what age will a daughter be allowed to date or to get her ears pierced? Decisions about family rules usually are determined by the parents' own experiences and beliefs developed in their own families of origin (Baum & Page, 1991; Clement, 1991; Jacobs, 1991; Papero, 1990; Schwab, Stephenson, & Ice, 1993).

Examples of times when family rules may form the basis of conflict in the health care system are decisions about the care of elderly, infirm relatives or the care of children or adults with severe handicaps (home care vs. institutionalization), moral choices about an unwed daughter's pregnancy, sterilization, and choice of treatment of specific illnesses. When one branch of an extended family chooses a form of care that conflicts with the family's "normal" rules, the result can be conflict with one or more other branches of the family. Depending on the lack of differentiation in the family, the conflict can extend into the entire family and result in the rulebreakers being forced out of the family (Baum & Page, 1991; Burns et al., 1993; Donley, 1993; Harrison & Cole, 1991; Herth, 1993).

BOUNDARIES

All people define themselves as they relate to others (Aponte, 1976). Within a family system, boundaries are the rules that keep the role of one family member separate from another. Boundaries are the unwritten principles that tell who belongs to a subsystem and how that participation is supposed to take place. Boundaries come into being because of family rules (Baum & Page, 1991; Burr, 1991; Clement, 1991; Fisher et al., 1992; Smith & Thelen, 1993).

Actually, it is the development of boundaries that creates subsystems or subdivisions within the family that promote effective family functioning. For example, it is important that the mother-father dyad be able to maintain its separateness from the children subsystem for effective relations within the family. If the father, for example, consistently functions as a child within the family and abdicates his leadership role, an elder son may move into the void to serve as an authority figure for

younger siblings. This creates confusion in family boundaries and can lead to family dysfunction. The outcome of physical illness can, at times, create these types of boundary disruptions within family subsystems (Baum & Page, 1991; Burr, 1991; Clement, 1991; Fisher et al., 1992; Smith & Thelen, 1993; Woods, Habaerman, & Packard, 1993).

In the hospital, patients and family members may appear to be either overfunctioning or underfunctioning in their roles within their families. They may be functioning within the roles that the dynamics of their own intrapsychic and family system have created for them, however. The hospital care system has very little power to change these dynamics during a hospital admission. It is preferable to work with them and design care to include these idiosyncrasies rather than discounting or ignoring them.

> Clarity of boundaries within a family provides a barometer of how well the family is functioning. To function adequately subsystem members must have contact with one another, but must not interfere with each other's functioning. . . . The two pathological extremes are disengaged (where there is no contact between family members) or enmeshed (where there is too much control) families [Jones, 1980, p. 64].

FUSION

The concept of fusion was introduced earlier as it related to the undifferentiated ego mass that can exist in highly emotional families (Bowen, 1974; Papero, 1990). Another aspect of fusion exists in many families: when two or more people consistently relate to one another on a more emotional level than they do with other family members, and form their own subsystem. Minuchin, Montalvo, and Guerney (1967) have called this phenomenon *enmeshment*. These relationships can be either positively or negatively charged. They can be dominated by feelings of closeness or of conflict. The fusion between two or more members implies that there is "tight interlocking" in the relationships (Minuchin, Montalvo, & Guerney, 1967). Fusion is essentially a problem caused by poor boundaries within a family (Clement, 1991; Donley, 1993; Jacobs, 1991; Papero, 1990; Smith & Thelen, 1993).

The system effect of a tight relationship between two or more people in a family is that other members are automatically excluded. These other members may join together in a form of alliance as well in order avoid feeling excluded. Generally, however, they instead remain outside, waiting for an "opening" so that they may join the fused subsystem (Clement, 1991; Donley, 1993; Jacobs, 1991; Papero, 1990; Smith & Thelen, 1993).

Fusion can exist to some degree in any normal family. It becomes a problem, however, in many families in which there is chronic physical or mental illness. One family member may overreact and do too much for the sick member, frequently a child. The sick role of the ill member is reinforced by the reaction of the member with whom he or she is enmeshed.

> Their quality of connectedness is such that attempts on the part of one member to change elicit fast complementary resistance on the part of others [Minuchin, Montalvo, & Guerney, 1967, p. 368].

In the hospital or outpatient setting, situations may be observed in which an overbearing parent, spouse, or some other family authority figure encourages sickness behavior in the ill family member. The efforts of the chronically ill member to move toward healthy rehabilitation may be thwarted and undermined by the other member of the fused dyad, who unconsciously needs the ill person to remain sick.

The process of enmeshment or fusion takes place during the early developmental years of the marriage and becomes more pronounced as children enter the family. Jones (1980, p. 65) describes the effects of this process on a family when it reaches pathological levels:

> Enmeshment is essentially a weakening of the boundaries that allow family subsystems to function: the boundary between nuclear family and families of origin is not well maintained; the boundary between parents and their children is crossed frequently in improper ways; the roles of spouse and parent are insufficiently differentiated so that neither the spouse subsystem nor the parental subsystem

can operate; and finally, the children are not differentiated on the basis of age or maturational level so that the sibling subsystem cannot contribute properly to the socialization process.

CASE EXAMPLE

Danny is a 12-year-old boy with asthma. He has been asthmatic since age 2. He has an older brother and sister. His mother has always been overprotective of him. During Danny's elementary schooling, his mother refused to allow him to join the Boy Scouts or Little League because she feared that any strenuous activity could bring on an acute asthma episode. Danny acquiesced to his mother's wishes, and gradually became introverted and isolated from his friends and more attached to and dependent on his mother. His older sister's disposition, which had been sunny in childhood, slowly gave way to sullenness as her mother had less time to spend with her due to increased attentiveness to Danny.

Danny's father, an outdoorsman, had always enjoyed the camping trips that his wife and he had taken with their family. When Danny developed asthma, his mother decided that Danny and she would no longer accompany the family on the trips. Danny's father has come to resent his son's illness and his wife's decreased interest in their relationship as a couple.

While the effects of pathological fusion may be observed in a chronic care setting, a pediatric unit, a psychiatric unit, or an acute care medical-surgical unit, it will be a challenge to approach the family about the negative short- and long-term effects of their family interactions; they have been operating in this manner for years. When fusion is present in a dyad, there are potentially more serious implications when one member develops a chronic illness or becomes terminally ill. The process of loss involved in either instance causes a major shift in equilibrium in the relationship. In fact, the entire family system will feel the effects if the dyad becomes dysfunctional.

Being approached by one nurse who suggests that their relationship needs to change will not usually have an impact on such a patient and family. Instead, concerns can be shared with other caregivers. Using knowledge of general family systems theory, the negative interactional style of the family can be discussed and the negative long-term implications presented if this enmeshment is not modified. A psychiatric liaison nurse specialist or social worker can also be consulted for further system support. Such evaluation will further reinforce the nursing assessment.

Remedial work on a negative fusion process can occur in many ways, depending on the severity of the fusion. It is important to be aware that fusion occurs, develops, and is fostered because of underlying intrapsychic needs of all family members (Masterson, Tolpin, & Sifneos, 1991; Schwab, Stephenson, & Ice, 1993). The dominant people in the fusion process usually do not change easily.

If the process is not severe, the family can be interviewed by astute medical and nursing caregivers in the outpatient care system. If the process is deeply entrenched, referral to a skilled family therapist can be considered.

TRIANGLES

Another important concept in understanding how a social system operates is the phenomenon of triangling.

The triangle is a three-person emotional configuration, the basic building block of any emotional system, whether it is in the family or any other group. The triangle is the smallest stable relationship system. A two-person system may be stable as long as it is calm, but when anxiety increases, it immediately involves the most available third person to become a triangle (Burr, 1991; Donley, 1993; Papero, 1990; Schwab, Stephenson, & Ice, 1993). When tension in the triangle is too great for the threesome, it involves others to become a series of triangles [Bowen, 1976, p. 76].

As Bowen implies, the ability for a two-person relationship to remain static and calm decreases when any type of tension occurs. When one member of the dyad is under stress, his or her anxiety is reflected in the relationship. Unconsciously, in order to decrease the tension and restore stability, one or the other

member will bring in a third member. This causes a shift in the tension so that the stress "within" the dyad is reduced. Triangling can have both positive and negative outcomes depending on the developmental maturity of each of the members (Burr, 1991; Papero, 1990; Schwab, Stephenson, & Ice, 1993).

The previous case example describing fusion between Danny and his mother could also be an example of triangling if we added the information that before Danny developed his asthma, his parents' marital relationship had been deteriorating. There was increasing conflict and tension between them. Danny's mother in effect triangled-in Danny as a way of avoiding ongoing conflict with her husband. Indeed, the relationship between the mother and father now is distanced, and active conflict within the couple dyad has been rare. Underlying, unspoken conflict remains, however.

Awareness of the triangling process can be helpful to nurses in both their professional and personal lives. An underlying dynamic in many nurses is their desire to be helpful. This dynamic can unknowingly cause them to become involved as the third member of an interpersonal triangle. Patients, family members, and friends may ask a nurse for help, when, with encouragement, these individuals may have the ability to resolve the problem themselves.

POWER

Power is another important dynamic in any family or unified group. In families, it is normally assumed that the father or mother holds the most power. Similarly, in the case of a nursing unit, it may be expected that the head nurse is the most powerful figure. This is not always so. Power is the ability to do something or control others.

Within a family, a physical symptom in one member can have a strong effect on all the other members. For example, a child who is prone to asthma can ultimately control his family with his physical symptoms. If a physical symptom in one member does exert strong control in a family, it is usually because the normally expected balance of authority in the family has been temporarily or permanently disrupted (Feldstein & Rait, 1992; Halm et al., 1993; Harrison & Cole, 1991; O'Brien, 1993).

In the case of an asthmatic child, a mother may interact in a submissive way with the child in order to avoid precipitating an emotionally induced asthmatic attack. She may also insist that all other family members alter their normal responses to this child. Frequently, this type of change in family dynamics becomes permanent and may weaken normal family functioning.

If, in a nursing unit, the head nurse's leadership is weak, the power on the unit can be controlled by a disruptive patient. Unless the head nurse is able to maintain control of difficult situations, the staff nurses may emulate her and be unable to manage troublesome situations with patients effectively. This gives a highly manipulative patient a great deal of power. The nurses will feel angry and helpless and react in passive but negative ways (Feldstein & Rait, 1992; Halm et al., 1993; Harrison & Cole, 1991; O'Brien, 1993).

CODEPENDENCE

Codependence is a term used to describe relationships in families where the role of one family member is often highly related to the dysfunction of another family member (Bennett & LaBonte, 1993; Cleary, 1994). The term *codependence* was originally used to describe family relationships when a family member was substance-addicted (Cleary, 1994). It describes a range of family responses to substance addiction (Wegscheider-Cruse, 1985; Wegscheider-Cruse & Gruse, 1990). The term has been expanded to include all families in which one person is preoccupied with another family member to the point that other relationships become affected negatively (Cleary, 1994).

The codependent family may be described as one in which there are unwritten, unspoken rules. These rules include "don't talk," "don't trust," "don't feel" (Black, 1982). It is necessary to abide by these rules to be accepted in the family. Cassem (1985) explains that there are certain roles ascribed to by the

codependent type of individual: caretaker, people pleaser, workaholic, martyr, and perfectionist. These roles are taken on in order to support family survival; they also perpetuate the dysfunctional relationships.

Issues of codependence will be most frequently seen by nurses who are caring for patients and families where there are chronic health conditions, for example, in home care or hospice nursing. Nurses can reduce codependent behaviors by supporting respite care. This includes encouraging caregivers to plan times in which others can substitute for them. The quality of the caregiver's sleep, rest, and nutrition are reviewed; the caregiver and nurse develop care plans that support the caregiver, as well as the patient.

SCAPEGOATING

Family members often assign one another fixed roles. One of these roles is the *scapegoat*. Scapegoats are made the "victims" of the other family members because of their inability to tolerate specific aspects of their own functioning (Burr, 1991; Donley, 1993; Papero, 1990; Schwab, Stephenson, & Ice, 1993).

> The scapegoat role is determined by many factors, not the least of which is a subtle awareness on the part of the person filling it that playing this role is vital to the psychic balance of the family, and has its rewards and importance as well as its pains and handicaps. The scapegoat is always as much volunteer as victim, and the role is fulfilled out of love as well as fear [Skynner, 1979, p. 645].

Scapegoating is a specific type of triangling that brings in a third person when two other members are unable to mediate the tensions in their own relationship. The scapegoated member may be a child or sick person who differs in some way from the rest of the family. He or she may have a chronic mental or physical condition. By scapegoating, the parents or the entire family are able to avoid the deeper and more basic problems within the family structure (Baum & Page, 1991; Donley, 1993; Papero, 1990; Pierce, 1979; Skynner, 1979). Scapegoating also may be common on nursing units when troublesome patients are avoided by some nursing staff members.

FAMILY SECRETS

One dynamic in a family that gives it ongoing momentum is its tendency to have secrets. This dynamic is particularly strong in families with a high level of fusion and tightness.

CASE EXAMPLE

Jim is a successful, 51-year-old businessman with five children. After college he enlisted in the army and served in the Korean War. While stationed there he had an affair with a female officer. She became pregnant. They were both dishonorably discharged. They did not marry. She had the child after they returned to the United States. He sent her voluntary child support payments until the child was 18 years old. Meanwhile, he was married a few years after he returned from the war. He told his wife of the earlier relationship and the existence of his child.

As part of their family functioning, when the wife became angry she occasionally raised the issue of his illicit affair and berated her husband for the expense of the child support payments. Their children were never aware of this family "secret." As they grew older, they wondered about the bitter tone in their mother's voice when the family was under financial strain from time to time. The mother imposed very restrictive spending and dating policies on their adolescent children. The father, although forceful and confident in his business and social relationships, became helpless and silent about his wife's uncompromising attitude toward their children. When they appealed to their father for help in changing their mother's harsh policies, they became frustrated and puzzled by his response, "Your mother knows best."

Family secrets cause rigidity and anxiety in families. They can be the underlying reasons for perplexing behavior and reactions observed in patients. Probing and questioning will not usually bring the secrets out unless you know the patient well. Remember that

most people have spent years and sometimes decades burying these secrets. Instead, if you observe the detrimental effects of a suspected secret, recommend that the patient share the problem with a trusted person or professional who may be able to help the patient deal with it rather than continuing to have it undermine his or her well-being and that of the family (Clement, 1991; Donley, 1993; Papero, 1990).

Secrets can also be used within families during times of acute family stress when there is concern about "overloading the system."

CASE EXAMPLE

Linda and Gerry were expecting their second child. Their only daughter was 2 years old. During her eighth month of pregnancy, Linda was in a serious automobile accident. Although every effort was made to save her life, she died after 1 week of intensive care. A cesarean delivery performed before her death produced a son who quickly developed respiratory difficulties. He was diagnosed as having hyaline membrane disease and was struggling for life in the newborn intensive care nursery.

Grief-stricken, Gerry told his daughter about her mother's death. Gerry decided that unless his daughter asked about the baby, he would withhold news of the baby's birth until the baby's health had stabilized. Gerry feared that it would be too much for the child to learn of the arrival of a new brother, only to learn later of his death.

FEEDBACK

One of the essential qualities of a system is the relatedness of its units. The way each of the units relates to the other units is through *feedback loops*. Feedback is the communication that occurs between all members of the family system (Donley, 1993; Papero, 1990; Woods, Habaerman, & Packard, 1993).

A physiological example of a feedback loop is the essential mechanism the body uses in maintaining homeostasis. One cell will signal another cell that it needs more or less input in order to maintain its normal level of functioning; similarly, one body system will notify another system that it needs to accelerate or slow down its level of functioning in order to promote the well-being of the entire body system (Dohms & Metz, 1991).

Feedback is the process by which a system maintains itself. In social systems it can be positive or negative. *Positive feedback* from one unit of the system reinforces a particular action or behavior of another unit and promotes similar behavior in the future. *Negative feedback* from one unit to another discourages a particular action or behavior (Bertalanffy, 1968).

When an individual within the family or all members of a family are highly defensive, however, they are usually unable to hear and process the negative feedback they are receiving. For example, when people are under moderate to extreme stress, they typically cannot absorb any information that will further add to their stress level (Papero, 1990; Woods, Habaerman, & Packard, 1993).

CASE EXAMPLE

Ann is a 19-year-old college sophomore. Her 26-year-old brother was diagnosed with AIDS 2 years ago. Her family had not been aware that he was homosexual. The revelation, accompanied by the shock of learning that their son had a fatal illness, was devastating for Ann's parents. This occurred during Ann's senior year of high school. Her parents, who had been actively involved in her older siblings' college searches, were too emotionally involved in her brother's difficulty to become interested in her college decision. She applied to a school over a thousand miles from home, was accepted, and left for school in the fall, without ever having seen the school.

Her roommate and dorm mates found Ann to be distant and aloof. Gradually, she became more isolated, but continued her studies. When she returned home during the summer, the environment in her home was very depressing, and her parents did not notice her distress because of their own high level of distress. Ann returned to school that fall and was described by her acquaintances as "being in a fog." She seemed unable to par-

ticipate in discussions and could not concentrate in class.

In this example, Ann and her parents were under so much stress due to Ann's brother's illness that they were not able to process negative feedback: Ann from her dorm mates or Ann's parents from her.

HOMEOSTASIS

It is important to view the entire family as a system when trying to promote positive change in one family member. In every family a balance is created by the total contributing dynamics of each family member. This is called *family homeostasis*. If change occurs in one family member, it will create a major change in the family balance. This is caused by the differences in interactions between the person and other family members (Burr, 1991; Papero, 1990; Woods, Habaerman, & Packard, 1993).

Homeostasis is an essential concept in designing a treatment program for patients with many types of emotional and physical problems. It frequently is the underlying reason why treatment approaches that appear to be successful while the patient is hospitalized are dismal failures once the patient is discharged into his or her regular family system. The family will continue to interact with the patient as a "sick" member. The person will quickly fall into his or her original and accustomed role in the family because the family homeostasis depends on it (Burr, 1991; Harrison & Cole, 1991; Papero, 1990; Woods, Habaerman, & Packard, 1993).

Without intervention, the family will continue to promote the person's sickness, whether by a heightened reaction to his gastrointestinal symptoms of Crohn's disease or to another's symptoms of alcoholism. A systems approach that addresses the interactional style of the family and enlightens members about the ways they feed into and promote a continuation of the patient's problems is an essential aspect of the management of chronic physical or mental disease states (Burr, 1991; Clement, 1991; Donley, 1993; Fisher et al., 1992; Harrison & Cole, 1991).

CONCLUSION

The use of a general systems approach in the nursing process involves the assessment of all aspects of a patient's functioning: physical, psychological, and social. When an event occurs in one realm, it affects the other two.

Family systems are indeed complex. Most people, especially in their own families, feel the effects of family dynamics but often are unable to identify the specific forces occurring. This chapter was written to help you understand the response of a family to a loved one's illness and to lend insight into the social dynamics of your own nursing unit. (Remember that the social dynamics of a nursing unit can have a strong effect on patient care because of the overall general systems effect of a positive or negative working environment.)

Family dynamics are important in a patient's response to illness for many reasons. A person is often influenced by his or her family's response to the stressful experience of illness. If the family system goes into crisis, the patient's ability to maintain an adaptive level of coping can be seriously undermined. This is because the ability to support a given member is one of the family's most important functions. When the family system is severely stressed or in crisis, this function is seriously weakened. So, too, if the patient is unable to cope, his or her family will be more threatened by the illness. The anxiety of all members will be continuously interchanged. The effects of stress on families will be discussed further in Chapter 16.

BIBLIOGRAPHY

American Heritage college dictionary (3rd ed.). (1993). Boston: Houghton-Mifflin.

Aponte, H. (1976) Underorganization in the poor family. In P. Guerin (Ed.) *Family therapy: Theory and practice.* New York: Gardner Press.

Bateson, G., Jackson, D., & Haley, J. (1956). Toward a theory of schizophrenia. *Behavioral Science, 1,* 251–264.

Bennett, L.A., & La Bonte, M. (1995). Recent developments in alcoholism: Family systems. *Recent Developments in Alcoholism 11,* 87–94.

Bertalanffy, L. von. (1968). *General system theory.* New York: Braziller.

Black, C. (1982). *It will never happen to me.* New York: Ballantine.

Black, J. M., & Matassarin-Jacobs, E. (Eds.). (1993). *Luckmann and Sorensen's medical-surgical nursing: A psychophysiologic approach* (4th ed.). Philadelphia: W. B. Saunders.

Boykin, A., & Schoenhofer, S. (1993). *Nursing as caring: A model for transforming practice.* New York: National League for Nursing.

Boszormenyi-Nagy, I., & Framo, J. L. (Eds.). (1985). *Intensive family therapy: Theoretical and practical aspects.* New York: Brunner/Mazel.

Bowen, M. (1974). Toward the differentiation of a self in one's own family of origin. In A. Andres & J. Lorio (Eds.), *Georgetown Family Symposia.* Washington, DC: Georgetown University Medical Center.

Brazelton, T. B. (1973). *Neonatal behavioral assessment scale.* Philadelphia: J. B. Lippincott.

Bulechek, G. M., & McCloskey, J. S. (1992). Defining and validating nursing interventions. *The Nursing Clinics of North America, 27*(2), 289–299.

Burns, C., Archbold, P., Stewart, B., & Shelton, K. (1993). New diagnosis: Caregiver role strain. *Nursing Diagnosis, 4*(2), 70–76.

Carpenito, L. J. (1993). *Nursing diagnosis: Application and clinical practice.* Philadelphia: J.B. Lippincott.

Cleary, M. J. (1994). Reassessing the codependency movement: A response to Sorentino. *HealthCare Management Reviews, 19* (1), 7–10.

Clement, J. A. (1991). Psychiatric nursing phenomena and the construct of family boundaries. *Archives of Psychiatric Nursing, 5*(4), 236–243.

Dohms, J.E., & Metz, A. (1991). Stress—mechanisms of immunosuppression. *Veterinary immunology and immunopathology, 30*(1), 89–109.

Donley, M. G. (1993). Attachment and the emotional unit. *Family Process, 32*(1), 3–20.

Dossey, B. M., Guzzetta, C. E., & Kenner, C. V. (1992). *Critical care nursing: Body-mind-spirit* (3rd ed.). Philadelphia: J. B. Lippincott.

Edlin, G., & Golanty, E. (1992). *Health and wellness: A holistic approach* (4th ed.). Boston: Jones and Bartlett.

Eisenman, R. (1992). Birth order, development and personality. *Acta Paedopsychiatrica, 55*(1), 25–27.

Elliott, B. A. (1992). Birth order and health: Major issues. *Social Science and Medicine, 35*(4), 443–452.

Engel, G. (1962). *Psychological development in health and disease.* Philadelphia: W. B. Saunders.

Engel, G., & Morgan, W. (1973). *Interviewing the patient.* Philadelphia: J. B. Lippincott.

Felten, D., & Felten S. (1991). Innervation of lymphoid tissue. In R. Ader, D. Felten, & N. Cohen (Eds.). *Psychoneuroimmunology* (2nd ed.) San Diego: Academic Press.

Felten, D., Cohen., Ader, R., Felten, S., Carlson, S., & Roszman, T. (1991). Neurochemical links between the nervous and immune systems. In R. Ader, D. Felten, & N. Cohen (Eds.). *Psychoneuroimmunology* (2nd ed.) San Diego: Academic Press.

Fisher, L., Ransom, D. C., Terry, H. E., & Burge, S. (1992). The California Family Health Project: IV. Family structure/organization and adult health. *Family Process, 31*(4), 399–419.

Fogarty, T. (1975). Triangles. *The Family, 2,* 11.

Fogarty, T. (1977). Fusion. *The Family, 4,* 49.

Franks, P., Campbell, T. L., & Shields, C. G. (1992). Social relationships and health: The relative roles of family functioning and social support. *Social Science and Medicine, 34*(7), 779–788.

Frye, L. S. (1991). The evolving American family. *AAOHN Journal, 39*(9), 422–426.

Gaut, D. A. (Ed.). (1993). *A global agenda for caring.* New York: National League for Nursing Press.

Goldberg, R. J., & Novack, D. H. (1992). The psychosocial review of systems. *Social Science & Medicine, 35*(3), 261–269.

Green, R., & Framo, J. (Eds.). (1981). *Family therapy: Major contributions.* New York: International Universities Press.

Hackett, J.P, Cassem N.H., Stern, T.A., & Murray, G.B. (1991). Beginnings: Consultation psychiatry in a general hospital. In N.H. Cassem (Ed.), *Massachusetts General Hospital handbook of general hospital psychiatry* (3rd ed.) (pp. 1–8). St. Louis: Mosby Year Book.

Haley, J. (1984). *Ordeal therapy* (3rd ed.). San Francisco: Jossey-Bass.

Halm, M. A., Titler, M. G., Kleiber, C., Johnson, S. K., Montgomery, L. A., Craft, M. J., Buckwalter, K., Nicholson, A., & Megivern, K. (1993). Behavioral responses of family members during critical illness. *Clinics in Nursing Research, 2*(4), 414–437.

Harrison, D. S., & Cole, K. D. (1991). Family dynamics and caregiver burden in home health care. *Clinics in Geriatric Medicine, 7*(4), 817–829.

Herth, K. (1993). Hope in the family caregiver of terminally ill people. *Journal of Advanced Nursing, 18*(4), 538–548.

Jackson, D. (1967). The eternal triangle: An interview with Don D. Jackson. In J. Haley & L. Hoffman (Eds.), *Techniques of family therapy.* New York: Basic Books.

Jacobs, E. H. (1991). Self psychology and family therapy. *American Journal of Psychotherapy, 45*(4), 483–498.

Jones, S. (1980). *Family therapy: A comparison of approaches.* Bowie, MD: R. J. Brady.

Kaplan, H. I., & Sadock, B. J. (1994). *Synopsis of psychiatry: Behavioral sciences, clinical psychiatry* (7th ed.). Baltimore: Williams & Wilkins.

Kaplan, H. I., & Sadock, B. J. (1995). *Comprehensive textbook of psychiatry/VI* (6th ed.). Baltimore: Williams & Wilkins.

Lipowski, Z. J. (1991). Consultation-liaison psychiatry 1990. *Psychotherapy and Psychosomatics, 55*(2–4), 62–68.

Masterson, J. F., Tolpin, M., & Sifneos, P. E. (1991). *Comparing psychoanalytic psychotherapies: Developmental, self, and object relations: Self psychology, short-term dynamic.* New York: Brunner/Mazel.

McCarthy, S. M., & Gallo, A. M. (1992). A case illustration of family management style. *Journal of Pediatric Nursing, 7*(6), 395–402.

McDaniel, S. H., Campbell, T. L., & Seaburn, D. B. (1990). *Family-oriented primary care: A manual for medical providers.* New York: Springer-Verlag.

Minuchin, S. (1974). *Families and family therapy.* Cambridge, MA: Harvard University Press.

Minuchin, S., & Fishman, H. C. (Eds.). (1981). *Family therapy techniques.* Cambridge: Harvard University Press.

Minuchin, S., Montalvo, B., & Guerney, B. (1967). *Families of the slums: An exploration of their structure and treatment.* New York: Basic Books.

Minuchin, S., Rosman, B., & Baker, C. (1978). *Psychosomatic families, anorexia nervosa in context.* Cambridge, MA: Harvard University Press.

Newberry, B. H., Jaikins-Madden, J. E., & Gerstenberger, T. J. (1991). *A holistic conceptualization of stress and disease.* New York: AMS Press.

O'Brien, M. T. (1993). Multiple sclerosis: Stressors and coping strategies in spousal caregivers. *Journal of Community Health Nursing, 10*(3), 123–135.

O'Connor, S. (1991). Psychiatry liaison nursing in a changing health care system. In N.H. Cassem (Ed.), *Massachusetts General Hospital handbook of general hospital psychiatry* (3rd ed.) (pp. 611–618). St. Louis: Mosby Year Book.

Pierce, C. (1979). Personality disorders. In G. Usdin & J. Lewis (Eds.), *Psychiatry in general medical practice.* New York: McGraw Hill.

Potter, P. A., & Perry, A. G. (1993). *Fundamentals of nursing: Concepts, process, and practice* (3rd ed.). St. Louis: Mosby Year Book.

Richards, W. R., Burgess, D. E., Petersen, F. R., & McCarthy, D. L. (1993). Genograms: A psychosocial assessment tool for hospice. *Hospice Journal, 9*(1), 1–12.

Sadler, J. Z., & Hulgus, Y. F. (1992). Clinical problem solving and the biopsychosocial model. *American Journal of Psychiatry, 149*(10), 1315–1323.

Satir, V. (1983). *Conjoint family therapy* (3rd ed.). Palo Alto, CA: Science & Behavior Books.

Schopler, J. H., & Galinsky, M. J. (1993). Support groups as open systems: A model for practice and research. *Health and Social Work, 18*(3), 195–207.

Schultz, N. L. (1993). Leadership: Effects of birth order and education. *Nurse Manager, 24*(8), 64I–64J, 64N, 64P.

Skynner, R., (1979). The physician as family therapist. In G. Usdin & J. Lewis (Eds.), *Psychiatry in general medical practice.* New York: McGraw-Hill.

Smith, L. B., & Thelen, E. (Eds.). (1993). *A dynamic systems approach to development: Applications.* Cambridge: MIT Press.

Stanhope, M., & Lancaster, J. (Eds.). (1992). *Community health nursing: Process and practice for promoting health* (3rd ed.). St. Louis: Mosby Year Book.

Tennant, D. (1993). The place of the family in mental health nursing: Past, present and future. *Journal of Advanced Nursing, 18*(5), 752–758.

Thomas, C. L. (Ed.). (1993). *Taber's cyclopedic medical dictionary* (17th ed.). Philadelphia: F. A. Davis.

Timby, B. K., & Lewis, L. W. (1992). *Fundamental skills and concepts in patient care* (5th ed.). Philadelphia: J. B. Lippincott.

Toman, W. (1976). *Family constellation* (3rd ed.). New York: Springer–Verlag.

Wegscheider–Cruse, S., (1985). *Understanding me.* Health communications.

Wegscheider–Cruse, S., A. Gruse, J. R. (1990). *Understanding co-dependency.* Health communications.

Wolman, B., & Stricker, G. (Eds.). (1983). *Handbook of family and marital therapy.* New York: Plenum Press.

Woods, N. F., Habaerman, M. R., & Packard, N. J. (1993). Demands of illness and individual, dyadic, and family adaptation in chronic illness. *Western Journal of Nursing Research, 15*(1), 10–25.

CHAPTER 8

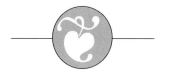

The Barry Holistic Systems Model

Patricia Barry

"Nursing is the only health care discipline that cares for the whole human being," said Dr. Gary Schwartz, former chairperson of the Department of Health Psychology at Yale University. Further, "nursing fills a unique position in the entire health care system because of its preparation in both the physical and social sciences."*

Nursing is a holistic discipline. It addresses the physical, psychological, and social needs of patients, working to promote health in each domain. Further, it embraces theories of psychosocial and physical functioning from other disciplines, incorporating many types of knowledge that are helpful in treating patients.

THE CHALLENGE OF STUDYING PSYCHOSOCIAL PHENOMENA

Testing psychosocial phenomena in the etiology, course, and treatment of physical illness involves a particular challenge that research in the physical sciences does not. In the social sciences it is more difficult to ensure a "controlled" research situation. For example, a researcher may be interested in determining the effects of touch on hypertension. Here the researcher cannot manipulate touch, the independent variable, because she has no control over the subject's emotional response to touch, which may then affect change in blood pressure rate, the dependent variable.

In spite of such challenges, theory development and research are becoming more and more vital to the nursing profession. They have been strongly enhanced by the North American Nursing Diagnosis Association (NANDA) movement, because each nursing diagnosis is developed based on review of many theoretical formulations. Nursing diagnosis as formulated by NANDA is a professional approach that has actively stimulated the testing of theory and the effectiveness of nursing interventions (Carpenito, 1993).

More research is needed. Because of the strong emphasis on psychosocial diagnoses in the NANDA list of approved nursing diagnoses, there is a need for more knowledge and research into the phenomena that cause psychosocial problems. In addition, there is a need for research into effective approaches to resolve or reduce these problems.

---

*Personal communication.

Patricia Barry: *Psychosocial Nursing: Care of Physically Ill Patients and Their Families,* 3rd ed.
© 1996 Lippincott–Raven Publishers

DEVELOPING A THEORETICAL PERSPECTIVE

Because of the abstract nature of social science theory, it is possible for a psychosocial response to be evaluated from many different perspectives, all of them well-founded in various psychological or related disciplines. The interventions based on these perspectives may be equally effective. The most critical question is "Did this approach resolve the problem?"

Nurses develop their own perspectives on clinical interventions with influence from a variety of sources. Three of the most important are the theoretical approach of the nurse's original nursing education institution; the nurse's own definition of nursing, which is a reflection of personal and professional values; and the availability of time. Certainly, in the health care environments of today, time is a strong factor in the nurse's prioritizing of nursing care options. Availability of time strongly impacts the first two factors.

Nursing is a biopsychosocial science that is developing and being defined by many nursing clinicians, researchers, and theorists. Regardless of their conceptual approaches, these nursing innovators describe nursing models with similar themes. The four themes most nursing models have in common are:

1. Person
2. Nursing
3. Environment
4. Health (Fawcett, 1984)

Within the descriptions of nursing theorists, the meaning and interpretation of these themes differ. Generally, however, each theme has an underlying central concept and a common core of beliefs.

The term *person* is viewed by the nurse as a human being comprised of biological, psychological, social, and spiritual needs. These needs are blended in a complex system that results in a unique individual (Fawcett, 1984; Leddy & Pepper, 1993; Parker, 1993; Stevens-Barnum, 1994).

Nursing is the role nurses take as they interact with patients. The role, regardless of the theoretical nursing model or the type of clinical practice, includes the following dimensions of care: comfort, including physical, psychological, and spiritual care, and the monitoring of hygiene (Fawcett, 1984; Leddy & Pepper, 1993; Parker, 1993; Stevens-Barnum, 1994).

Environment includes all the internal and external forces that affect the patient. These forces include biological, intrapsychic, spiritual, and social dynamics, as well as the external physical surroundings (Fawcett, 1984; Leddy & Pepper, 1993; Parker, 1993; Stevens-Barnum, 1994).

Health is a state of physical and mental functioning. It exists in a continuum ranging from wellness to death. This concept, perhaps more than the other three in the nursing paradigm, is the one most subject to value judgments. What is subjectively viewed as "good" or "bad" health by one person may be viewed differently by another. Also, the perception of what constitutes "health" by health care professionals may depend on the discipline of the caregiver.

SYSTEMS-ORIENTED NURSING MODELS

Systems-oriented models of nursing build on prior nursing theory by applying multidisciplinary perspectives about the meaning of *person*, the goal of attaining health, and the milieu in which the person functions. These models include the interactive effects of environmental stressors and the uniqueness of the individual stress responses in human psychological, spiritual, biological, and social systems. This is a natural development because of the evolution of a holistic nursing practice framework. The holistic approach is based on principles of interrelationship between the biological, psychological, spiritual, social, and physical environmental aspects of a human's functioning (Moyers, 1993; Nagel, 1993; Newberry, Jaikins-Madden, & Gerstenberger, 1991; Reeder, 1994).

NURSES' EXPECTATIONS REGARDING PSYCHOSOCIAL SUPPORT

Caring for patients' psychological, spiritual, and social needs can be one of the most challenging aspects of nursing. Much of the assessment in psychosocial nursing is based on deductive reasoning rather than on the concrete reasoning used in physical assessment; physical assessment most often relies on specifically measurable data. Perhaps it is the abstract nature of working with a patient's feelings and thoughts that makes some nurses feel uneasy and uncertain about whether their own perceptions are accurate.

At one time I worked as a psychiatric-mental health clinical instructor in an upper division baccalaureate nursing program. The students were registered nurses who ranged in age from 23 to 50. As part of their basic nursing educations, they all had spent 3 months working in psychiatric institutions. Most of them reported that they had felt uncomfortable talking with psychiatric patients during their original nursing education experience. They were not sure what to say to the patients or how the patients would respond. Many said they were frightened of the patients but did not acknowledge it to anyone. Because they were not sure what to do, they often played cards with the patients and engaged in superficial conversation.

The clinical setting used by the university for its mental health clinical experience was an inpatient drug and alcohol treatment hospital. The patients were coherent and rational. They were generally eager to share their thoughts and feelings with the nurses. Although the nurses were not in an acute psychiatric setting and the patients were not likely to have any psychotic episodes or to become violent, the nurses once again reported feeling uneasy. On reflection, the nurses discovered that they were not afraid of the patients, but of encounter between themselves and the patients. Perhaps, also, they feared what they did not know about themselves. One nurse said, "Usually when I'm with a general hospital patient there's something I have to do for him. I'm taking his blood pressure or checking a dressing or something; I may talk to him as I'm doing it, but at least I have something to do."

Sitting and talking intimately with a patient about major life issues was something most of the nurses in the class had rarely done before. Gradually, as they relaxed, they discovered that the patients were eager for someone to listen and care, not to utter magical words that would change the course of their lives.

The students learned that it was their listening and the skill of their questions, not their talking or recommendations, that was most therapeutic.

Chapter 2 describes many essential techniques for effective intervention with patients. Therapeutic nursing communication can make an important difference for patients and families. The following factors are important in determining the outcome of psychosocial nursing interventions:

1. Openness and warmth with a patient.
2. Ability to withhold judgment until an understanding of the patient's perceptions of himself, his illness, and his social system is clear.
3. Assessment skill.
4. Willingness to become involved when ineffective coping or the potential for it is observed.

In encountering a patient who is in emotional distress, many nurses believe they should be able to do something actively about this emotional pain, that they should be able to come up with a sentence or an idea that could eliminate this distress. This is not a fair or reasonable personal expectation for a nurse. A patient's emotional pain is usually the result of the combined effects of ineffective coping and, quite likely, an inadequate social system. These dynamics have been operating for years and possibly for a lifetime. It is unreasonable for a nurse to believe that a major change can be effected in a patient's thinking or feeling stage with just a few words.

IS IT REALISTIC TO TEACH PATIENTS AND FAMILIES NEW COPING SKILLS?

It is not unusual to see written on a patient's care plan "teach patient new coping skills." This expectation, which many nurses impose on themselves, may not be realistic. First of all, patients enter the hospital with a repertoire of defense or coping mechanisms that have been in use since childhood; most of the coping mechanisms are used unconsciously. They also utilize a series of conscious coping skills. When the stress of hospitalization occurs and gradually becomes more threatening, the patient's normal ability to cope regresses. Unconscious defense mechanisms progressively become more immature and are increasingly used by the ego in its effort to adapt. In most instances, patients are usually unaware of their use of defense mechanisms. They are automatic, unconscious responses as the ego works to protect the person.

If a patient is astute psychologically and has a high level of differentiation between thinking and emotions (see Chapter 7), a conscious stress management approach may be used as a response to most stresses of day-to-day life. Hospitalization for serious illness, however, usually removes the potential for conscious stress reduction techniques such as jogging, meditation, exercising, and so on. Coping ability may decrease in the hospital because of the inability to cope with stress in one's usual way. In addition, the threatening nature of the illness will decrease one's normal ability to cope consciously. The result is the ego's use of unconscious defenses to protect itself from unpleasant awareness of the environment and to lessen the patient's internal anxiety level.

The nurse may be conversant with many types of defense mechanisms and coping skills. Although an excellent teacher, the nurse cannot expect to *teach* someone who is under psychological stress a new way to use defense mechanisms. It is not possible to tell a patient to stop using unconscious, maladaptive denial or repression and, instead, to use a more adaptive defense against the threats he or she is experiencing. These defenses have been used unconsciously for most of an individual's life.

Instead of attempting to "teach" new defenses or coping mechanisms, the nurse can help to decrease the patient's level of anxiety by encouraging discussion about fears, providing reality testing, encouraging support from family members and other caregivers, and supporting problem-solving. These approaches can assist patients' egos to obtain a gradual awareness of reality, and open the way for more adaptive uses of defense mechanisms to occur. Gradually, patients may be able to apply their normal coping skills in order to reduce their level of anxiety and psychological or spiritual conflict.

NURSING INTERVENTIONS WITH PATIENTS AND FAMILIES

Helping patients to adapt to the stress of hospitalization and rehabilitation or chronic illness at home can be one of the most challenging aspects of nursing care. If ineffective coping or maladaptation occurs, it can have a profound and lasting effect on the patient's and family's quality of life. A nurse *can* have an effect on a maladapting patient. The nurse is a change agent, but change cannot be ordered or dictated. Adaptation and the changes required for it to occur greatly depend on the patient's mental state and customary family functioning. A nurse can be a catalyst in the process, but it is ultimately the patient and/or family that must change and adapt.

An essential aspect of being a change agent is providing emotional support to the patient or family member whose coping ability is weakened. The major causes of a weakened ego are:

1. *High levels of stress.* Stress due to hospitalization, fear of death, changes within family due to illness, and so on can alter coping ability.
2. *Characteristically weak personality style.* Dependent and inadequate personality styles in individual patients or family members, for example, have greater difficulty coping with hospitalization and illness.
3. *Cognitive mental disorder (CMD).* When brain tissue is affected by an organic dysfunction, it alters normal cognitive, sensory, and emotional responses, all of which are ego functions.

In most cases, these functions are weakened only temporarily due to either acute stress or physical dysfunction. When the nurse provides extra psychological or spiritual support by encouraging the patient to release emotion through talking, providing reality testing, and so on, this can help the patient to work through and resolve a potential crisis. This type of support can be compared to the use of sandbags as an extra support to the walls of a dike that are under strain of breaking because of a flood.

PROFESSIONAL VALUES RELATED TO THERAPEUTIC NURSING INTERVENTION

When ineffective coping with physical illness is present, the nurse can use a theoretical framework that assesses the various subsystems operating within and around the patient. Once the subsystems are assessed, they must be examined for their potential to change so that biopsychosocial and spiritual adaptation are the ultimate outcomes. Using such a framework implies the following belief about nursing interventions:

1. Professional nursing functions and activities are directed by a therapeutic purpose.
2. Underlying all nursing activity is a genuine caring and concern for the welfare of the patient.
3. Critical analysis of the patient and her condition is accompanied by respect for her as an individual whose dignity is always to be maintained.
4. When possible, the patient is an integral part of all planning and decision-making.
5. The nurse is the patient's advocate when she cannot be her own.
6. The nurse supports and promotes health and quality of life. Health is a subjective state of physical, psychological, spiritual, and social well-being, not solely the absence of disease or infirmity.

THE NURSE AS A CHANGE AGENT

Before a nurse can act as a change agent by assisting patients in adapting to illness or to long-lasting or permanent changes in body image, an internal change process may be important; learning to honor the patient's perceptions of health and how it can be achieved and stabilized.

The emotional and intellectual ability of the nurse to be less self-critical in the counseling process has perhaps not been emphasized enough. Nurses sometimes can feel a heavy responsibility in responding to the challenge of assisting a patient to cope effectively.

It is the rare nurse who is not self-conscious and cautious when talking with an emotionally overwhelmed patient. It can seem risky for a young nurse who feels inexperienced. When mindful of the theory presented in this text and with genuine concern for the patient's well-being, a nurse can be prepared to pull up a chair, sit down, and be *with* the patient.

The process of engaging in such a relationship can seem more threatening for the nurse than for the patient. A nurse can be aware of personal feelings, thoughts, and reactions; they should be evaluated gently, however. Above all, a nurse's involvement can, ideally, feel right for the nurse and the patient. If it is uncomfortable, there are other nurses available to the patient. If serving as a patient's primary nurse, however, hesitation can be discussed with a peer on the unit; an impartial supervisor (with whom one can be honest without fear of a negative evaluation); or a psychiatric liaison nurse whose clinical background can assist in understanding the response. It can be important to examine one's reaction to the situation so that such situations are not consistently avoided in the future. Future patients would perhaps miss some very valuable, special experiences.

FACILITATING PSYCHOSOCIAL CHANGE IN PATIENTS AND FAMILIES

Can the patient's biological subsystem be changed or modified? One hopes so, or hospitals would soon be empty. Can the psychological and spiritual subsystems be changed or modified? Yes. Although not fundamentally alterable, they can be supported in order to assist the patient to function at an improved level. It is the patient's conscious or unconscious resources that actually change the maladaptive process. The way the patient's intrapsychic subsystem operates is unique to that individual; it does not yield easily to change. If the patient is maladapting, it will be the unique individual responses to interventions that ultimately can produce change in maladaptation.

Remember, however, that it is not only the seriousness of illness that causes regression and potential psychological maladaptation; rather, it is the patient's perception of the threat of illness and its implications for the future that are a major cause of maladaptation because of the anxiety they generate.

Factors That Contribute to Change

Lewin has proposed that there are three main steps in the process of change. These can be helpful to keep in mind when attempting to bring about any type of change in a patient's belief system or behavior (Welch, 1979). Lewin's model is presented here with a focus on the patient or family member at risk for maladaptation.

   The unfreezing stage. The motivation to change must be put in motion. The patient or family member first must become aware that change is needed. The primary force in this process is the patient or family member's own emotional distress. At times, discussion with the nurse allows a more natural discovery in the event that the individual is not personally aware of ineffective coping. Talking with a few members of the family present in addition to the person who is coping poorly can sometimes increase self-awareness. It is important to remember the old adage, however, that a "horse can be led to water but cannot be forced to drink."

   The moving stage. Based on information received during the unfreezing stage, the patient or family member can choose a particular course of action from alternatives that he alone or he and the change agent develop together. The course of action is begun when a plan is agreed upon, supported, initiated, and subjected to ongoing evaluation by the patient, family members, and nurse.

   The refreezing stage. The action instituted by the change is in place and continues to be evaluated for its effectiveness. Blocks to success can be evaluated. Modifications or changes in the original plan may be needed to ensure the successful outcome of the change process.

Can the family system be changed? Yes, it can be modified. The functioning of a family is similar to each person's intrapsychic system; the family is made up of members who function in their own usually predictable ways. In addition, there are usually longstanding family dynamics involved, which can be evaluated in the assessment process (see Chapter 7). There can be more flexibility, however, in a group system than in an individual system because of the greater number of dynamics involved.

Can the other social relationships in the patient's environment be changed? Yes. This is a crucial concept when a patient is coping ineffectively. Social relationships include caregivers. It is important that caregivers be able to recognize the occurrence of maladaptation, assess it, and intervene or consult others to intervene. Caregivers can also evaluate and monitor the patient's continuing responses to illness and the interventions designed to promote adaptation. Caregivers can make an important difference if the patient's body, mind, or family are temporarily or permanently lacking the strength to overcome the problem. If no caregiver observes the patient's or family member's maladaptation, it is possible that discharge from the hospital, clinic, or home care system will occur without intervention. The longer a patient or family member responds with maladaptive defenses, the more likely that chronic maladaptation will be an ongoing part of their life.

In today's cost-conscious health care environments, the early, accurate assessment of problems that can impinge on a patient or family's well-being and quality of life is essential. If not assessed early in the inpatient or home care process, they may not be adequately treated, due to limited finances or limited access to the caregiving system. Use of the Holistic Systems Model presented in this chapter provides a systemic overview of the factors that can result in ineffective coping with physical illness, which can lead to chronic maladaptation. Such maladaptation is costly in terms of positive life outlook, as well as the economic cost of continued medical and nursing care that often accompanies it.

A CONCEPTUAL APPROACH TO NURSING INTERVENTION

The term *conceptual model* may be clarified by contrasting it to the word *idea*. An idea is actually an incomplete form of a concept. An idea is like a brick that has no mortar or glue to attach it to other bricks in order to form a wall. A conceptual model, on the other hand, is like a brick wall that has mortar to connect the bricks. An idea, when analyzed, may actually be unworkable because it is missing connectedness. A conceptual model has a framework or structure on which theory is built. Concepts are presented that build on each other and become the actual model.

THE BARRY HOLISTIC SYSTEMS ASSESSMENT MODEL: ASSESSMENT AND DIAGNOSIS OF HUMAN RESPONSES TO ILLNESS

My intention in presenting this model is that it be used as a guide. I encourage nurses to use flexibility rather than rigidity in applying it to the unique circumstances of patients and families.

This model proposes that a threatening, unresolved stressor can lead to a variety of problems in a person. These problems are interrelated biologically, psychologically, spiritually, socially, and environmentally. Stressors experienced within one of these domains with an accompanying stress response can have systemic effects on the remaining domains.

A MODEL FOR PROMOTION OF PSYCHOSOCIAL ADAPTATION

In keeping with traditional clinical nursing theory, it is important to have a formal conceptual model on which to base the nursing process. The model presented in this chapter is designed to promote patient's and families' adaptation to a change in health status. The emphasis in this model is to increase the nurse's awareness of the multiple subsystems and their forces that affect the patient's psychosocial response to the stress of illness. It was developed in the clinical environment using theoretical formulations from the physical and social sciences. It is a pragmatic model based on the practical experience of this author.

The nurse can promote the patient's and family's adaptation by constantly monitoring and assessing their responses to illness. As the nurse assesses the factors that have the potential to undermine individual and family adaptation, the factors may be modified or altered by nursing intervention to promote effective coping. As needed, the nurse can also change the approach used with the patient and family and temporarily give them appropriate support. When adaptation is at risk because of weakened intrapsychic defenses, organic failure, or temporary or chronic personal or family stress, there are intervention choices available to the nurse that can promote change and reverse ineffective coping processes.

This chapter presents the basic concepts of my approach to nursing care. The important concepts in this assessment approach are:

1. All people are constantly subject to stressors from many internal and external subsystems and systems. These stressors are sensed by one or more of these subsystems and then a protective or defensive response, called stress, is precipitated. Stress experienced in one subsystem can then create a cascade of sequential responses in that subsystem. Depending on the level of response in that subsystem, it can radiate into other subsystems, listed in Box 8-1.
2. The constancy of stress produces ever-changing dynamics in these subsystems and systems.
3. A person's responses to stress partially depend on the strengths and weaknesses in these same subsystems and systems; they continually feed into each other and are highly interdependent.
4. Personal and family dynamics (ways of operating) are fairly predictable and can be determined in the nursing assessment

BOX 8-1	Internal and External Subsystems Which Sense Stress
	1. Physiological 2. Psychological a. Cognition b. Emotion 3. Spiritual 4. Family 5. Other social relationships in the environment, such as: a. Friends b. Health care workers c. Work relationships d. Other social support individuals 6. The physical environment

process (normal coping style, personality style, physical responses to distress and so on).

5. The dynamics operating in the larger social system are the most flexible and subject to change. This is understandable considering the potential number of people in the environments to which a person is exposed.

If a person is maladapting to stress, it is important to examine the various subsystems and systems involved for their potential to contribute toward an adaptive response.

MAJOR CONCEPTS OF THE BARRY HOLISTIC SYSTEMS MODEL

Please note that the references related to the concepts described in this model are located in the specific chapters listed in the parentheses after each concept or definition.

PERSON

The following definitions apply to the concept of *person.*

A person is a biopsychosocial being who is an active participant in the nursing process.

A person is a being who is constantly interacting with the internal and external stimuli of his or her body and environment through sensory perception.

There is ongoing interactive and integrative feedback between the multiple subsystems that comprise the person. These subsystems include consciousness, unconscious processes, and the unique learned psychophysiologic responses to distress.

Risk factors, also known as threatening interactions, can result in physical or mental distress when the person's resources are not strong enough to neutralize or decrease them. Resources include the defensive, protective functions or strengths that are inherent in that individual. Resources can also include environmental factors such as social resources (i.e., family, caregivers, quality of physical environment).

A person is a biopsychosocial being who is born into a biological family and retains biological membership in that family through a lifetime. Social membership in a family is ongoing as the result of mutual election by the person and the family. Family homeostasis supports the physical and mental health of the person by providing an environment of physical, psychological, spiritual, and social support (1, 3–7, 9–11, 15–29).

ENVIRONMENT

The environment is the internal and external world of the person. The *internal environment* includes all physical, psychological, and spiritual functions. The *external environment* includes every external factor that impacts on and is sensed by a person's biological, psychological, spiritual, or social domains (Box 8-2).

HEALTH

Health is a state of homeostasis between a person's internal and external environments. Health is a state of subjective well-being in which the person experiences a positive qual-

BOX 8-2	Factors of the Personal Environment	
	Internal Environment	Values of the current national and state governments concerning needs of the society, health care spending, and so on
	Biological environment	
	All physiological body subsystems	
	Nutritional state	Physical environment
	Psychological environment	The immediate and local conditions in which the person lives and works, such as presence or absence of disease pathogens and available nutritional options
	Cognition	
	Emotion	
	Sensory processing	
	Spiritual environment	
		Cultural environment
	External Environment	The values held by the local, state, and national political and health care systems, country, religion, or ethnic group that affect a person's subjective sense of well-being and choices about health care
	Social environment	
	Includes family, nursing care, the health care system, work group, community, and so on	
	Economic environment	
	Level of income of individual and family	
	State of the economy	

ity of life. It is the absence of chronically threatening physical and/or psychological demands on a person.

Illness is a state that occurs when biological, psychological, spiritual, and/or social stressors result in a subjective feeling of distress with objective symptoms of physical or mental disorder. Homeostasis is disrupted by stressors that are stronger than the person's resources to defend against them (1, 3–7, 9–11, 15–28).

NURSING

Nursing is a process of care that is directed toward a person whose homeostasis is disrupted and potentially threatened by illness. Nursing care provides an environment in which health can occur or be restored. The goal of nursing care is to restore biopsychosocial and spiritual homeostasis of the person and the stability of the home caregiving system. It involves the following steps in an active decision-making process:

I. Assessment of the internal and external environments, (biological, psychological, social, spiritual, and physical envi-

ronment domains) in order to evaluate and describe the following factors related to health problems:

A. Subjective report of distress (in the biological, psychological, spiritual, social, or physical environment domains).

B. Objective presence of symptoms (symptoms are the physical or psychological signs of distress that can be observed by others).

C. Social system strengths and deficits.

D. Physical environment strengths and deficits.

E. The actual, potential, or possible causes and symptoms related to the problem (Alfaro-LeFevre, 1994; Carpenito, 1993; Gordon, 1987; McFarland, Wasli, & Gerety, 1992).

II. Nursing diagnosis of the problem (the naming of a problem that falls within the regulations of state nursing practice acts to identify and treat).

III. Care planning.

A. Analyzing the following factors within a biopsychosocial and spiritual framework in order to formulate a plan to resolve a problem:

B. The causes or contributing factors of the problem.

C. The symptoms or outward manifestations of the problem.

D. The subjective reporting by the patient or family member of distress related to the problem.

E. Problem-solving about these factors with the patient and caregiver when appropriate in order to develop:

1. A final measurable patient outcome or goal related to each problem whereby the original problem is resolved or therapeutically decreased, at DRG-established discharge date, as manifested by the patient's adaptive response, improved health status, and subjective change in feeling from distress to an increased sense of well-being.

2. Intermediate outcomes that demonstrate the patient's adaptive movement toward the goal of the final outcome within a specified period of time.

3. Measurable nursing interventions that are planned within specific time periods to bring about the intermediate and final patient outcomes.

4. Contracting with the patient to perform nursing care in order to bring about the final patient outcomes.

IV. Intervention (the actual performance of nursing functions designed to bring about the goals of the final and intermediate patient outcomes). Nursing interventions are designed to intervene at one or more of the following stages of problem development:

A. Primary

1. The problem has not occurred. The causative factors that can contribute to development of the problem are present or are perceived to be present by the person. There is a potential problem.

2. The goal of nursing intervention is to reduce or eliminate these causative factors. If they are incorrectly perceived to be present by the patient, the goal is to alter the perception.

B. Secondary.

1. The causative factors that can contribute to biopsychosocial or spiritual distress or crisis are present and increasing. There is a possible problem. Adaptive coping skills and social supports are available.

2. The goal of nursing intervention is to facilitate the use of physical treatment, adaptive coping skills, social supports, and the use of problem solving to reduce or eliminate the causative factors.

C. Tertiary

1. There is an actual problem. The patient is utilizing all available resources but is being overwhelmed by physiological, psychological, spiritual, and/or social stressors.

2. The goal of nursing intervention is to provide ongoing external support in one or more of the three domains until the person's resources are able to restore homeostasis.

V. Evaluation. The final step of the nursing process, evaluation involves reviewing the original problem with the patient or family members and assessing the intermediate and final outcomes to determine if the goals were realized within the expected time frame. If not, the problem should be redefined, if necessary, and the nursing process reinstituted by addressing the reformulated problem (1–30).

UNDERLYING CONCEPTS AND DEFINITIONS*

STRESSOR

An internal or external stimulus (demand) or risk factor that is perceived by the senses. It can be appraised by the psyche as nonthreat-

---

*The references related to the Barry Holistic Systems Model are included in the chapters whose numbers appear in parentheses following the presentation of each concept.

ening or threatening to the self. It can also be a physiological stressor that results in changes in physiological functioning (6, 9–11). When a physiologic demand or stressor results in physical pain, the cognitive, emotional, and spiritual domains are activated; coping is the adaptive response as stressors radiate from the biological state into the psychological and spiritual domains. When coping is ineffective, the individual stress is transmitted to the social environment.

There are four potential outcomes of a threatening stressor:

1. Health
2. Acute physical illness; if unresolved can lead to chronic physical illness
3. Ineffective coping; if unresolved can lead to mental or physical illness
4. Death

The response to the threatening stressor is a complex biopsychosocial and spiritual process that is dependent on the interactive response of some or all of the internal and external resources described below.

The potential health outcomes of the threatening stressor will be determined by:

1. The perceived level of threat of the stressor
2. The strength of the person's internal and external resources
3. The presence of risk factors that weaken the internal and external resources

STRESS

The subjective experience of a person who is responding to internal or external stimuli (stressors or demands).

DISTRESS

The subjective experience of a person who is responding to internal or external stimuli (stressors or demands) that are threatening or perceived as threatening to the self. These stressors can be felt as intrapsychic or physiological demands. Usually, the response to

stressors in one domain precipitates a stressful response in the other domains. The resources of the person are not strong enough to reduce or neutralize the stressor (3–7, 9–11, 15–29).

RESOURCES

The current state of internal and external elements that determine a person's capability to adapt to challenges, demands, and threatening stressors. The strength of these resources determines the level of a person's resistance to threatening psychosocial or physiological stressors. Resources assist in homeostasis. Internal and external resources are listed in Box 8-3.

RISK FACTORS

The actual, potential or perceived internal or external causes of stressful responses in the person. They are also known as *threatening stressors* or *demands*. They result in distress in the person.

A. Physical risk factors
   1. External—environmental factors that can produce disease or trauma, such as microorganisms, excessive temperature, impoverishment, and accidental injury
   2. Internal—inherent weakness of biologic body subsystem due to conditions such as genetic predisposition to disease of specific body system, malnutrition, immune suppression, infection, tumor
B. Psychological risk factors
   1. Presence of anxiety or depression-producing issues, including:
      a. Trust
      b. Self-esteem
      c. Shame
      d. Control
      e. Loss
      f. Guilt
      g. Intimacy (8)
   2. Ineffective coping or maladaptation caused by increase in risk factors and decreased resources leading to a de-

crease in cognitive, emotional, or perceptual functioning. Ineffective coping can also be caused by:

   a. Functional psychiatric disorder (3, 11)

   b. Cognitive mental disorder (11)

3. Developmental risk factors: The stage of life to which a person and family are currently responding and which imposes demands on a person's biological, psychological, spiritual, and social resources. These stages are listed in Box 8-5.

4. Situational risk factors: Events in a person's life that impose demands on biological, psychological, spiritual, and social resources. Such events can include loss of a spouse due to death or divorce, a job change, or moving to a new home (3–7, 9–11, 15–29).

SELF

The holistic integration of the biological, psychological, spiritual, and social subsystems of the person as they interact with the environment as a unified, whole, biopsychosocial being. The self includes the person's spirit. The spirit is an abstract entity that can encompass qualitative factors such as integrity, the will to live, identity, awareness of a universal force or God, and/or religious commitment. The effects of holism on

BOX 8-3	Internal and External Resources That Contribute to Homeostasis

Internal Resources
1. Overall nutritional state
2. Biological state of all body systems
  a. Cardiovascular
  b. Neurological
  c. Gastrointestinal
  d. Elimination
  e. Circulatory
  f. Immune
  g. Reproductive
  h. Musculoskeletal
3. Psychological State
  a. Cognitive
  b. Emotional
4. Spiritual state. The vital essence, unifying and animating force of the human being. The spirit is the connecting force with oneself; energy or will to live; other human beings; nature and the living elements of nature, such as animals, trees, plants; and God or some other higher power.
  a. Strengths and defenses
5. Genetic predisposition to health in each of the body subsystems (for instance, cardiovascular or psychological)
6. Current strengths and protective defenses
  a. Unconscious, automatic psychological defense mechanisms and
	conscious coping abilities
	  b. Physiological defenses
	7. Interpersonal style
	  a. Dependent, demanding
	  b. Orderly, controlled
	  c. Dramatizing, emotionally involved, captivating
	  d. Suspicious, guarded, complaining
	  e. Long-suffering, self-sacrificing
	  f. Superior
	  g. Uninvolved, aloof, distant
	  h. Antisocial
	  i. Inadequate
	
	External Resources
	1. Family coping style
	  a. During customary life stress
	  b. During acutely stressful conditions (i.e., acute illness of a family member)
	2. Availability of social support to patient and family
	3. Assessment skills of the health caregiving system
	4. The physical environment (i.e., hygiene, prevalence of pathogens, temperature)
	5. The economic environment
	6. The political environment of community, state, and nation
	7. The cultural environment
	  a. Complementarity of personal values with the norms of culture

the person are that the entire person-system responds when one of the subsystems is challenged (1–3, 10–12, 15).

HOLISM

The concept of a synergistic integration of biological, psychological, spiritual, and social subsystems into a dynamic person in a state of health (3–7, 9–11, 15–28).

BIOPSYCHOSOCIAL

A concept that describes the synergistic elements of a person that contribute to overall functioning and state of health. The term encompasses the systemic holism of biological, psychological, spiritual, and social functioning (Box 8-4). (9, 11)

HOMEOSTASIS

The state of a human being in which all subsystems or elements are in dynamic, constantly interacting balance. The elements include the biological, psychological, spiritual, and social domains. Each of these subsystems or elements contains subunits that are in states of ever-changing dynamism. The balance is maintained by feedback loop mechanisms between subunits and subsystems that regulate and maintain a state of health. This state of health is maintained by external systems that include the social and physical environments (3–7, 9–11, 15–29).

RESISTANCE

The synergistic integration of a person's resources that wards off threatening psychosocial or physiological stressors. Lack of resistance can lead to chronic physical or mental illness or death (3–7, 9–11, 15–29).

FINAL OUTCOME

The health goal established by mutual planning by nurse and patient (17, 18).

INTERMEDIATE PATIENT OUTCOME

Patient behaviors established by mutual planning of the nurse and patient that are preliminary steps to the final patient outcome (17, 18).

ADAPTATION/EFFECTIVE COPING

A positive adjustment to a threatening physical, psychological, spiritual, social, or physical environmental demand or risk factor. Homeostasis is maintained. The final outcome is health (3–7, 9–11, 15–28).

INEFFECTIVE COPING

The state of distress due to inadequate resources to meet the current biological, psychological, spiritual, or social challenges a person is experiencing (3–7, 9–11, 15–28).

BOX 8-4	Current State of the Ego/Psychological Functions
	The ego has many functions, including: Cognition Perception (sensory capacity) Regulation of mood/emotion/affect Interpersonal style Unconscious defense mechanisms (repression, denial, and so on) Coping (Conscious appraisal of perceived stressors) Judgment Memory

BOX 8-5	Stages of Life
	Individual
	Infant
	Toddler
	Preschool
	School-age
	Adolescent
	Young Adult
	Mid-life adult
	Older adult
	Infirm adult
	Family
	Courtship
	Early married
	Married without children
	Married with preschool or school age children
	Married with adolescent and separating children
	Mid-life
	Married with adult children
	Elderly, well functioning
	Elderly, infirm

MALADAPTATION

The result of chronic, ineffective individual or family coping. The health of the person is chronically or permanently altered. Mental or physical disorder can result. Maladaptation results in greater demands on the person's biological, psychological, social, and spiritual resources. Homeostasis is disrupted (3–7, 9–11, 15–28).

CRISIS

A state in which the normal resources of an individual are overwhelmed by stressors. Ineffective coping or physical illness occurs. Depending on the strength of the stressors and the strength of the resources, the following outcomes can occur (3–7, 9–11, 15–29):

1. Health (effective coping/adaptation and physical well-being) is restored.
2. Acute physical illness (leading to possibility of chronic illness) occurs.
3. Ineffective coping (leading to possibility of maladaptation) which can lead to mental disorder.
4. Death.

CONTINUUM OF HEALTH OUTCOMES

Figure 8-1 depicts the continuum of possible biopsychosocial primary and secondary outcomes to a threatening stressor.

When confronted by a threatening stressor, it is possible that the individual will cope effectively and health will result. Another possibility is that the internal and/or external resources will not provide adequate resistance. The body's resistance is decreased as the result of risk factors. The primary outcome of inadequate resistance is ineffective coping and the development or continuation of physical illness or death.

Nursing assessment, diagnosis, and intervention, as well as nurse-initiated collaborative diagnosis and treatment with other health care providers, is appropriate anywhere in the continuum of responses to threatening stressors. Each of the possible primary outcomes can respond to nursing intervention.

Ineffective coping and physical illness require assessment of and intervention with the patient and family. If stressors persist and are stronger than the resources and the interventions, secondary outcomes of maladaptation can occur in the form of continuing or secondary illnesses, ineffective coping that can lead to mental disorder in the individual and/or other family members, or death. If death occurs, intervention with the family can reduce the possibility of health changes in other family members.

The nursing assessment can be initiated with the Barry Psychosocial Assessment Interview Schedule, which is based on Gordon's Functional Health Patterns (see Chapters 12 and 13). When nursing problems are diagnosed, the documentation includes:

1. Manifestation or symptoms of the problems.
2. Risk factors contributing to each problem.
3. Nursing interventions that can support the resources and reduce or eliminate the risk factors.
4. Final patient outcomes that will indicate resolution of the problem.
5. Intermediate outcomes that will indicate progression toward the final outcome.

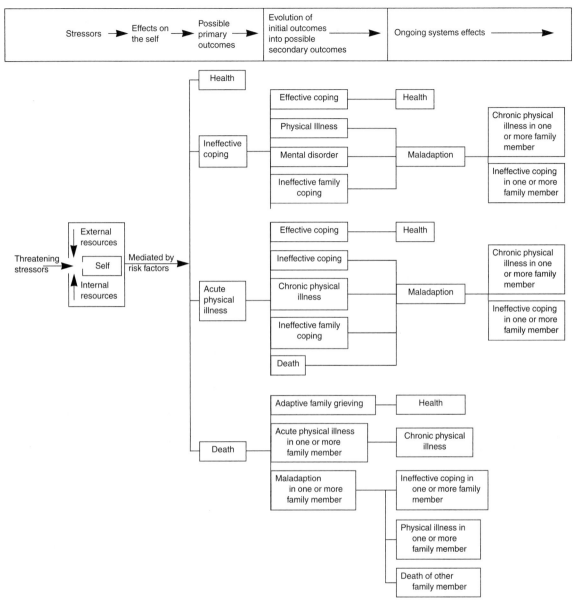

FIGURE 8-1. Continuum of human responses: Health outcomes of threatening stressors.

CONCLUSION

This conceptual model of the psychosocial nursing process with hospitalized and home care patients has been presented to give a formal structure on which to develop nursing assessment, diagnosis, care planning, intervention, and evaluation of outcome with patients and family members who are in the process of psychosocial adjustment to physical illness. It is a model that can help to connect and actualize the theory presented in other chapters.

Although time constraints in the actual clinical setting may prevent formal evaluation of each patient and family member in this step-by-step manner, this framework can assist in the development of patients' care plans using the nursing process, particularly when ineffective coping or maladaptation are potential or actual problems.

BIBLIOGRAPHY

Alfaro-LeFevre, R. (1994). *Applying nursing process*. Philadelphia: J. B. Lippincott.

American Heritage college dictionary (3rd ed.). (1993). Boston: Houghton-Mifflin.

Artinian, B. M. (1991). The development of the Intersystem Model. *Journal of Advanced Nursing Practice, 16*(2), 194–205.

Barry, P. D. (1994). *Mental health and mental illness* (5th ed.). Philadelphia: J. B. Lippincott.

Becket, N. (1991). Clinical nurses' characterizations of patient coping problems. *Nursing Diagnosis, 2*(2), 72–78.

Bock, G. R., & Whelan, J. (Eds.). (1991). *The childhood environment and adult disease*. New York: Wiley.

Boykin, A. (Ed.). (1994). *Living a caring-based program*. New York: National League for Nursing.

Boykin, A., & Schoenhofer, S. (1993). *Nursing as caring: A model for transforming practice*. New York: National League for Nursing Press.

Bulechek, G. M., & McCloskey, J. C. (1992). Defining and validating nursing interventions. *Nursing Clinics of North America, 27*(2), 289–299.

Burney, M. A. (1992). King and Neuman: In search of the nursing paradigm. *Journal of Advanced Nursing, 17*(5), 601–603.

Burns, C., Archbold, P., Stewart, B., & Shelton, K. (1993). New diagnosis: Caregiver role strain. *Nursing Diagnosis, 4*(2), 70–76.

Burns, N., & Grove, S. K. (1993). *The practice of nursing research: Conduct, critique and utilization* (2nd ed.). Philadelphia: W. B. Saunders.

Burr, W. R. (1991). Rethinking levels of abstraction in family systems theories. *Family Processes, 30*(4), 435–452.

Campbell, R. J. (1989). *Psychiatric dictionary* (6th ed.). New York: Oxford University Press.

Carboni, J. T. (1992). Instrument development and the measurement of unitary constructs. *Nursing Science Quarterly, 5*(3), 134–142.

Carpenito, L. J. (Ed.). (1991). *Nursing care plans and documentation: Nursing diagnosis and collaborative problems*. Philadelphia: J. B. Lippincott.

Carpenito, L. J. (Ed.). (1993). *Nursing diagnosis: Application to clinical practice* (5th ed.). Philadelphia: J. B. Lippincott.

Cassem, N. H. (1991). Depression. In N. H. Cassem (Ed.), *Massachusetts General Hospital handbook of general hospital psychiatry* (3rd ed.). St. Louis: Mosby Year Book.

Charney, D. S., Deutch, A. Y., Krystal, J. H., Southwick, S. M., & Davis, M. (1993). Psychobiologic mechanisms of posttraumatic stress disorder. *Archives of General Psychiatry, 50*(4), 295–305.

Chaska, N. L. (Ed.). (1990). *The nursing profession: Turning points*. St. Louis: Mosby Year Book.

Dewsbury, D. A. (1991). Psychobiology. *American Psychologist, 46*(3), 198–205.

Diagnostic criteria from DSM-IV. (1994). Washington, DC: American Psychiatric Press.

Donley, M. G. (1993). Attachment and the emotional unit. *Family Process, 32*(1), 3–20.

Edlin, G., & Golanty, E. (1992). *Health and wellness: A holistic approach* (4th ed.). Boston: Jones & Bartlett.

Estes, N., Smith-Dijulo, K., & Heinemann, M. (1980). *Nursing diagnosis of the alcoholic person*. St. Louis: C. V. Mosby.

Fawcett, J. (1984). The metaparadigm of nursing: Present status and future refinements. *Image: The Journal of Nursing Scholarship, 16*(3), 84.

Fitzpatrick, J. I., & Whall, A. L. (Eds.). (1989). *Conceptual models of nursing: Analysis and application* (2nd ed.). Norwalk, CT: Appleton & Lange.

Folkow, B. (1993). Physiological organization of neurohormonal responses to psychosocial stimuli: Implications for health and disease. *Annals of Behavioral Medicine, 15*(4), 236–243.

Friedman, M. M. (1992). *Family nursing: Theory and practice* (3rd ed.). Norwalk, CT: Appleton & Lange.

Frisch, N. (1993). Home care nursing and psychosocial-emotional needs. How nursing diagnosis helps to direct and inform practice. *Home Healthcare Nurse, 11*(2), 64–65, 70.

Gaut, D. A., & Boykin, A. (Eds.). (1994). *Caring as healing: Renewal through hope*. New York: National League for Nursing Press.

Gerteis, M., Edgman-Levitan, S., Daley, J., & Delbanco, T. L. (Eds.). (1993). *Through the patient's eyes: Understanding and promoting patient-centered care*. San Francisco: Jossey-Bass.

Goldberg, R. J., & Novack, D. H. (1992). The psychosocial review of systems. *Social Science and Medicine, 35*(3), 261–269.

Goldstein, M. G., & Niaura, R. (1992). Psychological factors affecting physical condition. Cardiovascular disease literature review. Part I: Coronary artery disease and sudden death. *Psychosomatics, 33*(2), 134–145.

Gordon, M. (1987). *Nursing diagnosis: Process and application*. New York: NcGraw-Hill.

Hall, L. E. (1963). Loeb Center for nursing. *Nursing Outlook, 11*, 805.

Hall, L. E. (1969). The Loeb Center for Nursing and Rehabilitation, Montefiore Hospital and Medical Center, Bronx, New York. *International Journal of Nursing Studies, 6*, 81–97.

Hall, L. E. (1964). Nursing: What is it? *Canadian Nurse, 60*, 150.

Halm, M. A., Titler, M. G., Kleiber, C., Johnson, S. K., Montgomery, L. A., Craft, M. J., Buckwalter, K., Nicholson, A., & Megivern, K. (1993). Behavioral responses of family members during critical illness. *Clinics in Nursing Research, 2*(4), 414–437.

Hartman, D., & Knudson, J. (1991). A nursing data base for initial patient assessment. *Oncology Nursing Forum, 18*(1), 125–130.

Harwood, A. (1981). *Ethnicity and medical care*. Cambridge, MA: Harvard University Press.

Heliker, D. (1992). Reevaluation of a nursing diagnosis: Spiritual distress. *Nursing Forum, 27*(4), 15–20.

Henderson, V. (1966). *The nature of nursing: A definition and its implication for practice, research and education.* New York: MacMillan.

Idill, S., Kelleher, K., & Shumaker, S. (1992). Psychosocial interventions in adult patients with coronary heart disease and cancer: A literature review. *General Hospital Psychiatry, 14*S: 28S–42S.

Johnson, E., Kamilaris, T., Chorous, B., & Gold, P. (1992). Mechanisms of stress: A dynamic overview of hormonal and behavioral homeostasis. *Neuroscience and Biobehavioral Reviews, 16*(2), 115–130.

Kaplan, H. I., & Sadock, B. J. (1994). *Synopsis of psychiatry: Behavioral sciences, clinical psychiatry* (7th ed.). Baltimore: Williams & Wilkins.

Kaplan, H. I., & Sadock, B. J. (1995). *Comprehensive textbook of psychiatry/VI* (6th ed.). Baltimore: Williams & Wilkins.

Kelly, M. P., & Sullivan, F. (1992). The productive use of threat in primary care: Behavioural responses to health promotion. *Family Practice, 9*(4), 476–480.

Lazarus, R. S. (1992). Coping with the stress of illness. *WHO Regional Publications, European Series, 44,* 11–31.

Leddy, S., & Pepper, J. (1993). *Conceptual bases of professional nursing.* Philadelphia: J. B. Lippincott.

Lederer, J. R., Marculescu, G. L., Mochik, B., & Seaby, N. (Eds.). (1991). *Care planning pocket guide: A nursing diagnosis approach* (4th ed.). Redwood City, CA: Addison-Wesley Nursing.

Leininger, M. (1991). Becoming aware of types of health practitioners and cultural imposition. *Journal of Transcultural Nursing, 2*(2), 32–39.

Leventhal, H., & Tomarken, A. (1987). Stress and illness: Perspectives from health psychology. In S. V. Kasl & C. L. Cooper (Eds.), *Stress and health: Issues in research methodology.* New York: John Wiley & Sons.

Levine, M. E. (1966). Trophicognosis: An alternative to nursing diagnosis. In *Exploring progress in medical surgical nursing practice.* New York: American Nurses' Association.

Levine, S. (1993). The influence of social factors on the response to stress. *Psychotherapy and Psychosomatics, 60*(1), 33–38.

Lipowski, Z. J. (1991). Consultation-liaison psychiatry 1990. *Psychotherapy and Psychosomatics, 55*(2–4), 62–68.

Loomis, M. E. (Ed.). (1992). *The Loomis/Wood model: Applying theory to nursing education, research, and practice.* New York: National League for Nursing Press.

Lundeen, S. P. (1992). Health needs of a suburban community: A nursing assessment. *Journal of Community Health Nursing, 9*(4), 235–244.

Malt, U. F., & Olafsen, O. M. (1992). Psychological appraisal and emotional response to physical injury: A clinical, phenomenological study of 109 adults. *Psychiatric Medicine, 10*(3), 117–134.

Mayer, G. G., Madden, M. J., & Lawrenz, E. (Eds.). (1990). *Patient care delivery models.* Rockville, MD: Aspen Publishers.

McCarthy, S. M., & Gallo, A. M. (1992). A case illustration of family management style. *Journal of Pediatric Nursing, 7*(6), 395–402.

McClowry, S. G. (1992). Family functioning during a critical illness: A systems theory perspective. *Critical Care Nursing Clinics of North America, 4*(4), 559–564.

McFarland, G. K., Wasli, E. L., & Gerety, E. K. (1992). *Nursing diagnoses and process in psychiatric mental health nursing* (2nd ed.). Philadelphia: J. B. Lippincott.

McGoldrick, M., & Gerson, R. (1985). *Genograms in family assessment.* New York: W. W. Norton.

McHaffie, H. E. (1992). The assessment of coping. *Clinics in Nursing Research, 1*(1), 67–79.

Moyers, W. (1993). *Healing and the mind.* New York: Doubleday.

Murray, B. B. (1991). Confusion, delirium, and dementia. In N. H. Cassem (Ed.), *Massachusetts General Hospital handbook of general hospital psychiatry* (3rd ed.). St. Louis: Mosby Year Book.

Nagel, T. (1993). What is the mind-body problem? *Ciba Foundation Symposium, 174,* 1–7.

Neuman, B. (1989). *The Neuman systems model* (2nd ed.). Norwalk, CT: Appleton & Lange.

Newberry, B. H., Jaikins-Madden, J. E., & Gerstenberger, T. J. (1991). *A holistic conceptualization of stress and disease.* New York: AMS Press.

Niaura, R., & Goldstein, M. B. (1992). Psychological factors affecting physical condition. Cardiovascular disease literature review. Part II: Coronary artery disease and sudden death and hypertension. *Psychosomatics, 33*(2), 146–155.

Orem, D. E. (1991). *Nursing: Concepts of practice* (4th ed.). St. Louis: Mosby Year Book.

Pagana, K. D., & Pagana, T. J. (1994). *Diagnostic testing and nursing implications: A case study approach* (4th ed.). St. Louis: Mosby Year Book.

Parker, M. (1993). *Patterns of nursing theories in practice.* New York: National League for Nursing Press.

Peplau, H. E. (1952). *Interpersonal relations in nursing.* New York: G. P. Putnam's Sons.

Pinkley, C. L. (1991). Exploring NANDA's definition of nursing diagnosis: Linking diagnostic judgments with the selection of outcomes and interventions. *Nursing Diagnosis, 2*(1), 26–32.

Pollock, S. E. (1993). Adaptation to chronic illness: A program of research for testing nursing theory. *Nursing Science Quarterly, 6*(2), 86–92.

Potter, P. A., & Perry, A. G. (1993). *Fundamentals of nursing: Concepts, process, and practice* (3rd ed.). St. Louis: Mosby Year Book.

Raya, A., Mantas, J., Priami, M., Andrea, S., Kalokerinou, A., Androulaki, O., Brokalaki, H., Halkiadaki, H., & Matziou, V. (1991). Psychosomatic nursing assessment of psychiatric patients. *Psychotherapy and Psychosomatics, 56*(1–2), 5–11.

Recker, D., & O'Brien, C. (1992). Using Gordon's functional health patterns to organize a critical care orientation program. *Focus on Critical Care, 19*(1), 21–25, 28.

Reeder, F. (1994). Rituals of healing: Ever ancient, ever new. In D. Gaut & A. Boykin (Eds.), *Caring as healing: Renewal through hope.* New York: National League for Nursing.

Rogers, C. (1961). *On becoming a person.* Boston: Houghton-Mifflin.

Rooda, L. (1993). Knowledge and attitudes of nurses toward culturally different patients: Implications for nursing education. *Journal of Nursing Education, 32*(5), 209–213.

Sadler, J. Z., & Hulgus, Y. F. (1992). Clinical problem-solving and the biopsychosocial model. *American Journal of Psychiatry, 149*(10), 1315–1323.

Savage, P. (1991). Patient assessment in psychiatric nursing. *Journal of Advanced Nursing, 16*(3), 311–316.

Smith, L. B., & Thelen, E. (Eds.). (1993). *A dynamic systems approach to development: Applications.* Cambridge: MIT Press.

Smolan, R., Moffitt, P., & Naythons, M. (1990). *The power to heal.* New York: Prentice Hall Press.

Stevens-Barnum, B. (1994). *Nursing theory: Analysis, application, evaluation.* Philadelphia: J. B. Lippincott.

Suddarth, D. S. (Ed.). (1991). *The Lippincott manual of nursing practice* (5th ed.). Philadelphia: J. B. Lippincott.

Thomas, C. L. (Ed.). (1993). *Taber's cyclopedic medical dictionary* (17th ed.). Philadelphia: F. A. Davis.

Timby, B. K., & Lewis, L. W. (1992). *Fundamental skills and concepts in patient care* (5th ed.). Philadelphia: J. B. Lippincott.

Toman, W. (1976). *Family constellation* (3rd ed.). New York: Springer-Verlag.

Tucker, S. M., Canobbio, M. M., Paquette, E. V., & Wells, M. F. (Eds.). (1992). *Patient care standards: Nursing process, diagnosis, and outcome* (5th ed.). St. Louis: Mosby Year Book.

Weber, G. J. (1991). Nursing diagnosis: A comparison of nursing textbook approaches. *Nurse Educator, 16*(2), 22–27.

Weisman, A. D. (1991). Coping with illness. In N. H. Cassem (Ed.), *Massachusetts General Hospital handbook of general hospital psychiatry* (3rd ed.). St. Louis: Mosby Year Book.

Welch, L. (1979). Planned change in nursing: The theory. *Nursing Clinics of North America, 14*, 307.

CHAPTER 9

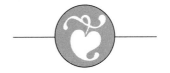

Major Coping Risks Associated With Physical Illness

Patricia Barry

Admission to a hospital is a threatening experience for most people. It can be an anxious time for family members, sometimes even more so than for the patient, who, because of the illness, may not be fully aware of what is happening.

Patients and families are understandably anxious about hospitalization or about coping with a threatening health condition. They are new experiences for most; the outcomes may be uncertain. Accordingly, they may need support in coping with the stress of illness or hospitalization. In order to help them in a meaningful way, nurses can be aware of the many underlying reasons for their emotional stress.

In understanding why people react as they do to becoming ill and being admitted to the hospital, it is helpful to be aware of the personality theories covered in the preceding chapters. Ideally, all people pass through the stages of personality development with no problem. Realistically, no one does. That is what makes each person unique. The personality traits a person carries into adulthood are the result of unconscious mental processes and psychological defenses within the personality that are the products of conflicts and crises that occurred in childhood and adolescence (Bock & Whelan, 1991; Noshpitz & Coddington, 1990; Pine, 1990; Smith & Thelen, 1993).

Patients and their family members have the potential to cope ineffectively with physical illness because of unresolved developmental conflicts. The risk of ineffective coping and possible maladaptation depends on a variety of factors:

1. The genetic disposition of the child, i.e., calm, hot-blooded, vigilant.
2. The degree of intrapsychic conflict the patient experienced during childhood development.
3. His or her normal coping style.
4. The level of stress experienced by the patient and family during the prior 1 to 2 years.
5. The level of threat this illness represents to the patient.
6. The way this illness and hospitalization awaken the old, unresolved emotional conflicts of childhood.

Patricia Barry: *Psychosocial Nursing: Care of Physically Ill Patients and Their Families,* 3rd ed.
© 1996 Lippincott–Raven Publishers

7. The way the hospital caregiving system responds to the patient.
8. The defensive ability of the patient's mind and body to help him or her cope with these experiences (Bock & Whelan, 1991; Dohms & Metz, 1991; Fisher et al., 1992; Woods, Habaerman, & Packard, 1993).

For example, a patient whose early personality development was frustrated at an important stage may, on admission, appear quite normal. If his illness can be easily treated, if his hospitalization is brief, if his family is supportive, if the hospital care system is able to meet his physical and emotional needs, and if his mind is able to cope with his experiences, this patient should have an uneventful hospitalization and adaptation can be ensured.

On the other hand, if one or more negative situations occur, such as a life-threatening illness, a complicated hospitalization, a demoralizing family, or an indifferent hospital care system, the risk of ineffective coping rises proportionately (Dohms & Metz, 1991; Fisher et al., 1992; Franks, Campbell, & Shields, 1992). It is as if the underlying and normally unobservable personality conflicts are similar to cracks in the foundation of a house. The cracks may never be a problem under normal conditions, but if the house is subjected to the stress of an earthquake, it may be seriously affected. So, too, can a normal person be seriously affected if the intensity of the stress he or she experiences as a result of physical illness is severe.

MAJOR DEVELOPMENTAL ISSUES

The unresolved conflicts referred to above occur as the individual's personality develops. These conflicts are left over from the major stages of early personality development. Erik Erikson's developmental theories were introduced in Chapter 3. He believed that there are major development hurdles one must work through in order to proceed to the next level of personality development. There can be varying degrees of frustration in working through each of these stages.

According to Erikson, the process of development does not stop when a partial block occurs. Instead, the personality proceeds to the next stage of development. The fixation remains, however, and may influence the succeeding developmental stages. When a stressful event occurs in adulthood and, because of its similarity to an earlier event, reawakens the original conflict, the psyche may have trouble adapting to the new demand. Being ill, obtaining medical attention, being admitted to the hospital, recovering from illness, and adjusting to the family's response, all events that occur in the illness continuum process, are stressors with the potential of awakening unresolved conflicts from earlier stages of development. The seriousness of the current coping response will depend on the seriousness of the earlier unresolved problem.

The potential areas of conflict that often present challenges in adaptation for the patient are trust, shame, self-esteem, control, loss, guilt, and intimacy. The cause of maladaptation can usually be traced to one or more of these major issues that continues to cause intrapsychic conflict for the individual or family member.

Two of the most common manifestations of ineffective coping and maladaptation are depression and anxiety (Cassem, 1991a; Rosenbaum & Pollock, 1991). It is important to be aware, however, that anxiety and depression are also adaptive processes when they are not prolonged or severe. They can motivate the patient to take action to resolve the underlying conflict causing the unpleasant feelings.

When ineffective coping develops into severe depression or anxiety in a patient, it is important to alert the attending physician that psychiatric consultation is indicated. Objective data, such as changes in sleep patterns, activity level, and vital signs, can be used to validate the recommendation. The physician can then request a formal psychiatric consultation. If the depression or anxiety is not severe, the nurse can intervene with the patient to promote a more positive coping outcome.

In order to work successfully with a patient's ineffective coping it is important to understand the nature of the patient's problem. Understanding the basic personality theories presented in earlier chapters—the use of defense mechanisms, normal personality styles, and underlying issues that confront the patient—is an important aid to developing insight about the dynamics involved and the probable cause of the problem (Groves & Kurcharski).

Effective or ineffective coping is related to more than developmental issues. Particular illnesses or conditions can, by their nature, impose severe stress on a person's coping ability (Feldstein & Rait, 1992; Halm et al., 1993; Harrison & Cole, 1991). For example, a person with severe burns has a condition that presents a significant coping challenge for anyone, no matter how psychologically "healthy" he or she may be (Welch, 1991). With severe illness, unresolved conflicts from earlier developmental stages can affect the patient's stress level (Groves & Kurcharski, 1991). Consider how coping with severe burns would impact the developmental issues of trust, shame, self-esteem, control, loss, guilt, and intimacy. Each of these issues is additionally compounded when family and caregiving staff relations are considered (O'Connor, 1991).

The major issues presenting adaptation challenges for patients are described in the order of their appearance during normal psychological development. Examples of patients' problems in each major area of development, and interventions to support and promote adaptation are included.

TRUST

When an adult has trouble trusting other people or dealing with new situations, the roots of distrust lie in the first year of life (Erikson, 1963). The child's first experience with trust is the way the environment responds to her. She does not know specifically who is doing something to make her feel good, but during the first few months of life she needs food and physical comfort, which includes being held and feeling loved. In fact, the food and physical comfort are inseparable in her mind. If these needs are consistently unmet, the child feels unsatisfied. Her brain is unable to reason, but the effect is that an adequate level of trust in the environment is never established (Bock & Whelan, 1991; Goodyer, 1990; Smith & Thelen, 1993).

Caregivers, one hopes, try to meet infants' needs. Sometimes, because of their own inability to give love or because of an infant's unusually high level of demand, the caregiver is not able to meet the needs of the infant that are basic to achieving an adequate level of trust (Bock & Whelan, 1991; Goodyer, 1990; Smith & Thelen, 1993). Erikson has described the developmental challenge of the first year of life as the achievement of trust. If it is not fully attained, the child will develop with a sense of distrust, a lack of hope, and a lack of drive (1963).

Mahler (1974) describes the developmental process of the infant's establishment of trust in her studies of the first 2 years of life. The infant's major hurdle in this process, the ability to trust her mother, occurs during the differentiation stage of ages 5 to 10 months. A child who feels comfortable with her mother will generalize these feelings to the environment at large.

When a person is hospitalized, his adaptation is challenged because he is repeatedly thrust into situations with which he has no experience. He is expected, however to have trust in each of these new situations (Groves & Kurcharski, 1991). He has to trust the people in his environment with his physical well-being. In many instances he places his life in their hands, despite the fact that he does not even know them.

In today's world of medical subspecialties, the patient's physician may be a specialist who is assigned rather than one chosen by the patient. Think for a moment what this means to a patient admitted for major surgery. The physicians in charge of the case perform many vital functions. They direct the patient's overall care, although the patient really does not know how competent they are. They prescribe medications. The patient may not know the contents of the pills prescribed, or the competency of the physician who orders them, the pharmacist who prepares them, or the nurse who administers them. The attending physician may ask other physicians to consult. The patient must trust these physicians' judgments as well.

The patient must trust his body's ability to get well. Most people rarely think about their body functions; they take them for granted until they fail to work. In addition, the patient must trust himself to cope psychologically with the stress of illness.

When the nurse gives care, the patient's ability to trust again is challenged. The nurse performs many procedures for the patient.

The patient really cannot be certain that the nurse knows her job. When a nurse says, "Roll over to the edge of the bed. Don't worry, I won't let you fall," how does a patient feel?

Another common example of a patient's uncertainty about trusting arises in the care of surgical patients. When the postsurgical thoracotomy or laparotomy patient is told that he must cough, he is frightened that his stitches will break loose. Yet he is reassured that they will hold. His ability to trust is difficult at this time. He is feeling very vulnerable. He will experience the same difficulty when he must ambulate for the first time.

The patient's ability to trust is also threatened when she is receiving care from other caregivers. For example, the recent stroke patient being supported by a physical therapist knows that if the therapist lets go she will fall and injure herself. Other examples are the patient with arthritis who is twisted into uncomfortable positions and left alone on a cold table in a dark room while the x-ray technician takes films, and the patient in acute respiratory distress who is intubated or has a tracheotomy with an automatic breathing device—she may apprehensively watch technicians and therapists manipulate dials to change her oxygen intake.

When a person is admitted to the hospital, there is little opportunity for gradual adaptation to the abrupt change in environment (Rosenbaum & Grove, 1991). Some hospital departments provide orientation programs for patients before they are admitted. For example, children anticipating surgery and parents anticipating birth are frequently taken on tours of the areas where they will be cared for as a way of reducing anxiety during hospitalization.

In most other instances, the patient and family members are suddenly thrust into a frightening, unexpected, and dependent situation. If an individual is admitted without warning for major surgery, his or her coping abilities may be severely stressed (Surman, 1991). The patient has lost the safety and security of home. The availability of known and trusted family members is interrupted. All patients are potentially at risk for ineffective coping because of difficulty in trusting. If a patient has defense mechanisms that assist his or her coping ability, there will be no outward signs of increased stress due to problems in trusting.

Most at risk for maladaptation due to distrust is the patient with a suspicious personality style. If the continuum of suspiciousness approaches paranoia, he will require strong support from the care system in order to tolerate the stress of hospitalization. The nursing care approaches described in Chapter 14 can be used with such individuals (Kahana & Bibring, 1964; Noshpitz & Coddington, 1990; Smith & Thelen, 1993).

SHAME

The experience of *shame* is one of the most painful emotions known by humans (Karen, 1992). The original psychic injury caused by shame is experienced in early childhood when a child is either unacknowledged by a parent or is reprimanded in a manner that implies that a child is "bad" (Kaufman, 1989; Morrison, 1989; Nathanson, 1987). Shame is a feeling about the self (Karen, 1992).

In most individuals primitive shame is a deeply repressed emotion. Indeed, most adults are not generally aware of the effects of shame in their lives. Most crucial life decisions are often made with unconscious vigilance about whether there are adequate inner resources to balance the resulting shame if failure occurs. When an adult experience causes the feeling of shame to occur, it may trigger repressed shame. When repressed shame is activated, the individual may feel psychologically and physically frozen, unable to defend against the powerful emotion.

Physical illness and hospitalization can sometimes activate old memories of shame. Certain physical conditions such as body-altering surgeries, congenital conditions, neurological or musculoskeletal conditions, and sexually transmitted diseases may evoke such a response.

CASE EXAMPLE

Rita is a 29-year-old, single female who experienced major conflict as a child with her father. He used a demeaning, abusive manner in talking with his wife and female children. Rita was offended by his behavior when she was a child; she frequently attempted to protect her mother and sister from his cruel remarks by actively challenging him. The result was that she experienced excessive emotional abuse from him.

As a young adult, Rita was exposed to herpes genitalia. She had a mild case and had been asymptomatic for 3 years. Although she was a beautiful and very pleasant young woman, she stopped dating after the initial symptoms occurred. She had also determined that "no one will ever marry me with this condition." She was unable to perceive herself other than as diseased and worthless. ❦

It is not uncommon for physical conditions that impact on sexuality to cause shame-related responses as described above. Some of these conditions include mastectomy, ostomy surgeries, infertility treatment, and impotence related to diabetes mellitus, prostatectomy, or antihypertensive medication. Caregivers who work in home-care settings can sensitively include questions about sexuality in their assessments. Partners are frequently affected by these issues as well. Strong avoidance patterns may occur in each member of a couple. Such avoidance is usually related to suppressed or repressed shame.

When shame occurs it is often concealed by the patient or family member. Sensitive discussion by the nurse can often begin the process of exploring and releasing the painful affect. Without intervention, such shame can have debilitating effects on a person's sense of worth as an individual and in relationships. Unacknowledged, it can severely inhibit future risk-taking and autonomy (Karen, 1992; Nathanson, 1987).

SELF-ESTEEM

Self-esteem is an essential issue that affects everyone. The personality characteristics that result from the other major issues discussed in this chapter remain fairly constant in the personality once they are formed in childhood. Self-esteem is more subject to temporary changes because of the patient's sensitivity to the reactions of family members and the larger social system. Others' reactions combine with the patient's own view of him or herself and can cause self-esteem to fluctuate (Baumeister,

Heatherton, & Tice, 1993; Epstein, 1992; Greenberg et al., 1992; O'Brien, 1993).

The development of self-esteem begins shortly after birth. The infant gradually becomes aware of her body; this helps to form the basis of her self-perception. The most important influence on the way a child perceives herself is how her parents and other important people interact with her (Buss, 1991). These important persons in a child's environment are called *objects* in some theoretical models of personality development (Buss, 1991; Pine, 1990). The way a child interacts with these significant persons forms the basis of all her future relationships. These early ways of relating with others are termed *object relations*. As she grows to toddlerhood, the way she behaves or appears influences the reactions of those around her. The child's ego develops as a result of her relationships with these important "objects."

If her family and friends are loving and approving, she will internalize their positive opinions and they develop into positive self-esteem. Accordingly, if these important individuals do not value her, but ignore, criticize, and reject her, this can lead to negative self-esteem. *Self-esteem* is the way a person feels about and values herself; it is a self-measurement of one's sense of worth.

Self-esteem is described as "being on good terms with one's superego" (Campbell, 1989). In addition to containing moralistic judgments about one's actions, the superego comprises one's own "positive stroking" ability, which enables a person to value herself even when criticized by others.

When people are able to value themselves in spite of others' input, they are described as having good *narcissistic supplies* (Pine, 1990). These are internal, intrapsychic sources of positive self-worth, primarily acquired during the first several years of life. The term is derived from Narcissus, a young man in Greek mythology who fell in love with his own reflection in a pool and was unable to love others because of his exaggerated self-love. Narcissism in toddlerhood is a normal and healthy occurrence. The child values herself very highly. Her behavior serves her own needs, and she is quite unaware of the needs of others. This gives way to normal, give-and-take social relationships as she grows older. When narcissism persists into adulthood, it is considered pathological (Pine, 1990).

There is a critical difference between being narcissistic and having good narcissistic supplies. The former is a negative personality style in adults; it denotes a self-centered, self-serving individual who has little or no awareness of the results of his actions on others. The latter helps to maintain self-esteem and is a desired ability. When a person's psyche is functioning properly, these supplies are usually present (Pine, 1990).

Self-esteem is maintained through drawing on one's own intrapsychic narcissistic supplies and, second, through looking to the social environment. The drawbacks to the second source of self-esteem maintenance are evident. What if no one in the environment gives positive feedback? Ideally all people have family, friends, and coworkers who are kind and complimentary; however, this is frequently not so. If a person lacks an internal ability to nourish his esteem, he becomes dependent on the people in his environment to do it for him. This can impose a burden on relationships. Think of acquaintances who are frequently "fishing" for compliments. They need to obtain from the environment what they lack in themselves. Unconsciously, they are trying to build up their self-esteem to a more comfortable level.

Self-esteem is not constant; it can change daily. There are usually not wide swings in self-esteem in the same person; however, external events, if seriously damaging to a person's sense of worth and stirring old feelings of shame, can temporarily undermine a normally good level of self-esteem. Narcissistic supplies, if strong, are usually able to help the person adapt to such an occurrence (Baum & Page, 1991; Buss, 1991; Goodyer, 1990; Lasky, 1993).

Persons with any type of illness experience such a challenge. Any type of illness is a threat to the self. The result can be a change in the way a person feels about himself. Physically ill people often experience a temporary change in their feelings about themselves and an accompanying decrease in their self-esteem (Feldstein & Rait, 1992; Halm et al., 1993; Harrison & Cole, 1991; O'Brien, 1993). Some conditions sparking lowered self-esteem are myocardial infarction and cardiac

surgery, cancer, amputation, chronic disease of any kind, stroke, diabetes mellitus, peptic ulcer, colitis, colostomy, skin disease, and burns. If patients do not overcome the negative potential of these assaults to self-esteem, it may be difficult to participate fully in life. Poor self-esteem is one of the main dynamics in depression (DSM-IV, 1994). Unless a person is able to achieve a more realistic view of himself, a chronic depressive state may result (Cassem, 1991a).

The unconscious or conscious need to maintain or improve self-esteem is the basic motivating force in human beings (Kaplan & Sadock, 1995). Abraham Maslow's theory, presented in Chapter 3, describes the drive of a person to achieve full potential (1970). The ability to pursue one's full development is closely associated with maintenance of self-esteem. The nurse's ability to detect the evidence of poor self-esteem in patients is important. Positive emotional support from the nurse may provide external stability for the patient's self-esteem until his or her own resources return.

Gates (1978) conceptualized self-esteem by dividing it into four separate components:

1. *The body self.* This component contains both the body image (how a person feels about the way his body looks, feels, and functions) and a person's thoughts and feelings about being able to perform basic functions.
2. *The interpersonal self.* This part of self-esteem contains a person's thoughts and feelings about the way he or she relates to others in both intimate and casual relationships.
3. *The achieving self.* This section includes a person's thoughts and feelings about his or her ability to obtain goals in family, work, and school environments.
4. *The identification self.* This aspect of self-esteem contains abstract feelings and behaviors that are involved with moral and spiritual concerns.

By considering the impact a specific illness can have on one or more of these components, it is possible to understand the threat of illness to the self-esteem of patients and their families. Some manifestations of poor self-esteem in hospitalized patients include the patient who is too compliant; she asks no questions about her care. Because of her poor self-worth, she may complacently accept all recommendations for treatment without being fully informed or understanding the justification for them. The patient may seem to view herself as a nonperson in the presence of authority figures (Epstein, 1992; Greenberg et al., 1992; O'Brien, 1993).

An example of a collective form of poor self-esteem is the family of a patient who is too ill or too young to become involved in his own care. For example, a patient with an unusual disease may be subjected to excessive tests or procedures that will provide little benefit, yet the family does not question caregivers about them. Another instance is a terminal patient in severe pain whose caregivers' highest priority is to avoid addiction (although the patient is close to death). The family members may not act to defend their loved one from an impersonal care system. Fortunately, most hospitals have caregivers who will promote the patient's rights if they see abuses. The role of patient and family advocate is frequently and unofficially filled by nursing staff members (Bouckoms & Hackett, 1991; Cassem, 1991b; Stewart, 1991; Weisman, 1991).

Poor self-esteem in families can sometimes be partially attributed to lack of knowledge about how to negotiate in a hospital care system. On occasion, when an acutely ill patient is not fully conscious or is too young to understand the aspects of his care, the attending physician may not communicate with family members about the patient's current clinical condition and short-term treatment plan. Family members have a right to obtain this information directly from the attending physician.

Occasionally, nurses may listen to family members who are angry that the attending physician is not informing them about their loved one's condition. When this occurs, the nurse should avoid becoming embroiled in the problem and refrain from making frequent excuses for the attending physician. Instead, the family's right to obtain this information directly from the physician who is overseeing the patient's care can be encouraged (Bouckoms & Hackett, 1991; Cassem, 1991b; Stewart, 1991; Weisman, 1991).

While caring for patients, the nurse can be aware of the potential short- and long-term damage to self-esteem that illness can cause. With the person who has positive self-esteem that has been temporarily lowered due to illness and a resulting change in self-image, the nurse has many opportunities to promote adaptation. If the patient is given the opportunity to talk about her feelings, she may be able to talk out her own doubts and resolve some of her concerns. By giving honest responses to her doubts and also by describing other patients who have successfully overcome the same conditions, you may help her to feel more self-confident (Epstein, 1992; Greenberg et al., 1992; O'Brien, 1993; Viemero, 1991).

BODY IMAGE

Body image, which is closely related to self-esteem, is the way a person thinks and feels about his or her body as a whole, its various parts, its functions, and the internal and external sensations associated with it. It also includes the person's perceptions of the way others see his or her body. It is possible that an infant's early awareness about his body causes the ego and all its functions to begin development (Freud, 1933; Mahler, 1974).

Body image development is a complex, lifelong process that is closely linked to the development of identity. In fact, it is impossible to separate the two. Body image theory is of great interest to nurses because it deals with the patient's view of his or her body and its functioning at every point of the health-sickness-recovery continuum. (Many theories have been combined to form this section: Engel, 1968; Erikson, 1963; Freud, 1933; Kaplan & Sadock, 1994; Mahler, 1974; Stewart, 1991; Surman, 1991; Weisman, 1991.)

Like self-esteem, body image begins to develop shortly after birth. The newborn infant is not aware of any separation between his own body boundaries and the environment around him. In infancy he becomes aware of where his body ends and, for example, his mother's body begins. A sense of separateness forms. The infant also is unconsciously aware that his mouth helps his body to feel pleasure (Buss, 1991;

Erikson, 1963; Goodyer, 1990; Smith & Thelen, 1993).

A very important factor in the child's development of positive body image and self-esteem is the amount of touching received from caregivers. The need to be touched continues throughout life. Most hospitalized patients have deep, unconscious needs to be touched caringly. Others, frequently as a result of abuse during childhood, are highly resistant to being touched (Bensman, Winters, & Kizilos, 1992; Herman, 1992). The sensitive nurse will be able to detect such resistance by observing eye and posture responses of the patient.

As the infant develops coordination during the second half of the first year, he becomes aware, again unconsciously, that he has a degree of control over his body. This awareness increases through toddlerhood. It has both conscious and unconscious elements (Erikson, 1963; Jensen, Turner, & Romano, 1991; Lasky, 1993).

There is strong interaction at this point between the child's body image and his self-esteem. If the social environment approves of the young child's efforts at body control, positive body image and positive self-esteem are bolstered. Body control efforts include sphincter control, walking, running, and manual dexterity.

Another important aspect of body control at this age is the reaction of authority figures—parents and relatives—to the child's exploration of his body. The child has insatiable curiosity about his own body and those of others. These are normal and healthy wonderings. As he feels the inside of his nose or discovers that it feels pleasant to touch his genitals, he is in the process of developing his body image (Bock & Whelan, 1991; Bullock, 1991; Goodyer, 1990; Smith & Thelen, 1993).

If the social environment is sternly disapproving, the child develops a sense that something is "bad" about his body. On the other hand, if no gentle constraints are placed on him, his ability to develop self-discipline and a sense of respect for his body will be distorted. If he is allowed to stand in the middle of a supermarket aisle picking his nose for 5 minutes, he will sense disapproval from the other shoppers without understanding why.

The child of 3 to 5 years is very aware of the physical differences between the sexes (Erikson, 1963; Smith & Thelen, 1993). Children are curious about who has and who does not have a penis. Little boys worry that they might lose their penis; little girls worry because they do not have one. The acceptance and approval of the parent of the opposite sex is important to the child's overall body concept. The same-sex parent's comfort with his or her own body is also very important to the child's overall body concept and forms the basis of gender identity.

The school-age child continues to be aware of sex differences, but predominately in a social way. Children's mastery of skills that were formerly stereotyped by sex helps them to feel good about their bodies. Cooking, ballet dancing, and figure skating were examples of typically female-role activities. For young boys, baseball, football, and ice hockey were and continue to be popular activities. Because of government mandates, all schools and public recreation programs today must offer equal opportunities to girls and boys. As a result, the opportunities for young girls to exercise actively and develop a healthy and confident sense of their bodies have increased markedly. With these changes in formal and physical education, there is an opportunity for children of both sexes to be exposed to many types of activities regardless of their gender identification (Berzonsky, 1992).

The adolescent's body image continues to develop as he has more opportunities to master skills. He learns to trust his body and feel that it is competent. The development of his body image is continually challenged by the physical changes of adolescence. He suddenly gains inches in height, his normally clear complexion begins to develop pimples, his facial and body hair is growing too quickly or too slowly and he feels different from his friends (girls share a similar type of anxiety in comparing their breast development), and changes in his genitals remind him that sexual activity is possible; his sexual drive is on a collision course with the values of his superego and authority figures.

All these changes cause an increase in self-doubt as his image of himself is alternately pleasing and then unacceptable. At various times he may accept or reject, love or hate, take for granted or be anxious about his body functions or overall appearance.

If a person of any age loses a body function that has always been taken for granted, it is quite common to go through a grieving process. The process is the same for the person adjusting to a change in his body: shock and denial, anger, bargaining, depression, and acceptance (Kubler-Ross, 1969). (These stages are described in this chapter in the subsection on loss.) Patients who experience the grieving process include those with burns, AIDS, cancer, cardiac disease, chronic illness, glandular disturbances, renal dialysis, hysterectomy, and amputations. If one part of the body is not functioning properly, it can color a person's feelings about his total body concept. If his image of only one part of his body is poor, it can also spill over and affect his self-esteem.

Another important concept in body image is a person's reaction to the aging process. The average person retains the appearance of youth until his or her mid-30s. After that, subtle changes in appearance and sensation signify that the aging process is underway: a few gray hairs, shortness of breath on exertion, joints that are not as limber, and muscles that ache after heavy exercise. There is a gradual loss of connective tissue; even a thin person develops a mild degree of flabbiness. There are changes in menstrual or sexual function. Wrinkles and other changes in appearance occur.

Awareness of these changes requires adjustment to a new image. This is another example of loss that requires adaptation. If the person's investment in his younger body image was strong, his reaction may resemble the grieving process described in the loss section of this chapter.

If a person maladapts to a major change in body image and develops low self-esteem, the result can be depression. One of the main dynamics in this depression is unresolved grief about the major change (Cassem, 1991a). This type of depression may begin in the hospital setting and can perhaps be averted by perceptive caregivers who allow the patient to talk about concerns (Surman, 1991). When the patient develops moderate to severe depression in the hospital as the result of a major change in body image, the nurse can suggest psychi-

atric consultation to the physician in order to help the person resolve his or her conflict.

Some patients are discharged home with no sign of depression, but it may develop as they become more aware of the loss of their normal functioning or appearance (Cassem, 1991a). Nurses who work in outpatient clinics, visiting nursing agencies, or physicians' offices can be watchful for clinically depressed patients and perform psychosocial assessment to determine the level of emotional dysfunction. If indicated, psychiatric referral can be recommended.

CONTROL

The ability to control what happens to oneself is important to most people: normal, independent adults know what they want and how to obtain it. Control also implies a certain sense of dominance over the environment. When a person is hospitalized, she defers much of her control to the dictates of the institution and various caregivers. Every patient therefore may be at risk for maladaptation because of lack of control over what is happening (Sherer, 1992; Small & Graydon, 1992; Terry, 1992; Weiner & Dodd, 1993).

Control becomes a major issue for the child between the ages of 2 and 3, the time when she is gaining mastery over her sphincters. A conflict occurs between the child and caregiver. The child wishes to maintain feelings of control over her urine and bowel movements. The needs of the caregiver and the environment at large are that she conform to social expectations. The way the caregiver ultimately wins the conflict will have a strong effect on the child's future perception of her control in new situations (Bock & Whelan, 1991; Engel, 1968; Kuhn, 1990; Smith & Thelen, 1993).

HELPLESSNESS (LACK OF CONTROL)

A related issue to control is lack of control, also called *helplessness* or *powerlessness*. The experience of helplessness has been described by Seligman (1991) as a learned state in which an individual experiences an inner response of defeat and powerlessness when challenged.

Barry (1991) hypothesizes that helplessness is a conditional physiological state that occurs as a response to an initial overwhelming and threatening event. The effect on the individual is a state of "freeze." The freeze state mimics the physiological responses of acute fear. Normal cognition and problem-solving skills are rendered powerless in the freeze state.

The experience of helplessness or powerlessness results either in a passive or dependent personality style when it is a pervasive personality characteristic. It also can be manifested when individuals are in emotionally overwhelming circumstances, such as being in a life-threatening situation or fearing the loss of a loved one.

When the characteristics of helplessness are present, regardless of whether the cause is an ongoing personality trait or a reactive state, it is important for the nurse to move into a more proactive, planning, interactive style. The patient or family operating in a helpless state will usually be unable to form plans that are fully self-supportive. When working with an individual or family who is experiencing helplessness, the nurse can assist in planning from an empathic posture. In exploring these options the nurse may recommend that specific aspects of the plan be followed. In other words, the nurse would take a stronger role in decision-making with this type of individual.

LOCUS OF CONTROL

Whether a person senses that events are under or outside of her control has been called locus of control. *Locus,* from the Latin, means *place* (*American Heritage College Dictionary,* 1993, p. 796). The term *locus of control* actually indicates the place to which a person attributes the cause and control of events in his or her life. Some people have an *internal locus of control.* They perceive events as within their control and believe that they have some power over their own response to events and at least some ability to modify environmental situations. Type-A individuals and people with controlled personality styles, as described in Chapter 14, have an internal locus of control. On the other hand, the person with an *external locus of control* perceives events as being outside his or her control and as being the result of fate, luck, chance, or powerful

others (Bullock, 1991). This is characteristic of people with dependent personality styles. The latter type of person tends to be more of a passive participant, believing that there is little he or she can do to change a situation.

Which type of person will be more at risk because of feeling that he or she has relinquished control? An internal locus of control person, who normally believes that she has control over events in her life, is potentially at risk because she has very little control in the hospital. Her diagnosis and prognosis, the outcome of hospitalization, and the actions of caregivers are all unpredictable. The following aspects of hospitalization are all ways in which the patient relinquishes control.

Relinquishing Clothes and Possessions

For some people, clothes and possessions are very important. Having to wear a hospital gown is a sudden, unexpected "leveler." They are unaccustomed to doing without this control factor. Remember that the way a person dresses often exerts a controlling influence on others' reactions to her.

Complying to New Schedules

The hospital system is notorious for disregarding people's normal schedules. The clock seems to control many aspects of a patient's care: when one must eat, sleep, urinate, and defecate; when one may or may not have pain medication, visitors, meals, and so on.

Being Subject to the Orders of Others

The patient is subjected to diagnostic tests of all kinds. Unless caregivers are sensitive to the patient's need to know what to expect, she may be ill-prepared for these events. Imagine the reaction of a frightened, mildly confused elderly individual to a bone marrow biopsy, or a computed tomography (CT) scan.

Undergoing Surgery

Anticipation of surgery is one of the most stressful times for all individuals, especially the orderly, controlled patient. Frequently, surgery is elective, so the patient must wait from a few days to several weeks for surgery to be performed. The waiting period can be very difficult. The patient is ambivalent. She wants to speed up the waiting period; at the same time she would like to forget the whole thing. The fear of anesthesia can be powerful. It signifies total loss of control. For some, it actively stirs fear of death. The patient cannot control events in the operating room. If something negative happens, she will not be awake to rectify it. Some patients worry that they may say something embarrassing as they emerge from anesthesia. Another realistic concern is when the surgery is exploratory or will involve a biopsy; the fear that a malignant tumor may be discovered and that while asleep parts of her body may be removed without full awareness can be very disturbing (Surman, 1991).

Being Subject to Invasive Procedures and Tubes

Another aspect of control that a patient loses is related to her own body boundary. When her normal body boundary is invaded, it may seem as if there no longer is a distinct sense of where her body begins and the environment ends; the tubes and other objects normally found in the environment are actually inserted into her body. They are inserted through the skin or the various natural or surgical openings in the body. Examples of these invasive lines are intravenous fluid and hyperalimentation, nasogastric and tracheal suctioning tubes, endotracheal tubes, central venous and arterial blood pressure lines, chest tubes, drainage tubes from various sites, gastrostomy and ureterostomy tubes inserted directly through the abdominal wall into internal organs, cardiac and other radiographic catheters, indwelling urinary catheters, and indwelling rectal temperature probes (Surman, 1991).

Some patients feel uneasy and insecure about the entrance of substances into their body. It is important to be aware of such uneasiness. In an intensive care unit, for example, it can be expected that this problem may contribute to a patient's anxiety, and the reason for the various tubes can be explained. The nurse can ask physicians for an appropriate

level of sedation if the patient maintains a high anxiety level. Without relief, high anxiety can develop into overwhelming panic or, occasionally, a paranoid psychotic reaction. In either case, the physiological state of the person is seriously compromised (Surman, 1991).

A patient who is permitted to control at least some aspects of the hospital environment may find it easier to accept his or her dependent status. With the patient who has a "controlling" type of personality, the nurse's sensitivity to anxiety over loss of control can make an important difference in whether adaptation or maladaptation to illness occurs.

LOSS

Loss is one of the most important issues any person has to adjust to during his or her lifetime. Object relations theory was discussed in Chapter 3 (Pine, 1990; Smith & Thelen, 1993). The emotional energy invested in an object originates with the pleasure-seeking and aggressive drives. For the young child, his original objects are his parents or other important caregivers. He forms affectionate bonds and attachments with them. As he matures, he is able to form relationships with others, the strength of which is based on the ability he demonstrated to form attachments with his parents. The strength of a person's attachment to an object will determine his reaction to the loss of that object (Bowlby, 1980).

The human being's normal goal is to establish bonds and relationships (Erikson, 1963; Freud, 1933). Accordingly, human behavior, from infancy through adulthood, is directed toward the goal of forming, maintaining, and defending against the loss of relationships.

Psychoanalytic theorists believe that only human beings can be classified as "objects." The energy invested in another person, the ability to relate to the other person, and the quality of that relationship are considered object relations (Pine, 1990). Other theorists consider any entity in which emotional energy is invested, not only other people, to be "objects." For example, a person can invest emotional energy in a job, a body that responds normally, a well-functioning heart, hair, a perfect baby, unmarked skin, working kidneys, or the ability to talk (Lasky, 1993; Smith & Thelen, 1993). In any case, whether the emotional investment is in another person, an aspect of one's self that is concrete or abstract, a job, or any other important entity, actual or threatened loss through the impact of illness can cause a maladaptive reaction.

> The goal of attachment behavior is to maintain an affectional bond; any situation that seems to be endangering the bond elicits action designed to preserve it; and the greater the danger of loss appears to be the more varied and intense are the actions elicited to prevent it [Bowlby, 1980, p. 42].

Grief and bereavement are closely related to loss, and sometimes the terms are used interchangeably. For clarification, *loss* is a change in status of a significant object. The loss can be actual or threatened; either way, the personality will organize itself to defend against its effects. A loss can be any change in the person's situation that reduces the probability of achieving implicit or explicit goals. These can be abstract, such as being able to marry; to obtain a promotion; or to have a well-functioning, attractive body.

Grief is the emotion experienced when a loss occurs. It is the affective result of a loss. It is the sadness a person feels when he anticipates losing something special or after he loses the valued object. The word *mourning* is sometimes used to refer to grief. It, too, means sadness in connection with a loss (Kaplan & Sadock, 1994, 1995). *Bereavement* is the actual process a person goes through after he experiences a major loss. It includes the various stages involved in the adaptation process of resolving the loss (Kaplan & Sadock, 1994, 1995).

Nurses should be aware of the process of adapting to loss and the potentially differing reactions to loss by the following people:

1. A dying individual who is working through the process of accepting his own death.
2. The family of the dying person.
3. A person who must resolve the loss of a body part, such as the uterus, or accept a change in normal body functioning. Both of these involve accepting a changed body image.
4. The family of the individual who is adapting to the loss of a body part or a change in normal functioning. The family's image of the patient has also changed and must be worked through so that they can accept the changes in their love one.
5. Individuals and families who are adjusting to the exacerbations and remissions of chronic illness.

Whether one works in an acute care, extended care, outpatient, or home care setting, it is possible to observe the effects if loss resolution does not occur. The nurse's recognition that the reaction to loss is maladaptive because of ineffective coping can be very important to patients and their families. Without appropriate intervention by you or by a referral you place in motion, the patient's and the family's quality of life can be seriously affected. Suggestions for appropriate nursing interventions when maladaptation is observed appear in Chapters 15 through 29. Many of the interventions presented are appropriate for patients and family members who are responding to any type of loss.

ANTICIPATORY GRIEF

Anticipatory grief is a concept that is helpful in understanding the responses of terminally ill patients and their families. It is the deep sadness experienced when a major loss is expected in the near future, as distinguished from the grief which occurs at or after the loss (Gordon, 1993). Lindemann (1944, p. 147) described the stages of anticipatory grief as "depression; a heightened preoccupation with the departed; a review of all the forms of death that might befall him; and anticipation of all the modes of readjustment which might be necessitated by it."

Lindemann described anticipatory grief in relation to the experiences of family members whose loved one entered the armed services and went to a dangerous battle zone. The anticipatory grief that operates with terminally ill patients is a more concrete experience because death is certain. There is a period during which all involved persons have an opportunity to "work through" the eventual death.

This helps to buffer the shock of the death when it occurs. It allows the person to prepare to cope with grief (Feldstein & Rait, 1992).

Conventional grief is differentiated from anticipatory grief by Aldrich (1974, p. 4), who states that "anticipatory grief is usually experienced (or denied) simultaneously by both the patient and his family, while conventional grief is experienced only by the family." Conventional grief is the grief occurring after a major loss (Bowlby, 1980; Kaplan & Sadock, 1994; Cassem, 1991b).

The process of adapting to loss can take a few days or a lifetime, depending on the meaning of the loss to the person experiencing it. If the loss is a significant one, such as a beloved spouse, it can take many years for the pain of the loss to be resolved. Bereavement is a normal response to the loss of a significant object. For many, the adaptation process is slowed and the quality of life of the grieving person is detrimentally affected for an extensive period of time. When this occurs, it is called unresolved grief or pathological bereavement (Bensman, Winters, & Kizilos, 1992; DSM-IV, 1994; Donley, 1993).

The best-known theory of the bereavement process is that of Elisabeth Kubler-Ross (1969). Her original book, *On Death and Dying*, describes the stages a dying person goes through before he finally is able to accept his own death. Remember that he is actually facing the loss of himself, that is, the loss of his own being. The stages are denial, anger, bargaining, depression, and acceptance. Although her book is written about the dying patient, these stages are the same for any person who is either anticipating losing or has already lost a valued entity or a valued object. This can be a woman reacting to the loss of a breast, a man who is adjusting to a severe myocardial infarct, an adolescent with diabetes mellitus, or expectant parents whose unborn child has died.

Family members will experience the loss in their own way. Accordingly, their process through the stages will usually be different. They will not be in the same stage at the same time as their husband, wife, or child. This dissimilarity of feelings can provoke serious coping problems for the family. These will be discussed more fully in later chapters.

Kubler-Ross Stages

In the *denial* stage, the person is shocked by his prognosis, and his mind may protect him with a cloak of denial. Within a few days he may become aware of the implications of his circumstances and move into the stage of *anger*. The anger may be rational; it can have a specific, reasonable focus. It can also be irrational and nonspecific, and the patient or family member may verbally strike out at anyone for any reason. People in this stage may unleash their anger at a "safe" person, one whom they trust not to retaliate against them. Frequently, nurses are the subject of this type of anger because they spend a great deal of time with the patient.

The next stage is *bargaining*. In this stage, the dying or grieving person actually is trying to postpone his dying or, in the case of someone who is responding to loss, his acceptance of the loss. He is not yet ready to accept it. The bargaining person may, for example, make "deals" with God. If God will allow him to live, he will make amends with his long-lost brother or will change his life. In another manifestation of bargaining, he may take risks in order to test the effects of his illness on his body. The bargaining stage is marked by frequent mood changes and ambivalence.

Depression is the fourth stage. It is as if the defenses of the earlier stages have failed. The patient or family member can feel overwhelmed by the loss. Its full impact hits him. He may be responding to losses he has already experienced with the current illness, or an old unresolved loss may resurface. He may also be responding to anticipated losses. A dying woman may never live to see her daughter married. The amputee will probably never ski again. The recently blinded man will never see his first grandchild's face.

The final stage is *acceptance*. The person begins to feel at peace about the loss. This stage involves a "letting go." The emotional ties to the lost object are loosened, and the person is able to invest in a new object. The dying person is able to say goodbye to his family and is ready to accept the peace of death. For the person responding to loss, he is able to consider allowing a new object to replace the old one.

In order to understand more fully the implications of loss, it is helpful to examine bereavement theory.

STAGES OF BEREAVEMENT

Bereavement is the actual state of experiencing a major loss, as contrasted with grief, which is the emotion experienced during the bereavement process. An important theory about the way people react to loss was presented by John Bowlby (1961). He describes three stages of bereavement:

1. *Beginning stage of protest*—characterized by denial, weeping, clinging to the lost object, and hostility.
2. *Middle stage of disorganization*—characterized by despair, apathy, and aimlessness.
3. *Termination stage of reorganization*—characterized by acceptance of the image of the lost object (the bereaved person "lets go" of the painful emotional attachment) and acceptance of new objects.

Bowlby's theory contains the same elements as that of Kubler-Ross; it differs only by using more emotional-sounding words to describe the process through which a bereaved person must pass in order for peaceful acceptance and resolution of a major loss to occur.

Beginning Stage of Protest

In Bowlby's first stage, the grieving person is not able to tolerate the loss of a valued object and still clings to the original memory of it. His emotional energy is invested in the person he anticipates losing or has lost, or in his formerly healthy heart, his formerly healthy spouse, and so on. He has not let go of the lost object; he continues to long for it.

An important phenomenon that occurs during the first stage of the bereavement process is ambivalence about the lost object; the bereaved will first feel love and yearning for the family member and then be shocked to feel anger toward him. Bowlby believes that the anger a person feels toward a lost object is part of the normal response during separation. Most separations a person experiences in life are temporary. For example, if a beloved pet "escapes" from its home, it usually is found. Similarly, when car keys are misplaced they are frequently found. There usually is an anxious response followed by anger about the loss. In fact, the anger usually results in increased energy and is the motivator behind the increased physical activity involved in retrieving the lost object.

Anger in each of these situations is a normal response, according to Bowlby. Anger serves the following functions: "first, it may assist in overcoming such obstacles as there may be to reunion; second, it may discourage the loved one from going away again" (Bowlby, 1973, p. 247).

God may be another focus of anger for people with a permanently changed health status or for dying patients and their family members and friends. The bereaved may think, "Why did God do this?" He may feel deep anger toward God. This type of anger is frightening and guilt-provoking to most people who have a normally strong religious faith. One of their underlying fears is that because of their anger, God may "strike" them again. The reaction of getting angry at God happens to many patients and their families, but because it seems abnormal, these feelings are often kept to themselves and they suffer silently (Carpenito, 1993). In working with bereaved or dying persons, it is helpful to mention that many people have these feelings. If the person seems particularly troubled by them, he can be referred to an understanding hospital chaplain or his own pastor, who may be able to relieve some of the guilt he is experiencing.

Ambivalence also occurs in anticipatory grief. Before the terminally ill person dies, the family member may find himself alternately wishing for the death, then for the survival, of the person. These feelings cause high levels of guilt and are rarely shared with others because they are so disturbing. When the course of a terminal illness is examined for its effect on remaining family members, we discover many factors that contribute toward these mixed feelings. A terminal illness puts heavy emotional demands on the family system. It is also possible that the ill person may be hospitalized frequently for long periods. The cost of these hospitalizations, even with insurance, can seriously undermine the family's financial stability.

Visits to the hospital by family members are time consuming, and the amount of time invested in the sick person may then create extra burdens on others. For example, a middle-aged woman who visits her seriously or terminally ill husband daily for several hours may need to take a leave from her job or be unavailable to her adolescent children who continue to need her support (Burns et al., 1993; Harrison & Cole, 1991). She may not be able to keep up her normal household responsibilities. Medical and nursing caregivers may believe that adult children should take over these responsibilities out of their concern and love for her and their father. This may not be the case, however. They may be experiencing anger about the impending loss of their father and may displace some of this anger onto their mother. She, in turn, may be repressing her anger toward her husband for leaving her and displace it onto her children because of their lack of support.

These extra pressures have an effect on all the spheres of a person's functioning: his relationships with others outside of the family system; his normal functioning at work, home, or school; his normal intrapsychic functioning, and so on. Accordingly, it is not uncommon, especially during times of fatigue, to wish that the difficult period caused by the chronic or terminal illness of the loved one could be over. In addition, the hope that the terminally ill person will die soon may be motivated by a genuine wish to end the loved one's suffering and pain (Burns et al., 1993; Carpenito, 1993; Harrison & Cole, 1991).

Middle Stage of Disorganization

The middle stage of bereavement is marked by disorganization. During this phase the emotional energy attached to the lost object is released; however, it has not been reinvested in another object. As a result, the emotion at times seems all-encompassing and overwhelming. The emotion that is being withdrawn from the lost object is not focused because the person's grief is not resolved enough to reinvest it in another object. This is a time of disequilibrium intrapsychically and within the family system. Everything may seem out of control. It is not unusual for persons in this stage of bereave-

ment to feel as though they are losing their sanity. Indeed, rather than experience the unpleasant emotional and cognitive reactions of this stage, many persons remain "stuck" in the first stage of bereavement. The loss is never fully resolved (Bowlby, 1973, 1980).

Termination Stage of Reorganization

In Bowlby's last stage of bereavement, the grieving person's mind allows his or her feelings to be attached once again to a new object. The new object never replaces the old; instead, the emotional energy that was invested in the original object is refocused and invested in a new object. In many instances, the acceptance of a new object begins before the letting go of the lost object is complete. In fact, it may facilitate the final acceptance of the loss. If a person is widowed, for example, there is a longing for the spouse. Ideally, a person should eventually begin to seek out other men and women friends. Sometimes this occurs before the person has totally resolved the loss.

By meeting and enjoying new people and eventually focusing on one of them, or by engaging in work or recreational pursuits that bring pleasure, the final acceptance of the original partner's loss may be resolved. This process is accompanied by feelings of hope for the future. The most important aspect of this last stage of bereavement and the one that indicates that the grief process is complete is that the bereaved is able to invest feelings in a replacement object. The person is able to feel emotional gratification from his or her new situation (Bowlby, 1973, 1980).

It is helpful to remember the various types of grief reactions that can be present in a general hospital with dying persons. The individual experiences grief in accepting the loss of self through death. His is an anticipatory grief. The final stage of acceptance for him occurs when he lets go of the emotional energy invested in his own life and accepts that he will no longer live. Many times, belief in some type of afterlife, or perhaps reunion with previously departed family members or God, becomes the new focus.

Family members may have many months to prepare for their loved one's death. In this case they may be able to work through some of the initial stages of grief before death occurs. The loss of a family member through accidental death presents a greater potential for challenge to effective coping failure because of its suddenness. Being able to prepare for the death of a loved one, if only for a few days, allows more coping mechanisms to develop in the family. For example, if an accident or coronary victim remains alive even a few days in an intensive care unit, it prevents the family members from having to cope suddenly with the shock of death with no warning. It can allow family members to say good-bye to their loved one.

Coping with loss is one of the most significant challenges facing physically ill people and their families. Serious illness in any family member poses threats to each family member no matter his or her age. Ineffective coping, if prolonged for more than 4 weeks or if severe, regardless of duration, should prompt the nurse to recommend referral to a mental health clinician who is knowledgeable about family systems (Carpenito, 1993; Feldstein & Rait, 1992; Halm et al., 1993; Harrison & Cole, 1991; Herth, 1993).

GUILT

Guilt is another major issue faced by physically ill patients and their families. The ability to feel guilt develops when the superego is formed, around the age of 4 or 5 (Kaplan & Sadock, 1994, 1995). People who have a strict and demanding superego can experience uncomfortable levels of guilt, in contrast to the guilt level people with normally or poorly developed superegos feel. Guilt is felt when a person violates his or her own conscience or moral code. Erikson (1963) has described guilt as the undesired personality trait that develops if the initiative stage in early childhood psychosocial development is not worked through successfully. Initiative is the amount of direction and purpose a person has. It is the outward and positive manifestation of the pleasure-seeking and aggressive drives.

During adolescence, the superego may initially be harsh, but gradually, as the adolescent matures, it softens and becomes more self-accepting. When this does not occur, the result is an adult who excessively displays some or all of the following behaviors: expresses guilt, rationalizes and intellectualizes, makes apologies when none are due, is depressed, denies sexual pleasure with resulting sexual dysfunction, uses avoidance behaviors to avoid guilt feelings, lacks realistic concern for self (masochistic behaviors), blames self for events that are beyond his or her control, and is hypersensitive to others' comments (Buss, 1991; Pine, 1990).

These manifestations of excessive guilt feelings may be observed in the following hospital situations:

1. The excessively apologetic person who finds it hard to let caregivers care for her.
2. The patient who refuses pain medication but displays pain behavior.
3. The individual who views his illness as a form of punishment.

When signs of excessive guilt are observed in a patient, attempts to decrease her guilt with strong counterarguments will only increase anxiety. The patient can be asked to talk about why she will not take pain medicine. The nurse can listen and respond by describing other patients who have felt the same way but were relieved when they took the medication.

Frequently, family members experience guilt when they must choose whether their loved one should have a cardiac alert or rush (each hospital has its own name for its response to a cardiac arrest) or whether the patient should be categorized as "no cardiac alert" and allowed to die if an arrest occurs. This is an example of a time when caregivers, the physician in this case, can make a recommendation to the family rather than arousing the family's guilt by leaving the entire decision to them (Gordon, 1993).

The young person in an intensive care unit whose brain death has been verified also poses a poignant dilemma for family members. At times, a physician favors discontinuing life support systems, but the family has a difficult time agreeing with the physician's decision. Usually the family needs a day or two to live with the gravity and hopelessness of their loved one's condition before they can accept the finality of the situation and make a decision. The nurse can encourage them to talk about their guilt.

Gradually, most families are able to work through this guilt, and their decision can be made. Consultation with a member of the hospital's pastoral care team or with their own pastor can assist them with this difficult decision (Dossey, Guzzetta, & Kenner, 1992; Halm et al., 1993).

Another guilt-ridden time for some families occurs when a relative needs constant care because of physical or mental infirmity. Family members who believe that the person must be cared for at home will have strong guilt feelings at the thought of placing their loved one in a nursing home (Harrison & Cole, 1991; O'Brien, 1993). Other members of the same family may believe that, because of the effort and strain on the remaining members, the nursing home is the most realistic alternative.

Serious family conflict of a long-standing nature may arise at this time if all family members are not in agreement. The family member who takes the ill person into his or her own home may eventually feel "used" by other family members who do not have the responsibility, and become resentful.

This type of family conflict can cause permanent splits in relationships between families of the same generation with far-reaching consequences into subsequent generations (Baum & Page, 1991; Harrison & Cole, 1991). Ideally, this and similar types of conflicts can be referred for professional assistance to a family therapy professional. The underlying dynamic that precipitates many family conflicts is guilt: while jealousy of other family members can be another cause of conflict, one of the basic dynamics of jealousy is guilt (Freud, 1924).

When a patient or family member displays signs of excessive guilt, it is possible that the guilt-ridden person has a tendency to place herself in situations in which she feels oppressed. Encouraging a patient to talk about why she cannot take pain medication or why she cannot let others help her may give the nurse the opportunity to present a more realistic perspective than the patient's own. She may be assisted by a nurse's assurance, for example, that it is normal and acceptable to take pain medication (Bouckoms & Hackett, 1991). Additional information on pain management can be found in Chapter 21.

Some people maintain their suffering behavior no matter what approach is tried with them. In fact, they seem to enjoy the hovering effect it has on their families and other visitors. For such individuals, it is advisable not to reward their behavior by increased attention. If attention is limited, the patient's behavior may return to more normal limits (Bouckoms & Hackett, 1991).

INTIMACY

Intimacy is another important issue of illness and hospitalization that may present adaptation problems for some patients or family members. In the progression of personality development, intimacy is the major developmental hurdle of the young adult (Erikson, 1963). In Western culture the word *intimacy* often means the same thing as sexual closeness. However, this is only one aspect of intimacy. The young adult most needs to be able to tolerate closeness interpersonally—to be emotionally close to people. Closeness is the ability to be open and honest, to trust, and to take risks in a relationship. Mature intimacy means knowing the other person interpersonally: his dreams and hopes, what gives him joy, what makes him sad, his positive side, his negative side, and who he really is; and allowing one's self to be similarly known (Boykin & Schoenhofer, 1993; Masterson, Tolpin, & Sifneos, 1991; Pine, 1990).

In his book *The Transparent Self,* Jouard (1971, p. 6) writes that "no man can come to know himself except as an outcome of disclosing himself to another person." He also writes that self-disclosure requires courage, not only the courage to be and to do, but also the courage to be known as one knows himself to be (pp. 6 and 7).

Some examples of close, trusting relationships are those between husband and wife, parent and child, or childhood or college friends maintained through a lifetime. These types of relationships are mutually supportive and enriching. The emotional give and take in the dyad may be uneven at times, but is generally equal over an extended time.

The ability to form intimate relationships is considered an essential aspect of full personality development. The essential quality necessary for development of intimate relationships is the ability to form good object relations (Pine, 1990). The foundation of intimacy was formed as the young child gained experience in trusting others. The ability to trust is the building block of the ability to form an intimate relationship (Schwab, Stephenson, & Ice, 1993).

The capacity to form an intimate relationship is essential to a meaningful sexual relationship. Patients' sexual functioning is often affected when serious or chronic illness occurs. The subject of sexuality was generally avoided, until recently, in the curricula of many nursing and medical schools. In addition, it is a sensitive subject for many caregivers to broach with their patients. Accordingly, although it may be of strong concern to a patient about to return home, the subject may not be discussed. The issues of sexuality and illness are addressed in several chapters. The reader is referred to the Index section on sexuality for additional information.

Some patients have never had a close relationship with another person. When such a person is admitted to a hospital, suddenly all aspects of her privacy are invaded. She may feel very threatened and find it difficult to cope. The physical surface of her body is felt, examined, pushed, prodded, washed, rubbed, shaved, pricked, and incised. An artificial emotional closeness may suddenly be thrust on her by innumerable caregivers whom she has never met before. Questions are asked about many aspects of her functioning (social, physical, sexual, emotional) and about any history of substance use (medications, alcohol, illegal drugs). She is asked about the cause of death of family members. She is told to take off all her clothes. Her sense of body modesty seems violated by the body positioning required for many procedures.

An aspect of intimacy that can be troublesome to the very shy, aloof, or suspicious patient is the type of social history taking that may occur in some settings. This individual can be very uncomfortable revealing intimate information to anyone, even her own family members; she will probably have difficulty confiding intimate information about her functioning to her primary caregiver. Some-

times caregivers who repeatedly ask for such information forget about the emotional impact on the patient, who may experience these questions as an invasion of privacy. Although these questions may be important, they can be asked in a supportive manner that acknowledges and empathizes with the patient's embarrassment. Frequently, it is helpful for the nurse to explain how this information will be used in designing the patient's care. If she understands the beneficial effects of her disclosures, her discomfort may be decreased, and her motivation to share this information can be more positive.

CONCLUSION

The issues of trust, shame, self-esteem, control, loss, guilt, and intimacy are important underlying dynamics in a patient or family member's capacity to adapt to illness. When ineffective coping occurs, usually one or more of these issues is implicated. The success of a nursing intervention plan designed to resolve or lessen a crisis can depend in part on the nurse's ability to identify a major underlying issue and its dynamics. It is also important to recognize that specific illnesses or conditions automatically threaten some of these issues. Diabetes, for example, raises control issues due to required changes in lifestyle, eating habits, scheduling, and so on. Chronic illness threatens each of the control issues discussed in this chapter. Add to that the unique, individual, personality responses to each of these issues, and the risk of ineffective coping is significantly increased. When a nursing diagnosis is established, the underlying dynamic or cause of the ineffective coping should be described if it can be identified.

BIBLIOGRAPHY

Aldrich, C. K. (1974). Some dynamics of anticipatory grief. In B. Schoenberg et al. (Eds.), *Anticipatory grief.* New York: Columbia University Press.

Arieti, S. (1967). *The intrapsychic self.* New York: Basic Books.

Barry, P. (1991). An investigation of cardiovascular, respiratory and skin temperature changes during relaxation and anger inductions. *Dissertation Abstracts International, 52-09-B,* 5012.

Baum, M., & Page, M. (1991). Caregiving and multigenerational families. *Gerontologist, 31*(6), 762–769.

Baumeister, R. F., Heatherton, T. F., & Tice, D. M. (1993). When ego threats lead to self-regulation failure: Negative consequences of high self-esteem. *Journal of Personality and Social Psychology, 64*(1), 141–156.

Bensman, A. S., Winters, J., & Kizilos, P. (1992). The effects of childhood trauma upon adult recovery from injury and illness. *Minnesota Medicine, 75*(11), 11–13.

Berzonsky, M. D. (1992). Identity style and coping strategies. *Journal of Personality, 60*(4), 771–788.

Bock, G. R., & Whelan, J. (Eds.). (1991). *The childhood environment and adult disease.* New York: Wiley.

Bouckoms, A., & Hackett, T. P. (1991). The pain patient: Evaluation and treatment. In N. H. Cassem (Ed.), *Massachusetts General Hospital handbook of general hospital psychiatry* (3rd ed.). St. Louis: Mosby Year Book.

Bowlby, J. (1961). Processes of mourning. *International Journal of Psychoanalysis, 42,* 317.

Bowlby, J. (1973). *Attachment and loss. Vol. 2: Separation.* New York: Basic Books.

Bowlby, J. (1980). *Attachment and loss. Vol. 3: Sadness and depression.* New York: Basic Books.

Boykin, A., & Schoenhofer, S. (1993). *Nursing as caring: A model for transforming practice.* New York: National League for Nursing.

Bullock, M. (Ed.). (1991). The development of intentional action. *Contributions to Human Development, 22.*

Burns, C., Archbold, P., Stewart, B., & Shelton, K. (1993). New diagnosis: Caregiver role strain. *Nursing Diagnosis, 4*(2), 70–76.

Buss, D. M. (1991). Evolutionary personality psychology. *Annual Review of Psychology, 42,* 459–491.

Cassem, N. H. (1991a). Depression. In N. H. Cassem (Ed.), *Massachusetts General Hospital handbook of general hospital psychiatry* (3rd ed.). St. Louis: Mosby Year Book.

Cassem, N. H. (1991b). The dying patient. In N. H. Cassem (Ed.), *Massachusetts General Hospital handbook of general hospital psychiatry* (3rd ed.). St. Louis: Mosby Year Book.

Daum, A. L., & Collins, C. (1992). Failure to master early developmental tasks as a predictor of adaptation to cancer in the young adult. *Oncology Nursing Forum, 19*(10), 1513–1518.

Dohms, J.E., & Metz, A. (1991). Stress—mechanisms of immunosuppression. *Verterinary immunology and immunopathology, 30*(1), 89–109.

Donley, M. G. (1993). Attachment and the emotional unit. *Family Processes, 32*(1), 3–20.

Dossey, B. M., Guzzetta, C. E., & Kenner, C. V. (1992). *Critical care nursing: Body-mind-spirit* (3rd ed.). Philadelphia: J. B. Lippincott.

Draucker, C. B. (1991). Coping with a difficult-to-diagnose illness: The example of interstitial cystitis. *Health Care for Women International, 12*(2), 191–198.

Engel, G. (1968). *Psychological development in health and disease* (2nd ed.). Philadelphia: W. B. Saunders.

Epstein, S. (1992). Coping ability, negative self-evaluation, and overgeneralization: Experiment and theory. *Journal of Personality and Social Psychology, 62*(5), 826–836.

Epstein, S., & Katz, L. (1992). Coping ability, stress, productive load, and symptoms. *Journal of Personality and Social Psychology, 62*(5), 813–825.

Erikson, E. (1963). *Childhood and society* (2nd ed.). New York: Norton.

Feldstein, M. A., & Rait, D. (1992). Family assessment in an oncology setting. *Cancer Nursing, 15*(3), 161–172.

Fisher, L., Ransom, D. C., Terry, H. E., & Burge, S. (1992). The California Family Health Project: IV. Family structure/organization and adult health. *Family Process, 31*(4), 399–419.

Franks, P., Campbell, T. L., & Shields, C. G. (1992). Social relationships and health: The relative roles of family functioning and social support. *Social Science and Medicine, 34*(7), 779–788.

Freud, S. (1924). Certain neurotic mechanisms in jealousy, paranoia, and homosexuality. In *Collected Papers, Vol. 22.* London: Hogarth Press.

Freud, S. (1933). *New introductory lectures on psychoanalysis.* New York: Norton.

Gattuso, S. M., Litt, M. D., & Fitzgerald, T. E. (1992). Coping with gastrointestinal endoscopy: Self-efficacy enhancement and coping style. *Journal of Consulting Clinical Psychology, 60*(1), 133–139.

Goodyer, I. M. (1990). *Life experiences, development, and childhood psychopathology.* New York: Wiley.

Gordon, M. (1993). *Manual of nursing diagnosis.* St. Louis: C. V. Mosby.

Groves, J. E., & Kurcharski, A. (1991). Brief psychotherapy. In N. H. Cassem (Ed.), *Massachusetts General Hospital handbook of general hospital psychiatry* (3rd ed.). St. Louis: Mosby Year Book.

Halm, M. A., Titler, M. G., Kleiber, C., Johnson, S. K., Montgomery, L. A., Craft, M. J., Buckwalter, K., Nicholson, A., & Megivern, K. (1993). Behavioral responses of family members during critical illness. *Clinics in Nursing Research, 2*(4), 414–437.

Harrison, D. S., & Cole, K. D. (1991). Family dynamics and caregiver burden in home health care. *Clinics in Geriatric Medicine, 7*(4), 817–829.

Herman, J. (1992). *Trauma and recovery.* New York: Basic Books.

Herth, K. (1993). Hope in the family caregiver of terminally ill people. *Journal of Advanced Nursing, 18*(4), 538–548.

Jensen, M. P., Turner, J. A., & Romano, R. M. (1991). Self-efficacy and outcome expectancies: Relationship to chronic pain coping strategies and adjustment. *Pain, 44*(3), 263–269.

Jouard, S. (1971). *The transparent self* (rev. ed.). New York: Van Nostrand Reinhold.

Kaplan, H. I., & Sadock, B. J. (1994). *Synopsis of psychiatry: Behavioral sciences, clinical psychiatry* (7th ed.). Baltimore: Williams & Wilkins.

Kaplan, H. I., & Sadock, B. J. (1995). *Comprehensive textbook of psychiatry/VI* (6th ed.). Baltimore: Williams & Wilkins.

Karen, R. (1992). Shame. *The Atlantic Monthly, 2,* 40–70.

Kaufman, G. (1989). *The psychology of shame: Theory and treatment of shame-based syndromes.* New York: Springer Publishing Co.

Kopp, R. G., & Ruzicka, M. F. (1993). Women's multiple roles and psychological well-being. *Psychological Reports, 72*(3 Pt. 2), 1351–1354.

Kubler-Ross, E. (1969). *On death and dying.* New York: Macmillan.

Kuhn, D. (Ed.). (1990). *Developmental perspectives on teaching and learning thinking skills.* New York: Karger.

Lasky, R. (1993). *Dynamics of development and the therapeutic process.* Northvale, NJ: J. Aronson.

Lindemann, E. (1944). Symptomatology and management of acute grief. *American Journal of Psychiatry, 101*(2) 141–148.

Maslow, A. (1970). *Motivation and personality* (2nd ed.). New York: Harper & Row.

Masterson, J. F., Tolpin, M., & Sifneos, P. E. (1991). *Comparing psychoanalytic psychotherapies: Developmental, self, and object relations: Self psychology, short-term dynamic.* New York: Brunner/Mazel.

McDaniel, S. H., Campbell, T. L, & Seaburn, D. B. (1990). *Family- oriented primary care: A manual for medical providers.* New York: Springer-Verlag.

Moran, P. B., & Eckenrode, J. (1992). Protective personality characteristics among adolescent victims of maltreatment. *Child Abuse and Neglect, 16*(5), 743–754.

Morrison, A. (1989). *Shame: The underside of narcissism.* Hillsdale, NJ: Analytic Press.

Nathanson, D. L. (1987). *The many faces of shame.* New York: Guilford Press.

Newberry, B. H., Jaikins-Madden, J. E., & Gerstenberger, T. J. (1991). *A holistic conceptualization of stress and disease.* New York: AMS Press.

Noshpitz, D., & Coddington, D. (Eds.). (1990). *Stressors and the adjustment disorders.* New York: Wiley.

O'Brien, M. T. (1993). Multiple sclerosis: The relationship among self-esteem, social support, and coping behavior. *Applied Nursing Research, 6*(2), 54–63.

O'Connor, S. (1991). Psychiatric liaison nursing in a changing health care system. In N. H. Cassem (Ed.), *Massachusetts General Hospital handbook of general hospital psychiatry* (3rd ed). St. Louis: Mosby Year Book.

Pine, F. (1990). *Drive, ego, object, and self: A synthesis for clinical work.* New York: Basic Books.

Rosenbaum, J. F., & Grove, J. E. (1991). Accident proneness and accident victims. In N. H. Cassem (Ed.), *Massachusetts General Hospital handbook of general hospital psychiatry* (3rd ed.). St. Louis: Mosby Year Book.

Rosenbaum, J. F., & Pollock, M. H. (1991). Anxiety. In N. H. Cassem (Ed.), *Massachusetts General Hospital handbook of general hospital psychiatry* (3rd ed.). St. Louis: Mosby Year Book.

Schussler, G. (1992). Coping strategies and individual meanings of illness. *Social Science and Medicine, 34*(4), 427–432.

Schwab, J. J., Stephenson, J. J., & Ice, J. F. (1993). *Evaluating family mental health: History, epidemiology, and treatment issues.* New York: Plenum Press.

Small, S. P., & Graydon, J. E. (1992). Perceived uncertainty, physical symptoms, and negative mood in hospitalized patients with chronic obstructive pulmonary disease. *Heart and Lung, 21*(6), 568–574.

Smith, L. B., & Thelen, E. (Eds.). (1993). *A dynamic systems approach to development: Applications.* Cambridge: MIT Press.

Stewart, T. D. (1991). The spinal-cord injured patient. In N. H. Cassem (Ed.), *Massachusetts General Hospital handbook of general hospital psychiatry* (3rd ed.). St. Louis: Mosby Year Book.

Surman, O. (1991). The surgical patient. In N. H. Cassem (Ed.), *Massachusetts General Hospital handbook of general hospital psychiatry* (3rd ed.). St. Louis: Mosby Year Book.

Terry, D. J. (1992). Stress, coping and coping resources as correlates of adaptation in myocardial infarction patients. *British Journal of Clinical Psychology, 31*(Pt. 2), 215–225.

Viemero, V. (1991). The effects of somatic disability or progressive illness on psychological and social well-being. *Psychotherapy and Psychosomatics, 55*(2–4), 120–125.

Weisman, A. (1991). Coping with illness. In N. H. Cassem (Ed.), *Massachusetts General Hospital handbook of general hospital psychiatry* (3rd ed.). St. Louis: Mosby Year Book.

Welch, C. (1991). Psychiatric care of the burn victim. In N. H. Cassem (Ed.), *Massachusetts General Hospital handbook of general hospital psychiatry* (3rd ed.). St. Louis: Mosby Year Book.

Wiener, C. L., & Dodd, M. J. (1993). Coping amid uncertainty: An illness trajectory perspective. *Scholastic Inquiry Into Nursing Practice, 7*(1), 17–31.

Woods, N. F., Habaerman, M. R., & Packard, N. J. (1993). Demands of illness and individual, dyadic, and family adaptation in chronic illness. *Western Journal of Nursing Research, 15*(1), 10–25.

Wykle, M. L., Kahana, E., & Kowal, J. (Eds.). (1992). *Stress and health among the elderly.* New York: Springer Publishing Co.

CHAPTER 10

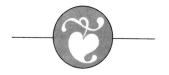

Assessment and Interpretation of Mental Status Changes

Patricia Barry

The ability to perform a formal mental status examination is essential for all professionals in the field of mental health. A *mental status examination* determines if there are abnormalities in the thinking, feeling, or behavior of the person being "examined." It is not necessary to carry out a formal question-and-answer mental examination in order to evaluate most aspects of a person's mental status, however. Instead, assessment of a newly admitted patient's mental status can be done by being attentive to his or her style of thinking, expressing feelings, and behaving during the regular nursing assessment process.

One of the challenges of assessing a patient's psychosocial functioning is that it involves processing nonverbal clues as well as integrating other information. Recognition of mental dysfunction is especially important in the general hospital setting because of the possibility that changes in normal functioning are caused by physiological factors.

FUNCTIONAL AND COGNITIVE MENTAL DISORDERS

There are two main types of mental dysfunction. A *functional psychiatric disorder* is caused by a dysfunction in the abstract psychic structures of the mind. For example, defense mechanisms may not adequately help a patient cope after she has had an unexpected amputation. Defenses may overprotect her so that denial shuts out reality, or the mind may be so overwhelmed that normal defense mechanisms fail.

A *cognitive mental disorder* (DSM-IV, 1994) previously called *organic mental disorder*, is caused by an organic dysfunction in the actual anatomical structures or the biochemistry of the brain. It is possible for medications, infec-

Patricia Barry: *Psychosocial Nursing:*
Care of Physically Ill Patients and Their Families, 3rd ed.
© 1996 Lippincott–Raven Publishers

tion, elevated temperature, or any other factor that affects anatomical or physiological functioning to cause a change in mental functioning (Geary, 1994; Murray, 1991). Chapter 11 discusses cognitive mental disorder in detail. The ability to recognize this important, yet underrecognized, syndrome is essential for all nurses working in acute or home care settings.

Because of the great variety of new stressors with which hospitalized individuals are bombarded, they are at risk for mental dysfunctioning due to coping failure *and* physiological failure. Regardless of the cause, there are usually methods available to resolve the dysfunctional state (Carpenito, 1993; McFarland, Wasli, & Gerety, 1992). No remedies can begin, however, if the subtle clues of mental dysfunction are missed by caregivers. Chapter 11 explains the differences in symptoms between these two main causes of psychiatric dysfunction.

THE IMPORTANCE OF MENTAL STATUS OBSERVATION

Making notations about the status of a patient's thinking ability, feelings, and behavior during the admission process and ongoing nursing care is an important element of a nurse's responsibilities. The patient's mental status is an essential aspect of overall psychosocial functioning. As the patient's history is developed with the subjective data he or she describes, it is important to be aware of the nonverbal data being given about mental functioning. Observations of thinking style, feelings, and behavior, when based on a sound understanding of normal and abnormal mental functioning, will form a solid basis for psychosocial nursing assessment.

It is important to note the difference between mental status assessment and psychosocial assessment. The former is an evaluation of the functioning of the patient's intrapsychic system. Psychosocial assessment includes this information plus an evaluation of the patient's social system, and investigates the interaction between the two.

Observations of thinking style, feelings, and behavior can be gathered while giving routine nursing care. The importance of obtaining a thorough baseline mental status on admission cannot be overemphasized. Even more important is the notation of changes observed from the mental state seen on admission and the time it was recorded. If, for example, mental dysfunction is noted on the third day after admission, and the patient was normal on admission, the contributing factor may be physiological in origin (Kaplan & Sadock, 1994, 1995; Murray, 1991). This type of organic dysfunction is frequently reversible.

In order to determine if mental status changes are occurring, the current mental status can be compared to the patient's mental status on admission as well as his or her prehospitalization level of mental functioning. This can be done in several ways:

1. Compare the data and time of the patient's mental status on his or her first day of admission to the date, time, and mental status on ensuing days.
2. Ask the patient if his or her current feelings, types of thoughts, manner of thinking, and memory are similar to what they were before the illness. If they are different, the patient can be asked to describe how they are different and why he or she thinks they are different. Frequently, the patient may have good insight into the cause of changes in physical and mental functioning.
3. If the patient is disoriented and confused, the family can be asked about premorbid (presickness) mental functioning. For example, with an 83-year-old patient who is disoriented, the nurse should not assume that it is the result of senility due to aging. It is possible that this patient was alert and articulate before hospitalization, but that toxicity due to an undiagnosed systemic infection has temporarily affected organic brain functioning. Unless the patient's prehospitalization mental status is obtained from the family, caregivers could lose valuable time in correctly arriving at possible causes of the mentally toxic physical disease process.

4. Use any extra information available about the patient in assessing his or her current status.

The nurse's social awareness, coupled with deductive reasoning skills, can often assist in investigating a patient's current mental response to illness.

The assessment process is similar to that of a detective. It can be challenging and creative to think through the available clues. When the preadmission history includes depression or anxiety that has lasted more than a few weeks, there are probably complex factors of long-standing duration present (Cassem, 1991; Rosenbaum & Pollack, 1991). In such cases, psychiatric referral of the patient can be recommended to the attending physician. When recommending psychiatric referral, it is essential to document precisely the symptoms observed in the patient and include the patient's observations (and those of the family if the patient is not reliable) of his or her preadmission emotional state.

When a preexisting, maladaptive emotional state is compounded by the stress of hospitalization and recuperation, the task of adaptation is seriously jeopardized. The astute nurse's observations and patient advocacy in recommending psychiatric referral and outpatient psychiatric follow-up care can have a profound effect on the future quality of life for the patient and all members of the family (Lipowski, 1992; O'Connor, 1991).

THE CATEGORIES OF MENTAL STATUS EVALUATION

The categories in Box 10-1 describe aspects of a patient's mental status. These mental status categories are assessed in the process of obtaining general information at admission or throughout hospitalization. The date and exact time of the assessment should always be recorded.

Use of the appropriate psychiatric terms to describe the various abnormal mental states observed is important in communicating with other members of the care team and other shifts.

LEVEL OF AWARENESS AND ORIENTATION

Level of Awareness

Level of awareness is one of the more observable aspects of brain functioning. It serves as an important indicator of mental status, especially for hospitalized patients. Usually the first sign that a toxic physiological state is developing is a change in a patient's level of consciousness and orientation. Nurses should be alert to subtle changes in these brain functioning indicators. Their early observations, when presented in an articulate manner to physicians, will usually result in prompt diagnostic

---

BOX 10-1	Mental Status Categories for Admission Assessment

1. Level of awareness and orientation
2. Appearance and behavior
3. Speech and communication
4. Mood or affect (feeling state)
5. Disturbances in thinking process, disorganization of thought process, disturbance in content of thought (delusions, phobias, obsessions), problems with memory and concentration
6. Problems with perception (hallucinations or distortions of reality associated with any of the senses)
7. Abstract thinking and judgment
8. Risk of suicidality or homicidality

and treatment measures that can reverse the cause of the toxic condition causing a cognitive mental disorder. The levels of awareness range on a continuum from unconsciousness and frank coma to drowsiness and hypersomnolence; to alertness, hyperalertness, or suspiciousness; to frank paranoia or mania. Figure 10-1 shows the range of levels of consciousness observable in general hospital patients.

At the opposite end of the continuum from the comatose individual is the patient who is hypervigilant and hyperaware of the environment. Hyperalert awareness is seen in a person who is moderately anxious, one with a suspicious, paranoid personality style, or one who is manic. It is most commonly seen in the intensive care units of general hospitals, when otherwise normal individuals may be prepsychotic from interactions between organic causes, frequently medication-related; environmental factors, such as sensory deprivation and sleep loss; or impairment of normal mental functioning due to the stress of illness, preexisting personality conflicts, or both (Dunner, 1993; Goldberg, Faust, & Novack, 1992; Kaplan & Sadock, 1994, 1995).

Orientation

Orientation is the patient's ability to identify who he is, where he is, and the approximate date. These three indicators of orientation are frequently termed *orientation to time, person, and place.* They may be abbreviated to *orientated x 3.* The approximate date is accepted because it is quite easy for any well-functioning person who has been hospitalized for several days to confuse the date by one day. Individuals who are postsurgical or with admissions extending beyond 1 week often lose the points of reference for days of the week and dates that they would generally be aware of in their normal environments.

The list in Box 10-2 contains terminology commonly used to describe level of consciousness and orientation.

APPEARANCE AND BEHAVIOR

A patient's appearance and behavior include any observable characteristics. They are listed by category in Box 10-3. Following each category is a partial list of words that describe the characteristic. One or more words can be used in describing each category.

SPEECH AND COMMUNICATION

Verbal Communication

Evaluating a patient's speech and communication means observing how she is communicating rather than what she is communicating. *What* the patient is communicating is the content. The content of a person's speech is actually a reflection of her thought process, which is described later in this chapter. The following aspects of a person's speaking style should be observed:

1. Rate
2. Volume
3. Modulation and flow
4. Production

The *rate of speech* is usually consistent with the patient's overall psychomotor status. If a person is depressed, speech, as well as activity level, is usually slowed. Conversely, a rapid rate of speech usually indicates elation or, in some cases, a manic mental state. In the same way, the volume or loudness of speech will range from almost inaudible in very depressed patients to loud in manic, confused, or suspicious patients.

Modulation and flow of speech pertain to the range of speech. Does the person talk in a dull monotone, or is there a spirited and lively quality? There is cause for concern if a patient is observed displaying a lively speech rate that alternates with a subdued pattern within a few hours. This may be the first indicator of the development of a cognitive mental disorder.

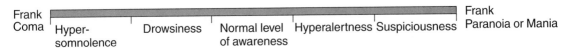

FIGURE 10-1. Continuum of levels of consciousness.

BOX 10-2	Levels of Orientation and Consciousness
	1. Confusion—Disorientation to time, person, or place
	2. Clouding of consciousness—Slight to moderate disturbance in perception or thought
	3. Stupor—Shock-like inability to recognize or react to environment
	4. Delirium—Moderate to severe disturbance in perception, thought, and emotion. Accompanied by marked fear
	5. Dreamy state—Hallucinatory type of disturbed consciousness
	6. Coma—All consciousness is lost

Speech production is the ability to produce words. A patient may be mute. A patient may display *pressured speech*, a rapid rate of speech usually associated with extreme anxiety or mania. Speech may be slurred; the words are then poorly formed.

Nonverbal Communication

Communication can occur nonverbally as well as verbally. The types of nonverbal communication include eye contact, gestures, and posture. Poor eye contact is a signal of lack of engagement with the other person. *Engagement* is the state of association or emotional connectedness that one person demonstrates toward another. Lack of engagement often indicates a lack of trust in oneself or the other person; this distrust may be caused by a variety of personality difficulties. Certain cultural and ethnic beliefs can also be manifested in avoidance of eye contact.

Posture and gestures are further indicators of a person's level of engagement. A person may sit facing or turned away from another. His arms and hands may rest comfortably in his lap, or he may rapidly fold and unfold them, or fold them across his chest, implying, "I am not open to you or anything you are saying to me." Likewise, a person may stand comfortably and at ease or may express tension by moving frequently or pacing.

An important assessment device is to evaluate the match between a person's verbal and nonverbal communication. For example, a person may be saying he is sad, but may not sound or appear sad. When such a disparity is observed, it should be recorded.

AFFECT (MOOD)

Affect is how a person feels and the way he or she appears to observers. The term *mood* is used to describe the patient's subjective feelings (Campbell, 1989). The terms are frequently used interchangeably in the clinical setting; this has become an acceptable practice.

Disturbances in affect that may be observed in patients are listed below. Only those feelings considered abnormal and indicative of mental status dysfunction are included.

A. Inappropriate affects
   1. A patient who is not responding as expected in a given situation
   2. Content of a discussion that does not fit with the emotions accompanying a patient's statements
B. Pleasurable affects
   1. Euphoria: excessive and inappropriate feeling of well-being
   2. Exaltation: intense elation accompanied by feelings of grandeur
C. Unpleasurable affects (dysphoria)
   1. Depression: hopeless feeling
   2. Grief or mourning: prolonged and excessive sadness associated with a loss
   3. Anxiety: feeling of apprehension caused by conflicts of which the patient is not aware
   4. Fear: excessive fright resulting from consciously recognized danger
   5. Agitation: anxiety associated with severe motor restlessness
   6. Ambivalence: alternating and opposite feelings occurring in the same person about the same object
   7. Aggression: rage, anger, or hostility

BOX 10-3	Appearance and Behavior Aspects	

	A. Dress
	  1. Neat
	  2. Careless
	  3. Eccentric
	B. Faces or facial expression
	  1. Animated
	  2. Fixed
	  3. Sad
	  4. Angry
	  5. Color of face (pale, reddened)
	C. Posture
	  1. Relaxed
	  2. Tense
	  3. Erect
	  4. Sitting, lying
	D. Motor activity
	  1. Agitated, restless
	  2. Tremors: coarse or fine
	  3. Motor retardation: slow movement
	    a. Catatonic: immobile
	    b. Waxy flexibility: body maintains position in which it is placed
	  4. Apraxia: inability to carry out purposeful movement to achieve a goal
	  5. Echopraxia: mimicking the body movements of the interviewer
		6. Abnormal (dystonic) movement
		  a. Akathisia: extreme restlessness
		  b. Akinesia: complete or partial loss of muscle movement
		  c. Dyskinesia: excessive movement of mouth, protruding tongue, facial grimacing (a common side effect of the major tranquilizers)
		  d. Parkinsonian movement: fine tremor accompanied by muscular rigidity
		7. Hypomania: increased motor activity accompanied by a mild to moderate level of emotional excitement
		E. Physical characteristics
		  1. Unusual appearance of any part of body
		F. Reaction to interviewer (requires subjective judgment of the interviewer)
		  1. Friendly
		  2. Suspicious
		  3. Hostile
		  4. Indifferent
		  5. Dependent
		  6. Passive

that is excessive or seems unrelated to a person's current situation

  8. Mood swings (also called lability): alternating periods of elation and depression or anxiety in the same person within a limited time

D. Lack of affect: blunted or flat affect: a normal range of emotions is missing. Commonly seen in people with depression, some forms of schizophrenia, and some types of cognitive mental disorder; it also can be seen in people whose personalities are tightly controlled (in such a case the person's feelings—indeed, his or her whole personality—is called constricted).

E. *La belle indifference*: a French term that, translated literally, means "the beautiful unconcern." It is used to describe the lack of worry an ordinary person would customarily feel in a difficult situation (Campbell, 1989).

THINKING PROCESS

A person's thinking process is the way she functions intellectually. It is sometimes also called cognitive style or state. It is the way she thinks, the reasoning she uses about the world, and the way she connects or associates these thoughts. When talking with a patient, abnormalities may be noted in speed of thinking: thoughts may be presented slowly or may tumble out quickly (*racing thoughts*).

Another important observation is about thought process, the association or connection between a patient's thoughts. As the patient is speaking it may be difficult for the nurse to understand how her thoughts relate to one another. A patient's thoughts may seem so unconnected that they are similar to a bouncing ball in a confined space. It is uncertain where thoughts are going next.

The process of thinking is ongoing for most people. Normal thinking occurs whenever a logical sequence of thoughts results in a reality-oriented conclusion. When this process is abnormal, you may see any of the following disturbances (Kaplan & Sadock, 1994, 1995):

SYMPTOMS OF THINKING DISORDER

A. Disturbances in thought process (also known as *disturbance in associations or connections between thoughts*).
  1. *Loose associations*: when a patient's thoughts are poorly connected and do not make logical sense to a listener.
     a. *Circumstantiality*: a flow of spoken thoughts that results in a patient's eventually getting to a conclusion after many digressions to associated ideas. It can be compared to someone starting out on a journey from New York to Los Angeles and stopping off in Montreal and Anchorage on the way.
     b. *Tangentiality*: a flow of spoken thoughts that results in many digressions, but in which a conclusion is never reached. It can be compared to a someone who starts a journey with a vague idea of where he wants to go, but who stops in so many other places that he eventually forgets his original destination.
  2. *Neologism*: a new word that a person makes up. It may sound like a nonsense word.
  3. *Flight of ideas*: rapid speaking with a quick shifting from one idea to another. Unlike the process of loose associations, these ideas do have a logical connection. Frequently seen in manic patients.
  4. *Perseveration*: repetition of the same thought or word in response to different questions.
  5. *Word salad*: disconnected mixture of unrelated words.
  6. *Blocking*: a stoppage in the train of thought or in the midst of a sentence.
B. Disturbances in content of thought.
  1. *Delusion*: a false belief, not consistent with a person's intelligence and cultural background, that cannot be corrected by reasoning.
     a. *Delusion of grandeur*: an exaggerated belief about one's abilities or importance.
     b. *Delusion of reference*: false belief that one is the center of others' attention and discussion.
     c. *Delusion of persecution (paranoia)*: false belief that others are seeking to hurt or damage a person either physically or by insinuation.
  2. *Preoccupation of thought*: connection of all occurrences and experiences to a central thought, usually one with strong emotional overtones. For example, someone who was injured while escaping from a fire may continue, even while safe in the hospital, to fear being trapped again. This preoccupation is evident in frequent discussion of the event.
  3. *Obsessive thought*: an unwelcome idea, emotion, or urge that repeatedly enters a person's consciousness.
  4. *Phobia*: a strong fear of a particular situation.
     a. *Claustrophobia*: fear of being in an enclosed place.
     b. *Agoraphobia*: fear of being in an open place, such as outdoors or on a highway.
     c. *Acrophobia*: fear of high places.
C. Other disturbances of thought.
  1. *Memory impairment*: any type of change in ability to accurately recall thoughts from the unconscious into consciousness.
     a. *Amnesia*: complete or partial inability to recall past experiences.
     b. *Confabulation*: the filling in of gaps in memory with untrue statements. This is done by the patient unconsciously because he is unable to recognize his intellectual deficits. It is most frequently seen in cognitive mental disorder. It is common in alcoholic persons with Korsakoff's syndrome (Kaplan & Sadock, 1994, 1995). Lay people may describe that the individual is making up stories or telling "white

lies." It is actually an unconscious attempt to compensate for memory deficits.

  c. *Déjà vu*: translated literally from French, this means "already seen." A feeling that one has experienced a new situation on a previous occasion. (This can normally occur in anyone who is fatigued or under stress.)

MEMORY

Human beings possess two types of memory: recent and long-term memory. *Recent memory* is the ability to recall events in the unconscious that have occurred in the immediate past and up to 1 or 2 weeks previously. *Long-term memory* is the ability to recall events from the distant past: names of schools attended, dates of siblings' birthdays, the sequence of U.S. presidents, and so on. When memory fails, recent memory is the first to be affected. Memory deficits can most often be seen in patients with chronic cognitive mental disorder (the irreversible senile dementias such as arteriosclerosis), acute cognitive mental disorder (the usually reversible toxic brain syndromes), and depressed individuals whose cognitive abilities are temporarily slowed by the depression.

  Clients with recent memory deficits will demonstrate confusion about recent events but are usually able to describe the names of their grandparents, their places of birth, or who was president when they graduated from grade school, and so on. The process of memory storage of recent events is fully or partially dysfunctional due to the presence of organic or functional pathology; however, the long-term memory is unaffected.

  In order to test a person's long-term memory, he can be asked specific questions about his childhood and early adulthood. When inquiring about recent events, it is essential that the correct answers are known in order to validate the accuracy of the patient's responses. If answer(s) to the following questions are correct, a patient's mental status is within normal range. If there are many gaps in his ability to answer these questions, there is a greater likelihood that brain dysfunction due to a physiological disorder is present.

The patient can be asked to describe:

1. The present illness: when it began, the symptoms, names of doctors involved (recent memory).
2. The past: birthdate, date of high school graduation or marriage, names of siblings or children (long-term memory).
3. Significant events in a topic that the patient acknowledges interest in, for example, politics, baseball, a job, during the past 5 years (recent and long-term memory).

These types of questions can all be asked conversationally without causing the patient to feel he or she is being "examined."

PERCEPTION

Perception is the way a person views herself, the environment, and her relationship with others in the environment. Perception is derived from the senses of vision, hearing, touch, and smell. The input from the senses is mediated by the mind and its defenses.

  In determining whether a person's perception is normal, there can be behavioral manifestations that the patient is distorting reality. If, for example, a patient appears to be picking things from her bed, body, or the wall, there is a strong possibility that visual hallucinations are occurring. The patient thinks she is seeing insects or other objects (a common type of hallucination in hospitalized patients with cognitive mental disorder) (Campbell, 1989; Kaplan & Sadock, 1994, 1995).

  The major type of perceptual dysfunction observed in hospital patients is *hallucinations*. Hallucinations are false sensory perceptions that do not exist in external reality. The types of hallucinations are listed below:

1. *Visual hallucination*
   The person sees objects that are nonexistent. This is one of the most common symptoms of mental disorder caused by delirium tremens (DTs), drug toxicity, or delirium resulting from any other physiological imbalance. Visual hallucinations are rare

in people with schizophrenia or other forms of functional psychiatric disorder.

2. *Tactile hallucination*

    The person feels objects or sensations that are nonexistent. This is also common in cognitive or other toxic-induced psychoses and is rare in functional disorders.

3. *Auditory hallucination*

    The person hears voices, bells, or other sounds that are nonexistent. The identification of auditory hallucinations usually signifies that there is no physical or toxic cause to the dysfunction. Auditory hallucinations are most common in schizophrenia, manic-depressive illness, and other transient psychiatric functional states.

4. *Hypnagogic hallucination*

    The person has any type of false sensory perception during the twilight period between being awake and being asleep. This type of experience can also occur in normal individuals, especially during times of severe fatigue or acute stress.

Another form of perceptual dysfunction is called an *illusion*. An illusion is a distortion or misinterpretation of an actual stimulus. For example, a person in the intensive care unit may distort the image of the intravenous tubing and report that he has snakes crawling on his arm. Illusions may be present in both cognitive mental disorder and the functional psychoses.

Two other forms of mental dysfunction are related to perception of oneself and the environment:

1. *Depersonalization:* a loss of sense of control over oneself, and a feeling of detachment from one's surroundings.
2. *Derealization:* a sense of unreality, a distortion, or a frank loss of reality about the environment.

Depersonalization and derealization are signs of many types of psychiatric disorders. They also may be experienced by normal persons during times of acute stress or extreme fatigue.

ABSTRACT THINKING AND JUDGMENT

Abstract Thinking

Abstract thinking is a person's ability to derive a conclusion from a logical reasoning process. *Concrete thinking* is in contrast to abstract thinking. When a person thinks concretely, he interprets what he sees and hears in a rigid way. He will perceive things exactly as they are sensed, rather than applying abstract judgment to decide the actual meaning. For example, when a patient is asked, "How did you happen to come to the clinic today?" he may reply, "By bus," rather than by telling you the health problem that caused him to come to the clinic. Concrete thinking in a person of normal to high intelligence is often an indication of cognitive mental disorder. People with a low level of intelligence may routinely think in a concrete manner. Concrete thinking may also be seen in schizophrenics (Campbell, 1989; Kaplan & Sadock, 1995).

Judgment

Judgment is evidenced by a person's ability to behave in a socially appropriate manner. In a formal mental status examination, this ability can be determined by asking a person what he would do if he found a wallet containing a large sum of money lying in the street. Another question that could be asked is, "What would you do if you discovered a fire burning in a building?"

Informally, in the hospital setting, a person's social judgment can be observed by the way he acts in his room, with health care team members, or with other patients. For example, the individual discussed below was a major concern to the nurses on his unit:

CASE EXAMPLE

Joe is a 38-year-old married man. His father is a prominent lawyer (this information can be used to infer that, under normal conditions, Joe should be aware of socially appropriate behavior). Joe's hospital room was located near the entrance of a busy surgical unit. Joe's normal attire was a loosely tied bathrobe. He declared that he did not like to wear underwear or pajamas; they were too constricting. He always wore a baseball hat with wings protruding from each side. Joe refused to lie under the covers; his lack of modesty was suggestive of socially poor judgment and a potential indicator of mental disorder. ❦

Poor social judgment is frequently seen in persons with mental dysfunction caused by cognitive mental disorder, schizophrenia, or severe depression.

ASSESSMENT OF SUICIDE POTENTIAL

Another aspect of the mental status evaluation is assessment of suicide potential. Because mention of the word *suicide* gives most medical-surgical caregivers an unpleasant feeling, the word can rarely be mentioned. Instead, phrases such as "doing oneself in," "ending it all," or other euphemisms are acceptable for caregivers in the general hospital setting to use with physically ill patients. Although the concept of suicide may be unpleasant to caregivers, suicides do occur in the general hospital and its potential must be evaluated.

Many nurses in inpatient or outpatient settings come into contact with seriously depressed individuals. Their depression and hopelessness may be due to preexisting personality disorders or may be the result of living with a chronic illness that has permanently disrupted the quality of their lives. Hopelessness from either source can eventually cause a person to want to die.

Chapters 17 and 18 describe specific recommendations to use in assessing and caring for depressed and potentially suicidal patients. Most professionals who are not specifically trained in clinical psychiatric theory are concerned that if they ask a seriously depressed person if he or she has ever thought about committing suicide, the person may make the idea a reality.

Actually, when severe or prolonged physical or emotional pain are occurring, many normal persons can experience fleeting wishes to be dead in order to no longer experience their distress. A person may wish that death would claim him, or he may think about killing himself in order to escape from his distress. In either case, if such ideas are present, it can be a relief for them to be acknowledged. In fact, when patients have such thoughts, they are usually troubled by them but are afraid to share them with professionals (Hackett & Stern, 1991; Kaplan & Sadock, 1994, 1995).

The following dialogue can be a guide to discussing this topic.

"Have you ever wished it would all be over or that you were dead?" If the answer is yes, continue on.

"What would you do to make that happen?" If the patient says "Nothing" or denies that he would do anything actively to kill himself, but would want the disease to kill him, then continue.

"What is it that keeps you from wanting to die?" Listen for him to tell you that his family needs him, or one or more other specific reasons why he could not commit suicide. If he has no reason, then he is at greater risk. If he tells you that he wants to kill himself, it is important for you to find out how he would do it.

"How would you kill yourself?" If he has no suicide plan, his risk for suicide is less than that of a person who has one. His intention to commit suicide must be taken seriously, however. If he has a suicide plan, he is at strong risk for suicide.

The assessment process may reveal that the patient has occasional or persistent thoughts of suicide. These thoughts are called *suicidal ideation.* He wants to die; his physical or emotional distress has caused him to give up hope. The only way that he sees out of his difficulty is to kill himself. If a suicide plan has been developed, he is at greater risk for self-inflicted harm. Whether suicidal thinking or an active plan has been developed, the attending physician should be notified at once. A notation about this assessment should be made in the clinical notes. If the patient has an active plan, a psychiatric consultation should be ordered without delay to protect the patient.

Another important consideration in recommending psychiatric consultation is your legal responsibility as a caregiver to this patient. The nurse can be held accountable if a patient harms himself. If the patient is considered to be a strong suicidal risk, then constant surveillance of the patient should occur until the psychiatric consultant arrives. Care of the suicidal individual is addressed more fully in Chapters 17 and 18.

ASSESSMENT OF HOMICIDAL POTENTIAL

When a patient demonstrates strong hostility toward another individual, an assessment of actual or potential harm to another is necessary. It becomes more urgent if the patient has a history of prior violence to another or if current or past behavior demonstrates poor impulse control (Kaplan & Sadock, 1994, 1995).

CONCLUSION

An evaluation of mental status of all patients is strongly recommended. It is possible for any patient to develop a cognitive mental disorder when the physiological functioning of the brain is impaired by the toxic effects of illness or medications. A mental status exam requires only a few minutes of time to assess and record. The original assessment of mental status will be important if organic causes or ineffective coping brings about changes in mental status. It will provide an important point of comparison.

Unlike functional psychiatric disorders, the psychiatric symptoms of cognitive mental disorder can vary markedly within the hour (Dossey, 1994; Frazier, Molinoff, & Winokur, 1994; Strub & Black, 1993). With documentation of a changing mental status caused by maladaptation or organic dysfunction, medical intervention can be initiated to diagnose and treat the underlying cause.

BIBLIOGRAPHY

Anderson, B., & Holmes, W. (1993). Altered mental status: An algorithm for assessment of delirium in the cancer patient. *Current Issues in Cancer Nursing Practice, 2*(5), 1–9.

Bassett, S. S., & Folstein, M. F. (1991). Cognitive impairment and functional disability in the absence of psychiatric diagnosis. *Psychology and Medicine, 21*(1), 77–84.

Bruera, E. (1991). Severe organic brain syndrome. *Journal of Palliative Care, 7*(1), 36–38.

Carpenito, L. J. (1993). *Nursing diagnosis: Application and clinical practice.* Philadelphia: J. B. Lippincott.

Cassem, N. H. (1991). Depression. In N. H. Cassem (Ed.), *Massachusetts General Hospital handbook of general hospital psychiatry* (3rd ed.). St. Louis: Mosby Year Book.

Coyle, M. K. (1987). Organic illness mimicking psychiatric episodes. *Journal of Gerontological Nursing, 13*(1), 31–35.

Diagnostic and statistical manual of mental disorders (4th ed.). (1994). Washington, DC: American Psychiatric Press.

Dossey, B.M. (1994). Dynamics of consiousness and healing. *Journal of Holistic Nursing, 12*(1), 5–7.

Dossey, B. M., Guzzetta, C. E., & Kenner, C. V. (1992). *Critical care nursing: Body-mind-spirit.* Philadelphia: J. B. Lippincott.

Dunner, D. L. (1993). Diagnostic assessment. *Psychiatric Clinics of North America, 16*(3), 431–441.

Easton, C., & McKenzie, F. (1988). Sensory-perceptual alterations: Delirium in the intensive care unit. *Heart and Lung, 17*(3), 229–237.

Fleishman, S., & Lesko, L. (1989). Delirium and dementia. In J. Holland & J. Rowland (Eds.), *Handbook of Psycho-oncology: Psychological care of the patient with cancer.* New York: Oxford University Press.

Frazier, A., Molinoff, P. B., & Winokur, A. (Eds.). (1994). *Biological bases of brain function and disease.* New York: Raven Press.

Geary, S. M. (1994). Intensive care unit psychosis revisited: Understanding and managing delirium in the critical care setting. *Critical Care Nursing Quarterly, 17*(1), 51–63.

Goldberg, R. J., Faust, D., & Novack, D. (1992). Integrating the cognitive mental status examination into the medical interview. *Southern Medical Journal, 85*(5), 491–497.

Groves, J. E., & Kurcharski, A. (1991). Brief psychotherapy. In N. H. Cassem (Ed.), *Massachusetts General Hospital handbook of general hospital psychiatry* (3rd ed.). St. Louis: Mosby Year Book.

Hackett, T. P., & Stern, T. A. (1991). Suicide and other disruptive states. In N. H. Cassem (Ed.), *Massachusetts General Hospital handbook of general hospital psychiatry* (3rd ed.). St. Louis: Mosby Year Book.

Hamilton, L. W., & Creason, N. S. (1992). Mental status and functional abilities: Change in institutionalized elderly women. *Nursing Diagnosis, 3*(2), 81–86.

Harper, R. G., Chacko, R. C., Kotik-Harper, D., & Kirby, H. B. (1992). Comparison of two cognitive screening measures for efficacy in differentiating dementia from depression in a geriatric inpatient population. *Journal of Neuropsychiatry and Clinical Neuroscience, 4*(2), 179–184.

Huber, M., & Kennard, A. (1991). Functional and mental status outcomes of clients discharged from acute gerontological versus medical/surgical units. *Journal of Gerontological Nursing, 17*(7), 20–24.

Kaplan, H. I., & Sadock, B. J. (1995). *Comprehensive textbook of psychiatry/VI* (6th ed.). Baltimore: Williams & Wilkins.

Kokmen, E., Smith, G. E., Petersen, R. C., Tangalos, E., & Ivnik, R. C. (1991). The short test of mental status. Correlations with standardized psychometric testing. *Archives of Neurology, 48*(7), 725–728.

Lipowski, Z. (1992). Update on delirium. *Psychiatric Clinics of North America, 15*(2), 335–346.

McFarland, G., Wasli, E., & Gerety, E. (1992). *Nursing diagnosis and process in psychiatric mental health nursing.* Philadelphia: J. B. Lippincott.

Menza, M. A., Murray, G. B., Homes, V. F., & Rafuls, W. A. (1988). Controlled study of extrapyramidal reactions in the management of delirious medically ill patients: Intravenous haloperidol versus intravenous haloperidol plus benzodiazapines. *Heart and Lung, 17*(3), 238–241.

Murray, G. B. (1991). Confusion, delirium, and dementia. In N. H. Cassem (Ed.), *Massachusetts General Hospital handbook of general hospital psychiatry* (3rd ed.). St. Louis: Mosby Year Book.

O'Connor, S. (1991). Psychiatric liaison nursing in a changing health care system. In N. H. Cassem (Ed.), *Massachusetts General Hospital handbook of general hospital psychiatry* (3rd ed.). St. Louis: Mosby Year Book.

Parker, G., Hadzi-Pavlovic, D., Hickie, I., Boyce, P., Mitchell, P., Wilhelm, K., & Brodaty, H. (1991). Distinguishing psychotic and non-psychotic melancholia. *Journal of Affective Disorders, 22*(3), 135–148.

Rosenbaum, J. F., & Pollack, M. H. (1991). Anxiety. In N. H. Cassem (Ed.), *Massachusetts General Hospital handbook of general hospital psychiatry* (3rd ed.). St. Louis: Mosby Year Book.

Strub, R. L., & Black, F. W. (1993). *The mental status examination in neurology* (3rd ed.). Philadelphia: F. A. Davis.

Sullivan, N., & Fogel, B. S. (1986). Could this be delirium? *American Journal of Nursing, 86*(12), 1359–1363.

Tesar, G. E. (1993). The agitated patient, Part I: Evaluation and behavioral management. *Hospital and Community Psychiatry, 44*(4), 329–331.

Trzepacs, P. T., & Baker, R. W. (1993). *Psychiatric mental status examination.* New York: Oxford University Press.

Zimberg, M., & Berenson, S. (1990). Delirium patients with cancer: Nursing assessment and intervention. *Oncology Nursing Forum, 17*(4), 529–553.

Zimberg, M., & Mahon, M. (1992). Understanding delirium: An impediment to quality of life. In L. Powell (Ed.), *Quality of life: A nursing challenge.* Philadelphia: Meriscus Publications.

CHAPTER 11

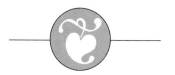

The Physical Causes of Cognitive Mental Disorders

Patricia Barry

Cognitive mental disorders (CMD) are frequently overlooked and underdiagnosed in the general hospital as a significant disease entity. CMD is a constellation of observable psychiatric symptoms caused by a dysfunction of the physical structure or the physiological functioning of the brain. The dysfunction results in emotional or intellectual changes in the patient's mental state. Another name for any type of organic brain dysfunction is *encephalopathy*.

Nurses and physicians in the general hospital are not alone in their lack of awareness of the etiology and symptoms of CMD. Lipowski, one of the best-known U.S. experts on CMD, has said that cerebral dysfunction and disease have remained a no-man's land straddling the boundaries of psychiatry, neurology, and neuropsychology (1975).

Mental disorders due to cerebral disease and dysfunction constitute an integral yet conspicuously neglected area of psychiatry. Lipowski, a psychiatrist, states that psychiatry has done little to investigate the syndrome, and the diagnosis of CMD falls squarely on the shoulders of psychiatry (1980). This is because

the psychiatric symptoms displayed by the patient with CMD usually motivate puzzled attending physicians in other medical-surgical specialties to refer the patient for psychiatric consultation if symptoms become acute and psychosis occurs.

NURSES AS OBSERVERS OF EARLY SYMPTOMS

Because nurses spend more time with patients than do all other members of the health care team, they are the caregivers most likely to notice a change in a patient's mental status over several hours. The symptoms of acute CMD occur rapidly. For example, at 10:30 AM a nurse may give morning care to an alert patient who displays normal levels of energy, intellectual ability, and emotional stabil-

Patricia Barry: *Psychosocial Nursing: Care of Physically Ill Patients and Their Families,* 3rd ed.
© 1996 Lippincott–Raven Publishers

ity. By 1 PM, the patient may be lethargic, confused, and not able to remember seeing the nurse in the morning. Or, in another example, he may be restless, hyperalert, and suspicious of any treatment or medication you wish to give him, and by 2 PM he may tell you that the television set in the room is actually a camera spying on him.

In both cases the patient's mental state has changed markedly from what it was on admission, earlier in his hospitalization, and as recently as a few hours ago. It is essential that these specific changes be noted, with the exact time observed.

When a change in mental state is observed, it is important to watch closely for the variations and specific changes in functioning mentioned in the previous chapter. When slight differences in mental status occur, they can indicate the possibility of development of cerebral dysfunction due to physical causes (Murray, 1991; Strub & Black, 1993). The patient's brain function may be deteriorating as the result of a new or worsening physical complication. Early detection by the nurse with an alerting call to the patient's physician may make a critical difference.

COMPARISON OF FUNCTIONAL AND COGNITIVE MENTAL DISORDERS

The psychiatric symptoms observed in the patient with CMD may appear to be the same as the symptoms in a hallucinating schizophrenic (Dunner, 1993; Murray, 1991; Strub & Black, 1993). Many nurses and physicians miss the symptoms of early and acute CMD because of lack of knowledge concerning the difference between functional and organically caused psychiatric disorders. A functional psychiatric illness is one with no active physical abnormality related to it (although researchers continue to search for relationships between neurobiology and functional diseases such as schizophrenia and depression). CMD is caused by specific, measurable deterioration in the physical structures or in the chemical functioning of the nervous system.

For this reason, one may hear a nurse remark, "Oh, Mr. Thomas is having hallucinations again. Let's give him some more haloperidol (Haldol)." The nurse may not be aware that Mr. Thomas's hallucinations may actually be caused by a fluctuating mental state due to toxicity from an undiagnosed medical problem or even from the haloperidol itself. She may incorrectly believe that Mr. Thomas may be a former psychiatric patient who must be controlled with medication.

In patients with either organic or functional disorders, psychosis is present at the severe end of the continuum. How then, does one tell if the psychotic symptoms observed are more likely to be of organic origin and therefore medically treatable and potentially reversible? There are some basic differences between the two, which the following chart will help to clarify (Table 11-1).

TYPES OF COGNITIVE MENTAL DISORDER

DELIRIUM

The most commonly observed acute form of CMD in general hospital patients is *delirium*. It can develop rapidly, in even a few hours. It is also called *toxic brain syndrome* (Kaplan & Sadock, 1994, 1995; Strub & Black, 1993). Delirium frequently is associated with an already existing physical illness that may have precipitated the toxic brain reaction. The most important distinguishing characteristics of delirium are fairly rapid changes in the patient's wakefulness, alertness, attention span, and ability to perceive the environment accurately. If the organic process continues, symptoms will gradually increase to a psychotic state.

Visual hallucinations are common when the patient is delirious. This is in contrast to functional psychiatric disorders such as schizophrenia, in which auditory hallucinations are far more common than visual ones. When the delirious patient develops inaccurate ideas and thoughts, the delusional thoughts are usually paranoid. When the pa-

TABLE 11-1
Differences Between CMD Pyschosis and Functional Psychosis

Differentiating Factors	CMD Psychosis	Functional Psychosis
Etiology (the cause should be traceable to one of the categories noted)	Metabolic disorder Electrical (convulsive) disorder Neoplastic disease Degenerative brain disease Arterial (cerebrovascular) disease Mechanical (structural) disease Infectious disease Nutritional disorder Drug toxicity (Goldberg, 1980)	Schizophrenia Manic–depressive illness Psychotic depression
Past history	Evidence of recent infection, head trauma, metabolic disorder, or other incident related to categories above	Usually reveals past psychiatric disturbances; recent history of an emotionally stressful precipitating event
Level of consciousness	Usually affected	Rarely affected
Orientation to time (usually first affected), place (less affected), person (least affected)	Usually one or more are affected	Rarely affected
Recent Memory	Usually affected	Rarely affected
Distant Memory	Less affected than recent memory	Rarely affected
Intellectual functioning (thinking and judgment)	Usually affected	Usually affected
Emotional functioning	Usually affected	Usually affected
Perception	Usually affected (hallucinations are more often visual)	Usually affected (hallucinations are more often auditory)
Neurological changes	Usually present	Rarely affected
Laboratory findings	Usually abnormal	Rarely affected

Adapted from Kaplan & Sadock, 1994, 1995; Lishman 1987; Goldberg, 1980.

tient is stimulated to alertness, his intellect remains relatively unchanged (Donner, 1993; Kaplan & Sadock, 1994, 1995; Strub & Black, 1993).

A change in the patient's activity level usually occurs. Most often the change is toward a slowing of movement, ranging to total stupor; however, toxic CMD may cause psychomotor restlessness and overactivity. Another characteristic of both acute and chronic CMD is a worsening of psychiatric symptoms at night. This syndrome is called *sun-downing*. When this occurs, the use of a night light in the patient's room can be a help as the patient tries to orient himself. If it is diagnosed promptly, and the cause of the toxic brain reaction is removed or treated properly, acute CMD reactions can frequently be reversed with no permanent effects.

DEMENTIA

Dementia is a chronic form of CMD. It develops over an extended time, in contrast to acute CMD. The predominant characteristic of dementia is a gradual deterioration in a person's intellectual functioning; cognitive deficits slowly become evident. Most notable are decreases in the ability to reason accurately, remember recent events, and use good social judgment. The patient remains fully oriented until the condition progresses. Although delusions, primarily of a paranoid nature, may occur, they are usually not as severe as in the patient with the delirium form of acute CMD (Dunner, 1993; Lishman, 1987).

Other common symptoms of dementia are changes in personality or an exaggeration of previously existing personality characteristics. For example, if the person had been thrifty in her buying habits, she might become obsessed with finding the cheapest possible item or refuse to spend her money at all as the dementia progressed. Any type of new situation may be frightening to the patient because she is not able to process observations accurately; she may feel overwhelmed by her helplessness. Marked anxiety ranging to panic level may occur unless emotional support is available to relieve her fears. The term used for this overwhelming state is *catastrophic reaction*.

Table 11-2 describes the differences between delirium and dementia. Specific nursing interventions with both delirious and demented patients are presented in Chapter 19.

CAUSES OF COGNITIVE MENTAL DISORDER

There are hundreds of possible causes of CMD. It would be impossible to try to remember each of these etiologies. However, a classification system arranged in a mnemonic, devised by Richard Goldberg (1980), can help to simplify the list of conditions that may lead to brain dysfunction. The mnemonic is MEND A MIND (see Box 11-1). The letters represent etiologies of CMD. Each of these categories will be presented in this chapter, with a description of its most common conditions or disorders.

It is important to note that there are complex neurological changes as well as overt psychiatric symptoms present in CMD. Only the psychiatric manifestations of each of the organic brain conditions are described in this chapter. The psychiatric changes are emphasized because the neurological changes are well described in most nursing and medical neurology textbooks. The psychiatric symptoms are frequently less well defined.

When a nurse knows what psychiatric changes to look for, these observations can make a critical difference in the data the physician uses to make a diagnosis. Delay in determining the diagnosis results in extreme emotional discomfort and sharply increased physical risk to the patient. The increased physical risk has two causes. The first is the potential lethality of an undiagnosed, underlying, physical disease condition affecting the central nervous system. The second is the increased risk of injury to a delirious patient, who may accidentally injure himself or caregivers.

Another consideration of the risks of CMD is the sequela of psychological discomfort related to the delirium episodes. Often, caregivers assume that the CMD patient will have no recollection of the terrors caused by hallucinations or delusions. In reality, many patients experience unpleasant after-effects once the underlying cause is treated. Although these patients were delirious, an awareness of their thoughts, feelings, and surroundings during the episodes is stored in their unconscious memory (Dunner, 1993; Strub & Black, 1993).

One of the emotional sequela that can occur is frightening nightmares related to the event (or events). There also may be persisting fears. These puzzle the patient and family because there is no conscious awareness of the cause. These fears may include fear of the dark, fear of strangers, fear of hospitals, and so on. There also may be a vague awareness of having experienced an unpleasant event. Such a memory may be mildly haunting (Goldberg, Faust, & Novack, 1992; Murray, 1991).

One of the best ways to relieve these after-effects is to allow the patient to recall what happened after he has returned to his normal

TABLE 11-2
Two Types of Cognitive Mental Disorder

Variables	Delirium	Dementia
Onset	Usually rapid; waxes and wanes abruptly	Usually slow: 1 month or more
Level of awareness	Increased or decreased	Normal or decreased
Orientation	Disoriented	Usually not affected until late in course
Appearance and behavior	May be semicomatose; agitated	Usually slowed responses
Speech and communication	Incoherence; degree of change based on severity of delirium	Usually slowed because of cognitive deficits
Mood	Labile; anxiety or panic common	Constricted affect or depression
Thinking process	Markedly altered	Mildly altered; decreased intellectual ability
Memory	Partial or full loss of recent memory; remote memory intact	Partial loss of both recent and remote memory
Perception	Usually markedly altered	Usually intact or mildly affected
Abstract thinking and judgment	Markedly decreased	Mildly decreased
Sleep-wakefulness cycle	Disrupted	Usually not affected
Treatment	Identify and remove underlying cause; symptomatic treatment	Symptomatic treatment
Prognosis	Reversible in most cases	Usually irreversible

Adapted from Bauer, Roberts, & Reisdorf, 1991; Fleishman & Lesko, 1989; Kaplan & Sadock, 1994, 1995.

state. For example, the nurse can inquire, "Mr. Smith, you've been very sick for the past few days. Do you remember anything that happened?" Because CMD is usually marked by a fluctuating mental status, there probably were periods when the patient was oriented. He will usually be able to remember some routine hospital events, for instance, speaking with his daughter or receiving medications. He may also recall some disturbing events. He may say, "I remember I saw bugs crawling all over my bed" or "I remember that I thought all of you were trying to capture me." If he remembers any disturbing thought or hallucination, he can be asked *how he felt at that time.* This is very important in releasing the unpleasant emotion that accompanied the event. Cues to exploring the disturbing memory with the patient can be deduced from the content being discussed. Questions can be asked that allow him to express the negative feelings fully.

In this example, Mr. Smith can be reassured that his reactions (seeing bugs, having paranoid ideas, and so on) are very common when someone has a physical crisis such as he experienced. It is the *physical* disease that caused his problems, not a mental illness. This reassurance can bring tears of relief to the patient, who has been silently suffering with fears that he may be crazy. The patient may also be

BOX 11-1	Mend A Mind
	M Metabolic disorder **E** Electrical (convulsive) disorder **N** Neoplastic disease **D** Degenerative (chronic) brain disease
	A Arterial (cerebrovascular) disease
	M Mechanical disease (disease of the actual physical structures of the brain) **I** Infectious disease **N** Nutritional disease **D** Drug toxicity
	Goldberg, R. (1980). *Psychiatry for the primary physician.* Darien, CT: Patient Care Publications.

afraid that it might happen again after he gets out of the hospital. You can tell him that unless all the conditions are duplicated (high fever, septic shock, or whatever his specific etiology was), it is highly unlikely.

In addition, you can explain that he may have dreams about what happened during his delirium or may remember aspects of it when he is awake. Unless the dreams become more severe, they should go away in time. You can recommend that talking about his feelings about these unpleasant events with supportive family members or friends can help to relieve the unpleasant memories.

In the remainder of this chapter, many conditions known to have the potential to change a person's mental status will be described. The psychiatric symptoms presented with them are typical examples of a broad range of symptoms. The way a person actually responds to an organic change will vary depending on his or her premorbid personality style (Lishman, 1987). Accordingly, this guide should not be rigidly adhered to. It is written to introduce the many types of organic disease that can result in broad ranges of psychiatric dysfunctioning.

METABOLIC

The metabolic etiology of CMD can include changes in functioning in the endocrine glands (the thyroid, parathyroid, adrenals, or Langerhans' islets [insulin-producing cells] in the pancreas) and deficiencies in electrolyte blood levels (calcium, sodium, potassium, and base bicarbonate levels).

Endocrine Gland Disorders

Table 11-3 presents the most commonly occurring metabolic conditions caused by dysfunctions of the endocrine glands.

Electrolyte Imbalance

Another major metabolic cause of CMD is electrolyte imbalance. Table 11-4 includes a list of electrolytes, their normal laboratory values, and the psychiatric symptoms that occur when the electrolyte level is either too high or too low.

Sudden increases or decreases in these electrolytes are more likely to result in observable CMD symptoms than gradual, prolonged increases or decreases. Brain tissues are able to adapt gradually to slight changes that may become surprisingly high or low after an extended period.

ELECTRICAL

The second major category of CMD etiologies is electrical disturbance, in which there is an excessive neuronal discharge within the brain (Kaplan & Sadock, 1994, 1995). The result is an epileptic seizure. Although there are four main classifications of seizures, only two are frequently accompanied by changes in psychiatric functioning: partial and generalized. The *partial seizure* classification involves two main types of disorder, simple and complex. Partial and generalized types of epilepsy, with their possible psychiatric effects, are presented in Table 11-5. Note that although mental status

TABLE 11-3
Mental Status Changes in Metabolic Conditions: Endocrine Gland Disorders

Name of Condition	Cause of Disorder	Changes in Mental Status
Addison's disease (hypoadrenalism)	Deficiency in adrenocortical hormones of the adrenal cortex due to disturbed hypothalamic, pituitary, or adrenal functioning	Depression Negativism Suspiciousness Apathy
Cushing's syndrome (hyperadrenalism)	Excessive amounts of adrenocortical hormones of the adrenal cortex due to diseases of the hypothalamus or pituitary that produce excessive amounts of adrenocorticotropic hormone or to hyperplasia of the adrenal cortex; can also be caused by steroid drugs	Excitement Acute anxiety Emotional instability Depression (when disorder is result of internally caused elevated levels) Euphoria (when disorder is result of steroid drugs)
Hyperthyroidism	Excessive secretion of thyroid glands; basal metabolic rate is elevated	Nervousness Excitability Emotional instability Insomnia Psychosis (in acute stages)
Hypothyroidism (myxedema)	Deficiency of thyroid secretion; basal metabolic rate is decreased	Apathy Sluggishness Irritability Delusions and paranoid thinking (in acute stage); can sometimes persist for months
Hyperparathyroidism	Excessive secretion of parathyroid glands results in increased levels of calcium and phosphorus	Mixed levels of anxiety and depression Weakness Irritability Psychosis
Hypoparathyroidism	Deficient parathyroid secretions	Apathy (if onset is rapid) Depression (if onset is slow) Psychosis
Hyperinsulinism	Adenoma of Langerhans' islets; excessive insulin in bloodstream due to overdosage or undereating	Anxiety attacks Confusion Emotional lability
Pituitary problems of any kind, depending on etiology and course; can also cause psychiatric symptoms		Mixed, depending on etiology course of the disease

Adapted from Kaplan & Sadock, 1994, 1995; Lipowski, 1992; Lishman, 1987; Stoudemire & Fogel, 1993.

TABLE 11-4				
Mental Status Changes in Metabolic Conditions: Electrolyte Imbalance				
Name of Electrolyte	Normal Level	Abnormal Level	Cause	Changes in Mental Status
Calcium	8.5 to 10.5 mg/dl	+Hyper-calcemia	Hyperparathyroidism	Loss of energy Depression Irritability
		−Hypocal-cemia	Hypoparathyroidism; deficiency of calcium or vitamin D in the diet	Psychosis in acute CMD caused by surgical removal of gland; nutritional deficiency results in less acute symptoms: ↓ concentration, ↓ intellectual functions, emotional lability, depression
Sodium	135–145 mEq/L	+Hyperna-tremia	Dehydration due to excessive water loss from body (vomiting, diarrhea) Diabetes insipidus Restricted fluid intake Excessive diuresis	Irritability Hyperactivity in intellectual ability Stupor
		−Hypona-tremia	Severe dietary restriction of sodium Addison's disease Excessive water consumption (polydipsia)	Depression Lethargy Withdrawal Anorexia
Phosphorus	2.6–4.5 mg/dl	−Hyophos-phatemia	Gram-negative septicemia Alcohol withdrawal Hyperalimentation Poor nutritional status	Apprehension Irritability Numbness Stupor
Potassium	3.5–5 mEq/L	+Hyper-kalemia	Renal disease Potassium-sparing diuretics Level of potassium in intravenous fluids	Weakness Dysphasia
		−Hypoka-lemia	Renal disease Cushing's syndrome Loss of potassium due to diuretics Self-induced vomiting Gastroenteritis	Changes in mood and personality Tearfulness Hopelessness Helplessness
Base bicarbonate	Blood pH 7.38–7.42, bicarbonate level 24 mEq/L	+Alkalosis	Prolonged vomiting Taking large amounts of bicarbonate Hyperventilation	↓ Intellectual functioning Apathy Delirium Stupor
		−Acidosis	Severe respiratory illness: emphysema, status asthmaticus Renal failure Diabetes mellitus with ketosis	↓ Intellectual ability Drowsiness Confusion Delirium

---

TABLE 11-5
Mental Status Changes of Different Types of Epilepsy

Type of Seizure	Changes in Mental Status
Simple partial (no loss of consciousness)	Perceptual hallucinations Dizziness Nonsensical speech (Brunner & Suddarth, 1988)
Complex partial (temporary loss of consciousness)	Catatonia or inappropriate movement Emotions of fear, anger, elation, or irritability No memory of seizure (Brunner & Suddarth, 1988)
Generalized seizures	↑ Irritability before seizure May be ↑ aggressive or emotional before seizure, confusion after seizure May demonstrate no confusion but may have transient episode of schizophrenia-like symptoms of psychotic affect, disturbances in thinking, or perceptual distortion (Kaplan & Sadock, 1994, 1995; Lipowski, 1992; Lishman, 1987; Stoudemire & Fogel, 1993.)

---

changes can and do occur in these conditions, their severity will depend on the patient's underlying personality style as well as on the severity of the electrical disturbance (Lishman, 1987). The majority of persons with epilepsy experience little or no emotional disturbance.

Epileptic disorder is a complex medical illness that requires the astute diagnostic ability of a neurologist. If emotional symptoms are present as well, the fine points of differential diagnosis should be evaluated by a psychiatrist. Psychiatric consultation will help to determine which aspects of the psychiatric symptoms are due to the physiological dysfunction and which are caused by a separate but concurrent functional psychiatric disorder (Kaplan & Sadock, 1994, 1995; Lishman, 1987).

NEOPLASTIC (BENIGN OR MALIGNANT TUMORS)

Any neoplasm within the brain, benign or malignant, can produce psychiatric symptoms. At least half of all patients with primary sites of brain neoplasms demonstrate changes in psychological functioning. In addition to tumors originating within the brain, the brain is also a common site of metastasis from other body sites, most commonly from the lungs, breast, gastrointestinal tract, prostate, and pancreas. The most frequent type of metastasis to the brain originates from the lungs (Kaplan & Sadock, 1994, 1995; Lishman, 1987).

In some instances, psychiatric symptoms may appear before existence of the primary cancer is known. Various psychiatric syndromes can occur. Depending on the location, size, and type of tumor, dementia, delirium, or progressive changes in personality can be observed. The major reason for the changes in psychiatric function is the increase in intracranial pressure, which applies pressure to all the brain structures (Capwell & Carter, 1991). Loss of ability to interpret sensory perceptions of vision, hearing, and so on (*agnosia*) and loss of ability to perform complex tasks or loss of motor control of all or specific parts of the body (*apraxia*) may occur.

In addition to intracranial tumors, psychiatric symptoms have been closely associated with another type of neoplasm, pheochromocytoma. *Pheochromocytoma* is a tumor of the adrenal medulla that, in most cases, is benign and can be treated. The tumor releases increased levels of epinephrine. The predominant symptom of this patient is a high level of anxiety, or "panic" attacks (Usdin & Lewis, 1979).

Another neoplastic illness with a high incidence of associated psychiatric symptoms is pancreatic carcinoma. Patients with this illness frequently become despondent and apathetic. Their mental state is that of a very depressed person (Usdin & Lewis, 1979).

DEGENERATIVE

The next possible cause of cognitive mental disorder includes diseases that lead to deterioration of the tissues of the brain. The diseases included in this category, and the type of neurological deterioration that occurs, include:

Multiple sclerosis—widespread destruction of myelin in the sheath of nerve fibers.
Systemic lupus erythematosus—antibodies attack neurons; cerebral vasculitis.
Alzheimer's disease—premature degeneration of neurons.
Huntington's chorea—frontal lobe atrophy.
Creutzfeldt-Jakob disease—motor neuron involvement; cerebellar, pyramidal tract damage.

These diseases are accompanied by marked changes in neurological status and, depending on the illness, gradual to marked changes in psychological functioning. Creutzfeldt-Jakob disease is suspected to be transmittable (Moller et al., 1994; Strub & Black, 1993).

For a full description of the pathological process, as well as accompanying neurological symptoms of each of these conditions, refer to any standard neurology textbook. Table 11-6 presents the psychiatric symptoms that are commonly seen as these illnesses progress.

ARTERIAL

The type of mental status symptoms that develop as the result of failure of blood supply to the brain depends on the disease process that causes the normal blood supply to be changed. Depending on the location and extent of the disease process, there can be a continuum of mental status changes ranging from no changes in mental functioning to loss of consciousness.

Cerebrovascular Accident

Cerebrovascular accidents (CVAs) are the third most common cause of death in the western hemisphere (Kaplan & Sadock, 1994, 1995; Lishman, 1987). CVAs are caused by atherosclerosis or hypertension that ultimately results in either infarction or hemorrhage. Infarction outnumbers hemorrhage 3:1.

Thrombosis, caused by the atherosclerotic process, is the most common cause of obstruction to the cerebral arteries that eventually results in CVA. In a CVA there is a loss of blood supply to particular regions of the brain. The specific region affected and the functions it performs usually determine the range of psychiatric symptoms observed.

The mental status symptoms that accompany the profound neurological symptoms fall within both the *delirium* and *dementia* categories. There can be fluctuating mental confusion and visual hallucinations or mental slowing, permanent personality changes, and other symptoms of dementia caused by permanent changes in the structures of the brain. Characteristics common in some stroke patients are emotional lability and hostility. Such patients can demonstrate mild paranoia, as well as aggressiveness in the face of new experiences, new medical regimens, and so on. Approximately half the patients with subarachnoid hemorrhage show mental status changes, including mental confusion, loss of drive, irritability, and anxiety (Kaplan & Sadock, 1994, 1995; Lishman, 1987).

Degenerative Changes of Cerebral Arteries

A second arterial cause of CMD is the chronic, gradual changing of mental functioning caused by degenerative changes of cerebral arteries. This category includes people with cerebral arteriosclerosis, or "hardening of the arteries." People in this category have no history of CVA but demonstrate chronic changes in mental functioning, typically during the seventh and eighth decades of life but sometimes as early as the sixth decade. The changes in mental status are the same as in senile dementia, including increasing loss of memory regarding recent events, poor social judgment, decreases

---

TABLE 11-6
Mental Status Changes of Degenerative Brain Diseases

Disease	Changes in Mental Status
Multiple Sclerosis Age of onset: 20 to 40 years Incidence: 50:100,000 (more common in women) Prognosis: long course; early symptoms may cause diagnostic confusion	Changes in mental status occur in 50% of patients; personality changes include lability, euphoria, decreased intellectual ability, progressive to gross mental deterioration (Kaplan & Sadock, 1995)
Systemic Lupus Erythematosus Age of onset: 20 to 40 years Incidence: women 8:1 Prognosis: long course; early symptoms may cause diagnostic confusion	Changes in mental status occur in 15% to 50% of patients; varied changes possible; thought disorder, depression, confusion (Kaplan & Sadock, 1995)
Alzheimer's Disease Age of onset: 40 to 60 years Incidence: 2 or 3:1 (women:men) Prognosis: death within 2 to 5 years	First phase (lasts 2 to 3 years): ↓ memory, ↓ general functioning, ↓ emotional stability Second phase (lasts approximately 1 year): ↓ intellectual ability, personality deterioration, dysphasia, apraxia, agnosia, acalculia, symptoms of Parkinson's disease (gait and muscular changes) Third phase (lasts approximately 6 months): profound dementia, grand mal seizures, delusions and hallucinations (Kaplan & Sadock, 1995; Lishman, 1987)
Huntington's Chorea Age of onset: 25 to 50 years Incidence: 6:100,000 Prognosis: death within 10 to 20 years	Initial phase: involuntary movements, changes in personality; quarrelsome or apathetic, paranoid, anxious, depressed Later phase: dementia, ↓ intellectual ability (memory may be impaired), psychotic episodes (Kaplan & Sadock, 1995; Lishman, 1987)
Creutzfeldt-Jacob Disease Age of onset: 40 to 50 years Incidence: 1:1 (women:men) Prognosis: death within 9 months to 2 years	Early phase: fatigue, insomnia, anxiety, depression, mental slowness, unpredictable behavior, slowly developing ↓ memory and ↓ concentration Later phase: ↓ intellectual ability, uncontrollable laughing or crying, clouding of consciousness or delirium, auditory hallucinations or delusions, eventual profound dementia (Kaplan & Sadock, 1995; Lishman, 1987)

Adapted from Kaplan & Sadock, 1994, 1995; Lipowski, 1992; Lishman, 1987; Stoudemire & Fogel, 1993.

in general intellectual ability, and anxiety in new social situations (Kaplan & Sadock, 1994, 1995; Lishman, 1987).

Multiple Infarct Dementia

Multiple infarct dementia is usually caused by hypertension. The mental status changes are similar to those of degenerative cerebral arteriosclerosis, described above.

MECHANICAL

Head trauma, subdural hematoma, and normal-pressure hydrocephalus fall within the mechanical CMD etiology. In these conditions, a force or pressure exerted on the brain results in changes in the patient's psychiatric functioning.

Head Injury

The most common after-effect of moderate to severe head injuries is loss of consciousness and amnesia about the accidental event. The cause of these two phenomena is possibly related to the rapidly accelerating or decelerating brain tissue that impacts on the inside of the cranium during the accident (Lishman, 1987).

A head injury results in structural changes as well as major changes in neurological functioning caused by differences in the circulatory, electrical, and biochemical functions of the brain. It has been suggested that the shock of the injury produces a sudden and very great neuronal discharge at the moment of injury, resulting in the release of large amounts of acetylcholine into the cerebrospinal fluid (CSF), which normally contains no acetylcholine. The effects of the neuronal discharge may continue to be present for days or weeks. They usually are present in proportion to the changes in brain electrical status as measured by electroencephalograph (EEG). Acetylcholine is also found in proportion to the degree of change in level of consciousness. As the level of acetylcholine in the patient's CSF decreases, overall mental and physical status usually improves (Lishman, 1987).

Following head injury, the patient may be unconscious for several hours, yet recover spontaneously with no ill effect. Generally speaking, prolonged coma of one or several days is the result of more serious injury to brain tissues. (See Chapter 10 for assessment methods to identify the level of consciousness of the patient with an acute head injury.) Mild to severe cognitive, behavioral, or physical deficits may be permanent when unconsciousness lasts more than a month. Cases do occur, however, in which people regain consciousness after a prolonged period and progressively return to their previous level of functioning (Lishman, 1987).

No matter what part of the brain receives a direct blow or what causes the injury, the most life-threatening aspect of head injury is caused by the resulting stress on the brain stem. The brain stem contains the life-supportive centers of respiration, cardiac rate, and blood pressure regulation as well as the swallowing reflex and the reflex that causes the iris to contract in response to light and regulate the pupil's size (Black & Matassarin-Jacobs, 1993).

The acute psychiatric effects of head injury are *loss of consciousness* and *amnesia* about the accident as well as *loss of memory* about events following the accident. In mild to moderate head injury, the cognitive functions of the ego, such as reasoning, problem solving and judgment, can be affected. It is not unusual for mild perceptual disturbances to occur in the form of decreased spatial relationship perception. Another outcome of this sudden change in ego functioning is a decrease in the ego's ability to control emotion. Increases in the range of emotion normally experienced are due to a decrease in ego defensive capability. As a result of these changes, the patient may experience mild to severe episodes of anxiety or panic (Carpenito, 1993; Lishman, 1987; Strub & Black, 1993). These changes in psychiatric functioning may last anywhere from 4 weeks to 6 months or longer, depending on the severity of the blow to the head. Exaggeration of preinjury personality characteristics can also occur. Recent memory is frequently impaired. Confabulation to cover up the memory deficits is another potential outcome.

In severe head injury, mental status changes can include coma, delusions, hallucinations, and marked disorientation to time, person, and place. These changes are caused by physical stresses on the brain structures from the accident. This type of CMD can be further complicated by biochemical, circulatory, infectious, or other sequelae of the injury (Lishman, 1987; Strub & Black, 1993).

In addition to the acute effects of head injury, patients with complex head injuries may experience chronic psychiatric dysfunction after they are discharged from the hospital. If the psychiatric dysfunction is specifically related to the accident, rather than a preexisting personality disorder, the patient may be depressed, experience high levels of anxiety, or become phobic. Some patients also demonstrate mild to marked permanent changes in personality or in cognitive functions. There is a low tolerance for effects of alcohol consumption for a few weeks to many months (Lishman, 1987; Strub & Black, 1993).

Subdural Hematoma

Subdural hematoma may or may not be present in the patient admitted for acute head trauma. If the patient has acute subdural hematoma accompanying a head injury, the psychiatric changes viewed in the patient will be similar to those presented in the previous section on head injury. The discussion of subdural hematoma in this section will be limited to the psychiatric effects of subdural hematomas that are undiagnosed at the time of injury, but develop slowly and are not diagnosed until weeks or months after the injury occurred. This type of chronic subdural hematoma is most commonly seen in the elderly patient who does not remember the precipitating fall or head injury.

The symptoms of chronic subdural hematoma usually begin with a vague headache. There may be mental slowness characterized by poor concentration and lethargy. This gradually progresses to fluctuating levels of consciousness, that is, changes from wakefulness to drowsiness that may occur as often as every 1 or 2 hours. Without medical attention the patient will eventually lapse into a coma. Because of its chronic and slow progression, the patient with subdural hematoma may be mistakenly diagnosed as having senile dementia. Brain scan examination is an important diagnostic aid in differentiating between the two conditions (Lishman, 1987; Strub & Black, 1993).

Normal-Pressure Hydrocephalus

Normal-pressure hydrocephalus (NPH) has been recognized only during the last two decades. The complex and sophisticated diagnostic screening advances of this period have helped to diagnose and treat this brain condition, which can sometimes be reversed if an early diagnosis is made. In hydrocephalus, the ventricles of the brain enlarge because of increased amounts of cerebrospinal fluid. It differs from other forms of hydrocephalus because there is no increase in spinal fluid pressure (Kaplan & Sadock, 1994, 1995).

The symptoms of NPH can be confused with those of senile dementia. Again, brain scanning will help to differentiate the two conditions. The specific symptoms of NPH are ataxia (abnormal gait), urinary incontinence, and dementia. The dementia associated with NPH includes symptoms of depression, agitation, changes in organization of thoughts, and forgetfulness (Lishman, 1987; Murray, 1991). With early diagnosis and surgical treatment, the prognosis for the patient with NPH is excellent (Gilroy & Meyer, 1975).

INFECTIONS

Several infectious diseases of the brain can result in psychiatric changes. They are AIDS, encephalitis, meningitis, cerebral abscess, and late-stage syphilis.

AIDS Dementia Complex

Human immunodeficiency virus type 1 (HIV-1) is a devastating physical condition that causes system failure in many body systems. This section will address the AIDS dementia complex. AIDS dementia complex (ADC) is usually a late complication of HIV-1 infection.

Clinical symptoms are related to these spheres of functioning: cognition, behavior, and motor. Brew (1993) describes three concepts that assist in understanding the progression of the disease pathology: *time locking*, the phenomenon of symptom occurrence related to the degree of disease development; *parallel tracking*, the concurrent involvement of different parts of the neurological system; and *layer-*

ing, the occurrence of multiple pathological processes within one part of the nervous system.

Symptoms of AIDS Dementia. The symptoms of ADC usually occur late in the disease progression. The early symptoms, which gradually progress into the more advanced late symptoms, are described in Table 11-7.

Nursing Intervention With ADC. Nursing assessment and intervention with the individual who has ADC can be based on addressing the specific symptoms presented. Sensitivity to the changing mental and motor state of the patient should first address the need for providing a safe external environment and developing a self-plan for care that includes personal safety.

Addressing emotional distress can be similar to assessing general coping effectiveness and supporting a sense of personal control, as well as emotional release when indicated.

As the symptoms of ADC become more pronounced, addressing personal safety becomes a higher priority. If the mental state at various times becomes psychotic or delirious, antipsychotic medication can be available on a PRN or ongoing order basis. If chronic demen-

tia becomes more pronounced, all aspects of safety will require ongoing monitoring and intervention (Sadler & Hulgus, 1992).

Support of the family and education regarding safety measures is an important nursing measure during this late stage of disease progression. The grief of the patient and family as the terminal phase advances can be addressed based on their expressed or implied needs.

Encephalitis

Encephalitis means inflammation of the brain. It can occur as a complication of viral diseases such as mumps, infectious hepatitis, herpes zoster and simplex, and rabies. It can also develop as a result of a further inflammatory reaction to brain abscess or meningitis. In addition to the physical symptoms of central nervous system (CNS) disease, the psychiatric symptoms include changes in level of consciousness. Seizures or delirium or both may also occur, depending on the type of encephalitis. The delirium symptoms can include general confusion and disorientation, hallucinations, or delusions.

After the acute phase of encephalitis is over, there usually is a prolonged recovery period of several months. If the patient is a child, it is not

---

TABLE 11-7
SYMPTOMS OF AIDS DEMENTIA COMPLEX

Cognition/Emotion	Behavior	Motor
Early		
Forgetfulness	Social isolation	Clumsiness
Decreased concentration	Apathetic	Tremor
Slowed thinking	Irritability	Poor balance
Decreased stress tolerance		Visuospatial confusion
Depression		Loss of fine motor coordination
Anxiety		Speech disturbance
Late		
Loss of insight	Mute	Loss of gait control
Global dementia	Disinhibition	Incontinence
Psychosis		
Severe memory impairment		

uncommon, especially in boys, for there to be personality changes and behavioral problems (Lishman, 1987). Studies of children after recovery from infectious brain disease have shown that there usually is no change in intellect, but there are problems of impulsiveness, restlessness, poor concentration, and antisocial behavior. These symptoms are similar to the personality changes noted with electrical disturbances in the brain (Kaplan & Sadock, 1994, 1995; Lishman, 1987; Strub & Black, 1993).

Meningitis

Meningitis is an infectious disease of the meninges, the three layers of membranes that surround the brain and the spinal cord. There are three different etiologies of meningitis: pyogenic, with meningococcal and pneumococcal causative organisms predominating; aseptic, which is usually caused by a virus; and tubercular, which is caused by the tubercle bacillus.

Pyogenic meningitis has a rapid onset with high temperature, severe stiffness of the neck, and CNS symptoms. In addition, the psychiatric disturbance is that of an acute, delirious brain reaction. There is a change in consciousness, and coma may occur. Disorientation, excitability, and hallucinations may also be present. Following treatment, psychiatric sequelae such as depression and low energy level may last for several months in adults. Permanent changes in intellectual functioning or in personality are rare. Usually people recover with no complications (Lishman, 1987).

Aseptic meningitis is the mildest form of meningitis. The patient displays symptoms similar to those of pyogenic meningitis. The course of the illness is usually rapid, and there are no negative psychiatric effects.

Tuberculous meningitis is the most severe form of meningitis. Its symptoms differ from those of the other two forms of meningitis; accordingly, the diagnosis may be delayed. The physical symptoms may develop over a 2- to 3-week period. There is vague malaise and a low-grade temperature. There may be no neck stiffness at the onset, then it may develop slightly.

Mild psychiatric symptoms are usually present at the beginning of the illness. These in-

clude poor attention and minor memory deficits. Gradually, changes in consciousness occur and drowsiness becomes prominent. Disorientation may proceed into frank organic psychosis. With delirium, the patient may be terror-stricken by hallucinations or delusions. Once the acute phase is over and the disease is treated, there are usually no consistent personality changes other than amnesia, which may improve slowly over several months (Lishman, 1987; Strub & Black, 1993).

Cerebral Abscess

The most common presenting symptom of a brain abscess is a change in mental status. It is rare for a brain abscess to develop as a primary lesion. Usually it is preceded by infection elsewhere in the body; frequently this infection is in the ears or the facial sinuses. Another cause is a penetrating head injury. The onset of symptoms may occur immediately or may be delayed if the abscess is dormant.

An abscess in the frontal lobe will produce more pronounced psychiatric symptoms than one in the temporal or occipital lobe. Frontal lobe symptoms include a decrease in concentration and memory as well as obvious changes in personality. If the development of the abscess is slow, regardless of the site of infection, mild delirium may be present. There also can be general changes in neurovegetative functioning. These include low energy level and loss of appetite. Depression and irritability may also be included in the clinical findings.

The prognosis regarding psychiatric complications after the acute stage depends on the extent of the infectious process and the time before diagnosis occurred as well as the duration of the acute stage.

Syphilis

Because of public information programs and the availability of penicillin, cases of syphilis in the western world rarely advance to the later stages. Psychiatric complications can be severe during the third and last stages of syphilis. There are three different ways syphilitic CNS involvement can occur: meningitic disease, tabes dorsalis, and general paresis. The meningitis form takes approximately 1 to 5 years to develop. The psychiatric symptoms begin in a mild form and gradually worsen. They are intellectual slowness, poor concentration, failing memory, dementia, and occasional psychotic episodes.

General paresis is a form of syphilis in which the syphilis spirochetes actually invade the brain tissue. With general paresis the mental status changes of meningitis syphilis are present. In addition, marked changes in temperament and personality occur. Poor social judgment, mania, depression, or schizophrenia-like symptoms may dominate the personality. If treatment is begun early in the clinical course, it is possible to reverse the disease process and restore the person to a more acceptable level of physical and mental health (Kaplan & Sadock, 1994, 1995; Lishman, 1987).

Tabes dorsalis is another form of syphilitic disease that occurs in approximately 20% of cases of general paresis. It may not occur until 8 to 12 years after the primary infection. It results in severe neurological disease but rarely causes mental status changes. Severe depression has been reported in some cases of tabes dorsalis. This depression could also be the result of the severe physical disabilities the person with advanced syphilis experiences (Lishman, 1987; Strub & Black, 1993).

NUTRITIONAL

The etiology of nutrition includes many types of vitamin deficiencies. The vitamins that are most important in promoting psychological well-being are the B-complex vitamins. These vitamins are essential to adequate brain metabolism and are also involved in the brain neurotransmitter process. The mental effects of B-vitamin deficiencies will appear before physical manifestations of malnutrition. The symptoms include fatigue, weakness, and emotional disturbances.

Vitamin B$_{12}$

The vitamin implicated in pernicious anemia is B$_{12}$. People with pernicious anemia cannot absorb vitamin B$_{12}$ in the stomach. Such patients are known to have an increased incidence of mental disorder in as high as 64% of

the cases. Included in the mental status changes are depression and lethargy progressing to confusion, paranoid delusions, and schizophrenia-like psychotic symptoms. (It is noteworthy that gastrectomy patients are at risk for pernicious anemia [Geaga & Amanth, 1975].)

Folic Acid

A common result of malnutrition is folate deficiency due to inadequate intake of folic acid. The psychiatric manifestations of this B-vitamin deficiency are depression, progressive dementia, or epilepsy. It is noteworthy that studies of patients in homes for the elderly and in psychiatric institutions frequently find that the folic acid levels of the elderly patients are subnormal. When the folic acid level returns to normal after treatment, it may take several months for the patient's mental status to return to normal (Huber & Kennard, 1991; Lishman, 1987; Strub & Black, 1993).

Nicotinic Acid

A deficiency in nicotinic acid (niacin) is the cause of pellegra. The initial mental changes of pellegra are weakness, nervousness, and memory disorder. There are swings in mood; emotional instability is common. Serious depression usually accompanies the illness. As the deficiency progresses, dementia occurs; confabulation to cover the mental deficits is common. In the later untreated stages, organic psychosis and delirium of a hallucinatory or delusional type occurs. Replacement nicotinic acid restores the patient to normal functioning very rapidly (Lishman, 1987).

Thiamine

Thiamine deficiency results in Wernicke's encephalopathy. It is commonly seen in patients with chronic alcoholism but may occur in those with carcinomas of the digestive tract, toxemia, or tuberculosis. The mental effects of this syndrome are general disorientation and confusion. Replacement of thiamine in these patients may improve their mental status but does not change the often terminal underlying illness.

Beriberi is another disease caused by thiamine deficiency. Patients present with psychiatric symptoms similar to those of Wernicke's encephalopathy. The condition can be reversed with thiamine replacement (Lishman, 1987).

DRUGS

This category includes toxic reactions to drugs or other substances that cause changes in normal brain functioning. These include alcohol, hallucinogens, heavy metals, and prescribed medications such as CNS depressants, digitalis, quinidine, and steroids. Actually, any drug can be suspected of causing a CMD.

Alcohol

Alcohol can cause CMD in several ways. The most commonly recognized is the immediate effect of excessive alcohol intake, in which the drunk person may develop poor social judgment, excitability, and mild disorientation. When alcohol abuse is chronic and addiction occurs, the withdrawal from alcohol results in the hallucinations and seizures of delirium tremens. The specific symptoms of alcohol withdrawal are presented in Chapters 17 and 18.

Nutritional deficiencies associated with chronic alcoholism may result in Wernicke's encephalopathy (see section on thiamine deficiency, above.) Korsakoffs syndrome is another alcohol-related CMD, in which patients display prominent psychiatric symptoms of delirium, including disorientation, insomnia, hallucinations, delusions, and incoherent muttering (Thomas, 1993). Liver disease is a physiological sequela of alcoholism and contributes toward the development of CMD because of the progressive inability of the liver to metabolize toxins. In addition, there can be permanent brain degeneration because of the excessive exposure of brain cells to alcohol (Kaplan & Sadock, 1994, 1995; Renner & Gastfriend, 1991; Strub & Black, 1993).

Hallucinogens

Many hallucinogenic drugs are available for illegal sale in the United States. Generally speaking, the population has become more wary of these substances because of massive information campaigns warning of long-term ill effects from using them. One of the most commonly used hallucinogenic drugs during the 1970s was lysergic acid diethylamide (LSD-25) It continues to be abused, but by fewer people.

LSD causes a wide variety of mental status changes. Large doses produce vivid hallucinatory experiences and marked changes in perception and body image. There is an accompanying strong sense of unreality. Unlike other CMD conditions, there usually is no change in intellectual functioning. This allows the person to maintain an awareness of the unreality he or she is experiencing. This awareness can lead to strong anxiety and panic in people who are unprepared for the severe perceptual distortions that can occur (Lishman, 1987). After the acute reaction is over, there can be unexpected psychiatric after-effects of the drug. These include acute depressive reactions, hallucinations, overwhelming nightmares, and a schizophrenia-like mental state.

Heavy Metals

In the Western world, occupational exposure is the most common source of CMD caused by heavy metals. The metals that may cause problems are lead, mercury, manganese, cadmium, and arsenic. People employed in chemical plants, the photoengraving industry, ore refining, steel or battery manufacture, electrowelding, insecticide production, the glassmaking industry, and lawn care products factories are at risk for heavy metal poisoning (Lishman, 1987). Children are at risk for lead poisoning by ingestion from chewing if they are exposed to old woodwork or furniture painted with a lead-based paint. It should be noted that lead-based paint is no longer manufactured.

Prescribed Medications

A detailed description of the types of psychiatric symptoms that can be drug-induced could fill a volume. Most prescription and over-the-counter drugs can have psychiatric side effects (*Physicians' Desk Reference, 1994*). As discussed above, people metabolize drugs in different ways. Psychiatric side effects are surprisingly common with many drugs. It is very important for nurses to be aware of the possible negative psychiatric effects of drugs because of their liability in administering them to patients, as well as the need to observe for negative side effects.

The most notable changes in mental status are found with steroids, belladonna derivatives, bromides, digitalis preparations, and all CNS depressants. In addition, there are hundreds of reports of negative psychiatric effects of commonly prescribed drugs used for medical, surgical, and obstetrical conditions. Table 11-8 lists commonly prescribed medications and the mental status changes they can cause.

Another medication-related phenomenon that can cause toxic side effects is called synergism. Synergism is the action of two or more drugs that, when taken together, produce a total effect that is stronger than if either was taken alone. The synergistic effects of even low doses of medication can produce either a delirium or dementia type of CMD (Karch, 1996). Nurses who work with patients with chronic illness or the elderly are likely to see patients with this type of encephalopathy.

PREVALENT OCCURRENCES OF COGNITIVE MENTAL DISORDER

POSTOPERATIVE

A phenomenon that has not been well described in medical literature but has been reported nonempirically by many people after all types of general surgery is a subtle but changed mental status that can last up to 6 weeks. The cause of this changed mental functioning can possibly be attributed to the medications and drugs administered during the immediate preoperative and postoperative periods as well as during the surgery itself.

Most people who undergo surgery are not accustomed to medications that have psychotropic alteration potential. The surgical patient's pharmacological regimen usually includes preoperative and intraoperative tranquilizing agents, curare-like paralyzing medications, general anesthetic, around-the-clock postoperative narcotics, and sedation at bedtime. Although the time of exposure to these

drugs may only last a few days, it is important to remember that they are not normally present in the brain. Brain tissues respond to a change in their normal homeostasis. It appears to take some people several weeks to return to their normal preoperative mental status.

The following changes in functioning have been reported:

Changes in cognitive functioning
  Decreased problem-solving ability
  Tendency toward more concrete than abstract reasoning
  Distractibility
  Decrease in recent memory retention
  Egocentrism; less aware of needs of others (ego is protecting the self during the recuperation period)
Changes in mood
  Increased emotionality
  Unexpected mood swings
Changes in neurovegetative functioning
  Changes in sleep patterns
  Difficulty falling asleep

As noted, these changes are mild and usually disappear 4 to 6 weeks after surgery. They appear to be part of the normal response to the acute surgical period.

Another factor that can contribute to the mental status changes of postoperative patients is the perception of surgery as a threat, one that requires a major coping effort of the ego. One of the results of this effort may be the temporary egocentrism identified above. It causes the person to focus on herself and her rehabilitation at a time when she lacks the physical energy to support the well-being of others.

Because of the possibility of these slight changes in mental functioning, it is advisable that patients follow their physician's recommendations on the length of their recuperation period before returning to work, even though they may feel physically well enough to return to work earlier.

COMMON EXAMPLES

The following case examples of CMD are presented in order to increase your awareness of its potential and prevalence.

TABLE 11-8
Some Drugs That Cause Psychiatric Symptoms

Drug	Reaction	Comments*
Amantadine (Symmetrel)	Visual hallucinations, nightmares	Occasional; more frequent in elderly[1]
Aminocaproic acid (Amicar)	Acute delirium with auditory, visual, and kinesthetic hallucinations	Immediately following bolus injection[2]
Amitriptyline (Elavil; others)	Anticholinergic psychosis	See Atropine
Amphetamines	See Dextroamphetamine	
Amphotericin B (Fungizone)	Delirium	IV and intrathecal use[3]
Anticonvulsants	Tactile, visual, and auditory hallucinations, delirium, agitation, depression, paranoia, confusion, aggression	Usually with high doses or high plasma concentrations[4]
Antihistamines	Anxiety, hallucinations, delirium	Especially with overdosage
Asparaginase (Elspar)	Confusion, depression, paranoia, bizarre behavior	Occur frequently in some studies[5,6]
Atropine and anticholinergics	Confusion, memory loss, disorientation, depersonalization, delirium, auditory and visual hallucinations, fear, paranoia	More frequent in elderly and children and with high doses[7]
	Sudden incoherent speech, delirium with high fever, flushed, dry skin, visual and tactile hallucinations	From eye drops, with high or repeated doses, and particularly when confusion with nose drops leads to overdosage[7]
Baclofen (Lioresal)	Visual and auditory hallucinations, paranoia, insomnia, nightmares, mania, depression, anxiety, confusion	Sometimes with treatment, but usually after sudden withdrawal[8]
Barbiturates	See Phenobarbital	
Belladonna alkaloids	See Atropine	
Benztropine (Cogentin)	See Atropine	
Bromocriptine (Parlodel)	Mania, delusions, visual hallucinations, paranoia, aggressive behavior	Occasional, not dose-related;[9] symptoms may persist 6 weeks after stopping the drugs[10]
Chlordiazepoxide (Librium)	Probably same as diazepam	
Chloroquine (Aralen)	Confusion, agitation, violence, personality change, delusions, hallucinations	Several cases, one within 2 hours of single 1-g dose[11]
Cimetidine (Tagamet)	Visual and auditory hallucinations, paranoia, bizarre speech, confusion, delirium, disorientation, depression	Many reports; usually with high dosage, more frequent in elderly and with renal dysfunction[12]
Clonazepam (Clonopin)	Probably same as diazepam	

* Frequency is unknown with many drugs; adverse effects are usually underreported.

(continued)

| | TABLE 11-8 (Continued) | |
| | Some Drugs That Cause Psychiatric Symptoms | |

Drug	Reaction	Comments*
Clorazepate (Azene; Tranxene)	Probably same as diazepam	
Contraceptives, oral	Depression	15% in one study[13]
Corticosteroids (prednisone, cortisone, ACTH; others)	Mania, depression, confusion, paranoia, visual and auditory hallucinations, catatonia	More common with high dosage or rapid increase but can also occur with low doses for short periods[14]
Cyclopentolate (Cyclogyl)	See Atropine	Eye drops
Cycloserine (Seromycin)	Anxiety, depression, confusion, disorientation, hallucinations, paranoia	Common
Dapsone (Avlosulfon)	Insomnia, irritability, uncoordinated speech, agitation, acute psychosis	Occasional, even with low doses[15]
Desipramine (Pertofrane)	Anticholinergic psychosis	See Atropine
Dextroamphetamine	Bizarre behavior, hallucinations, paranoia Depression	Usually with overdose or abuse[16] but can occur with lower doses On withdrawal
Diazepam (Valium)	Rage, excitement, hallucinations, depression, suicidal thoughts	Can occur with usual doses; depression and hallucinations can occur on withdrawal[17]
Diethylpropion (Tenuate)	See Dextroamphetamine	
Digitalis glycosides	Nightmares, euphoria, confusion, delusions, amnesia, belligerence, visual hallucinations, paranoia	Usually with excessive dosage or high plasma concentrations; more frequent in elderly[18]
Disopyramide (Norpace)	Agitation, depression, paranoia, auditory and visual hallucinations, panic	Within 24 to 48 hours after starting treatment[19]
Disulfiram (Antabuse)	Delirium, depression, paranoia, auditory hallucinations	Not related to alcohol reactions[20]
Doxepin (Adapin; Sinequan)	Anticholinergic psychosis	See Atropine
Ephedrine	Hallucinations, paranoia	Excessive dosage[21]
Ethchlorvynol (Placidyl)	Agitation, confusion, disorientation, hallucinations, paranoia	Continued use or on withdrawal[22]
Ethosuximide (Zarontin)	See Anticonvulsants	
Fenfluramine (Pondimin)	See Dextroamphetamine	
Halothane (Fluothane)	Depression	Postoperative period[23]
Imipramine (Tofranil; others)	Anticholinergic psychosis	See Atropine
Indomethacin (Indocin)	Depression, confusion, hallucinations, anxiety, hostility, paranoia, depersonalization	Especially in elderly[24]

* Frequency is unknown with many drugs; adverse effects are usually underreported.

TABLE 11-8 (Continued)
Some Drugs That Cause Psychiatric Symptoms

Drug	Reaction	Comments*
Isoniazid (INH; others)	Depression, agitation, auditory and visual hallucinations, paranoia	Several reports[25]
Ketamine (Ketalar; Ketaject)	Nightmares, hallucinations, crying, delirium, changes in body image	Frequent with usual doses[26]
Levodopa (Dopar; others)	Delirium, depression, agitation, hypomania, nightmares, night terrors, visual and auditory hallucinations, paranoia	More frequent in elderly; risk increases with prolonged use[27]
Lidocaine (Xylocaine)	Disorientation	
Methamphetamine	See Dextroamphetamine	
Methyldopa (Aldomet)	Depression, hallucinations, paranoia, amnesia	Several reports[28]
Methylphenidate (Ritalin)	Hallucinations	In children[29]
Methysergide (Sansert)	Depersonalization, hallucinations	Occasional[30]
Metrizamide (Amipaque)	Confusion, disorientation, hallucinations, depression	Can occur frequently[31]
Nalidixic acid (NegGram)	Confusion, depression, excitement, visual hallucinations	Rare
Niridazolle (Ambilhar)	Confusion, hallucinations, mania, suicide	More likely with higher doses[32]
Nortriptyline (Aventyl)	Anticholinergic psychosis	See Atropine
Pentazocine (Talwin)	Nightmares, hallucinations, disorientation, panic, paranoia, depersonalization, depression	During treatment[33]
Phenelzine (Nardil)	Paranoia, delusions, fear, mania, rage, aggressive behavior	Symptoms may resolve quickly after drug is stopped[34]
Phenmetrazine (Preludin)	See Dextroamphetamine	
Phenobarbital	Excitement, hyperactivity, visual hallucinations, depression, delirium-tremens-like syndrome	On withdrawal, or with usual doses in some children and the elderly, or with overdosage in epilepsy
Phentermine (Fastin; others)	See Dextroamphetamine	
Phenylephrine (NeoSynephrine)	Depression, visual and tactile hallucinations, paranoia	Overuse of nasal spray[35]
Phenytoin (Dilantin; others)	See Anticonvulsants	

* Frequency is unknown with many drugs; adverse effects are usually underreported.

(continued)

TABLE 11-8 (Continued)
Some Drugs That Cause Psychiatric Symptoms

Drug	Reaction	Comments*
Primidone (Mysoline)	See Anticonvulsants	
Procainamide (Pronestyl)	Paranoia, hallucinations	Uncommon[36]
Procaine Penicillin G	Terror, hallucinations, disorientation, agitation, bizarre behavior	Probably due to procaine; occurs occasionally; 33 patients in 1 report[37]
Propoxyphene (Darvon)	Auditory hallucinations, confusion	Usually with high doses[38]
Propranolol (Inderal)	Depression, confusion, nightmares, visual and auditory hallucinations, paranoia	Several reports, with usual doses and after dosage increases[39]
Protriptyline (Vivactil)	Anticholinergic psychosis	See Atropine
Quinacrine (Atabrine)	Bizarre dreams, anxiety, hallucinations, delirium	Can occur with usual doses but more common with high doses[40]
Rauwolfia alkaloids (reserpine—Serpasil, others; rauwolfia—Raudixin, others)	Depression	Occurs commonly with doses higher than 0.5 mg daily, may continue for months after drug is stopped[41]
Scopolamine (Hyoscine)	See Atropine	
Sulindac (Clinoril)	Paranoia, rage, personality change	Reported in 5 patients[42]
Thiabendazole (Mintezol)	Hallucinations	Occasional
Tricyclic antidepressants	Anticholinergic psychosis	See Atropine
Trihexyphenidyl (Artane)	See Atropine	
Trimipramine (Surmontil)	Anticholinergic psychosis	See Atropine
Vinblastine (Velban)	Depression	Occasional
Vincristine (Oncovin)	Hallucinations	Less than 5% of patients; high doses[43]

* Frequency is unknown with many drugs; adverse effects are usually underreported.

1. Borison RL. Am J Psychiatry 136:111, 1979; Harper RW, Knothe BUC, Med J Austr 1:444, 1973
2. Wysenbeek AJ et al. Clin Toxicol 14:93, 1979
3. Winn RE et al. Arch Intern Med 139:706, 1979
4. Franks RD, Richter AJ. Am J Psychiatry 136:973, 1979; Tollefson G. J Clin Psychiatry 41:295, 1980; Woodbury DM et al (eds): Antiepileptic Drugs, pp 219, 377, 449, New York, Raven Press, 1972; Stores G. Dev Med Child Neurol 17:647, 1975
5. Carbone PP et al. Recent Results Cancer Res 33:236, 1970
6. Moure JMB et al. Arch Neurol 23:365, 1970
7. Greenblatt DJ, Shader RI. N Engl J Med 288:1215, 1973; Adcock EW Ill. J Pediatr 79:127, 1971

8. Skausig OB, Korsgaard S. Lancet 1:1258, 1977; Lees AJ et al. Lancet 1:858, 1977; Jones RF, Lance JW. Med J Austr 1:654, 1976; Arnold ES et al. Am J Psychiatry 137:1466, 1980
9. Vlissides DN et al. Br Med J 1:510, 1978; Parkes D. N Engl J Med 302:1479, 1980
10. Caine DB et al. Lancet 1:735, 1978
11. Torrey EF. JAMA 204:867, 1968; Bomb BS, et al. Trans R Soc Trop Med Hyg 69:523, 1975
12. Adler LE et al. Am J Psychiatry 137:1112, 1980; Barnhart CC, Bowden CL. Am J Psychiatry 136:725, 1979; Arneson GA. Am J Psychiatry 136:1348, 1979; Flind AC, Rowley-Jones D. Lancet 1:379, 1979; Agarwal SK. JAMA 240:214, 1978; Nouel O et al. Gastroenterology 79:780, 1980; Jefferson JW. Am J Psychiatry

Continued

TABLE 11-8 (Continued)
Some Drugs That Cause Psychiatric Symptoms

136:346, 1979; Basavaraju NG et al. NY State J Med 80:1287, 1980; Beraud J-J et al. Nouv Presse Med 7:2570, 1978

13. Leeton J. Aust NZ J Obstet Gynaecol 13:115, 1973
14. Sullivan BJ, Dickerman JD. Pediatrics 63:677, 1979; Baloch N. Br J Psychiatry 124:545, 1974; Clark LD et al. N Engl J Med 246:205, 1952
15. Sahu DM. Indian J Dermatol 17:47, 1972
16. Petursson H. Aust NZ J Psychiatry 13:67, 1979
17. Floyd JB Jr, Murphy CM. J Ky Med Assoc 74:549, 1976; Ryan HF, et al. JAMA 203:1137, 1968; Karch FE. Ann Intern Med 91:61, 1979
18. Shear MK, Sacks MH. Am J Psychiatry 135:109, 1978; Sodeman WA. N Engl J Med 273:35, 1965; Volpe BT, Soave R. Ann Intern Med 91:865, 1979; Riesman D. Am J Med Sci 161:6, 1921
19. Falk RH et al. Lancet 1:858, 1977; Padfield PL et al. Lancet 1:1152, 1977; Ahmad S et al. Chest 76:712, 1979
21. Herridge CF, Brook MFA. Br Med J 2:160, 1968
20. Rainey JM Jr. Am J Psychiatry 134:371, 1977; Quail M, Karelse RH. S Afr Med J 57:551, 1980
22. Garza-Perez J et al. Med Serv J Can 23:775, 1967; Heston LL, Hastings D. Am J Psychiatry 137:249, 1980; Flemenbaum A, Gunby B. Dis Nerv Syst 32:138, 1971
23. Davison LA et al. Anesthesiology 43:313, 1975
24. Gotz V. Br Med J 1:49, 1978
25. Kiersch TA. US Armed Forces Med J 5:1353, 1954
26. Hawks WN Jr. et al. J Pediatr Ophthalmol 8:171, 1971; Dundee JW et al., Lancet, 1:1370, 1970
27. Shader RI (ed): Psychiatric Complications of Medical Drugs, p. 149. New York, Raven Press, 1972; Presthus J, Holmsen R. Acta Neurol Scand 50:774, 1974; Moskovitz C et al. Am J Psychiatry 135:669, 1978; Birkmayer W. J Neural Transam (Suppl) 14:163, 1978

28. Kellaway GSM. Drugs (Suppl) 11:91, 1976; Hawkins DJ. Miss Med 73:476. 1976; Riddiough MA. Am J Hosp Pharm 34:465, 1977; Endo M et al. Psychoneuroendocrinology 3:211, 1978
29. Lucas AR, Weiss M. JAMA 217:1079, 1971
30. Persyko I. J Nerv Ment Dis 154:299. 1972
31. Richert S et al. Neuroradiology 18:177, 1979; Schmidt RC. Neuroradiology 19:153, 1980
32. Calloway SP. Med J Zambia 10:70, 1976
33. Kane FJ Jr, Pokorny A. South Med J 68:808, 1975; Wood AJJ et al. Br Med J 1:305, 1974; Miller RR. J Clin Pharmacol 15:198, 1975; Hamilton RC et al. Br J Anaesth 39:647, 1967
34. Sheehy LM, Maxmen JS. Am J Psychiatry 135:1422, 1978
35. Snow SS et al. Br J Psychiatry 136:297, 1980
36. McCrum ID, Guidry JR. JAMA 240:1265, 1978
37. Bjornberg A, Selstam J. Acta Psychiatr Neurol Scand 35:129 1960; Green RL et al. N Engl J Med 291:223, 1974; Eggleston DJ. Br Dent J 148:73, 1980
38. Fraser HF, Isbell H. Bull Narc 12:9, 1960
39. Fleminger R. Br Med J 1:1182, 1978; Steinert J, Pugh CR. Br Med J 1:790, 1979; Gershon ES et al. Ann Intern Med 90:938, 1979; Greenblatt DJ, Koch-Weser J. Am Heart J 86:478, 1973; Hinshelwood RD. Br Med J 2:445, 1969; Voltolina EJ et al. Clin Toxicol 4:357. 1971
40. Engel GL. JAMA 197:515, 1966
41. Goodwin FK, Bunney WE Jr. Semin Psychiatry 3:435, 1971; Freis ED. Am Fam Physician 11:120, 1975
42. Thornton TL. JAMA 243:1630, 1980; Kruis R, Barger R. JAMA 243:1420, 1980
43. Holland JF et al. Cancer Res 33:1258, 1973 (Abramowicz M [ed]: Some drugs that cause psychiatric symptoms. Med Lett Drugs Ther 23:9, 1981)

CASE EXAMPLES

While dieting, and just before mealtimes, Ann notices that she is tremulous, anxious, and dizzy. She is irritable with her roommates. She finds her thinking "fuzzy" rather than clear. Ann's low blood sugar (hypoglycemia) has resulted in inadequate glucose availability to her brain cells (Kaplan & Sadock, 1994, 1995). ✾

Jerry is normally a shy person who lacks confidence and does not enjoy being with people. After having two drinks at a party, he notices that he has no trouble finding things to talk about and feels comfortable being with people. He finds almost every conversation amusing. The effects of alcohol have relaxed Jerry's normal ego and superego functioning. ✾

Stephanie experiences depression, irritability, and poor emotional control during the few days before her menstrual period each month. She believes it must be "all in my head." Actually, Stephanie is partially correct, except that she is not imagining these emotional changes. They are due to temporary premenstrual changes in physiology, which are caused by retention of fluid (resulting in slight swelling of all body tissues, including the brain) and rapid electrolyte and hormonal changes. Once her period begins, Stephanie's hormone and electrolyte levels return to normal and her symptoms disappear (Kaplan & Sadock, 1994, 1995). ✾

CONCLUSION

CMD occurs far more commonly than is normally recognized. When CMD results in a delirious episode, patients, families, and caregivers are frightened by the event. By being alert for subtle changes in mental status, it is possible to reverse or reduce progression to delirium by rapid nursing and medical intervention. Knowledge of the complex symptoms of CMD can help you in your nursing assessment and ongoing evaluation of patients. Another important point to remember in determining your patients' nursing diagnoses is that CMD is a potential etiological consideration in each of the nursing diagnosis categories.

BIBLIOGRAPHY

Albert, M., & Cohen, C. (1992). The Test for Severe Impairment: An instrument for the assessment of patients with severe cognitive dysfunction. *Journal of the American Geriatrics Society, 40*(5), 449–453.

Anderson, B., & Holmes, W. (1993). Altered mental status: An algorithm for assessment of delirium in the cancer patient. *Current Issues in Cancer Nursing Practice, 2*(5), 1–9.

Baron, D. A. (1991). Dementia in patients with the acquired immunodeficiency syndrome. *Journal of the American Osteopathic Association, 91*(8), 772–776.

Bassett, S. S., & Folstein, M. F. (1991). Cognitive impairment and functional disability in the absence of psychiatric diagnosis. *Psychological Medicine, 21*(1), 77–84.

Bauer, J., Roberts, M. R., & Reisdorff, E. J. (1991). Evaluation of behavioral and cognitive changes: The mental status examination. *Emergency Medicine Clinics of North America, 9*(1), 1–12.

Brew, B. J. (1993). HIV-1-related neurological disease. *Journal of Acquired Immune Deficiency Syndromes, 6*(Suppl. 1), S10–S15.

Bruera, E. (1991). Severe organic brain syndrome. *Journal of Palliative Care, 7*(1), 36–38.

Capwell, R., & Carter, R. (1991). Organic anxiety syndrome secondary to metastatic brain tumor. *Psychosomatics, 32*(2), 231–233.

Carbey, M. (1967). Serum folate values in 423 psychiatric patients. *British Medical Journal, 4*, 512.

Colombo, G., Perini, G. I., Miotti, M. V., Armani, M., & Angelini, C. (1992). Cognitive and psychiatric evaluation of 40 patients with myotonic dystrophy. *Italian Journal of Neurological Science, 13*(1), 53–58.

Coyle, M. K. (1987). Organic illness mimicking psychiatric episodes. *Journal of Gerontological Nursing, 13*(1), 31–35.

Easton, C., & McKenzie, F. (1988). Sensory-perceptual alterations: Delirium in the intensive care unit. *Heart and Lung, 17*(3), 229–237.

Fleishman, S., & Lesko, L. (1989). Delirium and dementia. In J. Holland & J. Rowland (Eds.), *Handbook of psycho-oncology: Psychological care of the patient with cancer.* New York: Oxford University Press.

Forstein, M. (1992). The neuropsychiatric aspects of HIV infection. *Primary Care, 19*(1), 97–117.

Frazier, A., Molinoff, P. B., & Winokur, A. (Eds.). (1994). *Biological bases of brain function and disease.* New York: Raven Press.

Geaga, K., & Amanth, J. (1975). Responses of a psychiatric patient to vitamin B$_{12}$ therapy. *Diseases of the Nervous System, 36*, 343.

Geary, S. M. (1994). Intensive care unit psychosis revisited: Understanding and managing delirium in the critical care setting. *Critical Care Nursing Quarterly, 17*(1), 51–63.

Gilroy, J., & Meyer, J. *Medical neurology* (3rd ed.). (1975). New York: Macmillan.

Goldberg, R. J. (1980). *Strategies in psychiatry for the primary care physician.* Darien, CT: Patient Care Books.

Goldberg, R. J., Faust, D., & Novack, D. (1992). Integrating the cognitive mental status examination into the medical interview. *Southern Medical Journal, 85*(5), 491–497.

Hales, R., & Yudofsky, S. (Eds.). (1987). *The American Psychiatric Press textbook of neuropsychiatry.* Washington, DC: American Psychiatric Press.

Hamilton, L. W., & Creason, N. S. (1992). Mental status and functional abilities: Change in institutionalized elderly women. *Nursing Diagnosis, 3*(2), 81–86.

Harper, R. G., Chacko, R. C., Kotik-Harper, D., & Kirby, H. B. (1992). Comparison of two cognitive screening measures for efficacy in differentiating dementia from depression in a geriatric inpatient population. *Journal of Neuropsychiatry and Clinical Neuroscience, 4*(2), 179–184.

Huber, M., & Kennard, A. (1991). Functional and mental status outcomes of clients discharged from acute gerontological versus medical/surgical units. *Journal of Gerontological Nursing, 17*(7), 20–24.

Kaplan, H. I., & Sadock, B. J. (1994). *Synopsis of psychiatry: Behavioral sciences, clinical psychiatry* (7th ed.). Baltimore: Williams & Wilkins.

Karch, A. M. (1996). *Lippincott's nursing drug guide.* Philadelphia: J. B. Lippincott.

Katz, A. (1994). AIDS dementia complex. *Journal of Palliative Care, 10*(1), 46–50.

Kelly-Hayes, M., Jette, A. M., Wolf, P. A., D'Agostino, R. B., & Odell, P. M. (1992). Functional limitations and disability among elders in the Framingham Study. *American Journal of Public Health, 82*(6), 841–845.

Lipowski, Z. (1975). Organic brain syndromes: Overview and classification. In D. Benson & D. Blumer (Eds.), *Psychiatric aspects of neurologic disease.* New York: Grune & Stratton.

Lipowski, Z. (1980). A new look at organic brain syndrome. *American Journal of Psychiatry, 137*(4), 6–13.

Lipowski, Z. (1980). A new look at organic brain syndrome. *American Journal of Psychiatry, 137*(6), 674–678.

Lipowski, Z. (1985). Delirium. In J. Frederiks (Ed.), *Handbook of clinical neurology* (Vol. 2). New York: Elsevier Biomedical Press.

Lipowski, Z. (1992). Update on delirium. *Psychiatric Clinics of North America, 15*(2), 335–346.

Lishman, W. A. (1987). *Organic psychiatry: The psychological consequences of cerebral disorder* (2nd ed.). Boston: Blackwell Scientific.

Menza, M. A., Murray, G. B., Homes, V. F., & Rafuls, W. A. (1988). Controlled study of extrapyramidal reactions in the management of delirious medically ill patients: Intravenous haloperidol versus intravenous haloperidol plus benzodiazapines. *Heart and Lung, 17*(3), 238–241.

Moller, A., Wiedemann, G., Rohde, U., Backmund, H., & Sonntag, A. (1994). Correlates of cognitive impairment and depressive mood disorder in multiple sclerosis. *Acta Psychiatrica Scandinavica, 89*(2), 117–121.

Murray, G. B. (1991). Confusion, delirium, and dementia. In N. H. Cassem (Ed.), *Massachusetts General Hospital handbook of general hospital psychiatry* (3rd ed.). St. Louis: Mosby Year Book.

Parker, G., Hadzi-Pavlovic, D., Hickie, I., Boyce, P., Mitchell, P., Wilhelm, K., & Brodaty, H. (1991). Distinguishing psychotic and non-psychotic melancholia. *Journal of Affective Disorders, 22*(3), 135–148.

Pincus, H., & Pardes, H. (Eds.). (1985). *The integration of neuroscience and psychiatry.* Washington, DC: American Psychiatric Press.

Pincus, J., & Tucker, G. (1985). *Behavior neurology* (3rd ed.). New York: Oxford University Press.

Price, R. W. (1994). Understanding the AIDS dementia complex (ADC). The challenge of HIV and its effects on the central nervous system. *Research Publications-Association for Research in Nervous & Mental Disease, 72,* 1–45.

Racagni, G. (Ed.). (1992). *Treatment of age-related cognitive dysfunction: Pharmacological and clinical evaluation.* New York: Karger.

Renner, J. A., & Gastfriend, D. R. (1991). Drug addiction. In N. H. Cassem (Ed.), *Massachusetts General Hospital handbook of general hospital psychiatry* (3rd ed.). St. Louis: Mosby Year Book.

Sadler, J.Z., & Hullgus, Y.F. (1992). Clinical problem-solving and the biopsychosocial model. *American Journal of Psychiatry, 149*(10), 1315–1323.

Sidtis, J. J. (1994). Evaluation of the AIDS dementia complex in adults. *Research Publications-Association for Research in Nervous & Mental Disease, 72,* 273–287.

Skerritt, P. (1991). The mental state examination: An iconoclastic comment. *Australian and New Zealand Journal of Psychiatry, 25*(1), 31–33.

Stoudemire, A., & Fogel, B. S. (Eds.). (1993). *Psychiatric care of the medical patient.* New York: Oxford University Press.

Sullivan, N., & Fogel, B. S. (1986). Could this be delirium? *American Journal of Nursing, 86*(12), 1359–1363.

Teri, L., Truax, P., Logsdon, R., Uomoto, J., Zarit, S., & Vitaliano, P. P. (1992). Assessment of behavioral problems in dementia: The revised memory and behavior problems checklist. *Psychology and Aging, 7*(4), 622–631.

Tesar, G. E. (1993). The agitated patient, Part I: Evaluation and behavioral management. *Hospital and Community Psychiatry, 44*(4), 329–331.

Thomas, C. L. (Ed.). (1993). *Taber's cyclopedic medical dictionary* (17th ed.). Philadelphia: F. A. Davis.

Trzepacz, P. T., & Baker, R. W. (1993). *Psychiatric mental status examination.* New York: Oxford University Press.

Usdin, G., & Lewis, J. (Eds.). (1979). *Psychiatry in general medical practice.* New York: McGraw-Hill.

Zimberg, M., & Mahon, M. (1992). Understanding delirium: An impediment to quality of life. In L. Powell (Ed.), *Quality of life: A nursing challenge.* Philadelphia: Meriscus Publications.

PART III

APPLICATION
OF THE
PSYCHOSOCIAL
COMPONENT
OF THE
NURSING PROCESS

The following 18 chapters, Chapters 12 through 29, are the "how to" part of this book. Nursing textbooks often urge nurses to intervene with patients who are coping ineffectively or are at risk for psychosocial maladaptation. However, nurses often feel uncertain about *how* to intervene with these patients. Traditionally, recommendations for intervention have included encouragement of "verbalizing," "support of coping," promotion of "ventilation," and so on.

The recommendations for care planning and intervention guidelines in Part 3 were developed in working with physically ill patients and their families, who were struggling to cope with the effects of illness.

THE NURSING PROCESS

The process of assessing patients' and family members' responses to illness can be carried out effectively using the structure of the nursing process. The nursing process is a flexible approach to patient care that can be used in any type of setting. It is not intended to be a rigid process or one that imposes restrictions on a nurse's creativity in designing care. Rather, it is intended to give the nurse a structure on which to develop the nursing care plan. It allows for the uniqueness of patients and nurses and is intended to meet the needs of both.

The steps of the nursing process are briefly reviewed here.

1. *Assessing and diagnosing.* Assessing involves collecting information about the patient and family to compile a nursing history and diagnosis, including information about physical, intrapsychic, and social functioning. The nursing diagnoses are based on the approved list of nursing diagnosis categories presented in Box 12-1.
2. *Planning.* The planning phase uses the nursing diagnosis or diagnoses as its base. When a general plan is being formulated, the patient should be included in the process whenever possible. Appropriate aspects of the care plan can be reviewed and developed with the patient's opinions and recommendations.
3. *Implementing.* Implementing is the action phase of the nursing care plan. It should be used by all nursing team members so that the caregiving system approaches the patient in the same or similar ways. This phase is strongly interactive, involving the patient, family members, caregivers from other disciplines, and nurses.

   The implementation phase includes ongoing assessment of the interactions described above and the flexibility of the nurse in modifying the original care plan.
4. *Evaluating.* Evaluating involves assessing the patient's response to the nursing intervention. Has the problem identified in the nursing diagnosis been resolved? Is it still present? Is it worse? Depending on your assessment, the care plan will be subject to modification, and new approaches may be necessary. The evaluation phase can actually be the first phase in a circular nursing process that is continually responding to patients' and families' needs.

CHAPTER 12

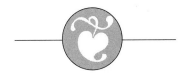

Clinical Decision Making

Patricia Barry

Nursing assessment is the systematic and continuous collection of data about the health status of the patient. *Data collection* is the assembling of all information about the patient's physiological, psychological, and social functioning. The sources of information include the patient, family, physician, and laboratory and other test findings.

As part of the nursing process, the nurse is the data processor who pulls together these bits of information. In the assessment process, this information will be integrated and applied to theories of normal and abnormal human functioning. Data about physiological, psychological, and social functioning are formulated to develop a list of the patient's problems. These concepts are integrated by using a systems approach in evaluating and analyzing data. It has been shown that if psychosocial assessment intervention and ongoing patient evaluation is carried out by nurses, it can and does result in fewer physiological and psychosocial emergencies for patients and families both in the hospital and after discharge (Frisch, 1992; Hartman & Knudson, 1991; McFarland, Wasli, & Gerety, 1992; Pinkley, 1991; Potter & Perry, 1993).

JUSTIFICATION FOR PSYCHOSOCIAL ASSESSMENT

The importance of nursing assessment of psychosocial status can be understood when one considers that the North American Nursing Diagnosis Association (NANDA), in conferences held biennially from 1974 to 1994, has identified that two-thirds of the disorders that nurses are capable of independently diagnosing and treating are in the psychosocial categories (Carpenito, 1993). Clearly, priority setting in delivering professional patient care may be shifted as nursing diagnoses become more widely utilized.

Nurses have the potential to identify patients and family members who are at risk for ineffective coping and are beginning the process of emotional maladaptation to physical illness. If intervention does not occur and the process continues, two responses are probable:

Patricia Barry: *Psychosocial Nursing: Care of Physically Ill Patients and Their Families,* 3rd ed.
© 1996 Lippincott-Raven Publishers

The patient may experience an in-hospital crisis and the problem may continue after his or her discharge.

The patient and family will experience a decrease in the quality of their lives because of the patient's ongoing postdischarge ineffective coping and maladaptation. Usually, the effects will eventually be experienced by all members of the family system (McFarland, Wasli, & Gerety, 1992).

With astute nursing assessment, the precrisis types of maladaptive processes such as depression, anxiety, and other signs of ineffective coping can be reversed. The maladaptive process can be recognized and properly treated when an adequate psychosocial assessment is part of the admission and ongoing evaluation data base. *I strongly recommend including in all nursing histories questions that will give the nurses who care for a patient a thorough personality and coping profile of that patient.*

Nursing has taken many of its clues about what data to include on an admission assessment from the medical model and frequently performs minimal psychosocial assessment. It is important to remember that nursing and medicine are different caregiving disciplines with different objectives in their care delivery to patients. Nursing is the only primary caregiving discipline prepared to monitor the psychosocial as well as the physical responses of the patient and family to illness.

THE NURSE AS ASSESSOR

Psychosocial nursing assessment calls on many of the nurse's abilities. Each patient is unique. So is each nurse. There will be many subjective and objective cues, or data, perceived by the nurse during assessment of the patient. The physical cues are usually assessable by the nurse's senses of sight, touch, hearing, smell, and taste. These cues are clear-cut, objective, identifiable, and less subject to interpretation that could be colored by the nurse's own beliefs, values, or knowledge of the theory of physiological functioning.

Psychosocial assessment cues, on the other hand, are not so concrete. The way a patient speaks and behaves is subject to the nurse's interpretation. The nurse's psychological state may influence perception of the patient and alter his or her ability to make an appropriate inference. An *inference* is the judgment or interpretation the nurse makes about the cue. The ability to make correct judgments about cues is dependent on the knowledge and experiential base of the nurse (Alfaro-LeFevre, 1994).

For example, a nurse who is emotionally guarded will have a number of defense mechanisms operating during the patient interview. Accordingly, the patient's responses to illness will be filtered through the nurse's own defenses; the nurse may not be able to recognize the symptoms of distress being manifested by the patient or family. A similar response can occur if a nurse is highly stressed. Individuals under stress have decreased cognitive and problem solving abilities (Creamer, Burgess, & Pattison, 1992).

On the other hand, a nurse who is recovering from a major loss and gradually working through grief, in working with a patient experiencing a major loss, may project subjective feelings or concerns onto the patient or family. Once again, this raises the possibility of bias in the assessment/judgment ability of the nurse (McClowry, 1992).

Psychosocial care planning is dependent primarily on accurate assessment of the overall response of the patient and family to illness (Alfaro-LeFevre, 1994; Carpenito, 1993). When patterns of normal, expected functioning are compared with the current response or state of the patient, it is possible to identify discrepancies and areas that require effective care planning. The discrepancies may take two major forms:

1. Alterations in the way the person functioned before this illness from usual functioning patterns (e.g., nutrition, sadness).
2. Differences in the way this person functions from the way the normal individual functions, where the functioning is customary for this individual (e.g., limping, being emotionally withdrawn) (Alfaro-LeFevre, 1994; Carpenito, 1993).

These discrepancies can be described using the terms *state* or *trait*. A *state* is the current condition of an individual. In the psychological realm, this would include any currently present cognitive, emotional, or behavioral state. A *trait* is a cognitive, emotional, or behavioral characteristic that is the person's customary and long-standing response (Campbell, 1989; Kaplan & Sadock, 1994, 1995). In order to determine which conditions are being observed, the following questions can be asked of the patient or family members.

1. Is this a normal response for this person?
2. Is this a response to the stress of this hospitalization or illness?
3. Is this response related to another recent event?

These questions are important whether assessing physical or psychosocial cues. They are especially important in the latter because they provide objective data that are less subject to the emotional or psychological bias of the interviewer.

PSYCHOSOCIAL VS. PHYSICAL ASSESSMENT

There are a number of published nursing assessment, diagnosis, and intervention guides available to assist nurses in the nursing process. Many of them are included in the bibliography at the end of this chapter. The majority are structured to be used with the NANDA nursing diagnosis model. These guides contain questions that can be helpful in determining whether the criteria for particular nursing diagnoses are present.

In the physical assessment process these questions are based on specific aspects of physical functioning that are observable and usually measurable. For example, a person is either drinking fluids or is not, and is either moving his or her bowels or is not. These questions in the assessment process are clear and understandable to both the nurse and the patient.

The nursing diagnoses that are psychosocial in origin, such as "Coping, ineffective individual," or those with contributing psychosocial factors, such as "Altered nutrition: Less than body requirements" are open to increased bias on the part of the nurse who is assessing the patient and the family. Many of the data on which psychosocial assessment are based are not objectively measurable, as are most physical data. Some of the reasons are:

1. Psychological or psychosocial functioning is usually not quantifiable or measurable in pure, scientific numbers. (Note: Certain aspects of psychological functioning can be measured by psychological tests administered by psychologists. Even those test results, however, are often subject to the interpretation of the psychologist.) Because of this, social science data are considered to be "soft" data, that is, not as reliable as the "hard" data of scientific measurement based on quantifiable numbers, such as blood pressure, pulse, and so on (Kerlinger, 1986).
2. The patient's assessment of her own functioning is subjective. For example, she might say "I am adjusting well," when, indeed, she is not. The nurse may not have enough clinical data to indicate otherwise, or may accept the word of the patient as accurate.
3. Assessment by family members is subjective; they may be inaccurately reporting the psychological state of the patient (McCarthy & Gallo, 1992).
4. The nurse's assessment is subjective; there may be a lack of awareness or knowledge of the ways psychosocial distress or dysfunction is manifested (Dossey, Guzzetta, & Kenner, 1992).
5. Dissimilar values or cultural beliefs between the patient and nurse can contribute to oversight of problems or identification of circumstances that may not be problems (Bushy, 1992).

Because of these and other reasons, assessment of psychosocial functioning will always be less reliable than assessment of physical findings. It is possible, however, for nurses to become quite skilled at psychosocial assessment. In fact, many nurses find it to be the most challenging and rewarding aspect of nursing.

CATEGORIES OF FUNCTIONING ASSESSED IN THE INTERVIEW

The data-gathering process described in this chapter and the accompanying psychosocial assessment scale have been categorized according to the functional health patterns identified by Marjorie Gordon (1987; Carpenito, 1993). They are grouped in this manner to facilitate the identification of corresponding nursing diagnosis categories.

The categories included in the assessment process are:

1. Health perception–Health management
2. Nutritional–Metabolic
3. Elimination
4. Activity–Exercise
5. Sleep–Rest
6. Cognitive–Perceptual
7. Self–perception
8. Role–Relationship
9. Sexual–Reproductive
10. Coping–Stress tolerance
11. Value–Belief

Within each of these patterns are diagnostic categories that make up the approved NANDA list of nursing diagnoses. Before beginning the nursing assessment it is important to be familiar with the nursing diagnosis categories (see Box 12-1). This will assist in focusing on specific aspects of the assessment where problems are identified. As these problem areas of functioning become apparent, a more specific form of assessment can be initiated.

Focus assessment is a narrowing of the general assessment process that provides a depth of information related to the specific problems.* Accurate identification of these etiologies ensures more accurate care planning and achievable outcomes of nursing care (Alfaro-LeFevre, 1994; Carpenito, 1993).

---

*When a problem surfaces during the general assessment process, the nurse can shift the questioning so that specific information about the causes of the problem and its effect on the patient and family can be more fully explored.

THE PRAGMATIC APPROACH TO PSYCHOSOCIAL NURSING ASSESSMENT

Many factors appear to contribute to a patient's and family's coping responses, including: perception of the illness and how it will affect life-style; sleep-rest patterns; current mental status; major coping issues of the illness (the way the illness strikes at the patient's own developmental issues); psychosocial family history and normal role functioning; normal interpersonal style; perceived changes in sexual functioning related to illness; level of stress experienced by the individual and family during the year before admission; normal coping patterns; and congruence between goals of patient, family, and caregivers.

It is possible to discern aspects of psychosocial functioning that do not fit within a normal range by using the questioning format presented in the next chapter, the Barry Psychosocial Assessment Interview schedule, or one adapted from it. Although distress or dysfunction related to the 11 functional health pattern categories (Carpenito, 1993; Gordon, 1987) discussed earlier is not measurable using "hard" science techniques, it can be systematically observed and analyzed by recording objective data. Early identification of areas of actual, potential, or possible psychosocial problems can result in:

1. Identification of distress-causing, *trait*-type psychosocial responses to the stress of illness.
2. Identification of distress-causing, *state*-type psychosocial responses to the stress of illness.
3. Effective, goal-directed care planning to alleviate the distress and to comply with diagnosis-related group (DRG) discharge requirements.

The psychosocial assessment scale that appears in Chapter 13, Figure 13-1, has been designed to assess the overall psychosocial functioning of an individual and family. The questions in the scale have been grouped according to the health patterns identified by

BOX 12-1	Nursing Diagnoses With Psychosocial Factors That Contribute to Defining Characteristics*

Activity Intolerance
Activity Intolerance, Risk for
Adaptive Capacity: Intracranial, Decreased
Adjustment, Impaired
Airway Clearance, Ineffective
Altered Nutrition: Less than body requirements
Altered Nutrition: More than body requirements
Altered Nutrition: Potential for more than body requirements
Anticipatory Grieving
Anxiety
Aspiration, Risk for
Body Image Disturbance
Body Temperature, Risk for Altered
Bowel Incontinence
Breastfeeding, Effective
Breastfeeding, Ineffective
Breastfeeding, Interrupted
Breathing Pattern, Ineffective
Caregiver Role Strain
Caregiver Role Strain, Risk for
Chronic Low Self-Esteem
Chronic Pain
Colonic Constipation
Communication, Impaired Verbal
Community Coping, Ineffective
Community Coping, Potential for Enhanced
Confusion, Acute
Confusion, Chronic
Constipation
Constipation, Colonic
Constipation, Perceived
Decisional Conflict (Specify)
Decreased Cardiac Output
Defensive Coping
Denial, Ineffective
Diarrhea
Disorganized Infant Behavior
Disorganized Infant Behavior, Risk for
Diversional Activity Deficit
Dysfunctional Grieving
Dysfunctional Ventilatory Weaning Response
Dysreflexia
Energy Field Disturbance
Environmental Interpretation Syndrome, Impaired
Family Coping: Potential for Growth

Family Process: Alcoholism, Altered
Family Processes, Altered
Fatigue
Fear
Fluid Volume Deficit
Fluid Volume Deficit, Risk for
Fluid Volume Excess
Functional Incontinence
Gas Exchange, Impaired
Grieving, Anticipatory
Grieving, Dysfunctional
Growth and Development, Altered
Health Maintenance, Altered
Health Seeking Behaviors (Specify)
Home Maintenance Management, Impaired
Hopelessness
Hyperthermia
Hypothermia
Inability to Sustain Spontaneous Ventilation
Incontinence, Bowel
Incontinence, Functional
Incontinence, Reflex
Incontinence, Stress
Incontinence, Total
Incontinence, Urge
Individual Coping, Ineffective
Ineffective Family Coping: Compromised
Ineffective Family Coping: Disabling
Infant Feeding Pattern, Ineffective
Infection, Risk for
Injury, Risk for
Knowledge Deficit (Specify)
Loneliness, Risk for
Management of Therapeutic Regimen: Community, Ineffective
Management of Therapeutic Regimen: Families, Ineffective
Management of Therapeutic Regimen: Individual, Effective
Management of Therapeutic Regimen (Individuals), Ineffective
Noncompliance (Specify)
Memory, Impaired
Oral Mucous Membrane, Altered
Organized Infant Behavior, Potential for Enhanced
Pain
Pain, Chronic

(continued)

BOX 12-1	Nursing Diagnoses With Psychosocial Factors That Contribute to Defining Characteristics* *(continued)*

Parent/Infant/Child Attachment, Risk for Altered
Parental Role Conflict
Parenting, Altered
Parenting, Risk for Altered
Perceived Constipation
Perioperative Positioning Injury, Risk for
Peripheral Neurovascular Dysfunction, Risk for
Personal Identity Disturbance
Physical Mobility, Impaired
Poisoning, Risk for
Post-Trauma Response
Powerlessness
Protection, Altered
Rape-Trauma Syndrome
Rape-Trauma Syndrome: Compound Reaction
Rape-Trauma Syndrome: Silent Reaction
Reflex Incontinence
Relocation Stress Syndrome
Role Performance, Altered
Self-Care Deficit
    Bathing/Hygiene
    Feeding
    Dressing/Grooming
    Toileting
Self-Esteem, Chronic Low
Self-Esteem, Situational Low
Self-Esteem, Disturbance
Self-Mutilation, Risk for

Sensory/Perceptual Alterations (Specify) (visual, auditory, kinesthetic, gustatory, tactile, olfactory)
Sexual Dysfunction
Sexuality Patterns, Altered
Situational Low Self-Esteem
Skin Integrity, Impaired
Skin Integrity, Risk for Impaired
Sleep Pattern Disturbance
Social Interaction, Impaired
Social Isolation
Spiritual Distress
Spiritual Well-Being, Potential for Enhanced
Stress Incontinence
Suffocation, Risk for
Swallowing, Impaired
Thermoregulation, Ineffective
Thought Processes, Altered
Tissue Integrity, Impaired
Tissue Perfusion, Altered (Specify Type) (Renal, cerebral, cardiopulmonary, gastrointestinal, peripheral)
Total Incontinence
Trauma, Risk for
Unilateral Neglect
Urge Incontinence
Urinary Elimination, Altered
Urinary Retention
Violence, Risk for: Self-directed or directed at others

*It should be noted that the sympathetic nervous system activation resulting from the stress response causes a continuum of physiologic changes in all body systems.

Gordon. If a specific area of distress or dysfunction is identified by the nurse, a focus assessment of that area should be completed to determine the underlying causes, scope, and depth of the problem (Alfaro-LeFevre, 1994).

The rationale for decision-making leading to a nursing diagnosis will be presented in Chapter 13. All theory related to these assessment criteria appears in the chapters identified above.

THE SETTING FOR THE ASSESSMENT INTERVIEW

The psychosocial assessment interview presented in Chapter 13 takes approximately 30 to 45 minutes to complete. It can be modified to a shorter form, but none of the major categories should be deleted. Before beginning the interview, it is helpful to explain to the patient that one of the responsibilities of a nurse is to understand how a patient is feeling about and reacting to illness, in order to support the recovery. This introduction during the admission period helps the patient to feel understood. It can give a sense of security at a time when there usually are apprehensive feelings (but frequently there is no one in whom to confide). Patients often will hesitate to tell their fears to their family because they do not want to worry them.

Ideally, the interview should take place in a setting that affords privacy for the nurse and patient. The best option to ensure privacy is to pull the curtain between the patient and his or her roommate, but not completely around the bed. In an interview a completely closed curtain often leaves the patient with an uncomfortable feeling of being closed in. In addition, if one cannot see the door it is possible to wonder if someone other than a roommate has entered the room. By sitting on a chair close to the head of the bed, it is possible to maintain a fairly reasonable level of privacy.

In the actual interview, it is helpful to use the therapeutic communication skills recommended in Chapter 2, to promote trust and openness. The approach to the patient should primarily be that of a nonjudgmental listener. If the patient begins to ask for the nurse's opinion about the information being presented, the question can be returned by asking, "What do you think?" During the admission process the patient is essentially looking for acceptance, not the nurse's opinion.

Regardless of what is said, the patient's level of anxiety may cause an inability to hear the nurse's response fully. The patient may describe, for example, the usual way the family responds to trouble. There could be a question about difficulty falling asleep at night and what it might mean. By returning the question to the patient, the nurse can say, "Your own opinion about this situation is important. Tell me more about it." The nurse is validating the original response with this approach. Sometimes, nurses will respond to this type of patient question with the answer, "I don't know. Why don't you ask your physician?" If hearing this response in the patient's place, would a level of trust increase, or would there be a feeling of being avoided and put off?

Whether a family member can be present during this interview is left to the nurse's discretion. If the patient is a child or is not a reliable informant, a family member should give the information. It can be a valuable part of the assessment to have a family member (usually a spouse) present. The family member's presence can ensure a far more realistic impression of both the patient's and family's response to the stress of illness. It is understandable, however, that family members' visits and nurse's available time often do not coincide. An interview with the patient alone can provide adequate information.

CONCLUSION

Psychosocial nursing assessment is a challenging step in the nursing process because of the diversity of factors that contribute to cognitive, perceptual, emotional, and social functioning. In addition, the patient's psychosocial state is affected by the psychosocial state of the people around him or her during the illness, particularly family members and caregivers.

The major factors that can influence the response of an individual to illness are:

1. Perception of the illness and the way it will affect his or her lifestyle.
2. Sleep-rest patterns.
3. Current mental status.
4. Major coping issues of the illness (the way the illness strikes at the patient's own developmental issues).
5. Psychosocial family history and normal role functioning.
6. Normal interpersonal style.
7. Perceived changes in sexual functioning related to illness.
8. Level of stress experienced by the individual and family during the year before admission.
9. Normal coping patterns.
10. Congruence between goals of patient, family, and caregivers.

BIBLIOGRAPHY

Alfaro-LeFevre, R. (1994). *Applying nursing process* (3rd ed.). Philadelphia: J. B. Lippincott.
American Heritage college dictionary (3rd ed.). (1993). Boston: Houghton-Mifflin.

Appley, M. H., & Trumbell, R. G. (1986). *Dynamics of stress: Physiological, psychological and social perspectives.* New York: Plenum Press.

Becket, N. (1991). Clinical nurses' characterizations of patient coping problems. *Nursing Diagnosis, 2*(2), 72–78.

Bowlby, J. (1973). *Attachment and loss, Volume 2: Separation.* New York: Basic Books.

Bulechek, G. M., & McCloskey, J. C. (1992). Defining and validating nursing interventions. *Nursing Clinics of North America, 27*(2), 289–299.

Bushy, A. (1992). Cultural considerations for primary health care: Where do self-care and folk medicine fit? *Holistic Nursing Practice, 6*(3), 10–18.

Campbell, R. J. (1989). *Psychiatric dictionary* (6th ed.). New York: Oxford University Press.

Carpenito, L. J. (Ed.). (1991). *Nursing care plans and documentation: Nursing diagnosis and collaborative problems.* Philadelphia: J. B. Lippincott.

Carpenito, L. J. (Ed.). (1993). *Nursing diagnosis: Application to clinical practice* (5th ed.). Philadelphia: J. B. Lippincott.

Creamer, M., Burgess, P., & Pattison, P. (1992). Reaction to trauma: A cognitive processing model. *Journal of Abnormal Psychology, 101*(3), 452-459.

Dossey, B. M., Guzzetta, C. E., & Kenner, C. V. (1992). *Critical care nursing: Body-mind-spirit* (3rd ed.). Philadelphia: J. B. Lippincott.

Estes, N., Smith-Dijulo, K., & Heinemann, M. (1980). *Nursing diagnosis of the alcoholic person.* St. Louis: C. V. Mosby.

Frisch, N. (1992). Home care nursing and psychosocial-emotional needs. How nursing diagnosis helps to direct and inform practice. *Home Healthcare Nurse, 11*(2), 64–65, 70.

Gerteis, M., Edgman-Levitan, S., Daley, J., & Delbanco, T. L. (Eds.). (1993). *Through the patient's eyes: Understanding and promoting patient-centered care.* San Francisco: Jossey-Bass.

Gordon, M. (1987). *Nursing diagnosis: Process and application.* New York: McGraw-Hill.

Hartman, D., & Knudson, J. (1991). A nursing data base for initial patient assessment. *Oncology Nursing Forum, 18*(1), 125–130.

Kaplan, H. I., & Sadock, B. J. (1994). *Synopsis of psychiatry: Behavioral sciences, clinical psychiatry* (7th ed.). Baltimore: Williams & Wilkins.

Kaplan, H. I., & Sadock, B. J. (1995). *Comprehensive textbook of psychiatry/VI* (6th ed.). Baltimore: Williams & Wilkins.

Kerlinger, F. (1986). *Foundations of behavioral research.* New York: Holt Rinehart & Winston.

Lederer, J. R., Marculescu, G. L., Mochik, B., & Seaby, N. (Eds.). (1991). *Care planning pocket guide: A nursing diagnosis approach* (4th ed.). Redwood City, CA: Addison-Wesley Nursing.

Leventhal, H., & Tomarken, A. (1987). Stress and illness: Perspectives from health psychology. In S. V. Kasl & C. L. Cooper (Eds.), *Stress and health: Issues in research methodology.* New York: John Wiley & Sons.

Mayer, G. G., Madden, M. J., & Lawrenz, E. (Eds.). (1990). *Patient care delivery models.* Rockville, MD: Aspen Publishers.

McCarthy, S. M., & Gallo, A. M. (1992). A case illustration of family management style. *Journal of Pediatric Nursing, 7*(6), 395–402.

McClowry, S. G. (1992). Family functioning during a critical illness: A systems theory perspective. *Critical Care Nursing Clinics of North America, 4*(4), 559–564.

McFarland, G. K., Wasli, E. L., & Gerety, E. K. (1992). *Nursing diagnoses and process in psychiatric mental health nursing* (2nd ed.). Philadelphia: J. B. Lippincott.

Miers, L. J. (1991). NANDA's definition of nursing diagnosis: A plea for conceptual clarity. *Nursing Diagnosis, 2*(1), 9–18.

NANDA nursing diagnoses. (1995). Philadelphia: North American Nursing Diagnosis Association.

Pagana, K. D., & Pagana, T. J. (1994). *Diagnostic testing and nursing implications: A case study approach* (4th ed.). St. Louis: Mosby Year Book.

Pinkley, C. L. (1991). Exploring NANDA's definition of nursing diagnosis: Linking diagnostic judgments with the selections of outcomes and interventions. *Nursing Diagnosis, 2*(1), 26–32.

Potter, P. A., & Perry, A. G. (1993). *Fundamentals of nursing: Concepts, process, and practice* (3rd ed.). St. Louis: Mosby Year Book.

Shapiro, J. (1986). Assessment of family coping with illness. *Psychosomatics, 27*(4), 262–264.

Suddarth, D. S. (Ed.). (1991). *The Lippincott manual of nursing practice* (5th ed.). Philadelphia: J. B. Lippincott.

Thomas, C. L. (Ed.). (1993). *Taber's cyclopedic medical dictionary* (17th ed.). Philadelphia: F. A. Davis.

Timby, B. K., & Lewis, L. W. (1992). *Fundamental skills and concepts in patient care* (5th ed.). Philadelphia: J. B. Lippincott.

Toman, W. (1976). *Family constellation* (3rd ed.). New York: Springer-Verlag.

Tucker, S. M., Canobbio, M. M., Paquette, E. V., & Wells, M. F. (Eds.). (1992). *Patient care standards: Nursing process, diagnosis, and outcome* (5th ed.). St. Louis: Mosby Year Book.

Weber, G. J. (1991). Nursing diagnosis: A comparison of nursing textbook approaches. *Nurse Educator, 16*(2), 22–27.

CHAPTER 13

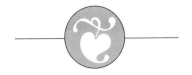

Integrating the Barry Holistic Systems and the NANDA Nursing Diagnosis Models

Patricia Barry

This section assists in analyzing the data from the psychosocial history obtained from a recently admitted patient and family member, if present. The nursing decision-making process involves these steps:

1. Collecting and identifying information.
2. Weighing and valuing that information based on the nurse's clinical knowledge.
3. Assembling the data into categories that are within the scope of independent nursing practice.
4. Identifying the data that indicates the presence of a collaborative patient problem. A *collaborative problem* is one that requires diagnosis and ordering of a treatment regimen by another caregiving group, most frequently, physicians.
5. Prioritizing identified problems based on the degree of risk each poses to the patient.

The nurse's ability to recognize the actual, possible, or potential seriousness of a psychosocial problem is directly related to knowledge about psychosocial risks for maladaptation

(Becket, 1991). This chapter presents the rationale for assessing each of the components of the psychosocial assessment interview schedule.

The Barry Psychosocial Assessment Interview schedule appears in Figure 13-1. It is based on the 11 functional health patterns identified by Gordon. The questions in the interview schedule are intended to be a general guide that can identify those areas of psychosocial functioning where the patient is currently experiencing difficulty or is at risk for ineffective coping. When problem areas are discovered, a shift to focus assessment should occur. A *focus assessment* is an information-gathering process that narrows the scope of questioning to a particular area of functioning where it appears that there may be an actual or potential health problem (Alfaro-LeFevre, 1994; Lederer et al., 1991).

(text continues on page 240)

Patricia Barry: *Psychosocial Nursing:*
Care of Physically Ill Patients and Their Families, 3rd ed.
© 1996 Lippincott–Raven Publishers

THE BARRY PSYCHOSOCIAL ASSESSMENT INTERVIEW SCHEDULE

All questions in italics should be subjectively assessed by the nurse, rather than asked of the patient directly. Bold-faced statements advise the assessor on how to proceed.

Admitting Information

Name _____ Age _____ Date of Admission _____
Date of Assessment _____
Marital Status   S _____M _____W _____D _____How long? _____
Occupation _____
Years of education completed _____
Admitting diagnosis _____

Health Perception–Health Management

Patient's Perception of Illness

What was the original problem that caused you to come to the hospital?
On what date did you first become ill?
What caused this illness?
How do you feel about being in a hospital?
How can the physicians and nurses help you most?
How will this illness affect you when you are out of the hospital?
Do you think it will cause any changes in your life?
How will it affect your family?
Potential for noncompliance? Yes _____ No _____ Possible _____
Related to: _____ Anxiety
                _____ Negative side-effects of prescribed treatment
                _____ Unsatisfactory relationship with caregiving environment or caregivers
                _____ Other
    Explain
Potential for Injury?   Yes _____ No _____Possible_____
    Explain

Nutritional–Metabolic

How does your current appetite compare with your normal appetite?
    Same _____ Increased _____ Decreased _____
    How long has it been different? _____
Has your weight fluctuated by more than 5 pounds in the last several weeks?
Yes _____ No _____
    How many pounds?
What is your normal fluid intake per day? _____ ml*
    Your current intake? _____ ml
Aspects of patient's illness or condition that could contribute to cognitive mental disorder?
    Yes _____ No_____
    Delirium type _____ Dementia type _____
    Possible cause:
    _____ Metabolic   _____ Arterial disease

FIGURE 13-1. The Barry Psychosocial Assessment Interview Schedule.

Electrolytes
Other metabolic or endocrine condition

_____ *Electrical disorder*	_____ *Mechanical disease*
_____ *Neoplastic disease*	_____ *Infectious disease*
_____ *Degenerative (chronic) brain disease*	_____ *Nutritional disease*
_____	_____ *Drug toxicity*

* Nurse can substitute estimate of ml for patient's reported fluid intake

Elimination

What is your current pattern of bowel movements?

Normal _____Constipated_____ Diarrhea _____ Incontinent _____

How does this compare to normal?   Same _____ Different _____

Explain

What is your current pattern of urination?

How does this compare to normal?   Same _____ Different _____ How is it different?_____

Explain

Possibility that emotional distress may be contributing to any change?

High_____ Moderate _____ Low _____

Activity–Exercise

What is your normal energy level?   High _____ Moderate_____ Low _____

Has it changed in the past 6 months?   Yes _____ No _____

To what do you attribute the cause?

How would you describe your normal activity level?

High _____ Moderate _____ Low _____

How may it change following this hospitalization?

What types of activities do you normally pursue outside the home?

What recreational activities do you enjoy?

Do you anticipate your ability to manage your home will be changed following your hospitalization? _____

Explain

Current self-care deficits?   Feeding _____ Bathing_____ Dressing _____ Toileting _____

Anticipated deficits following hospitalization?

Current impairment in mobility?

Anticipated immobility following hospitalization?

Alterations in the following?

Airway clearance _____How?

Breathing patterns _____How?

Cardiac output _____How?

Respiratory function _____How?

Potential for altered tissue perfusion as manifested by altered cognitive-perceptual patterns?

Sleep–Rest

Normal sleeping pattern

How many hours do you normally sleep per night? _____

From what hour to what hour?   _____ to _____

Changes in normal sleeping pattern
    Do you have difficulty falling asleep?
    Do you awaken in the middle of night?
    Do you awaken early in the morning?
    Are you sleeping more _____ or fewer _____ hours than normal? How many?_____

Cognitive–Perceptual

Are you feeling pain now?
    How severe?
    How often?
What relieves the pain?
What information does this client need to know to manage this illness/health state?
Ability to comprehend this information?   Good _____ Moderate _____ Poor _____
    If poor, explain

Mental Status Exam

Level of awareness and orientation _____
Appearance and behavior _____
Speech and communication _____
Affect (mood) _____
Thinking process _____
Related to: Inability to evaluate reality _____ *Aging* _____ *Other* _____
    Explain
If there is a distortion of the thought process, a focus assessment (see note at the end of scale) is indicated.
Perception _____
Abstract thinking _____
Social judgment _____
Memory _____
    Impairment in short-term memory_____ long-term _____
    Its there evidence of unilateral neglect? Yes _____ No _____ Does not apply _____

Self-Perception

Does the patient describe feelings of anxiety or uneasiness? _____
Is the patient able to identify a cause? Yes _____ No _____
    Cause?
If the patient feels anxious but cannot identify a cause, assess for the major coping risks of physical illness below.
Is there anything you are frightened of during this hospitalization or illness?
    Yes _____ No _____ What is it?
How will this illness affect your future plans?
Normally, do you believe that you control what happens to you *(internal locus of control)* or do you believe that other people or events control what happens *(external locus of control)*?
    Internal locus of control _____ *External locus of control* _____
Will this illness affect the way you feel about yourself?
    How?
    About your body?

Figure 13-1. (continued)

Psychosocial Risks of Illness

What are the major issues of this illness for this patient? For this family?

Use the following space to record patient and family comments illustrating how they are coping with these issues.

Trust	*Patient*	_____
	Family	_____
Self-esteem	*Patient*	_____
	Family	_____
Body image	*Patient*	_____
	Family	_____
Control	*Patient*	_____
	Family	_____
Loss	*Patient*	_____
	Family	_____
Guilt	*Patient*	_____
	Family	_____
Intimacy	*Patient*	_____
	Family	_____

Could one or more of these issues be contributing to feelings of anxiety, hopelessness, powerlessness, or disturbance in self-concept?

Yes _____ *No* _____ *Possible* _____

If so, explain which ones and proceed with focus assessment.

Role–Relationship

What is your occupation?

How many years have you been in this occupation? _____

Do you anticipate that this illness will have an effect on your ability to work?

Yes _____ No _____ How?

With whom do you live?

    Are they supportive?

Who are the most important people in your life?

Do you ever feel socially isolated?   Yes _____ No _____

    Explain

Is there any indication in this history of social isolation or impaired social interaction?

Yes _____ *No* _____

    Explain

Ability to communicate. Within normal limits _____ *Impaired* _____

    Describe

Family History

Who are the members of your immediate family? What are their ages and how are they related to you? Please include deceased members and when they died.

Name of family member	**Relationship to you**	**Age**	**Date of death**

What is your position in relation to your brothers and sisters? For example, are you the second oldest, the youngest...?

How often do you see your immediate family members?

What goes on in your family when something bad happens? What do most of the members do?

Have any of your relationships within your immediate and extended family changed recently?

    Which ones?

    How have they changed?

Is there any change in the way you parent your children? Yes _____ No _____

    If so, to what do you attribute the cause?

    _____ New baby

    _____ Death of family member

    _____ Illness in other family member

    _____ Change in residence

    Cause of change in residence

    _____ Other (describe)

What is your normal role within your family?

What role do the significant other people in your family play?

Potential for disruption of these roles by this illness? High _____ *Moderate* _____ *Low* _____

    Explain

While the patient is describing the family, is there indication of uncontrolled anger or rage?

    Yes _____ *No* _____

    Related to a specific issue or person?

    Explain

    Open (trusting) or closed (untrusting) communication style in family? (Can be initially determined by statements and emotional expression of patient.)

    Developmental stage of family

    _____ *Early married*

    _____ *Married with no children*

    _____ *Active childbearing*

    _____ *Preschool or school-age children*

    _____ *Adolescent children and children leaving home*

    _____ *Middle-aged, children no longer at home*

    _____ *Elderly, well-functioning*

    _____ *Elderly, infirm*

Is there any other aspect of your family or the way your family normally operates that you think should be added here? What is it?

If any item discussed in this section appears to be a current stressor for this patient or family it can be assessed using a focus approach with the other items under Coping–Stress Tolerance pattern.

Interpersonal style

    _____ *Dependent*

    _____ *Controlled*

    _____ *Dramatizing*

    _____ *Suspicious*

    _____ *Self-sacrificing*

    _____ *Superior*

    _____ *Uninvolved*

    _____ *Mixed (usually two styles predominate)*

Figure 13-1. (continued)

_____ *No predominant personality style*
Write a brief sentence explaining your choice.
Response to you as the interviewer. Guarded? _____ *Open?* _____
Is the patient able to maintain good eye contact?

Sexuality–Reproductive

Have you experienced any recent change in your sexual functioning? Yes _____ No _____
> How?
> For how long?

Do you associate your change in sexual functioning with some event in your life?

Do you think this illness could change your normal pattern of sexual functioning?
> How?

Is this change in sexuality patterns related to:
_____ *Ineffective coping*
_____ *Change or loss of body part*
_____ *Prenatal of postpartum changes*
_____ *Changes in neurovegetative functioning related to depression?*
Explain
Use focus assessment if necessary.

Coping–Stress Tolerance

Level of Stress During Year Before Admission

How long have you been out of work with this illness?

Have you experienced any recent change in your job?

Have you been under any unusual job stress during this past year?

What was the cause?
_____ Retirement
_____ Fired
_____ Same job, but new boss or working relationship
_____ Promotion or demotion
_____ Other; explain

Do you expect the stress will be present when you return to work?

The preceding questions should be adapted for students to a school situation.

Have there been changes in your family during the last 2 years? Which family members are involved? Include dates.
_____ Death
> Was this someone you were close to?

_____ Divorce
_____ Child leaving home
> Cause?

_____ Other

Has there been any other unusual stress during the last year that is still affecting you?
> Describe

Any unusual stress in your family?
> Describe

Normal Coping Ability

When you go through a very difficult time, how do you handle it?

_____Talk it out with someone   _____ Get angry and hit or throw something

_____ Ignore it   _____ Drink

_____ Withdraw from others   _____ Become anxious

_____ Get angry and yell   _____ Become depressed

_____ Get angry and clam up   _____ Other (Explain)

How often do you experience feelings of depression?

In the past, what is the longest period of time this feeling has lasted?

Have you felt depressed during the past few weeks?   Yes _____ No _____

To what do you attribute the cause?

If rape trauma is the cause of this admission, do not explore the psychological reaction with the patient until reading the report of the rape crisis counselor, who should have met with the patient within an hour of arrival at the emergency room. Either follow the recommendations in the report for ongoing assessment or proceed with gentle questioning about his or her current feelings.

What is the most serious trauma you have experienced?

What was the most difficult time you have experienced in your life?

How long did it take you to get over it?

What did you do to cope with it?

Potential for Self-Harm

This part of the assessment should be included if moderate to severe depression is present.

Have you ever thought of committing suicide? No _____ Yes _____

If yes, continue on.

What would you do to end your life? No plan _____ Plan_____

Describe

What would prevent you from committing suicide?

Note: The reader is strongly encouraged to read the section on suicide potential in Chapter 10 and the section on intervention with suicidal persons in Chapter 18 for further clarification of focus assessment guidelines.

Substances That May Be Used as Stress-Relievers

Smoking history

Do you smoke? _____ How long have you been smoking? _____ How many packs per day? _____

Alcohol use history

Do you drink? _____ How often? _____ How much? _____

Is there a history of alcoholism in your family? _____ Who? _____

Drug use

What prescribed medications are you currently using?

Name of medication	*Dose or schedule*	*Prescribing physician*

Figure 13-1. (continued)

Are you currently using any other drugs?   Yes _____ No _____
  What are they?
  How long have you been using it (them)?
  What is the usual amount?
  How often?
Have you ever been treated for drug abuse?

Value–Belief

What is your religious affiliation?
Do you consider yourself active or inactive in practicing your religion?
Active _____ Inactive _____
Is your pastor a supportive person? Yes _____ No _____
  Explain
What does this illness mean to you?
Are you experiencing spiritual distress? Yes _____ No _____
  Explain
What would you consider to be the primary cause of this spiritual distress (actual, possible, or potential)?
  _____ Inability to practice spiritual rituals
  _____ Conflict between religious, spiritual, or cultural beliefs and prescribed health regimen
  _____ Crisis of illness/suffering/death
  _____ Other (explain)
Do you expect there will be any disparity in your caregiver's approach that could present a problem for you? Please identify any problems in the areas of:
  _____ Spiritual rituals
  _____ Cause of illness
  _____ Perception of illness and sick role
  _____ Health maintenance
  _____ Communication
  _____ Problem solving
  _____ Nutrition
  _____ Family response
  Explain
How has this illness affected your relationship with God or the supreme being of your religion?
  Explain

The 11 functional health patterns were named by Marjorie Gordon (1987) in *Nursing diagnosis: Process and application.* New York: McGraw-Hill.

Note: This scale can be used in its entirety or to assist in developing psychosocial assessment criteria for individuals and families adapting to physical illness. When ineffective coping is occurring it can help the nurse to focus on the potential cause of the coping problem. The nurse's asking of specific questions about an issue is called *a focus assessment.* Effective nursing intervention and care planning can be enhanced by focusing on the cause of the problem.

ADMITTING INFORMATION

The admitting information includes basic data about the patient. Even this very basic information can trigger the nurse's analytical abilities if possible stressors are noted.

MARITAL STATUS

Whatever the patient's marital status, note that any marital status change during the previous year, including marriage, widowhood, or divorce, is a major stressor. Research has demonstrated that the rates of physical and mental illness and death are sharply increased in the recently bereaved (Maddison, 1968). The original research of Holmes and Rahe (1967) also found that marital separation, as well as the process of being married, were significant stressors in the lives of their research participants.

OCCUPATION

The patient's occupation can provide clues, such as how this illness is likely to affect his or her working status and personality style. For example, someone who works as an auto body repairman and has suffered a myocardial infarction will not be able to return to work as easily as an accountant. In this same example, the accountant is more likely to be a type A personality, for whom control may be more important, than the auto body repairman (Idill, Kelleher, & Shumaker, 1992). This need for control could potentially be identified early in admission, rather than after several days, when the level of anxiety may require sedation.

At this point in the assessment, it is important to consider the degree of threat this illness holds with regard to the patient's occupation. Some illnesses can leave a patient impaired so that return to a normal working role is not possible. This increases the risk of ineffective coping for both the patient and family (Frisch, 1993).

EDUCATION

For many patients, level of schooling serves as an indicator of intelligence and social class. It can indicate to the nurse what level of information may be appropriate when teaching the patient self-care procedures.

HEALTH PERCEPTION–HEALTH MANAGEMENT

PATIENT'S PERCEPTION OF ILLNESS

Questions asked in this part of the psychosocial assessment give information about how the patient perceives this illness and the potential threat it holds. Based on careful observation of verbal and nonverbal responses, this section of the assessment schedule can uncover any misperceptions the patient has about this illness. The nurse will want to develop care plans and teaching activities to address these issues. This section of the assessment also provides important information about other functioning categories, including mental status functioning; personality style; potential coping risks of this illness for this patient; and risks to role, family, and general relationships.

These questions are more complex for the patient to answer than those asked in other sections. Not only do they involve memory; they also require the patient to use complex thought processes such as problem solving, anticipatory reasoning, and judgment (Gerteis et al., 1993).

The question "What was the original problem that caused you to come to the hospital?" indicates how long the patient has had to prepare for the changes the illness is causing. Generally, the shorter the warning and the more serious the illness, the more strain will be put on a patient's and family's ability to cope.

Two other questions in this section should be judged subjectively by the nurse. The first regards the patient's potential for noncompliance. Noncompliance is caused by three major factors. The first is the negative side effects of prescribed treatment; the second is dissatisfaction with caregivers or the caregiving environment; and the third is denial, a defense mechanism that unconsciously blocks out the reality of a person's illness because it is too threatening to cope with consciously (Robinson, 1993).

NUTRITIONAL–METABOLIC

These questions yield information about current food and fluid intake. In addition, they can identify an important clinical symptom of depression: change in appetite with accompanying weight loss or gain. Appetite change is one sign of changes in neurovegetative functioning.

Neurovegetative functions are those aspects of physiological functioning affected by changes in neurotransmitters associated with depression. Neurovegetative signs include changes in appetite, sleep patterns, energy level, and sexual functioning (*Diagnostic Criteria from DSM-IV,* 1994). If depression is suspected, focus assessment of each of these areas of functioning should be included under the corresponding health patterns. Neurovegetative changes can be mentally noted by the nurse, and integrated with information obtained in the Coping-Stress Tolerance section to assess for the possibility of depression.

Questions about some neurovegetative functions may already be included in the nursing or medical assessment histories used in many institutions or agencies. *All* the functions should be assessed in order to have an accurate data base. If abnormal, they may indicate unresolved emotional conflict in patients, which is usually manifested as depression or anxiety. It is possible that this patient has been depressed or anxious for several months or longer. Emotional difficulties often progress to the physical symptoms included in this category. They occur as the result of changes in the autonomic nervous system, which are caused by ineffective coping (Kaplan & Sadock, 1994, 1995).

Frequently, mystified physicians admit their patients for diagnostic workups based on chronically occurring neurovegetative symptoms. They may not ask the patients if they are experiencing any emotional difficulty or unusual stress in their lives. If, in assessing neurovegetative functioning, it is learned that the patient is experiencing many physical changes from his or her functioning norm, it is possible that there is underlying emotional conflict. A shift to a focus assessment process will assist in determining if this is so.

ELIMINATION

Emotional distress is one of the underlying etiologies of alterations in normal bowel or urinary elimination. Because of neurotransmitter effects on smooth muscle, the sympathetic nervous system could be overstimulating or understimulating the bowel and bladder, changing their normal patterns. Anxiety, fear, adjustment disorders, and ineffective coping can cause overstimulation, resulting in diarrhea or frequent urination. Depression and prolonged grief can have the opposite effect, especially on the bowel, resulting in constipation (Leventhal & Tomarken, 1987).

ACTIVITY–EXERCISE

This section yields information about normal activity and home management levels. It also calls on the patient's decision-making and judgment abilities (Frisch, 1993). Responses to these questions can provide an opportunity for the nurse to note overall mental status functioning, which can be recorded in the Cognitive–Perceptual health pattern section.

ENERGY LEVEL

A person's level of energy can be an important indicator of normal functioning evident in activity and exercise. It can be used as a barometer for rehabilitation potential. A person who reports a chronically low level of energy will have a slower and possibly more complicated course of recovery than a higher-energy counterpart.

Energy level can be another neurovegetative sign of depression. A recent, gradual loss of energy accompanied by feelings of depression and low self-esteem can be warning indicators to the nurse that a possible depression may be occurring. Depression can complicate the outcomes of both hospitalization and rehabilitation (Cassem, 1991).

SELF-CARE SKILLS AND DISCHARGE PLANNING

One concern in the Activity–Exercise category is adjustment difficulties that the illness or condition could pose for the patient following discharge. Working with the family in assessing this impact can help to avert feelings of helplessness, loss of control, and unpreparedness that are avoidable with thoughtful planning. A step-by-step review of new or routine self-care skills that will be necessary on discharge can help all concerned to be aware of the challenges they will face (Frisch, 1993).

Knowledge deficits related to specific treatments associated with the illness or condition can be identified at this point in the assessment process, so that teaching strategies can be designed to alleviate them (Murray, 1991).

If the patient is hospitalized for long-term care, attention should also be paid to the potential for diversional activity deficit. This is especially important if the individual has a history of depressive responses to life adjustments. One of the most valuable aspects of using nursing diagnosis in care planning is that potential problems can be identified and interventions can be implemented to prevent their occurrence (Mayer, Madden, & Lawrenz, 1990).

RESPIRATORY FUNCTION

The possible alterations in respiratory function in the NANDA list share some common psychological etiologies. Some of them derive from neurotransmitter effects on the sympathetic nervous system and are triggered by fear, anxiety, or other types of ineffective coping. Some of these alterations are marked by rapid, shallow breathing. An additional form of respiratory dysfunction is hyperventilation. One of its etiologies is panic disorder, a frightening event in which the person's neurotransmitters trigger an acute physiological reaction of very rapid breathing and heart rate accompanied by a fear of imminent doom (*Diagnostic Criteria from DSM-IV,* 1994).

TISSUE PERFUSION

The final question in this section relates to difficulties with tissue perfusion pertaining to cerebral causes. Decreased cerebral tissue perfusion may manifest itself in a person of any age who has an alteration in mental status caused by cognitive mental disorder. The MEND A MIND assessment model used in the Nutritional–Metabolic section of Chapter 11 can be reviewed for any actual or potential cerebral tissue perfusion problems.

SLEEP–REST

This part of the assessment evaluates a person's normal sleeping patterns. Sleep disturbance is an important neurovegetative sign of depression. If changes in normal sleeping patterns are reported, a focus assessment can be used to determine the cause. For example, if a patient reports that she has had increasing difficulty falling asleep for the past six weeks, inquire why the patient thinks this is so. Listen and ask about changes in work or home relationships that could be contributing to the problem. Relationship changes will continue to affect her overall stress level and sleeping ability while hospitalized. Sleep patterns are often disturbed by the anxiety of hospitalization itself. Accordingly, the inability to sleep normally in the hospital will be compounded by the underlying sleep difficulty.

COGNITIVE–PERCEPTUAL

This is one of the most important sections for psychosocial assessment. It evaluates the patient's ability to perceive accurately what is currently happening. In addition, the patient's cognitive functioning can be determined. The assessment related to this question is covered in depth in Chapter 11.

Pain perception and response to pain are important cues to the nurse about underlying pathophysiological processes and the need for further assessment, as well as indicators of the need for pain management. Assessment of responses to pain is explained in Chapter 21, Pain Management in Acute Care and Home Care Settings.

MENTAL STATUS REVIEW

The "Knowledge deficit," "Sensory–perceptual alterations," and "Altered thought processes" diagnoses can all be evaluated using a standard mental status review. Specific information about mental status assessment and corresponding terminology can be found in Chapter 10. The categories of mental status include:

1. Orientation and level of awareness
2. Appearance and behavior
3. Speech and communication
4. Mood
5. Thinking process
6. Perception
7. Abstract thinking and social judgment
8. Short- and long-term memory
9. Potential for self-harm, self-abuse, suicide, trauma or violence to others

Orientation and Level of Awareness

If, during discussion with the patient, evidence of confusion is detected, it is recommended to question specifically if the patient knows who and where he is, as well as the day of the week, month, and year. Many times patients who appear oriented are actually masking mild to moderate confusion.

Appearance and Behavior

What is the patient's general appearance? Neat or disheveled? Is there anything remarkable about posture and overall behavior? Remember, in all these categories, if a normal range of responses is observed, it should be so recorded. If not recorded and there is any change later on, there will be no comparative data.

Speech and Communication

Is the patient's speech garbled, slurred, distinct, rapid, slow, accented? Is there anything remarkable about the patient's nonverbal communication?

Mood

What is the emotional state? Are a normal range of emotions evident as the patient discusses various issues, or is the range of emotions very constricted? Is there depression or anxiety? Does the patient display wide swings in emotions? Do the emotions match the topic of the discussion?

Thinking Process

Do the patient's statements make sense and proceed to logical conclusions? If so, they reflect a well-ordered thinking process. There are many abnormalities in this category, especially for patients with cognitive mental disorder (CMD) of either the dementia or delirium type. Refer to the thinking process section of Chapter 10 for specific references on situations in which abnormalities are observed. Abnormalities in thinking are subject to marked change in the patient with delirium over even a few hours. It is important to be as specific as possible and note the exact time of observations.

Perception

It is possible to assess the patient's perceptions with specific questions about whether things are seen or heard that are not really there. However, this is an inappropriate question for a nurse to ask the majority of general hospital patients, who function well perceptually. Unless a patient is being assessed who appears to be experiencing an organic or functional emotional disorder, the question need not be asked.

Abstract Thinking and Social Judgment

The evaluation of these categories is based on the manner in which the patient responds to the nurse's questions. As the patient's thoughts are being presented, the nurse can listen for examples of concrete thinking (see Chapter 10). If the patient is thinking concretely, this will be apparent at various points during the interview. Impairment in judgment may be seen in association with a concrete thinking style. Again, the patient's answers to the nurse's questions will indicate the level of social judgment.

Memory

A person's ability to recall information is essential to effective analytical thinking, problem solving, and judgment. There are two forms of memory impairment: short- and long-term memory loss. Short-term memory loss is more common. It involves loss of recall of some or all recent events. It occurs when people are anxious, depressed, coping ineffectively, or experiencing the delirium type of cognitive mental disorder (CMD). In these cases, the short-term memory loss is reversible. It is also present, but in a more severe form, in people with dementia-type CMD. Long-term memory loss is much less common. It is most common in people with advanced dementia-type CMD. In the dementia disorders memory loss is not reversible (Kaplan & Sadock, 1994, 1995; Murray, 1991).

SELF-PERCEPTION

This section of the psychosocial assessment interview schedule yields important information about the patient's perception of the stressors this illness will cause for her and her family. Responses to these questions can identify a number of actual, possible, or potential psychosocial diagnostic categories. The responses allow the nurse to further validate gathered information related to self-care, home management, and knowledge deficits.

This section can also assist the nurse in determining the patient's normal locus of control. Nurse decision-making about care planning can be more accurate with knowledge of a patient's need or lack of need for control. (See Chapter 9.)

PSYCHOSOCIAL RISKS OF ILLNESS

Evaluation of the coping risks of this illness for this patient yields important information about prime etiological factors in the nursing diagnoses. The nurse who is not experienced in psychosocial assessment may find it helpful to name all the possible etiological factors that could be contributing to the patient's problem. These factors can then be narrowed down to the possible causes. Interventions can then be clarified as to those that could reduce or eliminate the problem.

Coping risks of illness include the developmental issues every person faces. See Chapter 9 for a review of the developmental issues that are challenged by physical illness. All developmental issues are threatened by illness. Assessment of the threat of *this* illness to *this* patient will be based on the information obtained about this patient's unique personality. It is important to evaluate which psychosocial issues are most likely to contribute to the potential for ineffective coping that can lead to individual or family maladaptation (Mayer, Madden, & Lawrenz, 1990; Tucker et al., 1992).

Identifying the potentially most threatening issues will assist in identifying the challenges or threats the patient and family will experience in coping. One or all of the categories on the assessment scale can be highlighted. After checking it off, briefly justify the reasoning used.

It can be helpful to begin to identify the potential major issues of the patient's specific condition before beginning the assessment process. For example, a 38-year-old patient who is undergoing a mastectomy will probably experience a challenge adapting to the issues of self-esteem, changed body image, loss, and intimacy. During the assessment interview with the patient, it is possible to test this hypothesis based on her coping style, personality style, current life stressors occurring concurrently with this illness, and so on. The general guidelines in assessment of risk presented here should be integrated with the threats of the specific illness.

Although the nurse does not actively interview and formally assess the patient's family members, it is helpful to be aware of their potential for ineffective coping with each of these major issues. This can occur by listening astutely for cues during the patient's discussion about family members (Frisch, 1993). The issues which will challenge patients and their family members during a significant illness are:

TRUST
People who are most at risk for problems with trust:
   Dependent patients because of overly trusting and dependent behavior.
   Controlled patients because of their need to control all situations.

Suspicious patients because their ability to trust is minimal, yet they must follow caregivers' recommendations and accept their care.

Uninvolved patients because of their desire to be separate and independent of others.

SELF-ESTEEM

People who are most at risk for problems with a decrease in self-esteem:

Controlled patients because part of their need for control is related to self-esteem.

Persons with a type-A personality because there is often a great need to achieve; if the illness results in a change in their ability to work, it will present a greater threat.

Superior patients because their behavior is motivated by a need to bolster their self-esteem.

Body image change: With body image change, which is closely related to self-esteem, the degree of the perceived threat of a body change is a highly significant factor in the risk of the illness. The following example may help to clarify this point: a 24-year-old newly married woman must undergo a hysterectomy due to diethylstilbestrol (DES)-induced cancer, and a 48-year-old menopausal woman and mother of four children must undergo a hysterectomy because of frequent menorrhagia due to benign fibrosis. Of the two, the younger woman will likely perceive a greater threat of body image change than her older counterpart. The challenge to life goals in the younger woman can result in grieving about lost potentials.

CONTROL

People who are at risk for problems of control:

Controlled patients because of their lack of control in the hospital setting.

Suspicious patients because of an inability to trust caregivers' control of their care.

Self-sacrificing patients because their actions, behavior, and motivation seem

to be largely controlled by others' needs or by their own exaggerated perception of others' needs; these patients frequently overexert themselves physically after discharge because their own well-being and convalescence are sacrificed on behalf of others.

Superior patients because one common way they maintain control over others is by impressing them with their possessions, clothes, and so on; with hospitalization, the patient loses the reliance on these status symbols because of being socially "leveled."

Uninvolved, aloof patients because of their normally very independent state, which is threatened by hospitalization.

LOSS

People who are at risk for problems with loss:

All patients are at risk, however, this category is similar to body image changes, in that the degree of threat depends on the level of emotional investment in the lost person, body part, or function.

GUILT

People who are most at risk for problems with guilt:

Dependent patients whose normal way of interacting with others is passive, frequently because the person is motivated by guilt; if guilt is a major dynamic, the level of dependency may increase.

Controlled patients because their judgmental superegos (consciences) are already critical of themselves; extra guilt is a difficult burden.

Self-sacrificing patients because their behavior is often motivated by feelings of guilt and unworthiness.

INTIMACY

People who are most at risk for problems with intimacy:

Suspicious patients because closeness is threatening to them.

Uninvolved patients for the same reason.

All patients, to some extent, because of fear of self-disclosure related to impersonal hospital policies, need to discuss intimate types of information, loss of modesty and privacy, violation of body boundaries (tubing, catheters, endotracheal apparatus, and so on, imposed upon them).

All patients are also affected by the change in interpersonal relationships that hospital admission inflicts on them. They are removed from their normal social system; opportunities for privacy and closeness with loved ones are limited in the impersonal hospital environment.

ROLE–RELATIONSHIP

One of the most important factors in a person's capacity to rehabilitate to his or her former level of functioning is the ability to resume a normal working role. Anticipated difficulties here could be a strong etiological factor in many of the nursing diagnoses (Becket, 1991; Bulechek & McCloskey, 1992; Lazarus, 1992).

Available social support has been identified as a primary factor in avoiding crisis. In the event that this patient experiences ineffective coping and a high level of stress, knowing if someone is available and who that person is are important pieces of information.

FAMILY HISTORY

This section describes the pattern of family relationships and the normal way this patient interacts in the family. In addition, changes in the family that were affecting the family before their family member was hospitalized are identified. This can be important data in assessing the reserves, strengths, or challenges to effective coping that the family is bringing to the new stress of hospitalization (Burns et al., 1993). It can also spotlight the weaknesses of the family for whom the illness is the last straw, and disrupts the family's normal ability to relate to and support one another (Donley, 1993).

The first few questions here seek information about the quality and types of relationships that exist in the family: for example, the information could be "mother, father deceased, two sisters, and a brother." Ask the patient about deceased members of his or her immediate family and the dates they died. Observe also the emotional reaction in describing their deaths. This will provide information about this family's experience with major losses (Burr, 1991).

The position of the patient in relation to siblings, although not entirely predictable, can give you an idea of the patient's personality style. In general, oldest children tend to be more highly motivated and have more need for control than youngest children, who tend to be more dependent and passive (because many people met their needs in their original families). Middle children, on the other hand, tend to be more flexible and adaptable (McGoldrick & Gerson, 1985; Toman, 1976).

How often the patient sees parents and siblings and whether the patient has someone in whom to confide are very important pieces of information. They will tell you how able this person is to relate to others. If he develops a complication in the hospital, will he be able to receive support from someone close to him? People with suspicious or aloof personality styles are unlikely to have a close relationship with anyone (*DSM-IV,* 1994).

In many cases, the controlled person may also have difficulty with openness in a relationship. The patient's emotional response to the following relationship-related questions can be observed. Does he demonstrate pleasure, sadness, or anger? "What goes on in your family when a very bad event happens? What do most of the members do?" This answer describes the normal family coping style, an important clue to how the family system will respond if the patient faces a crisis. In some families, a member entering a hospital for any type of illness is a strong enough stressor to begin family maladaptation.

The patient's potential for violence, often expressed by rage and uncontrolled anger, can be most easily identified when a person is talking about individuals he is closest to. Distant relationships usually do not evoke the same level of emotion as do family relationships. The question about anger is included to assess the patient's level of impulse control. A person who erupts into rage with little provocation is demonstrating poor impulse control. Accordingly, he is more prone to violence when challenged (*DSM-IV*, 1994.)

COMMUNICATION STYLE

The communication style in the family may be difficult to discern. When assessable, however, it can help the nurse to judge the adaptability and adjustment potential of the family, particularly if the illness or condition will have long-term consequences. Generally, the open family is flexible and adaptable and has a good ability to trust outsiders. The need to rely on outside caregivers and the opinions of outside experts is important in chronic or long-term conditions. Closed families, on the other hand, are rigid and closed to outsiders; they have an inherent distrust of anyone who is not a member of the family (Guerin, 1976; McGoldrick & Gerson, 1985).

DEVELOPMENTAL STAGE

Knowing the developmental stage of the family is helpful in assessing the potential of this illness to disrupt the family's developmental process. For example, a young father diagnosed with cancer will respond differently, depending on his own stage of development and that of his spouse and family. A young husband and father of toddlers may have very different reactions from a married 57-year-old grandfather because of different levels of individual and family development.

(Additional information relating to patient and family functioning and responses to illness can be found in Chapter 3 in the section on defense mechanisms, and in Chapters 7, 9 and 15.)

INTERPERSONAL STYLE

The patient's normal interpersonal style can be evaluated by reflecting on communication patterns with health caregivers and family members. One clue is eye contact. Is the patient able to maintain eye contact consistently? Dependent people, for example, tend to main-

tain strong eye contact; they seem to be waiting for the other's response or looking for approval. On the other hand, the suspicious patient, the aloof patient, and sometimes the controlled patient will avoid eye contact.

Descriptions of feelings can be another strong indicator of interpersonal style. The suspicious or aloof patient typically avoids discussing feelings. In the controlled patient, emotions are constricted and lack a normal range. One of the controlled person's strong defense mechanisms is to overintellectualize. Using the defense of intellectualization, one is able to describe intellectual reactions to something in detail and, at the same time, repress feelings about the situation (Weisman, 1991). Patients who demonstrate normal to abnormally high levels of feelings typically have dependent personalities; dramatizing, emotionally involved personalities; and long-suffering, self-sacrificing personalities (guilt is a dominant feeling in these patients). The personality styles in which feelings seem dispensed with and in which the patients seem "above" having feelings are the antisocial and the superior personality types (*DSM-IV*, 1994).

Descriptions of relationships with other people are also strong indicators of the patient's normal interpersonal style and mode of interaction with others. Evidence of emotion can be noted as the patient describes his or her family's reaction to the illness or talks about the original family.

The way a patient responds to a nurse-interviewer is usually similar to his or her reactions to others. Is the patient comfortable and at ease, or anxious and tense? Is eye contact maintained, or do the patient's eyes consistently look around or at the floor?

SEXUALITY– REPRODUCTIVE

Questions about sexual functioning are significant because sexual functioning is an important indication of a person's ability to enjoy life. When people become chronically depressed or anxious, are involved in a conflict-riddled relationship, or have underlying personality disorders, diminished capacity for sexual enjoyment is of, en one of the first indicators of a problem.

In addition, many illnesses and different types of medications cause physiological changes that alter sexual functioning. The patient may associate a changed capacity for enjoyment with a myocardial infarction which occurred 3 years ago, the birth of a particular child, or the beginning of treatment for hypertension. Many of these causes can be potentially reversed with appropriate intervention. Information about the threat to intimacy caused by many diseases or conditions is presented in Chapters 17 and 18, which discuss psychosocial intervention with ineffective coping responses, and in Chapters 19 and 20, which discuss psychosocial aspects of selected physical conditions and chronic illness.

Alterations in sexuality patterns can be further assessed using a *focus interviewing technique.* Additional information that may assist in specific focus questions can be found in related sections in Chapter 3 (the section on the role of defense mechanisms in effective and ineffective coping), Chapter 7, Chapter 9, and Chapter 15.

COPING–STRESS TOLERANCE

This section is strategically placed at an important point in the interviewing process. The nurse has, by now, established rapport with the patient and family member, if one is present. Actual, possible, or potential problematic aspects of the patient's responses to illness are now known to the nurse. This section focuses the assessment on the ability of the patient and family to cope with these changes.

LEVEL OF STRESS DURING THE YEAR BEFORE ADMISSION

Research has demonstrated a strong correlation between high levels of stress and the development of illness. Newly admitted patients frequently report many changes in their lives during the year or so before admission. If questions about stress are asked on admission, the patient may attribute the development of his or her illness to one or more of these stressors.

The physician, using a medical model, may not obtain a comprehensive history of the patient's stress because the patient's psychosocial sphere is not the physician's major interest. The nursing diagnosis movement, however, has identified the psychosocial sphere as the major interest of the nurse. Nearly 70% of its diagnostic categories are in the psychosocial realm.

If information on stress is not routinely obtained, it is possible to overlook one of the original precipitants of the patient's illness. The patient's condition can be treated in the hospital; unless the patient's mode of dealing with stress is attended to, however, discharge may occur with the individual continuing to cope ineffectively with a preadmission stress level. The patient may also be discharged into the same social system that may have caused the stress that helped bring on the illness. If aware of the patient's stress history, interventions can be planned to promote more adaptive patient responses (Frisch, 1993).

Changes in Work or School

How long the patient has been out of work with the current illness will tell you the level of stress the patient and family may be experiencing because of economic hardship. If a breadwinner is out of work for several weeks or more, there are usually major strains in the relationships between all family members (Burr, 1991).

Changes in Family

Changes in the family, such as death, divorce, a child leaving home, a new baby, illness in another family member, a change in residence, and a change in job or financial state can all be profoundly stressful (McGoldrick & Gerson, 1985). Early research by Holmes and Rahe (1967) found that positive changes could be as stressful as negative changes because of the necessary adjustment process.

NORMAL COPING ABILITY

In this part of the history the patient's normal coping style is evaluated. This assessment includes the conscious coping strategies used when the patient is severely stressed. The word *conscious* implies that these are actual strategies that the patient is aware of using. Coping strategies are different from unconscious defense mechanisms, of which the patient is unaware. The care plan should support the patient's normal coping style.

Most patients know what coping method works best for them in reducing stress. It may be necessary to ask a few questions to discover what it is. When this information is obtained, assessment about whether these coping strategies may help during the current illness can be discussed. The following case examples clarify this point (McHaffie, 1992).

CASE EXAMPLES

Jim is 28 years old and a garage mechanic. One day, while he was working in the garage, a car fell on him. His neck was broken, and he was permanently paralyzed from the neck down. Jim's wife said that his normal way of handling stress was to pound his fist against the wall. Given this information and the overwhelming nature of his current situation, his normal coping ability cannot be used. Care planning regarding psychosocial support is an essential part of the early assessment and intervention process.

Diane is a 32-year-old schoolteacher. She and her husband were happily expecting their first child. During her fifth month of pregnancy the fetus was unexpectedly aborted. Diane says that when she is under stress, she normally shares everything with her husband, who is very understanding and caring. Given this information, what would be Diane's expected ability to cope adequately?

Obtaining information about normal coping strategies can assist the nurse in anticipating coping problems and the potential for patient maladaptation. As a further point, what would Diane's coping potential be if her husband was working in the Middle East for 6 months as a management consultant and would be given only a 2-week leave of absence to be with her?

When the question is asked, "When you experience stress in your everyday life, what do you do to decrease it?" or "When you go through a very difficult time, how do you normally handle it?" many patients are able to describe immediately their regular coping techniques. Others may need more help in finding their answer. If they should ask, "What do you mean?" the nurse can inquire, "What is the worst thing that ever happened to you? How did you get over it?"

Hospitalization for a serious or life-threatening illness can be a major crisis for the patient and family. Their normal, everyday stress responses may not work for them (Lazarus, 1992; McCarthy & Gallo, 1992). It is important to keep in mind that the way people respond to stress usually does not change significantly over a life-time. If, for example, the patient experienced a major crisis in his 20s and responded with serious depression, there is an increased possibility that depression can occur as the result of this current health crisis.

Usually patients are able to identify their normal response specifically if you describe some possibilities:

Talk it out with someone
Ignore it (actually, defense mechanisms of repression, denial, or avoidance are often being unconsciously used)
Withdraw from others
Get angry and yell
Get angry and clam up
Get angry and hit or throw something
Drink
Become anxious
Become depressed

It is important to elicit the patient's response to a major traumatic event or other serious crisis (Malt & Olafsen, 1992). The patient's answer to the question "How long did it take you to get over it?" will tell you about the person's adaptive ability. Remember, however, that major losses of significant people usually take over a year to begin to subside. The nurse is advised to be realistic in evaluating whether the patient's crisis resolution time is within normal limits (McClowry, 1992).

ASSESSMENT FOR DEPRESSION

There are several questions about depression in this interview schedule. They are included to assess for factors that could result in ineffective coping during this treatment period; maladaptation following hospital discharge; and, if not reversed, possible inability to return to normal roles in family and work, thereby causing long-term or permanent changes in lifestyle. Depression can also cause changes in sleep patterns and normal gastrointestinal functioning. It is believed to suppress the immune system in some individuals (Charney et al., 1993; Dewsbury, 1991; Folkow, 1993; Goldstein & Niaura, 1992; Johnson et al., 1992; Niaura & Goldstein, 1992; Solomon, 1985).

If the person is responding to a current trauma that caused the hospitalization, the patient may continue to be in a state of emotional numbness. If so, a focus assessment can be initiated to determine the level of shock, survival guilt, or need to discuss the event (Alfaro-LeFevre, 1994).

If rape trauma has occurred, the patient should have been seen by a rape crisis counselor in the emergency room. If possible, the counselor's report can be obtained and used as a guide to develop appropriate questions. If not, the comprehensive psychosocial assessment process can be delayed for 24 hours to allow the time of initial shock to pass. Questioning should be of a sensitive, but in-depth, nature to determine the individual's immediate concerns and needs.

If moderate to severe depression is evident, potential for self-harm should be evaluated. The questioning should be focused to determine if suicidal ideation is occurring or if, more seriously, it has progressed to an active plan for suicide. If a plan has been developed, ongoing questioning can reveal the full risk present. The reader is encouraged to review the sections on suicide assessment in Chapter 10, and the sections in Chapters 17 and 18 on psychosocial intervention with ineffective coping responses, to understand more fully the importance of careful questioning if such assessment is necessary.

SUBSTANCE ABUSE

Another indication of ineffective coping ability is the use of substances that are perceived by individuals with substance use disorders as stress relievers. This section includes questions about smoking, alcohol, and drug use. This is particularly significant information if these substances have been important to the patient and if continued use will impair future health status. For example, a chain-smoking person who has a severe myocardial infarction will be stressed by the major change in health functioning. Smoking, one of this individual's usual stress-relieving mechanisms, will be discouraged because it causes decreased cardiac perfusion. Losing the ability to smoke may further increase a patient's anxiety level.

Alcohol Use History

It has been reported that from 27% to 60% of all hospital admissions are alcohol related (Barcha, Stewart, & Guze, 1968; Gomberg, 1975; Kearney, 1968). The questions "Do you drink? How often? How much? Is there a history of alcoholism in your family? Who is that person?" are designed to explore the possibility that this illness is related to alcohol. Without obtaining information about the patient's drinking history, it is possible that the patient will receive full medical treatment, be discharged in an improved condition, and return to the hospital in 3 months because drinking problems have precipitated another disease process. Caregivers' lack of assessment regarding alcohol use is a costly omission. A patient who does have a drinking problem may not acknowledge it. By observing body language and evasive eye contact at the time of the question, the nurse can receive a better indication about the reliability of the obtained answer.

Many hospitals have alcohol counselors who work with patients and promote Alcoholics Anonymous concepts with alcoholic patients and family members. The question about history of alcoholism in the family is important because the child of an alcoholic parent is five times more likely to be an alcoholic as well (Estes, Smith-Dijulo, & Heinemann, 1980).

Medication History

This information is a necessary part of all hospital admission histories. In the psychosocial history it can also help to identify drugs that may be used to decrease anxiety or to manage some other type of mental distress. In the event of recent altered mental status, the medication history can aid in determining if one or more of currently prescribed medications are reported to have side effects of changes in mental status functioning.

Other Drug Use

When asking about drugs the patient can be told that it is important to his or her safety that this information be known, especially if surgery will be performed. Certain drugs, especially when chronically abused, cause changes in physiological and psychological functioning that can jeopardize the patient's health. They can also result in danger to caregivers if a toxic withdrawal from the drug occurs. For example, a young adolescent addicted to LSD may be seriously injured in an accident. When coming out of anesthesia he may experience a delirium with hallucinations and strike out at caregivers.

VALUE–BELIEF

The final section of the psychosocial assessment scale is related to the pattern of values and meaning that provide an inner source of strength to an individual. Three areas in the Value–Belief realm may be sources of conflict for hospitalized patients. They are the inability to practice spiritual rituals; conflict between religious or spiritual beliefs and the prescribed health regimen; and the crisis of illness, suffering, or death. Cultural disparity with the prescribed health regimen is an additional consideration in possible patient and family demoralization. Chapter 5 discusses these issues.

If spiritual distress is related to either of the first two or the last reasons, it can be help-ful to include a family member in the assessment discussion. This may relieve any discomfort the patient feels in describing religious or cultural beliefs stemming from fears that they will sound strange to the nurse.

On the other hand, if the spiritual distress is related to the crisis of illness, suffering, or death, it is best to ask about these issues when alone with the patient. These are usually very private thoughts or fears, which may never have been expressed or explored by them aloud. They fall into the realm of existential wonderings. What is the purpose of life? Of my life? My death? Is there really a God?

These questions lie deep within all people. When shared with another human being they evidence the important trust the confider is placing in the confidant. Such discussions do not typically happen in an initial encounter. Rather, they occur after a meaningful, trusting relationship has developed, as between a primary nurse and a dying patient who have known each other through many inpatient or home care admissions, or during a terminal admission.

The question "How has this illness affected your relationship with God or the supreme being of your religion?" is included because it can provide great relief to a patient or family member to talk about this. A person may have been a faithful believer in God, then developed a difficult disease, had a serious accident, or watched a family member suffer or die. It is not uncommon for the sufferer to become angry with God. This is a normal reaction. Anger is one of the stages in the normal adjustment to a loss of any kind.

Because the idea of being angry with God is contrary to religious beliefs, such anger can feel foreign to the patient. Even when the active anger passes, a person may continue to feel alienated from God. Accordingly, there can be a loss of a source of strength that has been drawn on for a lifetime. If a person is experiencing anger with God and associated alienation, it can be suggested that a pastor, other member of the clergy, or the hospital chaplain be called. Hospital chaplains are usually perceptive about the importance of resolving these psychological issues and can relieve the guilt that people may have been carrying for months.

CONCLUSION

This chapter gives a brief rationale for the questions asked in the psychosocial assessment interview schedule. A fuller explanation of the theory underlying these questions can be found in the chapters relating to the specific topics. The specific chapter numbers are listed in Chapter 12 and earlier in this chapter.

BIBLIOGRAPHY

See Chapter 12 for specific references related to clinical phenomena described in this chapter.

Alfaro-LeFevre, R. (1994). *Applying nursing process.* Philadelphia: J. B. Lippincott.

Artinian, B. M. (1991). The development of the Intersystem Model. *Journal of Advanced Nursing Practice, 16*(2), 194–205.

Barcha, R., Stewart, M., & Guze, S. (1968). The prevalence of alcoholism among general hospital ward patients. *American Journal of Psychiatry, 125*(5), 681–684.

Barry, P. D. (1994). *Mental health and mental illness* (5th ed.). Philadelphia: J. B. Lippincott.

Becket, N. (1991). Clinical nurses' characterizations of patient coping problems. *Nursing Diagnosis, 2*(2), 72–78.

Bock, G. R., & Whelan, J. (Eds.). (1991). *The childhood environment and adult disease.* New York: Wiley.

Bulechek, G. M., & McCloskey, J. C. (1992). Defining and validating nursing interventions. *Nursing Clinics of North America, 27*(2), 289–299.

Burns, C., Archbold, P., Stewart, B., & Shelton, K. (1993). New diagnosis: Caregiver role strain. *Nursing Diagnosis, 4*(2), 70–76.

Cassem, N. H. (1991). Depression. In N. H. Cassem (Ed.), *Massachusetts General Hospital handbook of general hospital psychiatry* (3rd ed.). St. Louis: Mosby Year Book.

Charney, D. S., Deutch, A. Y., Krystal, J. H., Southwick, S. M., & Davis, M. (1993). Psychobiologic mechanisms of posttraumatic stress disorder. *Archives of General Psychiatry, 50*(4), 295–305.

Dewsbury, D. A. (1991). Psychobiology. *American Psychologist, 46*(3), 198–205.

DSM-IV. (1994). Washington, DC: American Psychiatric Press.

Donley, M. G. (1993). Attachment and the emotional unit. *Family Process, 32*(1), 3–20.

Edlin, G., & Golanty, E. (1992). *Health and wellness: A holistic approach* (4th ed.). Boston: Jones & Bartlett.

Estes, N., Smith-Dijulo, K., & Heinemann, M. (1980). *Nursing diagnosis of the alcoholic person.* St. Louis: C. V. Mosby.

Folkow, B. (1993). Physiological organization of neurohormonal responses to psychosocial stimuli: Implications for health and disease. *Annals of Behavioral Medicine, 15*(4), 236–243.

Frisch, N. (1993). Home care nursing and psychosocial-emotional needs. How nursing diagnosis helps to direct and inform practice. *Home Healthcare Nurse, 11*(2), 64–65, 70.

Gerteis, M., Edgman-Levitan, S., Daley, J., & Delbanco, T. L. (Eds.). (1993). *Through the patient's eyes: Understanding and promoting patient-centered care.* San Francisco: Jossey-Bass.

Goldberg, R. J., & Novack, D. H. (1992). The psychosocial review of systems. *Social Science and Medicine, 35*(3), 261–269.

Goldstein, M. G., & Niaura, R. (1992). Psychological factors affecting physical condition. Cardiovascular disease literature review. Part I: Coronary artery disease and sudden death. *Psychosomatics, 33*(2), 134–145.

Gomberg, E. (1975). Prevalence of alcoholism among ward patients in a Veterans Administration hospital. *Journal of Studies in Alcohol, 36*(11), 1458–1467.

Guerin, P. (Ed.). (1976). *Family therapy: Theory and practice.* New York: Gardner Press.

Halm, M. A., Titler, M. G., Kleiber, C., Johnson, S. K., Montgomery, L. A., Craft, M. J., Buckwalter, K., Nicholson, A., & Megivern, K. (1993). Behavioral responses of family members during critical illness. *Clinics in Nursing Research, 2*(4), 414–437.

Hartman, D., & Knudson, J. (1991). A nursing data base for initial patient assessment. *Oncology Nursing Forum, 18*(1), 125–130.

Harwood, A. (1981). *Ethnicity and medical care.* Cambridge, MA: Harvard University Press.

Heliker, D. (1992). Reevaluation of a nursing diagnosis: Spiritual distress. *Nursing Forum, 27*(4), 15–20.

Holmes, R., & Rahe, R. (1967). The social readjustment rating scale. *Journal of Psychosomatic Research, 11*(2), 213–218.

Idill, S., Kelleher, K., & Shumaker, S. (1992). Psychosocial interventions in adult patients with coronary heart disease and cancer: A literature review. *General Hospital Psychiatry, 14S:* 28S–42S.

Johnson, E., Kamilaris, T., Chorous, B., & Gold, P. (1992). Mechanisms of stress: A dynamic overview of hormonal and behavioral homeostasis. *Neuroscience and Biobehavioral Reviews, 16*(2), 115–130.

Kaplan, H. I., & Sadock, B. J. (1994). *Synopsis of psychiatry: Behavioral sciences, clinical psychiatry* (7th ed.). Baltimore: Williams & Wilkins.

Kaplan, H. I., & Sadock, B. J. (1995). *Comprehensive textbook of psychiatry/VI* (6th ed.). Baltimore: Williams & Wilkins.

Kearney, T. (1968). Alcohol and general hospital patients. *American Journal of Psychiatry, 125*(10), 1451–1452.

Lazarus, R. S. (1992). Coping with the stress of illness. *WHO Regional Publications, European Series, 44,* 11–31.

Leininger, M. (1991). Becoming aware of types of health practitioners and cultural imposition. *Journal of Transcultural Nursing, 2*(2), 32–39.

Levine, M. E. (1966). Trophicognosis: An alternative to nursing diagnosis. In *Exploring progress in medical surgical nursing practice.* New York: American Nurses' Association.

Levine, S. (1993). The influence of social factors on the response to stress. *Psychotherapy and Psychosomatics, 60*(1), 33–38.

Lundeen, S. P. (1992). Health needs of a suburban community: A nursing assessment. *Journal of Community Health Nursing, 9*(4), 235–244.

Maddison, D. (1968). The health of widows in the year following bereavement. *Journal of Psychosomatic Research, 12*(4), 297–306.

Malt, U. F., & Olafsen, O. M. (1992). Psychological appraisal and emotional response to physical injury: A clinical, phenomenological study of 109 adults. *Psychiatric Medicine, 10*(3), 117–134.

Mayer, G. G., Madden, M. J., & Lawrenz, E. (Eds.). (1990). *Patient care delivery models.* Rockville, MD: Aspen Publishers.

McCarthy, S. M., & Gallo, A. M. (1992). A case illustration of family management style. *Journal of Pediatric Nursing, 7*(6), 395–402.

McClowry, S. G. (1992). Family functioning during a critical illness: A systems theory perspective. *Critical Care Nursing Clinics of North America, 4*(4), 559–564.

McGoldrick, M., & Gerson, R. (1985). *Genograms in family assessment.* New York: W. W. Norton.

McHaffie, H. E. (1992). The assessment of coping. *Clinics in Nursing Research, 1*(1), 67–79.

Murray, G. B. (1991) Confusion, delirium, and dementia. In N.H. Cassem (Ed.) *Massachusetts General Hospital handbook of general hospital psychiatry* (3rd ed.) St. Louis: Mosby Year Book.

NANDA nursing diagnoses. (1995). Philadelphia: North American Nursing Diagnosis Association.

Niaura, R., & Goldstein, M. B. (1992). Psychological factors affecting physical condition. Cardiovascular disease literature review. Part II: Coronary artery disease and sudden death and hypertension. *Psychosomatics, 33*(2), 146–155.

Parkes, C., Benjamin, B., & Fitzgerald, R. (1969). Broken heart: A statistical study of increased mortality among widowers. *British Medical Journal, 1*(646), 740–743.

Raya, A., Mantas, J., Priami, M., Andrea, S., Kalokerinou, A., Androulaki, O., Brokalaki, H., Halkiadaki, H., & Matziou, V. (1991). Psychosomatic nursing assessment of psychiatric patients. *Psychotherapy and Psychosomatics, 56*(1–2), 5–11.

Recker, D., & O'Brien, C. (1992). Using Gordon's functional health patterns to organize a critical care orientation program. *Focus on Critical Care, 19*(1), 21–25, 28.

Robinson, K. R. (1993). Denial: An adaptive response. *Dimensions in Critical Care Nursing, 12*(2), 102–106.

Rooda, L. (1993). Knowledge and attitudes of nurses toward culturally different patients: Implications for nursing education. *Journal of Nursing Education, 32*(5), 209–213.

Sadler, J. Z., & Hulgus, Y. F. (1992). Clinical problem-solving and the biophysical model. *American Journal of Psychiatry, 149*(10), 1315–1323.

Savage, P. (1991). Patient assessment in psychiatric nursing. *Journal of Advanced Nursing, 16*(3), 311–316.

Tucker, S. M., Canobbio, M. M., Paquette, E. V., & Wells, M. F. (Eds.). (1992). *Patient care standards: Nursing process, diagnosis, and outcome* (5th ed.). St. Louis: Mosby Year Book.

Weisman, A. D. (1991). Coping with illness. In N. H. Cassem (Ed.), *Massachusetts General Hospital handbook of general hospital psychiatry* (3rd ed.). St. Louis: Mosby Year Book.

CHAPTER 14

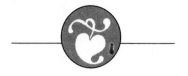

Nursing Diagnosis and Care Planning

Patricia Barry

One requirement of an occupation in order for it to be considered a profession is that its members use a specific body of knowledge in their practice. Since the inception of the North American Nursing Diagnosis Association (NANDA) in the 1970s, clinicians and educators have been clarifying the specific body of knowledge used in the nursing profession. In doing so they are identifying specific patient responses to illness that nurses are qualified to diagnose and treat within the scope of their practices (see Box 14-1).

Psychosocial nursing problems are abundantly evident in the diagnostic categories. Some categories have predominantly psychosocial dynamics in their etiologies. The other categories are customarily viewed as having physiological etiologies; actually, most typically have one or more psychosocial dynamics in their etiological course, because of being triggered by the sympathetic response in the autonomic nervous system.

Alfaro-LeFevre (1994) defines a nursing diagnosis as:

An actual or potential health problem (of an individual, family, or group) that nurses can legally treat independently, initiating the nurs-

ing interventions necessary to prevent, resolve, or reduce the problem.

SELECTING PSYCHOSOCIAL NURSING DIAGNOSES

Once the nurse has collected information about the patient's and family's psychosocial history using the assessment scale in Chapter 13, problems that need specific nursing intervention are ready to be identified. There are many ways to assemble the information in order to formulate nursing diagnoses. One of the most common is to make a list of the problems the patient or family is now experiencing. Following that, another list can be developed containing areas of functioning where the patient or family could be at risk if maladaptive trends continue or begin to occur, and areas of possible need that require further data to substantiate intervention.

Another way to identify problem areas is to review the Gordon health response patterns

Patricia Barry: *Psychosocial Nursing:*
Care of Physically Ill Patients and Their Families, 3rd ed.
© 1996 Lippincott–Raven Publishers

BOX 14-1	**NANDA-Approved Nursing Diagnoses**

Pattern 1: Exchanging

1.1.2.1	Altered Nutrition: More than body requirements
1.1.2.2	Altered Nutrition: Less than body requirements
1.1.2.3	Altered Nutrition: Potential for more than body requirements
1.2.1.1	Risk for Infection
1.2.2.1	Risk for Altered Body Temperature
1.2.2.2	Hypothermia
1.2.2.3	Hyperthermia
1.2.2.4	Ineffective Thermoregulation
1.2.3.1	Dysreflexia
1.3.1.1	Constipation
1.3.1.1.1	Perceived Constipation
1.3.1.1.2	Colonic Constipation
1.3.1.2	Diarrhea
1.3.1.3	Bowel Incontinence
1.3.2	Altered Urinary Elimination
1.3.2.1.1	Stress Incontinence
1.3.2.1.2	Reflex Incontinence
1.3.2.1.3	Urge Incontinence
1.3.2.1.4	Functional Incontinence
1.3.2.1.5	Total Incontinence
1.3.2.2	Urinary Retention
1.4.1.1	Altered (Specify Type) Tissue Perfusion (Renal, cerebral, cardiopulmonary, gastrointestinal, peripheral)
1.4.1.2.1	Fluid Volume Excess
1.4.1.2.2.1	Fluid Volume Deficit
1.4.1.2.2.2	Risk for Fluid Volume Deficit
1.4.2.1	Decreased Cardiac Output
1.5.1.1	Impaired Gas Exchange
1.5.1.2	Ineffective Airway Clearance
1.5.1.3	Ineffective Breathing Pattern
1.5.1.3.1	Inability to Sustain Spontaneous Ventilation
1.5.1.3.2	Dysfunctional Ventilatory Weaning Response (DVWR)
1.6.1	Risk for Injury
1.6.1.1	Risk for Suffocation
1.6.1.2	Risk for Poisoning
1.6.1.3	Risk for Trauma
1.6.1.4	Risk for Aspiration
1.6.1.5	Risk for Disuse Syndrome
1.6.2	Altered Protection
1.6.2.1	Impaired Tissue Integrity
1.6.2.1.1	Altered Oral Mucous Membrane
1.6.2.1.2.1	Impaired Skin Integrity
1.6.2.1.2.2	Risk for Impaired Skin Integrity
1.7.1	Decreased Adaptive Capacity: Intracranial
1.8	Energy Field Disturbance

Pattern 2: Communicating

| 2.1.1.1 | Impaired Verbal Communication |

Pattern 3: Relating

3.1.1	Impaired Social Interaction
3.1.2	Social Isolation
3.1.3	Risk for Loneliness
3.2.1	Altered Role Performance
3.2.1.1.1	Altered Parenting
3.2.1.1.2	Risk for Altered Parenting
3.2.1.1.2.1	Risk for Altered Parent/Infant/Child Attachment
3.2.1.2.1	Sexual Dysfunction
3.2.2	Altered Family Processes
3.2.2.1	Caregiver Role Strain
3.2.2.2	Risk for Caregiver Role Strain
3.2.2.3.1	Altered Family Process: Alcoholism
3.2.3.1	Parental Role Conflict
3.3	Altered Sexuality Patterns

Pattern 4: Valuing

| 4.1.1 | Spiritual Distress (distress of the human spirit) |
| 4.2 | Potential for Enhanced Spiritual Well Being |

Pattern 5: Choosing

5.1.1.1	Ineffective Individual Coping
5.1.1.1.1	Impaired Adjustment
5.1.1.1.2	Defensive Coping
5.1.1.1.3	Ineffective Denial
5.1.2.1.1	Ineffective Family Coping: Disabling
5.1.2.1.2	Ineffective Family Coping: Compromised
5.1.3.1	Potential for Enhanced Community Coping

(Continued)

BOX 14-1	**NANDA-Approved Nursing Diagnoses** *(Continued)*

5.1.3.2	Ineffective Community Coping
5.1.2.2	Family Coping: Potential for Growth
5.2.1	Ineffective Management of Therapeutic Regimen (Individuals)
5.2.1.1	Noncompliance (Specify)
5.2.2	Ineffective Management of Therapeutic Regimen: Families
5.2.3	Ineffective Management of Therapeutic Regimen: Community
5.2.4	Ineffective Management of Therapeutic Regimen: Individual
5.3.1.1	Decisional Conflict (Specify)
5.4	Health Seeking Behaviors (Specify)

Pattern 6: Moving

6.1.1.1	Impaired Physical Mobility
6.1.1.1.1	Risk for Peripheral Neurovascular Dysfunction
6.1.1.1.2	Risk for Perioperative Positioning Injury
6.1.1.2	Activity Intolerance
6.1.1.2.1	Fatigue
6.1.1.3	Risk for Activity Intolerance
6.2.1	Sleep Pattern Disturbance
6.3.1.1	Diversional Activity Deficit
6.4.1.1	Impaired Home Maintenance Management
6.4.2	Altered Health Maintenance
6.5.1	Feeding Self Care Deficit
6.5.1.1	Impaired Swallowing
6.5.1.2	Ineffective Breastfeeding
6.5.1.2.1	Interrupted Breastfeeding
6.5.1.3	Effective Breastfeeding
6.5.1.4	Ineffective Infant Feeding Pattern
6.5.2	Bathing/Hygiene Self Care Deficit
6.5.3	Dressing/Grooming Self Care Deficit
6.5.4	Toileting Self Care Deficit
6.6	Altered Growth and Development
6.7	Relocation Stress Syndrome

6.8.1	Risk for Disorganized Infant Behavior
6.8.2	Disorganized Infant Behavior
6.8.3	Potential for Enhanced Organized Infant Behavior

Pattern 7: Perceiving

7.1.1	Body Image Disturbance
7.1.2	Self Esteem Disturbance
7.1.2.1	Chronic Low Self Esteem
7.1.2.2	Situational Low Self Esteem
7.1.3	Personal Identity Disturbance
7.2	Sensory/Perceptual Alterations (Specify) (Visual, auditory, kinesthetic, gustatory, tactile, olfactory)
7.2.1.1	Unilateral Neglect
7.3.1	Hopelessness
7.3.2	Powerlessness

Pattern 8: Knowing

8.1.1	Knowledge Deficit (Specify)
8.2.1	Impaired Environmental Interpretation Syndrome
8.2.2	Acute Confusion
8.2.3	Chronic Confusion
8.3	Altered Thought Processes
8.3.1	Impaired Memory

Pattern 9: Feeling

9.1.1	Pain
9.1.1.1	Chronic Pain
9.2.1.1	Dysfunctional Grieving
9.2.1.2	Anticipatory Grieving
9.2.2	Risk for Violence: Self-directed or directed at others
9.2.2.1	Risk for Self-Mutilation
9.2.3	Post-Trauma Response
9.2.3.1	Rape-Trauma Syndrome
9.2.3.1.1	Rape-Trauma Syndrome: Compound Reaction
9.2.3.1.2	Rape-Trauma Syndrome: Silent Reaction
9.3.1	Anxiety
9.3.2	Fear

with the appropriate diagnostic labels categorized within each pattern. As an actual (*A*), potential (*Pt*), or possible (*Ps*) problem area is noted, check it off and place an *A*, *Pt*, or *Ps* next to the label. The NANDA nursing diagnoses categories are grouped by clinical patterns in Box 14-1.

ASSESSING AND PRIORITIZING PSYCHOSOCIAL PROBLEMS

If a patient is exhibiting acute psychosocial or physical distress, the admitting nurse will shift from a formal data-base assessment process to an immediate problem-solving approach designed to intervene with the acute presenting problem. The decision model is based on treating situations ranging from the most threatening (life-endangering), to psychosocial problems that are uncomfortable but not dysfunctional. The Hierarchy of Human Needs described by Abraham Maslow (1970) is often used in prioritizing the problems that need to be addressed. The levels of needs are:

1. Physiological needs
2. Physical safety
3. Belonging to a social group
4. Self-esteem
5. Self-actualization

If a patient is at high risk for self-harm or violence, these problems require immediate intervention. They should be considered in the same category as hemorrhage or acute cardiac distress. The situation becomes even more acute if the individual is in a delirious state or has otherwise lost contact with reality and the risk to self or other is acutely active.

Although the vast majority of psychosocial diagnoses do not fall into such emergency diagnosis or care planning categories, they are very important to health restoration. For example, a person who is 8 weeks post–cardiac bypass may be physically healed and in better physical condition than for many previous years. At the same time, there may be depression, fear, and lack of motivation to return to work; the partner relationship may have been disrupted by the ineffective coping of each partner with this major change in health status; and there also may be sexual dysfunction. Certainly, this individual, couple, and probably the family are in deep psychosocial distress.

During this cardiac patient's hospitalization, physical care was essential to maintain physiological homeostasis. In the early days following surgery it was properly prioritized ahead of psychosocial care.

It is most likely, however, that the cues and signs of potential psychosocial distress were present on admission. An abbreviated psychosocial history with a few questions about working history, normal coping patterns, history of recent stressors, and roles in the family would have helped to identify them. Following surgery, once the physical condition was stabilized, nursing care planning could have included active addressing of the underlying psychosocial problems. Such difficulties are best addressed in the acute care setting. Once discharge occurs, the individual and family fall into their former patterns, compounded by the stress of the changed health status.

COLLABORATIVE PROBLEMS

As the nurse assesses the problem list developed from the physical and psychosocial histories, there usually are two main categories of problems: those that fall within the province of independent nursing diagnosis and treatment, and those that require collaboration between the nurse and other health care disciplines. Both sets of clinical problems require nursing intervention. Carpenito has called this dual approach of nursing the *bifocal clinical nursing model* (1993).

One of the ways nurses' and physicians' roles overlap is in treating collaborative problems. Many pathophysiological states fall into this category. A *collaborative problem* is defined by Alfaro-LeFevre (1994) as:

> An actual or potential problem with structure or function of an organ or system requiring nurse-prescribed and physician-prescribed interventions. Nurses share accountability for treating these problems with the doctor [p. 88].

I would add to Alfaro-LeFevre's definition *problems that may occur from physical or mental disorders* that can be prevented, resolved, or reduced through collaborative interventions.

DIFFERENTIATING COLLABORATIVE PROBLEMS FROM NURSING DIAGNOSES

The nursing diagnosis categories describe many of the possible ways a person can demonstrate ineffective or impaired coping, adjustment, and relationship patterns. In most instances, there is a continuum of maladaptation that ranges from mild forms of distress to major forms of distress. These are depicted in Table 14-1.

In some instances, a dysfunctional form of psychosocial distress may be treatable by a nurse. For example, acute or prolonged grieving could be responsive to nurse intervention. When psychosocial functioning is altered to the point that it is dysfunctional, however, psychiatric consultation is always recommended. Conditions like dysfunctional grief meet the criteria of psychiatric disorders and are collaborative problems. The psychiatric diagnoses include:

Development disorders of childhood and adolescence
Anxiety disorders (traumatic stress, phobia, anxiety states, adjustment reactions)
Eating disorders (anorexia nervosa, bulimia)
Cognitive mental disorders (delirium, dementia)
Substance use disorders (alcohol, other drugs)
Affective disorders (depression, mania)
Schizophrenia (paranoid, catatonic, undifferentiated)
Somatoform disorders (hypochondriasis, somatization, conversion)
Dissociative disorders (dissociation, depersonalization, multiple personality)
Sexual disorders (paraphilias, sexual dysfunctions, sexual desire disorders, sexual arousal disorders, orgasm disorders, sexual pain disorders)
Sleep disorders (insomnia, hypersomnia, dream disorder)

Impulse control disorders (attention deficit, hyperactivity, explosive or other impulse control disorders) (*Diagnostic Criteria from DSM-IV*, 1994)

Figure 14-1 depicts the steps involved in identifying problems that require nursing care planning, regardless of their final categorization as nursing diagnoses or collaborative problems.

DIAGNOSTIC DESCRIPTIONS OF MAJOR PSYCHOSOCIAL OR PSYCHIATRIC COLLABORATIVE PROBLEMS

Collaborative psychiatric problems need to be formally diagnosed by the physician. If symptoms clearly indicate that a particular psychiatric diagnosis exists, it is acceptable to state the problem as Potential Complication: Eating disorder or Potential Complication: Major affective disorder, for example. It is strongly recommended, however, that medical-surgical nurses who may not be familiar with the diagnostic criteria of the various psychiatric disorders use the general term "psychiatric disorder," thus, Potential Complication: Psychiatric disorder.

Nurses should be careful not to overidentify problems as psychiatric in nature, because psychiatric labels are often negatively interpreted by general hospital caregivers. Worse, they may be improperly applied to a particular patient, thereby stigmatizing that individual with other staff members. A diagnosis of schizophrenia, for example, is particularly damaging, even when correctly applied. Even psychiatric professionals are reluctant to use the term until the differential diagnosis has been astutely identified over a period of several months of treatment (McFarland, Wasli, & Gerety, 1992).

In life-threatening situations it is essential that the nurse immediately initiate care planning to ensure the safety of the patient and staff members. The nursing diagnosis category of "Potential for violence: Self-directed or directed at others" is appropriate as the nurse designs interventions within the domain of nursing practice that can be instituted while waiting for psychiatric consultation.

TABLE 14-1
Continuum of Psychosocial Functioning Under Stress

Level of Distress	Psychosocial Response

Minor Forms of Psychosocial Distress	*Response within self:*
	    Realistic self-perception
	    Effective coping
	    Moderate grieving
	    Mild depression
	 Role performance:
	    Capable of fulfilling normal roles in family and work
	 Relationship with others:
	    Can be strained or distorted under stress
	 Capacity to function:
	    Normal social functioning
	 Potential for violence:
	    Low
	 Potential for injury or self-harm:
	    Low
	 Potential for noncompliance:
	    Low

Major Forms of Psychosocial Distress
 	
 (Depending on level of severity and capacity to function)
 	
 Psychiatric Disorders
	Response within self:
	    Unrealistic perception of self
	    Too acute, prolonged grieving
	    Major depression
	    Ineffective coping
	    Feelings of chaos and disorganization
	    Little or no tolerance for stress
	    Anxiety or fear most of time
	    Separated from external reality
	 Role performance:
	    Difficulty filling normal family or work role
	 Relationships with others:
	    Social isolation
	    Fear
	    Avoidance
	 Capacity to function:
	    Poor
	 Potential for violence:
	    High (in some individuals)
	 Potential for injury or self-harm:
	    High (in some individuals)
	 Potential for noncompliance:
	    High

REFERRAL OF COLLABORATIVE PROBLEMS FOR PSYCHIATRIC CONSULTATION

The most common psychiatric conditions found on medical-surgical units are cognitive mental disorders, primarily of the acute, reversible delirium type or of the chronic, irreversible dementia type. Another much less common psychiatric disorder seen in general hospitals is threatened or attempted suicide. Occasionally, a medical-surgical patient will reach a point of despair about the outcomes of illness and threaten suicide. If the individual is seriously physically ill, the decision is often made to continue to provide care in the physical care setting rather than transfer to the psychiatric unit. The person who has attempted suicide is most frequently treated in the intensive care unit, and transferred to a general medical-surgical unit once physiologically stabilized. (Assessment and intervention recommendations for suicidal patients appear in Chapters 17 and 18.)

For these and other collaborative psychiatric problems, it is essential that psychiatric consultation occur as soon as possible. In particular, the delirious patient must be given appropriate psychotropic medication without delay to ensure the safety of self and caregivers. Differential diagnosis of the psychiatric disorder should be done by the psychiatric physician, rather than medical-surgical attending physicians or house staff. The psychiatrist is most qualified to recommend care for the psychiatrically diagnosed medical-surgical patient. Before developing a formal nursing care plan, it is helpful to consult with a psychiatric staff nurse or clinical specialist either in person or by telephone.

WRITING NURSING DIAGNOSIS STATEMENTS

Alfaro-LeFevre (1994), Carpenito (1993), and McFarland, Wasli, and Gerety (1992) recommend the use of a standard format in describing nursing diagnoses. The acronym PES describes the recommended form of the statement:

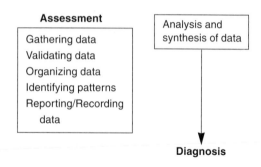

FIGURE 14-1. The diagnostic process. Alfaro-LeFevre, R. (1994). *Applying nursing process: A step-by-step guide* (3rd ed). Philadelphia: J.B. Lippincott, p. 81.

P—Name the problem (P) using the Nursing Diagnosis term

E—Name the etiology (E) using the words "related to"

S—Name the symptoms (S), cues, defining characteristics

For example, the nursing diagnosis could read:

Ineffective individual coping related to altered health status as manifested by depression; or

Altered family processes related to infertility as manifested by increased marital conflict

When the three elements of a clinical problem are identifiable—the problem + the etiology + the symptoms—the result is an *actual nursing diagnosis.*

In addition to the actual nursing diagnosis, there are two other categories of nursing diagnoses that can be stated following assessment of the data base. The first is a potential nursing diagnosis. A *potential nursing diagnosis* is a health problem that could occur. The etiological or risk factors are present; however, there are no identifiable symptoms (defining characteristics) at the time of the assessment. Examples of potential nursing diagnoses are:

Potential for violence: self-directed related to hopelessness; or

Potential for social isolation related to lack of significant other and immobility

The other alternative for nursing diagnosis statements is a possible nursing diagnosis. A *possible nursing diagnosis* is a health problem that may be present but requires more data to confirm or rule out the presence of etiological factors and symptoms. Usually, one or more etiological factors and symptoms are vaguely present, but not confirmed. Examples of possible nursing diagnoses are:

Possible altered thought processes related to side effects of medications; or
Possible altered parenting related to impaired parental-infant attachment (bonding)

The Center for Nursing Case Management has published recommendations for nursing care planning that list the risk factors for potential nursing diagnoses directly under the problem statement (Stetler & DeZell, 1987). Such a statement would look like this:

Potential for impaired social interaction
Risk factors
Dependent interpersonal style
Poor impulse control
Death of spouse within last 3 months
Retirement within last 9 months

The goal of writing a nursing diagnosis statement is that the reader be able to determine from it the nursing care problem, its cause, and the specific symptom the patient is manifesting. It is a clear description of the current state of the patient.

NURSING CARE PLANNING

Nursing care planning is a judgment process that calls on all aspects of nursing knowledge to identify the plan of nursing orders and actions that will restore the patient to optimum health status.

Carpenito says that the purpose of nursing orders is to:

direct individualized care to a patient. Nursing orders are different from nursing actions, which are standard interventions that can apply to any number of patients sharing a similar problem [1993, p. 71].

Examples of nursing actions include:

Increase fluid intake

Ambulate
Monitor for dysr

There are a vari
scribe the process of

Defining characteristi
or symptom of th
Etiology. The cause prob-
lem. It should be s in nursing terminology, not as a medical diagnosis term. This ensures the ability of nursing to act independently in planning to reduce the causative factor.
Evaluation. The final step of the nursing process in which the identified patient outcomes are assessed for achievement. Achievement is determined by the absence of the original symptoms or defining characteristics of the patient problem.
Intermediate patient goal. Patient behavior(s) or psychological state(s) that can be measured at particular times or dates during the hospitalization or recovery period.
Nursing care plan. A written document that includes information derived from the five steps of the nursing process: assessment, nursing diagnosis, care planning, intervention, and evaluation. In addition, it includes two outcome criteria that will be used for evaluation: intermediate patient goals and specific measurable outcomes describing the optimum behavioral or physiological state related to a patient's identified problems.
Nursing intervention (also called nursing action or nursing order). A nursing action that is designed to reduce or eliminate the problem identified in the nursing diagnosis. The determination of appropriate nursing interventions occurs as the result of problem solving, which identifies actions that will change or modify the etiological factors causing the problem.
Patient outcome. The optimum anticipated state of health of the patient at the end of hospitalization. The outcome should be related to the symptoms/defining characteristics of the patient's problem and be stated in measurable terms.

(Alfaro-LeFevre, 1994.)

...AND FAMILY PARTICIPATION ...N THE NURSING CARE PLAN

Development of the nursing care plan involves the patient and, ideally, the family through each step of the process. This is especially therapeutic when addressing psychosocial problems. One of the most important aspects of psychosocial nursing care is that the nurse relates with the patient using an adult-to-adult interpersonal style. She does not function as an "all-knowing" caregiver who unilaterally decides what the patient "needs."

Richards (1975), in an article titled "Caring About versus Caring For," describes the therapeutic effect of the attitude of a caregiver who respects the patient's right to maintain control of choices and work in a collaborative way with caregivers. This approach is contrasted with an authoritative nursing posture that places the patient in a passive, helpless role. Such behavior on the part of the nurse encourages patient dependence, just at the time assistance is needed to develop independence and the ability to make decisions related to current needs and desired health status.

The only time a patient should not be expected to participate in care planning is if the person is unconscious, semiconscious, or temporarily experiencing acute physical or mental disorder, or is an infant or toddler. Even a person who is cognitively or perceptually impaired should be included in psychosocial care planning; here care planning can be used as a therapeutic intervention to assist reality-testing. In situations where the patient cannot fully participate, a family member or other significant person should be included in the assessment and planning process.

Ideally, in the inpatient setting, a family member can be present during initial data-collecting, even for individuals who are not obviously impaired or unable to communicate. Home care assessments are usually more comprehensive with the primary caregivers in attendance, saving valuable time for the nurse over the course of time spent with the patient. The presence of a family member acknowledges the importance of social system responses to this illness or hospitalization in the data-gathering process.

Disparities in information about patient functioning or potential conflicts inherent in the family are usually identified much more easily when a family member participates. The reaction of the family system, especially the spouse, can be the primary factor in adaptation or maladaptation to illness. Physical healing can occur long before emotional well-being is restored. When emotional maladaptation to physical illness occurs there can be profound results in a family. These include:

1. Premature death of the ill member or other family member.
2. Development of physical or mental discord in another family member.
3. Divorce.
4. Permanent changes in family relationships.
5. Development of a related or new physical disorder in the patient as a response to stress and conflict within the family (Carpenito, 1993).

STEPS IN A NURSING CARE PLAN

The steps in the care planning process can ensure that joint planning with the patient and a family member occurs at the appropriate points in the planning process.

1. *Gather data* with patient and, if possible, with a family member or other significant person.
2. *Analyze* the data.
3. *Develop the problem list* with corresponding nursing diagnoses and collaborative problems.
4. *Clarify the problem list*, naming both physiological and psychosocial problems.
5. *Name the diagnoses with their related etiologies and symptoms.* These sequential steps can be done with the patient and family member unless the judgment of the nurse is to omit sharing some of this information. It should be emphasized, however, that unless there is some psychological impairment present, it can be calming to an anxiety-ridden person and family member to know that a caregiver is perceptive enough to know why he or

she is fearful, ineffectively coping, or experiencing other forms of psychosocial distress. Consultation with a clinical nurse specialist or other caregiving discipline may also be indicated at this point in the planning process.

6. *Prioritize the problems.* It is important during this process to employ the therapeutic communication skills that encourage trust and rapport between nurse, patient, and family members. These are described in Chapter 2.

   By discussing the problems, their causes, and the symptoms they are manifesting, the nurse is able to validate the initial cues and his or her interpretations of them. This is a critical step in a therapeutic nurse-patient-home caregiver planning conference. It allows the patient or family member to provide feedback about the nurse's interpretation. Perhaps the nursing judgment is based on incomplete information. If it is, interventions could be formulated that will not address the cause of the problem. The result can be further deterioration of that particular patient response.

   It takes more time to proceed in this manner, but the result can be a care plan that is on target with achievable physical and psychosocial outcomes. The patient and family are participants in those outcomes. Their anxiety about how they will manage following discharge can be allayed by their successful participation in the hospital experience.

   In today's health care system, diagnosis-related groups (DRGs) are an important dynamic. They can result in a rapid discharge for which patients and families do not feel prepared. Joint care planning with home caregiver(s), as described above, rather than unilateral nurse-directed care planning, can reduce much of this anxiety. Another aspect of such planning is that some problems that could delay discharge beyond DRG length of stay guidelines can be identified early in the hospitalization period. Prompt identification of these problems with appropriate goal-directed nursing interventions could result in fewer delays in discharge due to

complications (Gerteis et al., 1993; Mayer, Madden, & Lawrenz, 1990).

In my experience as a psychiatric liaison clinical specialist in the medical-surgical setting, many of the delayed discharges that occurred were related to psychosocial problems. This was so regardless of whether the delays were officially identified as physical or psychosocial complications. When I was asked to consult about these patients I found that the underlying psychosocial problems were present before admission, but neither the medical or nursing staff was aware of them. They included:

   a. Depression
   b. Highly dependent interpersonal style
   c. Highly controlled interpersonal style
   d. High level of individual or family stressors during preceding year
   e. Long-standing history of ineffective coping responses

   As priorities are being established, it is helpful for the nurse to present the rationale for priority setting. By doing so, the patient and family will be able to participate actively in the achievement of the intermediate patient goals and patient outcomes because they understand the reasons for doing so.

7. *Identify patient outcomes for each identified health problem.* The outcome should represent the optimum desired health status or behavior achievable by the time of discharge. A psychosocial outcome should be stated in the following domains:

   a. *Cognitive.* Health behavior or state related to changes in knowledge base or intellectual functioning.
   b. *Affective.* Health behavior or state related to changes in feelings, values, or attitudes.
   c. *Psychomotor.* Health behavior related to changes in physical skills.

   The patient outcomes become the evaluation criteria for identifying successful resolution or reduction of the patient health problem, indicating the patient's readiness for discharge, and, importantly, establishing criteria for nursing care audits.

8. *Develop measurable intermediate patient*

goals for each of the patient outcomes. The establishment of intermediate goals encourages the nurse to keep interventions specific and concrete. It also aids the evaluation process in that the markers indicate a progressive, measurable movement toward achievement of each of the patient outcomes.

9. *Describe the nursing interventions needed to meet the intermediate patient goals and patient outcomes.* The nursing interventions should be stated with active verbs and include the following information:
   a. *Who* is responsible for performing the intervention?
   b. *At what specific times* and/or dates?
   c. *For how long* a period of time?

10. *Document the nursing care plan.* A nursing care plan is successful when it communicates a systematic plan for achieving patient outcomes. It must be stated in language that is understandable to all nurses who will be caring for the patient and family.

    Use the nurses' notes section of the patient record to record information that does not appear in the nursing care plan. These notes may be in the form of a flow chart that includes preprinted nursing orders with boxes that can be checked to signify that the order was carried out. It may also contain factual information, like a record of vital signs. There will also be narrative space for nursing notes. Here the nurse can use objective, factual, and measurable terminology in describing the response of the patient to teaching, discussions about coping, and so on. For example:

    During discussion about coping, patient had poor eye contact, was agitated, and did not respond to most questions; or

    During discussion about coping, patient had good eye contact, appeared comfortable, and was able to answer questions in a manner that demonstrated insight into the cause of ineffective coping

    Avoid judgmental inferences in the nursing note, such as:

    Wife failed to meet at previously arranged time to discuss possible marriage conflict and discharge planning

Instead, the following should be noted:

    Wife did not arrive for arranged appointment at 3 PM to discuss possible alteration in family processes and discharge planning

11. *Evaluate the nursing care plan daily* to determine answers to the following questions:
    a. Are the prescribed nursing interventions achieving the intermediate patient goals?
    b. Are the original times and dates realistic?
    c. Is it necessary to modify the nursing interventions to ensure achievement of the intermediate patient goals?
    d. Is it necessary to modify the language of the nursing care plan or the communication method to ensure participation by nurses on other shifts?
    e. Is it necessary to consult with a nursing specialist or other health team member for more information that would assist in identifying the cause of problems, or developing appropriate interventions for goal achievement?
    f. Is there a change in condition of the patient that warrants the addition of a new nursing diagnosis or collaborative problem?
    g. Is there a need to reprioritize the original problem list?

    A daily review of the intermediate goals established for the previous day with the patient and family member continues to involve them in the rehabilitation process. It also allows them to realistically view their own responsibility for goal achievement and preparation for discharge. It ensures their own sense of control. It can also allay anxiety about discharge and their ability to manage the patient's state of health.

STANDARDIZED NURSING CARE PLANS

With computerized, standardized nursing care plans, there is an opportunity for nurses to type in individualized etiologies, defining characteristics, patient outcomes, intermediate patient goals, nursing orders and interventions, and evaluation criteria. These modifications can be added to meet the specific needs of the patient.

It is common for nurses who are using standardized care plans as a development of psychosocial nursing diagnoses to discover that the etiologies, defining characteristics, and nursing actions often require more individualization than many of the physical nursing diagnosis categories.

Nursing Care Plans 14-1 and 14-2 at the end of this chapter, which relate to specific nursing diagnoses, illustrate the principles explained in this chapter. As shown, it is possible to work on resolving more than one patient problem at the same time.

PROBLEM-ORIENTED RECORDS

Another format actively used in today's hospital is the problem-oriented record (POR). The POR concept was originally described by Dr. Lawrence Weed of the University of Vermont (Birmingham, 1978). It was developed as a method of ensuring a systematic record that integrated and documented the assessment, care planning, interventions, and outcomes of the combined efforts of the various care disciplines involved with one patient.

The original plan has been modified in many institutions to meet the unique needs of patient and caregivers. The original approach involves the following elements:

1. A data base
2. A problem list
3. A plan
4. Progress notes

The nursing contribution to the first three of these elements has been described in this and preceding chapters in this section. Figure 14-2 depicts the multiple sources of information that are part of the data base.

The fourth element, *progress notes,* includes three sections:

1. A narrative note

2. A flow sheet
3. A discharge summary

The narrative note includes the recording of information in a specific format called SOAP charting. These initials represent:

Subjective data—Statements of the patient about his or her problem

Objective data—Nurse's observations about the patient's problem

Assessment—Interpretation of the data base to determine presence of patient problems

Plan—Plan to reduce or resolve the patient's problems

The original SOAP format has further evolved into an acronym that incorporates the documentation criteria of the nursing process. It is called SOAPIE charting. The I and E represent:

Interventions—Nursing actions to reduce or resolve the patient's problems

Evaluation—Judgment about whether the identified problems are reduced or resolved

A narrative note should be included in the progress notes when changes occur in the original assessment. These changes include:

1. The addition of progressive steps in the resolution of a specific problem.
2. Occurrence of a new problem.
3. A new piece of pertinent information that affects the subjective or objective data base.

An example of SOAPIE charting is:

Problem: Impaired adjustment related to chronic illness as manifested by excessive sleeping and inability to resume work role *6/15*

S—"I just don't think I have it in me anymore to go back to the old grind. I'm too tired." *6/15*

O—Patient sleeps 10 to 12 hours a night and naps twice during the day *6/15*

A—Ongoing lethargy and refusal to consider returning to work *6/15*

P

1. The patient will return to work by 7/15 to 7/30
2. Visit home for half an hour twice a

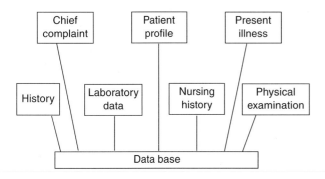

FIGURE 14-2. Data base in nursing assesment of patient problems.

week for 2 weeks for ongoing assessment and intervention

I

1. Discuss with patient and wife what they believe are the factors involved in husband's inability to return to work
2. Evaluate the possibility of depression as one of the causes of lack of rehabilitation, using changes in neurovegetative signs as evaluation criteria:
   Sleeping patterns
   Nutritional–Metabolic
   Elimination
   Activity–Exercise
   Sexuality–Reproductive

E

1. Home visits as planned *6/15 6/18 6/22 6/25*
2. Patient and wife identify the factors they believe are causing husband's inability to return to work *6/18 6/22 6/25*
3. Evaluation of neurovegetative signs to determine possibility of depression. Three of five are positive *6/18*

CONCLUSION

This chapter has presented information on the psychosocial nursing diagnosis and planning process. Analysis of data about patient problems allows the nurse to categorize problems as either nursing diagnoses that can be independently diagnosed and treated by nurses or collaborative problems requiring orders from another caregiving discipline, usually medicine.

Nursing diagnosis statements may be in the form of actual, potential, and possible diagnoses. Actual nursing diagnoses state the problem, identify the etiology, and name the symptoms that confirm the presence of the problem. Potential nursing diagnoses contain the etiologies as potential risk factors, but lack evidence of symptoms. Possible nursing diagnoses are those requiring more data to confirm or rule out the presence of etiologies or symptoms.

Once the problems are identified the nurse begins a care planning process that includes several additional steps:

1. *Establishing the patient outcome.* Stating the optimum measurable behavior or health state, as related to a specific problem, that the patient is anticipated to achieve on or before his or her scheduled discharge date.
2. *Setting intermediate patient goals.* Stating the measurable activities the patient will engage in to ensure achievement of the stated outcome. These include specific dates when the patient should achieve the goal.
3. *Nursing interventions.* The nursing actions that will promote the achievement of intermediate goals and outcomes.
4. *Evaluation.* Criteria that can be used to measure the achievement of intermediate patient goals, and outcomes signifying resolution or reduction of the patient problem.

Documentation of the nursing process is required by state law and is necessary to meet standards for nursing care imposed by state law, the American Nurses Association, and the Joint Commission on Accreditation of Hospitals. Documentation should be done using the expected format of the institution in which the nurse is employed.

BIBLIOGRAPHY

Alfaro-LeFevre, R. (1994). *Applying nursing process.* Philadelphia: J. B. Lippincott.

Birmingham, J. (1978). *The problem-oriented medical record: A self-learning module.* New York: McGraw-Hill.

Carpenito, L. J. (Ed.). (1991). *Nursing care plans and documentation: Nursing diagnosis and collaborative problems.* Philadelphia: J. B. Lippincott.

Carpenito, L. J. (1993). *Nursing diagnosis: Application to clinical practice* (5th ed.). Philadelphia: J. B. Lippincott.

Diagnostic criteria from DSM-IV. (1994). Washington, DC: American Psychiatric Press.

Frisch, N. (1993). Home care nursing and psychosocial-emotional needs. How nursing diagnosis helps to direct and inform practice. *Home Healthcare Nurse, 11*(2), 64–65, 70.

Gerteis, M., Edgman-Levitan, S., Daley, J., & Delbanco, T. L. (1993). *Through the patient's eyes: Understanding and promoting patient-centered care.* San Francisco: Jossey-Bass.

Gordon, M. (1987). *Nursing diagnosis, process and application.* New York: McGraw-Hill.

Lederer, J. R. (Ed.). (1991). *Care planning pocket guide: A nursing diagnosis approach* (4th ed.). Redwood City, CA: Addison-Wesley Nursing.

Maslow, A. (1970). *Motivation and personality* (2nd ed.). New York: Harper & Row.

Mayer, G. G., Madden, M. J., & Lawrenz, E. (Eds.). (1990). *Patient care delivery models.* Rockville, MD: Aspen Publishers.

McFarland, G. K., Wasli, E. L., & Gerety, E. K. (1992). *Nursing diagnoses and process in psychiatric mental health nursing* (2nd ed.). Philadelphia: J. B. Lippincott.

NANDA nursing diagnoses. (1995). Philadelphia: North American Nursing Diagnosis Association.

Pagana, K. D., & Pagana, T. J. (1994). *Diagnostic testing and nursing implications: A case study approach* (4th ed.). St. Louis: Mosby.

Parkes, C., Benjamin, B., & Fitzgerald, R. (1969). Broken heart: A statistical study of increased mortality among widowers. *British Medical Journal, 1*(646), 740–743.

Pinkley, C. L. (1991). Exploring NANDA's definition of nursing diagnosis: Linking diagnostic judgments with the selection of outcomes and interventions. *Nursing Diagnosis, 2*(1), 26–32.

Prescott, P.A., Dennis, K. E., & Jacox, A. K. (1987). Clinical decision-making of staff nurses. *Image: The Journal of Nursing Scholarship, 19*(2), 56–62.

Richards, F. (1975). Do you care for, or care about? *AORN Journal, 22,* 792–798.

Sadler, J. Z., & Hulgus, Y. F. (1992). Clinical problem-solving and the biopsychosocial model. *American Journal of Psychiatry, 149*(10), 1315–1323.

Tucker, S. M. (Ed.). (1992). *Patient care standards: Nursing process, diagnosis, and outcome* (5th ed.). St. Louis: Mosby Year Book.

Tucker, S. M., Canobbio, M. M., Paquette, E. V., & Wells, M. F. (Eds.). (1992). *Patient care standards: Nursing process, diagnosis, and outcome* (5th ed.). St. Louis: Mosby Year Book.

Weber, G. J. (1991). Nursing diagnosis: A comparison of nursing textbook approaches. *Nurse Educator, 16*(2), 22–27.

NURSING CARE PLAN 14-1.
Collaborative Nursing and Physical Therapy Care of a Patient With Amputation

History:

C.B. is a 28-year-old mechanic whose lower leg was amputated following a work-related accident in which his leg was crushed. Since the amputation he has been withdrawn, and has expressed feelings of being unable to cope. His ineffective coping is contributing to noncompliance with his rehabilitation program.

Nursing Diagnoses:

1. Individual Coping, Ineffective
2. Noncompliance With Rehabilitation Program

Evaluation: Circle dates when completed. If not completed by target date, repeat the nursing process and set dates. Date of assessment: 9/10

Nursing Diagnosis #1

Individual Coping, Ineffective

Related to:
 • Disfigurement due to surgery
As manifested by:
 • Verbalization of inability to cope

Final Patient Outcome	Intermediate Patient Outcome	Nursing Interventions	Evaluation
Verbalizes increased coping ability and describes feeling emotional relief 9/15	Relates feelings associated with his amputation with nurse and spouse 9/10, 9/11	Explore patient's current emotional responses to his amputation *for 15 minutes each day*	Specific feelings are named and described 9/10, 9/11
	Identifies losses or changes he anticipates as the result of his amputation 9/11	Ask patient to identify losses or changes he anticipates as the result of the amputation *between 9 AM and 12 Noon 9/11*	Losses are identified 9/11
	Describes his own positive and negative coping responses to nurse 9/11	Examine with patient the previous outcomes of his positive and negative coping responses and explore the ways he is currently using positive responses *for 10 minutes between 1 PM and 3 PM 9/11*	Outcomes of positive and negative coping patterns are identified 9/11

Nursing Diagnosis #2

Noncompliance With Rehabilitation Program

Related to:
 • Ineffective coping
 • Depression
 • Lack of motivation

As manifested by:
 • Refusal to go to physical therapy to learn crutch-walking

NURSING CARE PLAN 14-1. (Continued)
Collaborative Nursing and Physical Therapy Care of a Patient With Amputation

Final Patient Outcome	Intermediate Patient Outcome	Nursing Interventions	Evaluation
Ambulates with crutches and without other assistance *9/18*	Discusses feelings and fears about ambulation with nurse *9/11, 9/12, 9/13*	Explore patient's feelings and fears about ambulation for 10 minutes *between 9 AM and 12 Noon and again between 1 PM and 3 PM 9/10, 9/11*	Specific feelings and fears are named and described *9/11*
	Meets with physical therapist in own room to discuss safety during ambulation and to establish joint goals for physical therapy *9/12*	Discuss possibility of meeting with physical therapist *9/10*	Agrees to meet with physical therapist *9/11*
	Attends physical therapy on schedule agreed on with physical therapist *9/13*	Consult with physical therapy by telephone and discuss current patient problem and causes *9/11*	Contracts for and maintains physical therapy attendance schedule *9/12*
		Arrange meeting with patient and physical therapist *9/11*	
		Notify patient of approximate meeting time with physical therapist *9/11*	

NURSING CARE PLAN 14-2.
Collaborative Nursing and Medical Care of a Patient With Organic Mental Disorder

History:

M.B. is a 74-year-old patient admitted to the medical intensive care unit with acute obstructive pulmonary disease. During the admission she developed a delirium-type cognitive mental disorder as the result of toxic side effects of her medications.

Medical Diagnosis:

Cognitive Mental Disorder, Delirium Type

Nursing Diagnoses:

1. Sensory-Perceptual Alteration: Visual
2. Risk for Violence: Directed at Others
3. Risk for Violence: Self-directed

Evaluation: Circle dates when completed. If not completed by target date, repeat the nursing process and set new dates.

Date of assessment: 10/15

Nursing Diagnosis #1

Sensory-Perceptual Alteration: Visual

Related to organic mental disorder
As manifested by hallucinations, incoherent speech, disturbance of sleep-wakefulness cycle by insomnia

(Continued)

NURSING CARE PLAN 14-2. (Continued)
Collaborative Nursing and Medical Care of a Patient With Mental Disorder

Nursing Diagnosis #2

Risk for Violence: Directed at Others

Related to cognitive mental disorder
As manifested by statements indicating high level of paranoia about family and staff members

Nursing Diagnosis #3

Risk for Violence: Self-Directed

Related to cognitive mental disorder
As manifested by hallucinations, disorientation, lack of awareness of IV tubing and urinary catheter

Final Patient Outcome	Intermediate Patient Outcome	Nursing Interventions	Evaluation
Is oriented (can identify who she is, where she is, and the time and date *10/17*	Will discuss reality-based awareness of current situation *10/16*	Move patient to private rooms closest to nurses' station *10/15*	Patient in new location *10/15*
Demonstrates no harmful behavior *10/17*	Will discuss memory of delirious event and related fears *10/16*	Notify family of change in health status *10/15*	Family notified *10/15*
Describes no frightening impulses *10/17*		Use full bed rails *10/15*	Bed rails up and bed position lowered *10/15*
		Lower bed position *10/15*	
		Ask orderly to attend constantly	Orderly in constant attendance *10/15*
		Instruct orderly on safe care of patient in restraints *10/15*	Orderly instructed *10/15*
		Monitor patient *every 10 minutes until sedation is effective, then every half hour*	Monitoring as ordered *10/15*
		Medical orders	
		Use four-point restraints	Restraints in place *10/15*
		Give Haldol 5 mg IM *every hour or p.r.n.* when hallucinations, extreme anxiety, or agitation are present	Haldol given: *10/15* 5 mg IM *10AM* 5 mg IM *11AM* 5 mg IM *12:30PM* 5 mg IM *3:30PM*

PART IV

PSYCHOSOCIAL ASSESSMENT AND INTERVENTION WITH INEFFECTIVELY COPING PATIENTS AND FAMILIES

Stresses and fears associated with various illnesses and conditions, such as cancer, emergency surgery, and terminal illness, can make it even more difficult for patients and families to break out of pervasive maladaptive patterns. The chapters in this section incorporate Gordon's Functional Patterns of Human Responses to Illness and the Barry Holistic Systems Model into the development of nursing care plans that help arrest maladaptive coping, support effective coping, and promote healing in individuals and families. By integrating biopsychosocial theory into the nursing process, the nurse can help an individual develop healthy and effective coping and communication.

CHAPTER 15

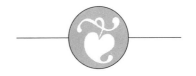

Effective Interventions With Difficult Patients and Family Members

Patricia Barry

In order to give appropriate treatment, it is helpful for hospital caregivers to have insight into patients' and family members' personalities and their psychosocial responses to the stress of illness. A number of authors have described a broad range of personality styles seen in normal individuals when they are physically ill.

Most persons display personality characteristics from each of several major personality styles described in this chapter. Some demonstrate certain characteristics to an excessive degree in their interpersonal relationships. They are responding outside of the normal range of behavior customarily seen in hospitalized individuals. Extremes of behavior can be due to a personality or character disorder or may be the result of the extreme stress experienced as a result of physical illness and hospitalization. Certainly persons who demonstrate excessive traits will challenge nurses' tolerance in caring for them.

When ill, the normal person experiences increases in the basic needs described by Maslow (1970): physiological needs, safety needs, love and belonging needs, esteem needs, and the need for self-actualization. Each of these needs is threatened by the implications of illness and hospitalization.

In individuals displaying extreme behavior and those whose responses to illness fall within the normal range, the basic operating dynamic is anxiety (Kaplan & Sadock, 1994, 1995). Patients or family members are under stress because their basic selves may be threatened by this condition. In this chapter, each of the major personality styles will be presented, with a discussion of how these styles evolve and their major characteristics or identifying traits. Suggestions for management will be presented. The approaches recommended for use with each personality style can also be used with family members who present prob-

Patricia Barry: *Psychosocial Nursing: Care of Physically Ill Patients and Their Families,* 3rd ed. © 1996 Lippincott-Raven Publishers

lems to the nursing staff because of their particular personality style responses to their loved one's illness.

STATE VS. TRAIT CHARACTERISTICS

When observing a patient's personality style, it is helpful to ask if these are the normal personality traits of this person or a temporary state brought on by acute stress (Kaplan & Sadock, 1994, 1995). For example, there is a difference between a person who is chronically anxious, no matter what is going on in his or her life, and a person who is normally serene but who becomes anxious the night before exploratory surgery for an unidentified tumor mass.

The psychosocial history will be helpful in determining whether these characteristics are personality states or traits. The patient can be asked how she normally responds to stress or to describe herself. A series of questions can be asked that describe various personality characteristics—for example, "Have you ever thought of yourself as being an anxious person (a depressed person, a person who has trouble trusting)?" If the patient says that she often is depressed or anxious, she is demonstrating a trait. If, on the other hand, her current response to illness is quite atypical of her normal personality characteristics, a temporary state is occurring (Kaplan & Sadock, 1994, 1995).

Personality traits develop as a result of the specific defense mechanisms used when the child's personality was developing. The total range of traits a person acquires in the maturing process determines his or her personality style (Oldham, 1991; Stone, 1993).

The following are major personality styles:

MAJOR PERSONALITY STYLES SEEN IN PERSONS WITH PHYSICAL CONDITIONS

Dependent, demanding
Orderly, controlled
Dramatizing, emotionally involved,
  captivating
Suspicious, guarded, complaining
Long-suffering, self-sacrificing
Superior

Uninvolved, aloof, distant
Antisocial
Inadequate

In implementing the suggested therapeutic approaches to patients or family members in each category, it is essential that the suggestions be recorded on the nursing care plan so that all members of the nursing staff, and ideally all other caregivers, use the same approach. If only a few members of the nursing staff use the approach, the result will be negligible or may even increase the patient's anxiety because of the mixed messages received from the staff.

MAJOR PERSONALITY STYLES

THE DEPENDENT, DEMANDING INDIVIDUAL

Most people's dependency increases when they are hospitalized. Nurses are aware of and are usually able to meet these increased requirements for attention (Cassem, 1991). However, some persons exhibit an unusual need for attention. Their personalities are normally very dependent; others may regress to an excessively dependent level.

Such individuals are clingy, needy, and demanding. They may be unaware of their excessive demands on the nurse, or may be superficially apologetic about their constant requests. They have a low tolerance for frustration and an underlying fear of abandonment, which motivates much of their behavior. While caring for the dependent and demanding patient, nurses may initially feel guilty about their own annoyance. Eventually, most nurses avoid going near the patient's door. This patient may have an increased tendency toward addiction (Aguilera, 1994; Stone, 1993). The addictive personality has strong dependency needs from the earliest years of life.

Nursing Intervention

The basic need of the dependent, demanding patient is to be attended to by an interested and caring staff. This patient's often excessive demands on nurses is a way of compensating for feeling unloved and unwanted.

It may be necessary with the patient making many demands to impose limits on those demands that are unrealistic. When setting limits with a demanding patient, it is important to do so in a supportive way by explaining the realistic expectations of care the patient is entitled to as well as the effects on the staff when demands are excessive. If, for example, he frequently calls for insignificant reasons, a wise approach can be to tell the patient, in a caring way, that he will be checked every half hour during the day. Although this individual may be severely demanding, a punitive tone should be avoided. He can be asked to save his requests until the nurse returns. It is then important to be reliable about arriving on time. When possible, the patient's needs can be anticipated so that fear of abandonment is minimized.

At least once a day it is helpful to pull up a chair next to the patient's bed to talk with him. When sitting down, nurses promote a stronger sense in the patient that they will not be "running out the door." A nurse can be there no longer than if standing, but to the patient the nurse appears more available and interested in him. Most demanding patients occupy the nurse's time with incessant requests to do things. The nurse is occupied rolling up the bed, getting a blanket, getting a bathrobe, and so on. These can be unconsciously manipulative devices used by a patient to ensure the nurse's presence and attention. They are often motivated by anxiety about being alone. Frequently, this patient's anxiety level will drop off dramatically when a nurse sits and asks about him and his needs.

THE CONTROLLED, ORDERLY INDIVIDUAL

The controlled, orderly personality is identified by compulsive character traits (Adler, 1990; Aguilera, 1994). The nonpathological manifestation of these traits can be observed in many successful peosple. They are self-disciplined individuals who maintain a high level of order in their lives. They are usually hard working and, in fact, may overwork in order to meet their own high expectations. Sometimes they seem "driven" to achieve. This tendency toward high self-expectations may spill over and be projected onto other people. As a result, their expectations of others may be very high as well.

Compulsive behavior can be observed in a person whose grooming, even when hospitalized, is very important. She may keep in frequent touch with her workplace to ensure that all is well. Her personality is typically rigid and inflexible, as seen in an obstinate behavior and belief system. Spontaneity in conversation or thinking is rarely seen.

The controlled, orderly person tends to think rather than feel. Her conversation is frequently intellectual; a listener may find it difficult to tell how she is really feeling. If she is very controlled, she may be unaware of her own feelings. Her emotional reactions to situations are usually split off from her intellectual awareness of them. This is the defense of *isolation*, also known as rationalization or intellectualization (see Chapter 3).

These compulsive traits develop as the result of events that occurred between the ages of two and four. The patient either was raised in a rigid, disciplined way and eventually incorporated the demands of her caregivers into her developing superego, or was raised by indulgent caregivers who gave in to her every whim. With the latter possibility, the *reaction formation* defense mechanism may have caused the ego to reverse the situation into its exact opposite, so that the person became very controlled (see Chapter 3). Many compulsive traits occur as a result of an internal voice that seems to say "I should . . . I should" (Kreitler & Kreitler, 1990; Stone, 1993).

In the hospital, where the patient is no longer in charge of herself or her schedule, she frequently feels anxious. This may or may not be observed by the nurse. Occasionally, such individuals control the outward appearance of their anxiety, and the character traits described here intensify. However, as the patient's anxiety increases, her control may eventually begin to fail.

Nursing Intervention

The most important point to remember in caring for the controlled, orderly person is that she needs to feel in control of herself and her environment at all times. An event that threatens her sense of control will provoke anxiety. Examples of such events are entry into a hospital setting where the rules are so inflexible that they preclude her input into her own schedule, and surgery of any type. Surgery provokes anxiety for two important reasons related to loss of control: anticipation of loss of consciousness while under anesthesia and inability to oversee the actions of the surgeon. Cancer or any other type of disease that is subject to unpredictable exacerbations and recurrences also provokes anxiety, as does any other type of chronic illness because of its unrelenting duration.

When caring for such a person, nurses find that she asks many questions about her illness, the medication she receives, and any procedures about to be performed on her. The best way to relieve this patient's anxiety is to answer all questions. She needs to know what is going on and why in order to feel that some control is being maintained.

Whenever a procedure is to be performed for any patient, it is important to explain in advance what will be done and why. With the controlled, orderly patient, it is especially important that she understands in advance what will be happening. The reason for and steps involved in the procedure can be carefully reviewed. This is important, especially in intensive care units, even with semiconscious or semisedated individuals who are suspected of having a controlled type of personality. When care is administered to the controlled type of person at night, she will react better when given an explanation, even if semiawake.

Teaching should be done by sitting with the patient and explaining in detail the different aspects of her illness. She may question certain aspects of her care. Once questions are answered, positive, firm reassurances may promote her sense of security. Another important intervention with this type of individual is to allow her, whenever possible, to determine bath schedule, medication schedule, and any other aspect of care that will not be compromised if her ability to make choices is permitted. Such an approach strongly enhances her feeling of control (Kahana & Bibring, 1964; Robinson, 1984).

THE DRAMATIZING, EMOTIONALLY INVOLVED, CAPTIVATING INDIVIDUAL

The dramatizing personality represents another type of person who may be seen in the hospital (Kahana & Bibring, 1964). One of this patient's characteristics is a more emotional response to events than is customary. This type of person, quite opposite from the orderly individual, seems to experience feelings more intensely and not be able to verbalize them in an intellectual ("thinking") way. In other words, he may tend to feel more than he thinks. He may, for example, say "I feel awful!" but may not be able to explain why. Emotion seems to flood his intellect. The increased emotionality presents itself in many ways, positive as well as negative. He usually becomes quickly engaged with caregivers and also has a warmth and appeal that can be described as "captivating" (Kahana & Bibring, 1964).

If these traits appear on the pathological end of the continuum, they are described as *hysterical* or *histrionic* (American Psychiatric Association, 1994). These traits may rarely be observed in hospitalized persons; instead, one may see patients who respond in a warm, personal, and eager way. These individuals may be somewhat dramatic in their statements and their behavior may, at times, seem to be attention-seeking. They may initially seem like the dependent type of person, but they can be differentiated by their emotionality, dramatic behavior, and engaging personality (Adler, 1990; Aguilera, 1994; Kreitler & Kreitler, 1990).

Nursing Intervention

It is important to remember in caring for the dramatizing, emotionally involved, captivating patient that his emotional response to stress may be strong and exaggerated. The intellectual, detailed, explanatory type of approach you would use with the controlled type of personality should be avoided; it could actually increase this person's anxiety. Instead, a simple, calm, straightforward explanation can be given. This type of individual may even say, "I don't want to know a thing. Just do it. Tell me when it's over." When such an individual is feeling a high amount of stress, it may be difficult to reason with him.

The anxiety these patients experience as a result of explanations or teaching may cause them to respond with the defense mechanism of repression. Consequently, they may forget what they are told. Whenever teaching such a patient, it is important to check his comprehension by asking him to repeat instructions. Does he understand what they mean? When necessary, it is helpful to repeat the instructions in a calm, reassuring way in order to allay his normally anxious response.

Whenever possible, he can be asked how he is feeling about his illness. His feelings tend to build up quickly, and, when he is particularly anxious, he may feel about to be overwhelmed by them. The opportunity to talk about his feelings will have an effect similar to releasing steam periodically from a pressure cooker. He will feel relieved, and his anxiety level may decrease markedly.

On occasion, this type of patient, because of his captivating qualities, may appear to be manipulative. If "caught up" by such a patient, it is important to set caring but firm limits on his demands. Many nurses unknowingly become overinvolved with this type of person because of their normal desire to help; they can then feel taken advantage of. If this occurs, it is important to avoid anger and not to withdraw and avoid him. These rejecting behaviors will increase his anxiety; his maladaptive traits may become more pronounced, and eventually the caregiver can feel even more manipulated and resentful. A caring, limit-setting approach can help to restore the balance in the nurse-patient relationship.

THE SUSPICIOUS, GUARDED, COMPLAINING INDIVIDUAL

The suspicious person who questions caregivers' intentions or frequently complains about her care may eventually undermine the best intentions of nursing staff members. One of this patient's greatest fears is to be in a vulnerable position, physically or mentally. The main defense mechanism used is projection. As she becomes more anxious, fault may be found with hospital policies, medical and nursing staffs, and various aspects of care or diet. The fault-finding that is projected onto the environment is actually a reflection of her own internal anxieties and self-dislike (Pervin, 1990; Stone, 1993). When these characteristics increase to the pathological end of the trait continuum, they form the basis of *paranoia*. The fixation that results in these character traits occurs between the ages of one and three.

The paranoid person is not usually observed in the general hospital setting. It is not uncommon, however, for an organically caused cognitive mental disorder to develop into a paranoid psychosis. It can be precipitated by the myriad of drugs given in intensive care units. This psychosis is usually a transient but terrifying experience for the patient as well as the nurse.

Nursing Intervention

Symptoms may vary in suspicious, complaining patients. These individuals fervently believe the statements they make. If their negative statements are contradicted by reassurances that the physicians are competent or that the hospital policies are reasonable, they are likely to respond by becoming impatient, frustrated, and angry. A placating reassurance will increase the patient's anxiety and lack of trust.

On the other hand, agreeing with the patient in order to halt the unceasing complaints adds credibility to his or her statements. For example, if a nurse agrees that another nurse is unpleasant, an intern is never available, or that the food is terrible, the cycle and intensity of complaints is strengthened.

The most therapeutic approach to use with the complaining person is to acknowledge his beliefs but not to offer an opinion about them. If either a positive or negative opinion is given, the situation can remain at an impasse. The patient will be provided with more fuel for his counterargument.

However, if the patient's feelings are acknowledged by mirroring them in words similar to his own, injecting no opinion, the patient's suspiciousness can be reduced. Just knowing that someone else understands a problem can be comforting. Usually when a patient feels understood, anxiety decreases.

When fear and suspiciousness are occurring, several approaches can be included in the care plan. Because the patient's level of trust is poor, simple explanations, rather than the technical, intellectual approach needed for the controlled patient, can be given. A complex explanation can increase anxiety because it can further increase wariness and suspicions. Touching this patient when being emotionally supportive and attempting emotional closeness should be avoided. He is unable to tolerate this type of closeness. Accordingly, his level of suspicion may rise uncomfortably if you demonstrate this type of normally supportive behavior.

All movement with a suspicious patient should be purposeful rather than rushed. A rushed approach can trigger fear. Also, if it is necessary to stand near the bed, it can be less anxiety-provoking if the nurse stands at the foot of the bed when talking. Ideally, it is best to sit rather than stand while engaged in discussion. This avoids imposing authority. Another approach that will minimize anxiety is to allow the patient access to the door. For example, a nurse can stand on the side of the bed away from the door; a suspicious individual can become even more so if he thinks that he cannot "escape" or get out the door because it is being blocked.

Other interventions that can promote a less suspicious response are the use of a primary nursing approach, maintenance of continuity of nurses on other shifts, and reviewing the daily schedule of events. Nurses on other shifts can be encouraged to do the same. This provides a consistent systems approach that is reassuring and can promote trust.

The following explanation by someone who underwent cardiac bypass surgery illuminates the experience of a person with a transient, drug-induced, paranoid psychosis:

When I woke up I forgot where I was. All I knew was that someone was trying to find me so that he could kill me. I had something (the endotracheal tube) in my throat, and I couldn't talk. I didn't know any of the people around

me, but I had to make them understand that someone was after me. Something told me that the only way they could understand me was if I spoke French to them, and I don't know how to speak French! I didn't even try to speak English.

The more I tried to make them understand, the more they told me there was nothing to be afraid of. The only way I could tell them was by using my hands and arms. Then they tied them down, and my feet too! [His hands and feet were restrained by intensive care personnel.] I was convinced at that point that I was going to be killed because no one understood what was going on!

After they took the tube out I kept trying to make them understand. They all ignored me. Finally, one nurse told me she understood and would help me. I felt so relieved! I trusted her. Shortly afterward my son came in, and he too told me that he would help me. Thank God that the two of them "humored" me along. I was so frightened before that, I didn't know what to do.

In imagining this person's terror, is it possible also to imagine his relief when, finally, one of the nurses told him she understood? If a nurse is with a patient who has this level of fear (psychotic though it may be, it is still very real to him), it is important that at least one caregiver allies himself or herself with the patient and remains available. Another situation in the general hospital during which this type of paranoid reaction may occur is when the central nervous system of an addicted individual is responding to the withdrawal of alcohol or drugs. This process is usually called *withdrawal* or *detoxification* (Aguilera, 1994; Kaplan & Sadock, 1994, 1995).

THE LONG-SUFFERING, SELF-SACRIFICING INDIVIDUAL

The long-suffering, self-sacrificing patient has a history similar to the overly dependent patient. There has frequently been a succession of illnesses or other disappointments in her life. The difference, to the observer, is in the person's behavior. The dependent person seems to expect someone to do something because she is so helpless. The long-suffering person needs the listener to feel something. There appear to be two types of long-suffering patients: the first suffers silently, is selfless, and shows no regard for her well-being because of her need to sacrifice and do for others; the second seems to enjoy relating the awfulness of her situation. At the pathological end of the spectrum, such a presentation becomes manipulative in attempting to win the listener's sympathy. The pathological form of these traits is called *masochism*.

The masochistic person is one whose childhood was usually marked by harsh discipline and strong guilt instilled by caregivers. The consequence of this upbringing is a bittersweet experience that associates pleasure with suffering. Because of a strong and constant sense of guilt, she can have a difficult time experiencing pleasure from events that people normally enjoy (Adler, 1990; Aguilera, 1994; Kahana & Bibring, 1964; Kreitler & Kreitler, 1990; Pervin, 1990; Stone, 1993).

Nursing Intervention

The basic need of the long-suffering, self-sacrificing person is to feel loved and cared for. However, she is unable simply to accept such care as offered because of her high guilt level. Instead, she denies herself and suffers, either silently or vocally. If the person is a silent sufferer, there may be many clues to poor self-esteem. With this type of individual it can help to reinforce that her needs are real and important, and to affirm her sense of self-worth. She may need firm reassurances that it is normal to take pain or sleep medication.

Frequently, it is important to do discharge planning and teaching with her spouse. She may have a strong tendency to overdo when she goes home, and to reassure family members that she is feeling fine. Many long-suffering patients' spouses and family members have become so accustomed to being overindulged that they have no awareness of the realistic needs of their family member. Accordingly, her exhaustive efforts come to be expected. In teaching this patient about ways to ensure her well-being after discharge, it is important to remember that she has a very low regard for her own needs and may not listen seriously to recommendations about health or rehabilitation. A successful tactic in talking with her is to remind her that her family will be without her services for a longer period if she has a physical setback because of overdoing activities after discharge.

If the patient is the manipulative type of long-suffering individual who seeks sympathy and complains about her pain, illness, and so on, she does not expect it to be cured. Instead, she needs acknowledgment that her discomfort is recognized. She frequently is not as distressed as the normal patient would be in similar circumstances because the illness is accepted as "just one more trouble"; it is acceptable, in a distorted way, because it relieves her guilt.

THE INDIVIDUAL WITH SUPERIORITY FEELINGS

The person who has an exaggerated sense of importance is not usually comfortable in the sick role. The development of illness is sensed as an assault against her own person; indeed, her body image is under strong attack. Accordingly, she is even more threatened when the illness is severe enough to require hospitalization. Actually, her air of confidence is a defense against conscious and unconscious feelings of poor self-esteem.

This individual may expect preferential treatment, may insist on care only from her attending physician, or may choose the chief of staff as her personal physician and attempt to devalue the care decisions of house officers and nursing staff. She may devalue their personal qualities as well. When the traits are extreme, this patient is described as *narcissistic*.

Narcissistic character pathology develops in the first years of life, when the child may have felt conflict about unmet needs or when conforming with her mother's wishes. It also can occur as the result of unconscious, deep-seated feelings of inferiority (Adler, 1990; Aguilera, 1994; Stone, 1993).

Nursing Intervention

In caring for the person with feelings of superiority, alienation between the nurse and patient can be diminished if the nurse reflects her statements and feelings back to her in a non-judgmental way. Negative reactions such as impatience or anger by the nurse will usually increase the patient's anxiety and feelings of superiority as she attempts to compensate and decrease her discomfort.

Frequently, such a patient experiences a decrease in her need to maintain superiority when she is able to talk with another "authority" figure. This sometimes helps her to feel she has an ally. In very difficult circumstances, the head nurse can acknowledge her expectations. If the head nurse becomes involved, the patient's behavior can be interpreted from his or her perspective, and recommendations for behavioral changes can be given to the patient. This discussion can be carried out in a positive, expectant manner rather than in a punitive one.

THE UNINVOLVED, ALOOF INDIVIDUAL

The uninvolved, aloof patient may appear distant and hermit-like and avoid encounters with other patients as well as caregivers. He may, for example, spend long periods alone in a sunroom or unit lobby. He may rarely have visitors; this is a reflection of his remoteness and lack of relationships outside of the hospital. He appears apathetic because of his bland emotional tone. He may lack the ability to show anger or express feelings. These personality traits can result from disappointments in early childhood in trying to establish loving relationships with the important persons in his life. When these traits are especially dominant, this personality is called *schizoid* (Kaplan & Sadock, 1994, 1995).

Nursing Intervention

The uninvolved, aloof person's inability to establish relationships during early childhood has resulted in a lifestyle characterized by avoidance of all persons and situations that could potentially reawaken early feelings of rejection and disappointment.

When hospitalized, he is forced into environmental closeness with others. This closeness raises his level of anxiety. He would be emotionally more comfortable in a single room, if possible. If it does not interfere with his care regimen, he can be allowed to spend as much time as desired sitting alone wherever he can find privacy. In talking with this patient, a nurse can be aware of the need to remain physically and emotionally distant. Touching should be avoided, other than when giving direct care. During teaching or other types of discussion, his statements can be acknowledged. There should be minimal probing for emotional responses. Although he may be aloof, there can be a middle ground in remaining available to him in a quiet, caring, nonintrusive way.

THE ANTISOCIAL INDIVIDUAL

The antisocial person can present difficult behavioral problems for the nurse. Initially, he is charming and appealing. Eventually, he may display many styles of unacceptable behavior. Some of these traits are unreliability, manipulativeness, lack of guilt, lack of responsibility in interpersonal relations, and superficial charm.

At times, the antisocial patient can be sexually aggressive. Some drug addicts present a mixture of the dependent and the antisocial personality types. They tend to be impulsive and have a poor tolerance for frustration. Their history often shows a lack of a positive relationship with a significant person in early childhood or the lack of a caregiver who gave consistent care. Antisocial traits are characterized by lack of superego control. Such a person also demonstrates a lack of tension, and his anxiety level may not appear to be affected in stressful situations (Aguilera, 1994; Kaplan & Sadock, 1994, 1995). When significant trait pathology is observed, this personality type is called *psychopathic* or *sociopathic*.

Nursing Intervention

Antisocial persons can be very trying to the nursing staff. These patients frequently are young and may enter the hospital as a result of accidental injury. No matter their age, their management can be problematic if firm but caring limits are not established early in the hospitalization. These limits should initially be explained by the head nurse, who is the official authority figure on the unit.

The limits must be maintained by all nurses and should be carefully outlined in the nursing care plan so that they are used uniformly by all caregivers. A person may single out one nurse who is not able to set firm limits and manipulate that nurse into compliance in meeting his needs. If uniformity in his care is not established, he may play two groups of nurses against each other: those who are "for" him and those who are "against" him.

Serious staff conflict can occur if he is hospitalized for an extended period. The process of dividing the staff into two groups is called *splitting*. These individuals usually have long-standing experience in splitting that they learned in their original families.

Antisocial persons usually are bright and articulate. They respond poorly to harsh rules and practices. Accordingly, if the nursing staff overreacts by imposing unfair, petty rules, the patient may act out even more. When limits are fair and explained well, they are most effective in curbing unacceptable behavior.

Frequently, these patients, if not already addicted before admission, seem to rely heavily on pain medication. For nursing staff who have concerns about overdependence on narcotic analgesia, an important nursing care consideration is the use of placebos. Placebos may be used as a way of decreasing dependence on narcotic analgesia. However, they should not be used deceptively as such use usually results in many more behavioral complications.

THE INADEQUATE INDIVIDUAL

The last type of patient to be considered in this chapter is sometimes referred to as having an *inadequate personality*, characterized by an immature response to physical, intellectual, or emotional stress. Her responses to stress are unstable and unpredictable. Adaptation to stressful events is poor, and, although she may be intelligent, her judgment is lacking. She may react to stress with an im-

pulsive, exaggerated response or may seem to "wilt" under pressure. The inadequate personality usually develops as a result of early emotional or experiential deprivation (Adler, 1990; Aguilera, 1994).

Nursing Intervention

In many ways, working with the inadequate individual is a tentative process. Because the patient's responses are unpredictable, it can be difficult to decide exactly what approach will be most effective. By determining how her coping inadequacies are being manifested, it is possible to supply extra support to obviously weak areas of the coping response. This may provide enough support to sustain the person's own limited emotional reserves.

The most common symptoms seen in this type of individual are regression, depression, overdependence, and demanding behavior. Sometimes one of these symptoms may be dominant; other individuals exhibit a mixed clinical picture.

The most helpful approach is to anticipate spending more time with the inadequate patient. She is emotionally needy and may feel abandoned and more anxious if interpersonal contacts are hurried and limited only to essential physical care. The extra periods of time spent with her from the beginning of her hospitalization will prove worthwhile. Without such an approach, the nurse could end up spending much more time later on responding to frequent call bells, giving extra reassurance, and solving other care-related problems. As the nursing member of the health care team, liaison work with caregivers in the other disciplines will ensure a more supportive team approach. The patient will sense this as reassuring and anxiety will often be lessened.

Family members can be another important support to this patient. If they are instructed about the rationale for the medical and nursing care the patient is receiving, they can in turn support her emotionally. In addition, they can be taught various aspects of her physical care and participate in her inpatient care. They are usually eager to help, and the patient can be comforted by their presence and concern.

If the patient seems significantly strengthened by the presence of the family members and they are not troublesome to the staff, the relaxation of normal hospital policies can allow someone to be with the patient to relieve her anxiety. This can include overnight stays with the patient until the physical crisis is over.

Once the emotional as well as physical crisis is over, the nursing staff can acknowledge that the family member's presence during the critical period was very helpful. It can then be suggested that the patient needs the time to rest and to become more independent. The nurse's "permission" may allow the family members to relinquish their own need to be with the patient.

The following points can be important when working with family members, especially when they have an unusual need to stay with the patient for most of the day or night, regardless of their family member's condition.

1. The family member who is constantly at the bedside is potentially at risk for exhaustion.
2. When the patient returns home, the family member may be too tired to give her the extra attention and time her care may require.
3. The patient's dependence may be reinforced if she has someone with her all the time.
4. When the patient is discharged, the caregiver may not be as available because of other demands on his or her time.
5. It is emotionally more adaptive for the patient to adjust to the lack of a family member's constant presence in the hospital rather than at home.
6. Once the patient has returned home, there is rarely a "good" time to curtail constant attendance. The longer the patient is accustomed to it in the hospital, the harder it will be to accept its loss when she returns home.
7. At times, the patient's "need" to have someone with her is actually a projection of the family member's need to be with the patient.

CONCLUSION

Knowledge about personality characteristics can be helpful in implementing the nursing process steps of assessment, diagnosis, planning, intervention, and evaluation. It can also provide an understanding of the dynamics causing patient responses to the illness and the nursing staff. Without awareness of personality traits, it is possible for nursing interactions to provoke higher levels of patient anxiety, depression, or other unpleasant feelings. However, with this knowledge, nursing interventions specific to the patient's personality style can be planned and implemented to promote psychosocial adaptation to the stress of illness.

These approaches may also prove helpful with family members whose personality styles can, at times, prove troublesome to their hospitalized relatives or to the nursing staff.

BIBLIOGRAPHY

Adler, D. A. (Ed.). (1990). *Treating personality disorders.* San Francisco: Jossey-Bass.

Aguilera, D. C. (1994). *Crisis intervention: Theory and methodology* (7th ed.). St. Louis: Mosby.

American Psychiatric Association. (1994). *Diagnostic and statistical manual of mental disorders.* (4th ed.). Washington, D.C.: American Psychiatric Association Press.

Barry, P. D. (1994). *Mental health and mental illness* (5th ed.). Philadelphia: J. B. Lippincott.

Brumback, R. A. (Ed.). (1993). *Behavioral neurology.* Philadelphia: W. B. Saunders.

Burgess, J. W. (1992). Neurocognitive impairment in dramatic personalities: Histrionic, narcissistic, borderline, and antisocial disorders. *Psychiatry Research, 42*(3), 283–290.

Carstairs, K. (1992). Paranoid-schizoid or symbiotic? *International Journal of Psychoanalysis, 73*(Pt. 1), 71–85.

Cassem, N. H. (Ed.). (1991). *Massachusetts General Hospital handbook of general hospital psychiatry* (3rd ed.). St. Louis: Mosby Year Book.

Davis, K., Klar, H., & Coyle, J. T. (Eds.). (1991). *Foundations of psychiatry.* Philadelphia: W. B. Saunders.

Eisenman, R. (1993). Living with a psychopathic personality: Case history of a successful anti-social personality. *Acta Paedopsychiatrica, 56*(1), 53–55.

Fenigstein, A., & Vanable, P. A. (1992). Paranoia and self-consciousness. *Journal of Personality and Social Psychology, 62*(1), 129–138.

Hurt, S. W., Reznikoff, M., & Clarkin, J. F. (1990). *Psychological assessment, psychiatric diagnosis & treatment planning.* New York: Brunner/Mazel.

Kahana, R., & Bibring, G. (1964). Personality types in medical management. In N. Zinberg (Ed.), *Psychiatry and medical practice in a general hospital.* New York: International Universities Press.

Kaplan, H. I., & Sadock, B. J. (1994). *Synopsis of psychiatry: Behavioral sciences, clinical psychiatry* (7th ed.). Baltimore: Williams & Wilkins.

Kaplan, H. I., & Sadock, B. J. (1995). *Comprehensive textbook of psychiatry/VI* (6th ed.). Baltimore: Williams & Wilkins.

Kreitler, S., & Kreitler, H. (1990). *The cognitive foundations of personality traits.* New York: Plenum Press.

Maslow, A. (1970). *Motivation and personality* (2nd ed.). New York: Harper & Row.

Mezzich, J. E., & Zimmer, B. (Eds.). (1990). *Emergency psychiatry.* Madison, CT: International Universities Press.

Moffitt, T. E. (1993). Adolescence-limited and life-course-persistent antisocial behavior: A developmental taxonomy. *Psychological Reviews, 100*(4), 674–701.

Neilson, P. (1991). Manipulative and splitting behaviors. *Nursing Standard, 6*(8), 32–35.

Oldham, J. M. (Ed.). (1991). *Personality disorders: New perspectives on diagnostic validity.* Washington, D. C.: American Psychiatric Press.

Pervin, L. A. (Ed.). (1990). *Handbook of personality: Theory and research.* New York: Guilford Press.

Reich, J. (1991). Using the family history method to distinguish relatives of patients with dependent personality disorder from relatives of controls. *Psychiatry Research, 39*(3), 227–237.

Rienzi, B. M., & Scrams, D. J. (1991). Gender stereotypes for paranoid, antisocial, compulsive, dependent, and histrionic personality disorders. *Psychological Reports, 69*(3 Pt. 1), 976–978.

Robinson, L. (1984). *Psychological aspects of the care of hospitalized patients* (4th ed.). Philadelphia: F.A. Davis.

Schwab, J. S., Stephenson, J. J., & Ice, J. F. (1993). *Evaluating family mental health: History, epidemiology, and treatment issues.* New York: Plenum Press.

Shaw, D. S., & Bell, R. Q. (1993). Developmental theories of parental contributors to antisocial behavior. *Journal of Abnormal Child Psychology, 21*(5), 493–518.

Stone, M. H. (1993). *Abnormalities of personality: Within and beyond the realm of treatment.* New York: Norton.

Stoudemire, A., & Fogel, B. S. (Eds.). (1993). *Psychiatric care of the medical patient.* New York: Oxford University Press.

Treatment outlines for avoidant, dependent and passive-aggressive personality disorders. The Quality Assurance Project. (1991). *Australian-New Zealand Journal of Psychiatry, 25*(3), 404–411.

Valerio, C., Santilli, V. B., Valitutti, C., Bianchi di Castelbianco, A., & Cesario, L. (1991). Hysterical personality and family: A clinical case. *Australian-New Zealand Journal of Psychiatry, 25*(3), 392–403.

Webb, C. T., & Levinson, D. F. (1993). Schizotypal and paranoid personality disorder in the relatives of patients with schizophrenia and affective disorders: A review. *Schizophrenia Research, 11*(1), 81–92.

CHAPTER 16

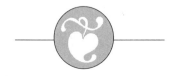

Crisis Intervention With Physically Ill Persons and Their Families

Patricia Barry

The concept of *crisis* has been discussed in earlier chapters. Major illness can be a crisis-precipitating event in the life of a person and his or her family. Maladaptation or ineffective coping are the result of an inability to work through the threat of illness. The degree of maladaptation depends on many factors, which will be presented in this chapter. In Chapter 6, crisis stress responses and ineffective coping were discussed in several contexts.

Crisis is a state of reaction within a person who is responding to a threatening event. Aguilera (1994) describes a crisis as both a danger and an opportunity. It is a danger because of its potential to overwhelm a patient or family. It is an opportunity because, when the crisis is overcome, with or without assistance, the person acquires a more adaptive coping potential for future crises (Auerbach & Stolberg, 1986; Carpenito, 1993; Cox & Davis, 1993; *Diagnostic and Statistical Manual* [DSM-

IV], 1994; Dixon, 1987; Duggan, 1984; Van der Kolk, 1987; Smith, 1990).

A crisis is a time-limited event. It may last anywhere from a few days to a few weeks (Smith, 1990). A crisis state is a period of disequilibrium. Because the ego is constantly attempting to adapt to intrapsychic or environmental stress, it eventually will find a way to relieve itself within a limited time, even if the result is maladaptive (Aguilera, 1994).

A person who is in crisis is, indeed, in a state of disequilibrium; his or her normal defense mechanisms are not working in their usual way. Because of this, crisis theorists suggest that the person is more able to accept intervention and to develop new types of coping responses than when he or she is under non-crisis conditions (Aguilera, 1994; Herman,

Patricia Barry: *Psychosocial Nursing:*
Care of Physically Ill Patients and Their Families, 3rd ed.
© 1996 Lippincott–Raven Publishers

1992; Kaplan & Sadock, 1994, 1995; Moos, 1979; Parad & Caplan, 1965; Rapaport, 1965; Smith, 1990). This belief is the basis of the idea that a crisis can actually be a *positive* learning experience for a person if effective coping occurs and the outcome is adaptation rather than maladaptation.

The event that leads to a crisis is usually one that is new to a person or family. They have no experience in knowing how to deal with it, and their coping ability with regard to this type of threat has never developed; it never was needed before. In working through the crisis, a higher level of coping skills usually develops. These become part of the person's coping repertoire when challenges occur in the future (Aguilera, 1994; Herman, 1992).

When a patient is under severe stress and copes effectively, *adaptation* occurs and the potential crisis is resolved. If the patient does not cope well but intervention by professionals or by supportive family or friends strengthens coping ability or helps in regaining equilibrium, maladaptation is reversed; adaptation is the outcome and the crisis is worked through and resolved. If the patient does not cope ef-

fectively and no one in the social system is alert to this coping failure, then the patient's unsuccessful continued defensive and coping attempts can result in *maladaptation*. The patient is unable to help himself or herself and is in crisis (Aguilera, 1994).

A crisis experienced by one person, because of family system effects, can ultimately affect the family. If family members are able to cope with the crisis of their member, it is possible that their support can reduce that member's crisis response (Brimblecombe, 1993; Pender, 1993). The major factors that determine whether a threatening event will become a crisis are summarized in Box 16-1.

COPING ABILITY IN A CRISIS

A person's ability to cope with a stressful and threatening event depends on many factors. One critical factor is the repertoire of coping skills the person already possesses and can use to adapt to the crisis. Figure 16-1 depicts the

---

BOX 16-1	**Crisis Potential of a Threatening Event**

Sequence of Developments After a Critical Event
1. Perception of event by person
2. Degree of threat as perceived by person to:
   a. Personal safety
   b. Life goals
   c. Normal role functioning
   d. Family stability
3. Accurate perception of the threat is strongly influenced by:
   a. Current mental status
   b. Normal personality style
   c. Normal ego strength
   d. A developmental issue that is triggered by the event: trust, threat to self-esteem, control, loss, guilt, or intimacy
   e. Coping skills during normal stresses of living
   f. Level of stress in the person's life during previous year
   g. Availability of support from:
      (1) Family
      (2) Friends
      (3) Caregivers
4. Outcome
   a. Adaptation (coping) or
   b. Maladaptation (crisis)

critical paths involved in the normal individual's response to a threatening event. If a person's normal coping abilities are temporarily overwhelmed or a chronically inadequate ego prohibits their use, it is possible to structure some of the coping abilities described below into the intervention plan. These coping abilities have been described as follows (Moos, 1979):

1. Denying or minimizing the seriousness of the illness
2. Seeking relevant information
3. Requesting reassurance and emotional support
4. Learning specific illness-related procedures
5. Setting concrete, limited goals
6. Rehearsing alternative outcomes
7. Finding a general purpose or pattern of meaning in the course of events

1. Denying or minimizing the seriousness of the illness. Until the ego is able to accept the implications of the illness fully, it will use many defense mechanisms to protect itself. Denial, projection, displacement, and avoidance are common. Another frequently used defense is *isolation*; the person intellectually accepts the meaning of the illness but does not feel the emotion related to it (Groves & Kucharski, 1991; Murray, 1991; Weisman, 1991).

The ability to deny or minimize the seriousness of an illness is a normal ego response to a very threatening event. It is not something that can be learned when a person is in a threatening situation. It is an effective coping device if it occurs automatically when a person comes under acute stress (Kruger, 1992; Pollin & Holland, 1992).

For this reason, for the first day or so after the patient has learned of a threatening diagnosis, the nurse should not intervene if the pa-

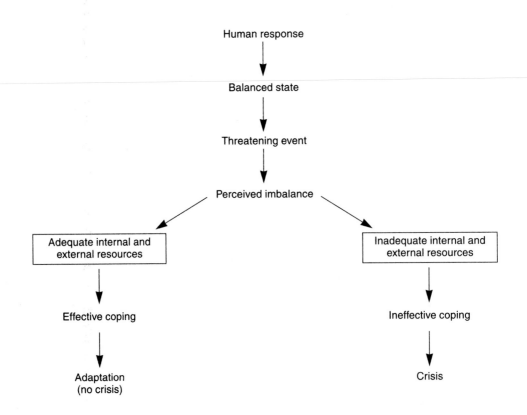

FIGURE 16-1. Critical paths of coping response.

tient copes by using denial. This statement does not imply that the caregiver should deny or minimize the seriousness of the illness. This would be ethically wrong and could seriously jeopardize the patient and family's trust in the caregiver and caregiving system at large. The patient should initially be able to use this denial mechanism.

Ideally, this coping mechanism should give way to a more realistic perception of the situation within a day or two. If it does not, it becomes *ineffective denial*. Nursing interventions for ineffective denial are found in Chapters 17 and 18.

2. Seeking relevant information. By learning more about the illness, its cause, treatment, prognosis, and other related information, the patient gains a sense of control. Intellectual understanding relieves some of the anxiety experienced by all patients, especially those with controlling personalities (see Chapter 15). Nurses can assist in this process but should not overwhelm the patient with excessive information. Initially, only the patient's specific questions should be answered; excessive detail should be avoided. Within a day or two, the patient will probably ask more specific questions. Let these questions be the guide.

3. Requesting reassurance and emotional support. Many patients automatically look to family, friends, and hospital caregivers for support when they are threatened by illness. However, anxiety can be aroused if too much support is given; patients with guarded (suspicious), uninvolved, and antisocial personality types can be threatened by too much nurse involvement. They can be encouraged to share their fears with family members and friends.

Occasionally, with highly anxious patients, it may be necessary for a few days to develop more flexible visiting hours or overnight rules so that trusted family members can provide extra emotional support for these patients in order to avoid crisis. Special attention should be given to the patient who withdraws. Observe this patient carefully for his or her reaction to a supportive approach.

4. Learning specific illness-related procedures. Patients and families are often threatened by

their lack of skills in providing self-care or care to their loved ones with newly acquired conditions. Formal inpatient teaching programs and informal teaching sessions with staff nurses can help patients and their family members acquire the technical skills required in illnesses such as diabetes, or skills involving catheter care, dressing changes, and so on.

Because of the trend toward rapid discharge from the hospital while the individual is physically weak and vulnerable, often requiring significant nursing care in the home setting, there are major psychosocial demands on patients and families during the discharge period. Home nursing visits during the initial adjustment stage of home discharge can also be very helpful to the patient and family who initially lack confidence (Aguilera, 1994; Pender, 1993).

5. Setting concrete, limited goals. For the patient who is adjusting to a catastrophic illness, or an illness that has a long recuperative period, it is important to help in structuring signs of progress into achievable objectives. For example, the goal of taking the first step is a positive and hopeful goal for an amputee. If this patient sets an initial goal of walking down the aisle with his daughter who will be married in 3 months, you can help him to set another, more easily achievable initial goal that can be mastered in a relatively short time. This approach helps the patient to maintain and continually restore hope. Hope is an essential element in the rehabilitative process (Aguilera, 1994; Kruger, 1992).

6. Rehearsing alternative outcomes. Rehearsing alternative outcomes is slightly more sophisticated than information-seeking. The patient thinks through, in advance, his concerns about future surgery, the recuperation period, and other events that create anxiety. In this way he confronts the feared event before it occurs, and works through some of the associated anxiety. When the threatening event occurs, some of the anxiety associated with it has already been released or unconsciously defended against by the ego.

For example, if a patient who is frightened about a cardiac catheterization can be encouraged to talk about her specific concerns and associated feelings, some of the unpleasant affect is discharged. In addition, it will be possible to correct any misconceptions that may be unnecessarily contributing to her fear.

7. Finding a general purpose or pattern of meaning. After the initial effects of the illness have been dealt with using the coping skills mentioned above, some thoughtful patients will continue to probe for the reason why the event occurred. Patients often ask, "Why?" It may take several days, weeks, or longer for the person to arrive at an existential answer, but if and when the person does, he or she may develop a peaceful acceptance of the illness.

The patient will usually answer this "why?" through a deep probing of self. Although the patient may ask you and other people "why," it is helpful to turn the question back gently and ask, "Why do you think this happened?" The person rarely will find the answer anywhere but inside himself or herself.

A crisis is a sequential event that occurs over a given time. Ballou (1980) has proposed four stages to a crisis. They are shown with their accompanying perceptual, emotional, and intellectual components in Table 16-1.

NURSING PROCESS IN CRISIS INTERVENTION

Crisis intervention is a collaborative attempt that involves the nurse and the patient, as well as the support of the patient's social system. An important factor in crisis intervention is the nurse's openness to the patient's response to illness. A nurse can be aware of the patient's psychological dynamics and actually anticipate a crisis if the threatening event has serious implications for the patient's or the family's well-being. Chronic, long-term illness or rehabilitation can have as much maladaptive potential as an acute, life-threatening illness.

Using the data in the Barry Psychosocial Assessment Interview Schedule in Chapter 12, it may be possible to predict those patients most at risk for crisis. Ideally, intervention should begin *before* a crisis actually occurs. An emotional crisis in a patient whose physical equilibrium is unstable presents more overall risk to the patient's physiological status. By intervening and

reducing psychological stress, there is increased probability that nursing intervention can:

Promote systemic well-being.
Decrease emotional stress.
Frequently, prevent prolonged hospitalization.
Reduce the risk of chronic maladaptation.
Support capacity for normal role functioning.
Promote adaptive family dynamics, because the averted crisis can no longer disrupt the family.

ASSESSMENT: INITIAL EVALUATION OF PATIENT'S RESPONSE

Two types of patient responses can prompt a crisis intervention approach by the nurse. The first is a *precrisis situation,* in which the threat of illness, the patient's personality style, the level of stress she has experienced in the past year, her normal coping ability, and her family dynamics are warning signals that her ability to cope will be under severe stress. The second is a *catastrophic illness or accident,* in which the patient and her family have had little or no time to prepare for this serious psychological trauma. When the immediate denial stage passes, intrapsychic crisis in the patient or a system crisis in the family may occur.

Anxiety or depression are the two most common presenting symptoms of poor coping and potential crisis (Cassem, 1991; Weisman, 1991). Ideally, the patient will be able to recognize his own psychological discomfort and work with you as you help him to adapt to the stress of illness. If he is unaware of his maladaptation because of a distorted or lost sense of reality and is unable to help himself with support from family and general caregivers, psychiatric consultation should be requested.

In the assessment process, it is important that the nurse understand the implications of the illness from the patient's perspective. Too often, nurses believe that they understand the effect that an illness may or may not have on a patient. Actually, what often occurs is that the nurse views the illness within the context of his or her value system and life goals. The nurse projects thoughts and feelings onto the patient's situation and assumes that they are cor-

	TABLE 16-1 **Stages of Crisis**		
Stage	**Intrapsychic Response**	**Intellectual Response**	**Emotional Response**
Shock; denial	Dulled responses	Cognitive blocking	Dulled emotion
Distress	Disorganization	Confusion	Anxiety; helplessness
Disequilibrium	Overwhelmed	Cognitive racing; disorganized thinking	High anxiety
Stabilization	Increased sense of control	Problem-solving ability is regained	Lower anxiety
Effective coping; adaptation	Integration of new coping abilities	Increased current choices for coping responses	Emotional equilibrium is restored

Adapted from Ballou, M. (1980). Crisis intervention and the hospital nurse. *Journal of Nursing Care, 13*(1), p. 18.

rect. It is essential to find out what *this* illness means to *this* patient (Brimblecombe, 1993; Pender, 1993).

In order to find out how the patient views the illness, it is helpful to use the "tree approach" of information gathering recommended in Chapter 2. When caring is demonstrated in questioning the patient, he or she may feel marked relief. I have been surprised at times by the rapid reduction of anxiety within 5 or 10 minutes of beginning this process with an overwhelmed patient. Nurses should not underestimate their therapeutic value. The counseling techniques recommended in Chapter 2 can assist in knowing how to talk appropriately with a patient or family member in distress.

A significant clue to the patient's anxiety or depression can be obtained by asking, "Have you ever known anyone else with this problem?" A large number of patients have indeed known someone; indeed, the person they knew usually had severe complications that resulted in death or permanent disability. The person can be anyone: the distant cousin of a high school classmate or a relative who may have died 30 years ago (in a much different medical environment). Ask the patient to describe the circumstances. Often, it will be learned that the person had a complex illness with a different etiology than the patient's own. There also may have been many other factors present that are not present in this patient's illness.

Frequently, there is an opportunity to correct the patient's misconceptions and identification with the other person. This may dramatically lower the patient's fears. The following case example illustrates this technique.

CASE EXAMPLE

Sarah is a 64-year-old woman with diabetes. An injury to her ankle resulted in a chronic ulcer that would not heal. A below-the-knee amputation was recommended, but Sarah adamantly refused to consider it. The active urging of caregivers to have the surgery resulted in a high level of anxiety. Her surgeons were fearful that ultimately they would have to remove more of her leg if further tissue deterioration occurred. Finally, psychiatric liaison consultation was requested to "persuade" the patient that amputation was in her best interest.

It was soon discovered that 15 years earlier, Sarah's uncle had been in an automobile accident. He had been in acute shock from severe hemorrhage; kidney failure and severe metabolic distress had resulted. Because of peripheral vascular failure, three of his limbs were amputated, one at a time, in an attempt to save his life. Eventually, he died. Sarah was convinced that the removal of her foot could lead to the same end for herself. With explanation, she was able to understand that her circumstances were different in many ways from those of her uncle. By nightfall she decided to proceed with the amputation recommended by the surgeons. ❧

Sometimes in attending to psychosocial distress with patients, it is believed that a high level of skill in psychiatric assessment is necessary to understand why a patient is so anxious or fearful. Nurses may devalue their own ability to help a troubled patient because of this misconception. Actually, the patient may be able to describe why she is reacting in such a way. Failing to ask what *she* thinks is causing her to react to the illness as she is leaves caregivers having to guess, or inaccurately assume, the cause. Many times the patient knows the answer, but until she talks about it and explores it out loud with a caring person, it remains a personal, abstract terror.

Until caregivers understand why a patient is threatened by a particular illness, they will not be able to develop a therapeutic intervention. There are no specific interventions that are guaranteed to help for certain types of maladaptation. Detective work in the assessment process and understanding of the dynamics underlying the specific type of this patient's distress will help in the design of an effective intervention.

PLANNING THE INTERVENTION

During the planning stage, it is important to evaluate the patient's reality testing about his or her reaction to the illness. For example, it may be obvious to you, the other caregivers, and the family that the patient's coping is not at an adaptive level. Initially, however, he may not be aware of his own inadequate coping. When this is so, this stage of crisis intervention can be a challenge, yet not an impossible one. Ballou (1980) has recommended the following techniques when the patient is defending himself from awareness of his own responses:

1. Reflecting the patient's feelings
2. Summarizing the content of messages
3. Helping the patient clarify feelings
4. Gently asking the patient to explain the consequences of an intended behavior

5. Not personalizing angry or hopeless feelings expressed by the patient but acknowledging his or her right to those feelings
6. Not avoiding dependency that might be manifest

As alluded to in recommendations 5 and 6 above, it is possible that the patient may temporarily direct some frustration and discouragement at the caregiver. These are often projections of the patient's own helplessness. The nurse should avoid feeling helpless or responsible for them, however. Instead, an attempt should be made to recognize where these feelings of helplessness originate. It is also helpful to recognize where these feelings originate in the patient. This can be valuable information. The patient's feelings will pass when his or her coping ability returns. As described in Chapter 8, it is not possible to make a person cope. In addition to projecting his or her own feelings onto the caregiver, the patient may temporarily need to rely on the caregiver's problem-solving ability until his or her own returns. This neediness and dependency may last only a day or two (Aguilera, 1994; Kruger, 1992; Pender, 1993).

During the admission assessment, it may have been determined that the patient has a dependent personality style. If so, it is wise not to allow overdependence to continue beyond a day or two. If dependency becomes a problem for nursing staff members, there is potential for yet another crisis to occur: the patient may have a crisis when he or she finds the nurse unwilling to continue meeting unreasonable demands. If marked dependency is occurring beyond the second day in a crisis, the limit-setting approach outlined in Chapters 17 and 18 can help to reduce the anxiety of both the patient and the nursing staff.

It is also important in the planning stage of the intervention process to evaluate the response of the family or of the patient's other significant person to the patient's illness. These people may be coping well and have the potential to support the patient while his or her coping ability is temporarily weakened. Another possibility is that their fear and immobilization may undermine the patient's ability to cope.

In a family whose dynamics are undermining the patient's coping ability, it may be necessary to modify one's approach. Some family dynamics are very rigid and may have been operating for decades and generations. The intervention approach may be unfamiliar and may be viewed as yet another threat to family equilibrium. The family's reality testing can be supported so that family members do not continue to undermine the patient's adaptive capacity (Brimblecombe, 1993; Kruger, 1992; Pender, 1993).

Referral sources of support for families include a family therapist with a medical, nursing, or social work background; a psychiatric liaison clinical nursing specialist; a clinical nursing specialist in the specialty field of the patient's illness (oncology, cardiac disease, obstetrics, and so on); a hospital social worker; or a member of the hospital pastoral care team. The family's priest, minister, or rabbi could also assist them. In addition, most families usually have extended family members who are respected as "elders" who can help during difficult family times.

In planning the intervention, the patient can be asked about trusted confidantes. If the patient describes positive relationships with one or more family members or friends and they live within traveling distance of the hospital, they can be included in the plan. One of the recommendations can be as simple as encouraging the patient to share concerns honestly with them.

Developing the actual steps to be used in the nursing intervention should involve the patient. In most cases, even if he is initially unaware of his ineffective coping, his concern and reality testing will result in a willingness to assist in the intervention plan.

When the nurse and the patient agree about the reasons why he is not coping well, the patient can be asked how he thinks the nurse and other staff members can help. He can be asked directly, "Is there something I can do to help?" or "What do you need from us [the nurses] in order to help you through this time?" The patient may be able to describe his needs directly, and these ideas can be incorporated into the plan. Then the nurse's ideas can be shared. Some of the proposals may appeal to the patient more than others. Allow him to describe the merit or lack of merit anticipated from the options that are presented. This step is called *reviewing the alternatives*. The patient should choose the approaches he believes would be most helpful.

INTERVENTION

Once an intervention plan is decided on, its success will depend on its use by all the nurses involved in the patient's care on all three shifts. This is called a *systems approach*. The plan will provide a consistency and security that can be very supportive to a patient whose ego defenses are weakened or overwhelmed. The plan is recorded on the nursing Kardex and its rationale and use verbally encouraged with the other staff members.

Nurses rarely share their crisis intervention plan with the house officers and attending physicians who are also caring for the patient. They mistakenly believe that physicians are not interested or would not be bothered to use their recommendations. The way they are approached can make a difference in their receptivity to the plan. Specific examples of the patient's symptoms of ineffective coping can be described: unusual levels of anxiety, depression, noncompliance, or other behaviors; shutdown of communication with spouse; frequent use of analgesics with excessive sleep as a way of avoiding the reality of the situation; or similar types of objective data.

Rather than suggesting to the physician that he or she follow these recommendations, the approach that has been devised can be described with the rationale for the plan. If the plan is having a positive effect, the nurse's observations can be described. It is then the physician's choice whether or not to use a similar approach. Many physicians are open to nurses' psychosocial recommendations and respect their opinions if they are articulate in presenting supporting data.

The key to successful crisis intervention in the general hospital is the consistency of caregivers in maintaining the crisis intervention plan that is developed. This will promote the patient's reality-testing ability. Most important, it will allow the patient to trust the nurses and his environment at a time when trust in himself may be faltering (Brimblecombe, 1993).

The goal of crisis intervention is to help the patient regain a precrisis level of functioning (Aguilera, 1994). This is an important point to remember. At times caregivers may expect more than that of themselves, and this can undermine their confidence in actively intervening with a maladapting patient. For example, a patient may have a type A (controlling) personality and become highly anxious because of the circumstances of hospitalization. The goal of crisis intervention will be to assist this patient to understand the source of his or her anxiety and to gain more of a sense of control of the environment. The outcome of intervention will be that the patient's personality style is unchanged. Ideally, however, the maladaptive anxiety will be reduced.

When a reduction in the patient's maladaptation is seen, it is important that the intervention process be continued. The continuity of this approach will be an essential factor in resolving the crisis.

EVALUATING THE INTERVENTION

The final stage of the nursing crisis intervention process is evaluating the outcome of the intervention. This is an ongoing process that should begin in the planning stage. During each interaction with the patient, his or her mental status should continue to be evaluated, with the nurse looking specifically for a reduction in anxiety, depression, or other maladaptive responses that were the original clues of ineffective coping with the illness. If a decrease in the patient's maladaptation response is not observed within 24 hours, another approach should be prepared. The original plan can continue to be used if the caregiver and patient believe it is helping.

A second type of intervention plan can be used as an extra support during the critical period. The choice of a second type of approach should be arrived at using the same process as the original intervention plan. An important factor in a complex crisis situation is the nurse's flexibility in objectively evaluating the patient's response to interventions. The nurse should be prepared to alter the original plan and be creative in developing different alternatives (Aguilera, 1994; Kruger, 1992).

WHEN NURSING CRISIS INTERVENTION IS NOT ENOUGH

Some patients have personality structures that are unable to tolerate normal levels of stress in their everyday lives (Aguilera, 1994). Accordingly, the stress that accompanies illness and hospitalization can quickly become very threatening. When this occurs, it is not a reflection on the adequacy of the caregiving system. Nurses should not personalize the patient's maladaptive reaction. Instead, they can view the patient's maladaptation as the consequence of developmental and environmental factors that were in process before hospital admission. Strong clues in the patient's admission psychosocial history as well as his or her interactions with hospital personnel can indicate a high crisis potential for this patient (Kruger, 1992; Pollin & Holland, 1992).

When patients experience major setbacks and complications in their hospitalization, nursing interventions may be of great importance to them; however, as yet another setback occurs, it may be "the straw that breaks the camel's back." The nurse may believe that he or she is no longer able to deal with the patient's response. Some patients' coping failure is due to the effects of a cognitive mental disorder. Because of actual deficits in brain functioning, the patient's normal defenses are weakened (Bassett & Folstein, 1991; Goldberg, Faust, & Novack, 1992).

Other patients' maladaptive responses, such as noncompliance, dysfunctional grieving, or disturbance in self-concept, can result in nurses' inability to be objective. Their frustration levels prevent them from being able to solve problems and be a support to the patient.

In all these circumstances, as well as others that contain multiple complicated factors, it is important to be able to recognize the need for assistance in knowing how to care for certain patients. Nurses in these circumstances are wise to be open to the need for formal psychiatric consultation (O'Connor, 1991). Attending physicians and house officers are usually alert to the patient who is not coping well and will themselves initiate formal psychiatric consultation to assist the patient. If they are not aware of the maladaptive response, they will usually be receptive to the specific data a nurse presents about a patient's inability to cope. When the supporting data is presented, psychiatric consultation can be recommended. The final decision is theirs, but physicians can be strongly influenced by an articulate nurse who has astutely assessed the patient.

If a psychiatric consultant is called in to work with the patient, it is important for the nurse to continue to maintain involvement. The nurse is a very important support person to the patient because of the amount of time spent with him or her, and the trust that usually has been established.

Most psychiatric consultants are willing to share their impressions of patients with nursing staff members. (If they are psychiatric liaison consultants, they usually will seek out the nurse to share their recommendations.) Talking to the consultant can be especially helpful when there is concern that the original nursing approach to the patient was not effective or if specific recommendations are sought about what can be done to help the patient.

POTENTIAL FOR CRISIS

Critical developmental periods and situational events can precipitate crisis. These periods and events usually occur in nonhospital environments and may initially seem to be unrelated to hospitalization and illness. It is possible that there is an association between developmental or situational crisis and the eventual development of physical illness.

The psyche (the mind) and the soma (the body) are constantly interacting; they are not two subsystems operating independently of each other (Kiecolt-Glaser & Glaser, 1991). There are times when the ego is no longer able to mediate and defend against intrapsychic stress. Through an action related to neurotransmitters, it is possible for the temporary overwhelming of the ego to result in failure of one of the body's subsystems. Physiological defense mechanisms are affected, and the body's ability to maintain homeostasis is temporarily overcome (Elliot, 1992; Everly, 1993; Kiecolt-Glaser & Glaser, 1992).

It is possible that the development of physical illness provides the severely stressed person with a means to restore psychological equilibrium. When someone becomes ill:

1. She has a temporary break from normal work or school pressures.
2. She is able to withdraw temporarily from her extended social system, which has multiple social dynamics and inherent stresses.
3. She retreats to the safety of family or to trusted support people at home.
4. Family members and support people rally and provide the ill person with extra physical as well as emotional care.
5. Work on job-related decisions, proposals, projects, or term papers is temporarily halted.
6. Any ongoing conflict in which she is involved is discontinued. The illness temporarily unsettles the adversary.

Often, the illness and its effect of removing the patient from the active psychosocial crisis present an opportunity for her to regain a sense of life goals, priorities, and personal objectivity. Actually, illness that develops out of these types of distressing circumstances may be adaptive.

Although nurses cannot be expected to help resolve preillness crises that the patient is still reacting to unconsciously when hospitalized, it is important to be aware of the possibility of their existence. It is important to take the time to find out how seriously this preillness stressor is affecting the patient (Brimblecombe, 1993; Kruger, 1992; Pender, 1993).

For example, a 52-year-old woman who is admitted with chronic obstructive pulmonary disease may tell you that she has been upset because her 25-year-old schizophrenic son has been in frequent crises because of his refusal to take medication. By using a problem-solving approach with this patient, it may be possible to devise some different approaches that can be used to help improve her difficult situation. It is also possible that there are no solutions. By helping her to work through to the reality of the situation, however, she may experience a lessening of guilt. She may feel a sense of relief that perhaps there really is no solution and she is not ultimately responsible.

By understanding the patient's preillness stressors, it will be possible to identify the potential of postdischarge stressors waiting at home. If the person has worked through to the reality of the situation, he or she can feel some hope about a chronic problem that may have seemed hopeless. In addition, a referral to a mental health professional with experience in family therapy to address the family problem may promote both the patient's psychological and physiological adaptation.

When patients are hospitalized who have been experiencing high levels of stress from developmental or situational crises, they are more vulnerable to an in-hospital crisis reaction to an illness-related problem. For example, if it is discovered during the assessment process that an older, single woman who was admitted with chest pain of undetermined origin has been retired from her job for 2 years, but has developed few outside interests and reports being chronically depressed since her retirement, part of the nursing intervention can be to discuss her preillness living situation and postdischarge plans for seeking meaningful interests.

Too many times patients are admitted, extensive physical histories are obtained, elaborate physical workups are carried out, physical ills are treated, and discharge occurs without clinicians being aware of preillness, maladaptive psychosocial circumstances. It is not unusual for patients such as the woman described above to be readmitted 2 months later with similar symptoms. Whether the patient is in crisis or in a precrisis state, it is important to take the time to find out what else is going on in his or her life.

STRESS AND FAMILY CRISIS

Stress is the greatest threat to healthy functioning of a family, both physically and socially. Stress has been identified as the link between psychiatric and physical illness (Felten et al., 1991; Goldstein & Niaura, 1992; Kiecolt-Glaser & Glaser, 1992).

The most important factor in a family's ability to tolerate stress is the coping ability of the family members. The actual use of coping responses was identified as more important than other factors, such as a sense of control or positive self-esteem, in studying the persistent life strains of marriage and parenting (Pearlin & Schooler, 1978).

The events that cause the most strain in families are:

Persistent life strains or deficits: Long-term types of problems that a person faces in a life role, such as marriage to a partner who has a chronic illness or being a parent or sibling of a premature infant who requires long-term hospitalization.

Crises: Suddenly occurring, upsetting events that threaten emotional and physical well-being and require maximum coping ability, such as accidental catastrophic injury to oneself or a family member or sudden death of a family member.

Transitions: The time following a crisis when adjustments are slowly made and equilibrium is regained, such as a young adolescent discharged after a severe head injury who requires an extended period of treatment to regain his previous level of functioning or a middle-aged mother who requires intermittent courses of chemotherapy after surgery for cancer.

Without intervention with the family, members will continue to promote the patient's sickness through a heightened reaction, whether to gastrointestinal symptoms of Crohn's disease or to symptoms of alcoholism. A systems approach that addresses the family's interactional style and enlightens members about ways they feed into and promote a continuation of the patient's problems is an essential aspect of the management of critical events related to chronic physical or mental disease states (Brimblecombe, 1993; Burns et al., 1993; Pender, 1993).

DEVELOPMENTAL CRISES

Developmental crises occur as the result of poor adaptation to the emotional, physical, or social challenges of the normal process of growth and aging (Aguilera, 1994; Smith, 1990). Because of the prevalence of material in other textbooks on the major adjustments required during the various developmental stages, this chapter will only briefly present the stages and their critical adaptive challenges (see Box 16-2). Be aware that the system effects within a family cause *all* family members to be affected by the developmental struggle of one member. For example, an adolescent's struggle to separate from the family has a marked effect on the mother, father, and siblings (Brimblecombe, 1993).

SITUATIONAL CRISES

Situational crises are crises resulting from stressful events that threaten a person's physiological, psychological, or social equilibrium. Many events have the potential to tax severely a person's adaptive capacity. When these experiences coincide with stressful developmental periods, or if two situational crises occur at or near the same time, they can be more disruptive. In addition, some persons have a lower-than-normal ability to adapt to stress and easily become at risk for crisis.

The following events are the most commonly encountered situational crises: separation from family, marriage, childbirth, divorce, life-threatening or chronic illness, and death. They are briefly reviewed below.

Separation From Family

The process of a young person's moving away from the nuclear family into an independent living situation can result in increased anxiety or depression for the young person and one or both parents. Whether the departure is caused by a move to another city for employment, the beginning of college, or enlistment into the armed services, the young adult may experience a period of self-doubt and fear about ability to cope with the many changes he or she is experiencing. If the family has had difficulty in promoting the young person's autonomy and allowing him or her to separate gradually from them psychologically during the middle years of adolescence, the young adult's actual physical departure from the home may be more complicated. Parents' expectations or overcautiousness are internalized and eventually may make it more diffi-

cult for the young person to individuate (Aguilera, 1994).

Marriage

Despite the tendency today for many young people to live away from home as singles before they marry, there are still many young men and women who do not move out of their parents' homes until they marry. These people also face the issues discussed above. Because of changing social mores and emphasis on the divorce rate, many young people approach marriage with more trepidation than was apparent in their parents' generation. This stress is added to a couple's concerns as they commit themselves to one another and are subject to the normal strains in an intimate relationship. In addition, they usually are confronted by the differences in their value systems and the expectations of their extended families. Sometimes, aspects of compromise that are essential to a healthy marital relationship do not arise as significant factors during their courtship. The idealization of the partner that is common during the courtship and "honeymoon phase" of early marriage gives way to the realities of coexistence (Aguilera, 1994; Hoff, 1989).

Childbirth

The birth of a child causes a major shift in the interpersonal dynamics between a husband and a wife. A study of 48 American couples' responses to their first child revealed some of the dynamics that contribute to the crisis potential of childbirth. In the study, all the couples were middle class and between 25 and 35 years of age, and all the husbands were college graduates. Thirty-eight of the 46 couples (83%) reported extensive or severe crisis in adjusting to their first child. The following data were obtained from the 38 couples (LeMasters, 1965):

1. Thirty-five of the pregnancies were planned or desired.
2. Thirty-four of the couples' marriages were self-rated as good, and 31 of them were rated as good or better by close friends.
3. The personality development of the 76 husbands and wives was considered aver-

BOX 16-2	Developmental Stages

Infancy and Early Childhood (birth to 3 years)

Major issues (progressive from birth): trust, dependency, awareness of separateness from mother, development of autonomy

When issues are not resolved: distrust, poor self-confidence, dependency, fusion of self with caregiver, poor self-control

Childhood (3 to 11 years)

Major issues: identification with significant elders; development of initiative, security, and acceptance within family and eventually within peer group; mastery of age-appropriate skills and intellectual challenges

When issues are not resolved: guilt, lack of direction and purpose, self-undermining behavior, feelings of inadequacy, self-concept disturbances

Adolescence (12 to 20 years)

Major issues: Idealization of significant others, resolution of loss of childhood, development of sexual identity, acceptance by peer group, psychological separation from family as adolescent develops own perceptions of the world; physical separation usually occurs a few years later

When issues are not resolved: inability to separate from family and assume independence, sexual confusion, self-consciousness, inability to form relationship with person of opposite sex, poor object relations

Early Adulthood (20 to 30 years)

Major issues: ability to develop intimacy and commitment within a relationship, commitment to employment, exploration, and clarification of societal norms as they pertain to self

When issues are not resolved: superficiality in relationships with others, poor goal setting, drifting in and out of relationships and employment, lack of responsibility to self and others

Adulthood (30 to 50 years)

Major issues: maintenance of life goals, creativity, and spontaneity; ability to maintain meaningful relationships; appropriate channeling of emotions

When issues are not resolved: inability to work or to feel pleasure, poor motivation, egocentrism in goal setting

Late Adulthood (50 years and older)

Major issues: ability to resolve losses of aging and to integrate ongoing losses, maintenance of hope, acceptance of uncertain future

When issues are not resolved: continual wishing to relive past experiences, inability to take pleasure in the present, loss of hope, depression

age or above average. They did not have psychiatric disabilities.

4. The 38 couples admitted that they had idealized the parenting role. They had not been prepared for the reality of taking care of an infant:
   a. The major adjustment reported by the mother was to constant fatigue from full-time care of the infant.
   b. The major adjustment of the father was related to the changes in his wife's roles of sexual partner and income earner.
5. Mothers with professional training (eight) experienced "extensive" or "severe" crisis in every case.

It is important to emphasize that despite the critical effect of childbirth in a young marriage, most couples adapt effectively within a reasonable time.

Divorce

Divorce is a disruptive event. It results in major role shifts and losses within the family. Some of the issues that divorced people experience are a disruption in role and normal family dynamics; reactions of children and extended family and friends; social stigma; rejection by former spouse, critical acquaintances, and possibly religious affiliation; loneliness; and anxiety about independent functioning. Many individuals also experience a major decrease in their self-esteem.

Because of the crisis potential in the process of divorce, there are many self-help groups offered by agencies in most communities. One of the risks inherent in the postadjustment phase of divorce is remarriage to a partner who is similar to the first spouse. It is common for neurotic needs to lead a person unconsciously into a second marriage with dynamics similar to the first (Aguilera, 1994).

Major Illness

A life-threatening or severe chronic illness poses many challenges to a person and his or her family: changes in body image and self-esteem, loss of control, issues of dependence and trust, separation from family, and changes in role functioning. Because of its usually ongoing nature, the illness continually presents new challenges to the person and the family. Coping ability may be constantly tested. See Box 16-3 for the challenges associated with major illness.

With caregivers' increased awareness of the psychological risks of major illness, patients and families can be assisted in adapting to this major life event. The following case example illustrates how developmental and situational crises were further compounded by a physical illness.

CASE EXAMPLE

John is a 67-year-old retired insurance adjustor. He is married and has three children. He was admitted to the hospital after a major myocardial infarction (MI). He had had

---

BOX 16-3	The Coping Challenge of Major Illness

Illness-Related
1. Coping with pain and helplessness
2. Coping with the hospital environment
3. Coping with different procedures
4. Coping with multiple caregiver relationships

General Coping Challenges
1. Maintaining emotional balance
2. Maintaining self-esteem
3. Maintaining meaningful relationships
4. Maintaining work productivity
5. Coping with unknown future

---

an earlier, less severe MI at age 59. Five years ago John developed a tumor of the spinal cord. As the result of surgery and radiation, he is paraplegic. John had to retire because of his disability. He has continued an active life and has many interests, including gardening, working with his tools, and traveling.

John had an unusually strong upper torso and arms and was able to move himself inside and outside by wheelchair. He drove a car and functioned independently. His adaptation to his paraplegia was very good. John's wife and family are strongly supportive. John was told by his physicians 1 year ago that the effects of the tumor would eventually result in loss of control of his bladder and bowels as he grew older. He had become increasingly depressed during the 9 months before admission as he envisioned himself eventually being unable to travel or attend the theatre. He believed that he would become an unbearable burden to his wife.

When the critical stage of MI treatment was over and his survival seemed probable, John became acutely depressed. Psychiatric liaison intervention was requested because he was rapidly losing his will to live.

Because of the severity of his myocardial damage, John was convinced that he would be unable to use his arms in order to maneuver himself in and out of his wheelchair. His concern about his impending bowel and bladder incontinence began to overwhelm him. Because he did not want to worry his wife, he withheld these overwhelming concerns from her. He was markedly anxious and was frightened by his inability to cope. ❦

John was indeed in a difficult situation. His nurses and physicians identified with him and soon lost their objectivity, believing that perhaps there was no possible resolution. John had demonstrated during earlier illnesses that he had strong adaptive ability. His adaptation had been weakened by his concerns of the previous several months. The depression was compounded by the severe MI. He was maladapting. Some of the psychiatric liaison interventions that were developed with John's approval were as follows:

1. Schedule an arm stress test as soon as possible in order to give him definite knowledge of his upper torso stress capability. (Stress test scheduling in the hospital is usually on a first-come, first-served basis. Physicians were asked to justify an earlier placement for this patient because of his critical need to know his future endurance and mobility potential.)

2. When John had talked out his overwhelming fears to the point that he felt ready to share them with his wife, he was encouraged to do so. The consultant pointed out that this might help relieve any loneliness she was feeling and give her the opportunity to voice her own unspoken fears from which she had perhaps been trying to protect him.

3. Consultation with a neurological rehabilitation clinical specialist was arranged so that the patient could gain a more realistic perspective of his future bowel and bladder state.

4. Daily sessions with the psychiatric liaison consultant had the following goals:
   a. Continual reality testing with supporting data.
   b. Encouraging patient to express his deepest fears regarding his future course.
   c. Giving patient choices in his care plan whenever appropriate.

5. Ongoing psychiatric liaison work with nursing and medical staff to hear their concerns and recommend appropriate caregiver interventions.

6. A session with John and his wife was held on the third day, when his anxiety level was lower and he agreed to a joint session. Intervention to reduce communication barriers that had developed in their normally open relationship was utilized.

When the results of the stress test were available, they provided a great relief for John. They demonstrated that his activity level could be increased gradually to his pre-MI level as soon as he was comfortable. He became less depressed, more relaxed, and optimistic.

Another crisis developed a few days later, however, when a urological consultant recommended "dye studies" to determine his current urological status. Twenty years earlier John had experienced a cardiac arrest as the result of dye used in a kidney study. The moment the urologist mentioned "dye," John shut out everything else. He was convinced he would die if he underwent such a study. John initially refused the study. He was asked by the psychiatric liaison consultant if he would be willing to allow the urologist to return. He was encouraged to write down specific questions about his concerns. On the physician's return visit, John learned that the dye was nontoxic and would be in his bladder, not his kidneys. John agreed to have the test. The results showed that he had a large retention capacity and strong sphincter control. His bladder condition was very good, and he was elated. He was discharged a few days later. His adaptation potential and that of his wife were positive.

Death

The potential loss of oneself or a loved one to death is another event that causes major adaptive stress in individuals and families. The effect of death on patients and families will be dealt with in depth in Chapter 24. Usually death is not a sudden, unexpected event. Both the dying person and his or her family and loved ones have a time before the death during which they can gradually accept the effects of the impending loss. At times, especially when the dying person is a child or a young or middle-aged adult, the strains of adaptation result in crisis (Baile et al., 1993; Halm et al., 1993). Unexpected deaths sometimes have a greater potential for crisis, however, because the ego has had no time to develop adaptive mechanisms to deal with the sudden loss.

In either case, families with open patterns of communication will usually respond with strong emotions. The members of an open family are receptive to these emotions and solidly support one another. Their interactions are in contrast to families where emotions are repressed and avoided, in which the typical way losses are dealt with is to avoid feelings or verbalized thoughts. This is a closed system of family relationship (Burr, 1991; Clement, 1991). When emotional dependence is denied in this type of family, the potential for crises within the family as a whole or in members is increased (Bowen, 1976; Papero, 1990).

CONCLUSION

The concepts in this chapter are important in understanding how people maintain psychosocial equilibrium during the threat of physical illness. When the stress of illness disrupts equilibrium, it is possible for nursing intervention to help restore it. By identifying the cause(s) of coping failure, an intervention can be designed to help avert or resolve a crisis. The theory presented in this chapter, when combined with the specific intervention approaches recommended in Chapters 17 to 29, can help promote psychosocial adaptation in both patients and families.

BIBLIOGRAPHY

Aguilera, D. C. (1994). *Crisis intervention: Theory and methodology* (7th ed.). St. Louis: Mosby.

Auerbach, S., & Stolberg, A. (Eds.). (1986). *Crisis intervention with children and families*. Washington, DC: Hemisphere Publishing.

Baile, W. F., DiMaggion, J. R., Schapira, D. V., & Janofsky, J. S. (1993). The request for assistance in dying. The need for psychiatric consultation. *Cancer, 72*(9), 2786–2791.

Ballou, M. (1980). Crisis intervention and the hospital nurse. *Journal of Nursing Care, 13*(1),15–19.

Bassett, S. S., & Folstein, M. F. (1991). Cognitive impairment and functional disability in the absence of psychiatric diagnosis. *Psychology and Medicine, 21*(1), 77–84.

Brimblecombe, N. (1993). Family crisis. *Nursing Times, 89*(44), 40–41.

Burns, C., Archbold, P., Stewart, B., & Shelton, K. (1993). New diagnosis: Caregiver role strain. *Nursing Diagnosis, 4*(2), 70–76.

Burr, W. R. (1991). Rethinking levels of abstraction in family systems theories. *Family Process, 30*(4), 435–452.

Carpenito, L. (1993). *Nursing diagnosis: Application and clinical practice*. Philadelphia: J. B. Lippincott.

Cassem, N.H. (1991). Depression. In N.H. Cassem (Ed.), *Masschusetts General Hospital handbook of general hospital psychiatry* (3rd ed.). St Louis: Mosby Year Book.

Clement, J. A. (1991). Psychiatric nursing phenomena and the construct of family boundaries. *Archives of Psychiatric Nursing, 5*(4), 236–243.

Coler, M. S., & Hafner, L. P. (1991). An intercultural assessment of the type, intensity and number of crisis precipitating factors in three cultures: United States, Brazil and Taiwan. *International Journal of Nursing Studies, 28*(3), 223–235.

Cox, R. P., & Davis, L. L. (1993). Social constructivist approaches for brief, episodic, problem-focused family encounters. *Nurse Practitioner, 18*(8), 45–49.

Diagnostic and staiistical manual of mental disorders (4th ed.). (1994). Washington, DC: American Psychiatric Press.

Elliott, B. A. (1992). Birth order and health: Major issues. *Social Science and Medicine, 35*(4), 443–452.

Erikson, E. (1963). *Childhood and society* (2nd ed). New York: Norton.

Evans, J. V. (1993). Crisis, grief and loss. *Canadian Nurse, 89*(8), 40–43.

Everly, G. S. (1993). Psychotraumatology: A two-factor formulation of posttraumatic stress. *Integrating Physiology and Behavioral Science, 28*(3), 270–278.

Goldberg, R. J., Faust, D., & Novack, D. (1992). Integrating the cognitive mental status examination into the medical interview. *Southern Medical Journal, 85*(5), 491–497.

Goldstein, M. G., & Niaura, R. (1992). Psychological factors affecting physical condition. Cardiovascular disease literature review. Part I: Coronary artery disease and sudden death. *Psychosomatics, 33*(2), 134–145.

Groves, J. E., & Kurcharski, A. (1991). Brief psychotherapy. In N. H. Cassem (Ed.), *Massachusetts General Hospital handbook of general hospital psychiatry* (3rd ed.). St. Louis: Mosby Year Book.

Halm, M. A., Titler, M. G., Kleiber, C., Johnson, S. K., Montgomery, L. A., Craft, M. J., Buckwalter, K., Nicholson, A., & Megivern, K. (1993). Behavioral responses of family members during critical illness. *Clinics in Nursing Research, 2*(4), 414–437.

Harrison, D. S., & Cole, K. D. (1991). Family dynamics and caregiver burden in home health care. *Clinics in Geriatric Medicine, 7*(4), 817–829.

Herman, J. (1992). *Trauma and recovery*. New York: Basic Books.

Hoff, L. A. (1989). *People in crisis: Understanding and helping* (3rd ed.). Redwood City, CA: Addison-Wesley Health Sciences.

Holmes, R., & Rahe, R. (1967). The social readjustment rating scale. *Journal of Psychosomatic Research, 11*(2), 213–218.

Kaplan, H. I., & Sadock, B. J. (1994). *Synopsis of psychiatry: Behavioral science, clinical psychiatry* (7th ed.). Baltimore: Williams & Wilkins.

Kaplan, H. I., & Sadock, B. J. (1995). *Comprehensive textbook of psychiatry/VI* (6th ed.). Baltimore: Williams & Wilkins.

Kiecolt-Glaser, J. K., & Glaser, R. (1992). Psychoneuroimmunology: Can psychological interventions modulate immunity? *Journal of Consulting Clinical Psychology, 60*(4), 569–575.

Krueger, D., & Krueger, G. R. (1991). How does the subjective experience of stress relate to the breakdown of the human immune system? *In Vivo, 5*(3), 207–215.

Kruger, S. (1992). Parents in crisis: Helping them cope with a seriously ill child. *Journal of Pediatric Nursing, 7*(2), 133–140.

Lynch, I., & Tiedje, L. B. (1991). Working with multiproblem families: An intervention model for community health nurses. *Public Health Nursing, 8*(3), 147–153.

McClowry, S. G. (1992). Family functioning during a critical illness: A systems theory perspective. *Critical Care Nursing Clinics of North America, 4*(4), 559–564.

McFarland, G. K., Wasli, E. L., & Gerety, E. K. (1992). *Nursing diagnoses and process in psychiatric mental health nursing* (2nd ed.). Philadelphia: J. B. Lippincott.

Moos, R. (1979). Coping with the crisis of physical illness. In A. Freeman, R. Sack, & P. Berger (Eds.), *Psychiatry for the primary care physician*. Baltimore: Williams & Wilkins.

Murray, G. B. (1991). Confusion, delirium, and dementia. In N. H. Cassem (Ed.), *Massachusetts General Hospital handbook of general Hospital psychiatry* (3rd ed.). St. Louis: Mosby Year Book.

O'Connor, S. (1991). Psychiatric liaison nursing in a changing health care system. In N. H. Cassem (Ed.), *Massachusetts General Hospital handbook of general hospital psychiatry* (3rd ed.). St. Louis: Mosby Year Book.

Papero, D. V. (1990). *Bowen family systems theory*. Boston: Allyn and Bacon.

Pender, S. B. (1993). Critical care unit family support sessions: Using postvention principles in a medical setting. *Crisis, 14*(1), 8–10.

Piaget, J., & Inhelder, B. (1969). *Psychology of the child*. New York: Basic Books.

Pollin, I. S., & Holland, J. (1992). A model for counseling the medically ill: The Linda Pollin Foundation approach. Introduction. *General Hospital Psychiatry, 14*(6 Suppl), 1S–2S.

Rambur, B. (1991). Human environments, phenomena, crises, and lifestyles. Unifying concepts of nursing curriculum. *Nursing and Health Care, 12*(9), 464–468.

Rosenbaum, J. F., & Pollack, M. H. (1991). Anxiety. In N. H. Cassem (Ed.), *Massachusetts General Hospital handbook of general hospital psychiatry* (3rd ed.). St. Louis: Mosby Year Book.

Schwab, J. J., Stephenson, J. J., & Ice, J. F. (1993). *Evaluating family mental health: History, epidemiology, and treatment issues*. New York: Plenum Press.

Smith, L. (1990). Crisis intervention: Theory and practice. In J. Mezzich & B. Zimmer, *Emergency psychiatry*. Madison, CT: International Universities Press.

Teasdale, K. (1993). Information and anxiety: A critical reappraisal. *Journal of Advanced Nursing, 18*(7), 1125–1132.

Weisman, A. D. (1991). Coping with illness. In N. H. Cassem (Ed.), *Massachusetts General Hospital handbook of general hospital psychiatry* (3rd ed.). St. Louis: Mosby Year Book.

CHAPTER 17

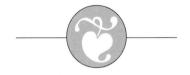

Psychosocial Intervention With Ineffective Coping Responses to Physical Illness: Anxiety-Related

Pamela Minarik

Physical illness, injury, and/or disability are important events in a person's life, whether catastrophic, acute, or chronic. These events may occur as an admission to a hospital, care received in an ambulatory setting, or care given at home. Such events are likely to be stressful or even provoke a crisis, severely taxing a person's coping abilities and resources. The way people respond and cope depends upon their perception of the situation and the meaning of it for the person and family members involved. Each family member is affected; the normal dynamics of the family are shifted temporarily or permanently by changes in functioning of one or more of its members.

THE COPING RESPONSE

Coping is a dynamic, constantly changing process serving two overriding functions: man-agement or alteration of the problem causing distress (*problem-focused coping*) and regulation of distress (*emotion-focused coping*). Coping effectiveness in a specific situation is based on both functions. A person who manages a problem effectively but at great emotional cost cannot be said to be coping effectively, nor is a person who regulates emotions successfully but does not deal with the source of the problem (Lazarus & Folkman, 1984).

Coping responses are cognitive and behavioral efforts—anything that the person thinks or does to manage specific external and/or internal demands, regardless of how well or badly it works. "Coping should not be equated with mastery over the environment; many sources of stress cannot be mastered, and ef-

Patricia Barry: *Psychosocial Nursing:*
Care of Physically Ill Patients and Their Families, 3rd ed.
© 1996 Lippincott–Raven Publishers

fective coping under these conditions is that which allows the person to tolerate, minimize, accept, or ignore what cannot be mastered" (Lazarus & Folkman, 1984, p. 140).

Coping is based on *appraisal*. Often not conscious, appraisal is an evaluative cognitive process that intervenes between the situation and the reaction. People appraise a situation based on what is important to them, their knowledge or experience with the situation, their beliefs, commitments, vulnerabilities, values, goals, and coping styles and capacities. The meaning of a situation to a person shapes the emotional and behavioral response; emotions shift as the meaning of the illness situation shifts. The two main evaluative issues are "Am I in trouble or being [benefited], now or in the future, and in what way?" and "What, if anything, can be done about it?" (Lazarus & Folkman, 1984, p. 31). Factors in a situation that make it stressful are unfamiliarity, uncertainty, ambiguity, physical characteristics of the setting, and the effectiveness of social support, including the staff. These factors affect the person's sense of control.

The nursing diagnosis of *ineffective individual coping* is defined as impairment of a person's adaptive behaviors and problem-solving abilities in meeting life's demands and roles (Kim, McFarland, & McLane, 1993). The effectiveness of a coping strategy depends on the extent to which it is appropriate to the internal and/or external demands of the situation. For coping to be effective, there also must be a good match or fit between coping efforts and the person's values, goals, commitments, beliefs, and preferred styles of coping.

Most people try to maintain control and manage the stress of physical illness or injury with their characteristic coping responses, such as maintaining hope, suppressing feelings, talking about feelings, seeking information, relying on experts, and using humor. If these mechanisms fail in a situation appraised as stressful, people may turn to more primitive mechanisms such as denial and aggressive behavior. If there is a tendency to use coping strategies that are inappropriate or a misfit, the person's adaptation over the long term could be affected (Lazarus & Folkman, 1984).

When the psychological stress of illness is too great, patients manifest emotions and behaviors that present difficulties for care providers. Then patients are said to be coping ineffectively and the responses seen as maladaptive. Automatic processes, such as defense mechanisms (see Chapter 3), may also lead to maladaptive response patterns. Because a person may cope effectively in one context and not in another, it is useful to ask, "Coping with what? Ineffectively according to whom?" Through the coping efforts of the person and the availability and strength of a support system, coupled with thoughtful interventions by care providers, coping can be more effective.

Ineffective coping responses related to anxiety are described in this chapter. These include unusual levels of anxiety; post-trauma response; maladaptive denial; demanding, noncompliant, or manipulative behavior; and cognitive disorder or "ICU syndrome." Anxiety is a normal albeit distressing response to the stress of physical illness. Cognitive impairment and ICU syndrome (delirium) will be described in this chapter because many of the associated behaviors mimic and are mistaken for problems in coping. Delirium, anxiety, and depression can increase the severity of physical illness, prolong hospital stay, complicate the course of treatment, increase the utilization of health services, and increase patient disability (Billings, 1990). Because of their continuous contact with patients, nurses can recognize the more subtle signs of these disorders and obtain needed diagnosis and treatment, thereby decreasing morbidity and cost.

Each section of the chapter includes a description of the anxiety-related response and recommended interventions. In all instances, if symptoms persist despite interventions, or are severe, psychiatric or psychiatric nursing consultation should be requested to ensure the patient's safety, emotional comfort, and future adaptation. Consultation may also be justified to reduce the stress of care providers in a prolonged, difficult situation. The consultant may be able to recommend alternative interventions that will be more helpful and promote effective coping for all concerned.

THE PATIENT WHO IS ANXIOUS

The experience of *anxiety* is a universal part of human existence, especially when someone is physically ill. Vague and without a known object or event, or out of proportion to known events, it is a feeling of apprehension, tension, and uneasiness (Maxmen & Ward, 1995). Anxiety is a normal alerting response that results from a real or perceived threat to a person's biological, psychological, or social integrity, esteem, identity, or status. It occurs in response to things that actually happen or in response to how we think about things happening in the past, present, or future. The greater the threat, the greater the anxiety response. People with a strong need for control may experience higher levels of anxiety during such situations. The anxious person is unaware of the specific cause of his or her feelings.

Fear is the same as anxiety except that it is caused by consciously recognized, realistic danger. Fear of dying often accompanies illness and treatment. Because anxiety is significantly associated with post-trauma disorder and denial is a defense against anxiety, these topics will be discussed following this section.

Anxiety may occur as a reaction to the psychological stress of illness. It may also occur as a symptom of a medical condition (see Box 17-1) or as an anxiety disorder secondary to the use, intoxication, or withdrawal from drugs (see Box 17-2), or as a primary psychiatric (anxiety) disorder. An anxiety disorder may predate the development of the physical illness. Anxiety is a prominent feature of delirium and is often a manifestation of depression (Badger, 1994).

A wide variety of signs and symptoms accompany mild, moderate, severe, and panic levels of anxiety. Especially in persons who use avoidance coping patterns, anxiety may escalate into an agitated, hypervigilant response. This is a *maladaptive coping response* that occurs in a situation appraised as highly dangerous and time-pressured, with no perceived escape. This response manifests itself as excessive attentiveness to the point of distractibility, severe anxiety, restlessness, morbid preoccupation with frightening images of what could go wrong, and a search for a way out of danger.

Overwhelmed with feelings of helplessness and loss of control, the person's problem-solving is impaired. Hypervigilant behaviors range from heightened alertness and repetitive, pressured questioning of anyone nearby to full-blown panic. A potent antecedent condition of hypervigilance is a "near-miss," a harrowing or life-threatening experience that overwhelms coping. The memory creates psychological havoc. Serious illness and its treatment, especially in the complex environment of the hospital, may foster a state of hypervigilance (Leavitt & Minarik, 1989).

Skill in early recognition of anxiety is essential so that care providers can intervene immediately to alleviate symptoms to prevent escalation and loss of control. Anxiety is highly

---

BOX 17-1	**Medical Conditions Associated with Anxiety**

Endocrine conditions: hyper- and hypothyroidism, hyper- and hypoparathyroidism, pheochromocytoma, hypoglycemia, hyperadrenocorticism (Cushing's disease)
Cardiovascular conditions: congestive heart failure, pulmonary embolism, arrhythmia
Respiratory conditions: chronic obstructive pulmonary disease, pneumonia, hyperventilation
Metabolic conditions: vitamin B_{12} deficiency, porphyria, hypomagnesemia
Neoplasms: Islet cell adenomas, pheochromocytoma
Neurological conditions: neoplasms, vestibular dysfunction, encephalitis, multiple sclerosis, myasthenia gravis, peripheral neuropathy

Information adapted from DSM-IV, 1994; Billings, 1990.

BOX 17-2	**Drugs That May Cause Anxiety**	

Associated with intoxication
  alcohol
  amphetamine and related
    substances
  caffeine
  cannabis
  cocaine
  hallucinogens
  marijuana
  nicotine
  inhalants
  phencyclidine and related
    substances
  other or unknown substances

Associated with withdrawal
  alcohol
  cocaine
  sedatives, hypnotics, and
    anxiolytics
  other or unknown substances

Medications reported to evoke anxiety symptoms
  anesthetics and analgesics
  sympathomimetics or other bronchodilators
  anticholinergics
  insulin
  thyroid preparations
  oral contraceptives
  antihistamines
  antiparkinsonian medications
  corticosteroids
  antihypertensive and cardiovascular medications
  anticonvulsants
  lithium carbonate
  antipsychotic medications
  antidepressant medications

Substances reported to evoke anxiety symptoms
  heavy metals
  toxins

Information adapted from DSM-IV, 1994.

contagious and easily communicated between people. In addition, therapeutic effectiveness can be severely compromised when nurses fail to recognize and manage their own anxiety.

Responses to anxiety can be *adaptive*. Anxiety can be a powerful motivating force for productive problem-solving and achievement. Talking, crying, sleeping, exercising, deep breathing, imagery, and relaxation techniques are adaptive strategies used to relieve anxiety. Responses to anxiety also can be *maladaptive*. Maladaptive patterns may include automatic psychological processes and behaviors such as obsessive-compulsive hand-washing rituals, aggressive acting out, withdrawal and isolation, overeating, drinking, gambling or spending, and drug use or sexual overactivity.

NURSING INTERVENTION

Recognition of Anxiety

Nursing intervention begins with recognition of the signs and symptoms of anxiety (see Table 17-1).

Anxiety occurs along a continuum. Lazarus and Folkman's (1984) differentiation of problem-focused coping and emotion-focused coping provides a framework for a discussion of intervention strategies matched to the continuum of responses. As a person moves along the continuum, the problem causing the distress is lost sight of and distress itself becomes the focus of attention. Intervention strategies can be divided into *preventive* and *treatment* strategies and can be used with patients and family members in a variety of settings (see Fig. 17-1).

Before assuming that anxiety is primarily psychological, review the patient's record for recent changes in medical condition and/or medications. Ask whether the patient was taking medications for "nerves," depression, or insomnia to determine whether drugs were inappropriately discontinued or whether anxiety symptoms predated the current illness. Also ask about over-the-counter medications, illicit drugs, alcohol intake, and smoking history. Document observations and findings and communicate them to other members of the treatment team (Badger, 1994).

TABLE 17–1
Responses to Anxiety

Anxiety level	Physiologic	Cognitive/Perceptual	Emotional/Behavioral
Mild	Vital signs normal. Minimal muscle tension. Pupils normal, constricted.	Perceptual field is broad. Awareness of multiple environmental and internal stimuli. Thoughts may be random, but controlled.	Feelings of relative comfort and safety. Relaxed, calm appearance and voice. Performance is automatic; habitual behaviors occur here.
Moderate	Vital signs normal or slightly elevated. Tension experienced; may be uncomfortable or pleasurable (labeled as "tense" or "excited")	Alert; perception narrowed, focused. Optimum state for problem solving and learning. Attentive.	Feelings of readiness and challenge, energized. Engage in competitive activity and learn new skills. Voice, facial expression interested or concerned.
Severe	Fight or flight response. Autonomic nervous system excessively stimulated (vital signs increased, diaphoresis increased, urinary urgency and frequency, diarrhea, dry mouth, appetite decreased, pupils dilated). Muscles rigid, tense. Senses affected; hearing decreased, pain sensation decreased.	Perceptual field greatly narrowed. Problem-solving difficult. Selective attention (focus on one detail). Selective inattention (block out threatening stimuli). Distortion of time (things seem faster or slower than actual). Dissociative tendencies, vigilambulism (automatic behavior).	Feels threatened; startles with new stimuli; feels on "overload." Activity may increase or decrease (may pace, run away, wring hands, moan, shake, stutter, become very disorganized or withdrawn, freeze in position/unable to move). May seem and feel depressed. Demonstrates denial; may complain of aches or pains; be agitated or irritable. Need for space increased. Eyes may dart around room or gaze may be fixed. May close eyes to shut out environment.
Panic	Above symptoms escalate until sympathetic nervous system release occurs. Person may become pale, blood pressure decreases, hypotension. Muscle coordination poor. Pain, hearing sensations minimal.	Perception totally scattered or closed. Unable to take in stimuli. Problem solving and logical thinking improbable. Perception of unreality about self, environment, or event. Dissociation may occur.	Feels helpless with total loss of control. May be angry, terrified; may become combative or totally withdrawn, cry, run. Completely disorganized. Behavior is usually extremely active or inactive.

From Fortinash & Holoday-Worret, 1995, p. 20. Used with permission.

If a readily treatable cause for the patient's anxiety is not apparent, calmly approach the patient and help him or her to recognize and label the anxiety. Start the conversation by simply asking, "How are you feeling?" or "Mr. Jones, you look very nervous. Are you worried about something?" and/or "What happened just before you had these feelings?" (Badger, 1994; Fortinash & Holoday-Worret, 1991).

Often patients are able to identify the cause of their anxiety and coping skills they have used in the past; when they do, their discomfort decreases. The patient's anxiety may be greatly reduced by opening up discussion of concerns believed to be painful, frightening, or shameful, such as being dependent or accepting help. Use open-ended questions, reflection, clarification and/or empathic remarks, such as "So you're discouraged about being here so long," "You believe your condition is worsening?," "This must be very difficult for you" (Badger, 1994; Fortinash & Holoday-Worret, 1991). Help the patient to identify and build upon previously successful coping methods and integrate them with new ones, using statements such as "What has helped you get through difficult times like this in the past? How can we help you use those methods now?" "Let's talk about some new strategies that may fit in your situation." Assist the patient in identifying significant supportive individuals who can help either with tasks or emo-

Anxiety Level	Interventions
Level 1 Mild ↓ to ↓ Moderate	**Preventive Strategies** • Concrete objective preparatory information. • Event warning. • Provide opportunity for control and participation (teach direct coping skills). • Acknowledge fears. • Explore near-miss events in patient's situation. • Control pain. • Reduce sensory deprivation, isolation.
Level 2 Moderate ↓ to ↓ Severe	**Treatment Strategies** • Use of regular support person as "emotional anchor." • Encourage expression of feelings, doubts, and fears. • Explore near-miss events, past and present. • Provide accurate information for realistic restructuring of fearful ideas. • Teach focusing, breathing, relaxation, imagery techniques for anxiety reduction. • Use massage, touch, physical exercise. • Control pain. • Evaluate use of anti-anxiety medications. • Delay procedures to promote patient control and composure. • Call on expert resources.
Level 3 Panic ↓	• Stay with the patient (take shorter shifts). • Maintain calm atmosphere, reduce stimulation. • Use anti-anxiety medications, monitor carefully. • Ensure adequate pain control. • Use focusing and breathing techniques. • Use demonstration. • Repeat realistic reassurances. • Repeat simple answers. • Call on expert resources.

FIGURE 17-1. Continuum of interventions for the anxiety response. (Adapted from Leavitt, M., & Minarik, P. [1989]. The agitated, hypervigilant response. In B. Riegel & D. Ehrenreich. *Psychological aspects of critical care nursing*. Rockville, MD: Aspen. Used with permission. Copyright © 1989 Aspen Publishers, Inc.)

tional support (Fortinash & Holoday-Worret, 1991).

Remember that personal presence and body language are powerful communicators and can be an effective treatment for anxiety. Convey calm attentiveness and interest. If possible, sit down, maintain eye contact, listen carefully, and do not hurry the patient. Explore the factors contributing to the situation and offer appropriate reassurance (Badger, 1994).

Preventive Strategies
(Leavitt & Minarik, 1989)

Provide concrete, objective preparatory information. Exaggerated fears or incomplete un-

derstanding about an illness, procedure, test, or medication may be the basis for the patient's anxiety. Expose the person to preparatory information that describes both the subjective and objective experiences of the specific health care event using concrete and objective terminology (Christman, Kirchhoff, & Oakley, 1992). Also known as mental rehearsal, stress inoculation, and preparatory sensory information, concrete objective preparatory information allows for the development of stress tolerance and coping mechanisms under less urgent and more supportive conditions.

The opportunity to prepare, however, should not be forced on those who prefer avoidance coping patterns. Encourage the patient to ask questions and provide preparatory information in as much or as little detail as requested. Anxiety hinders retention, so present information in understandable terms and continue to repeat and rephrase it until the patient retains it. Remember that too much information at one time may cause or worsen anxiety (Badger, 1994).

Provide stressful event warning. Notifying the person in advance of a stressful event allows the person time to prepare. In addition, information as to the person's role during procedures allows for mental rehearsal in advance.

Acknowledge fear. Be available and encourage the expression of feelings. Use an approach that is indirect and receptive to the patient's inner fears, rather than a confrontational one. The nurse's availability can be structured to match other responsibilities. Do not deny that problems exist or reassure anxious people that "everything will be fine." Do not avoid the anxious person. Avoidance increases vulnerability, isolation, helplessness, and anxiety. Early, structured intervention will save time in the long run.

Increase opportunities for control through decision making, activity, sensory stimulation, and interpersonal support. Physical illness can seriously disrupt a person's sense of control and increase anxiety. Constantly pushing the nurse call button or making telephone calls for trivial requests may be an attempt on the part of the anxious person to control the behavior of care providers or reassure themselves of the presence of others. Trying to meet the patient's every demand may frustrate the nurse, possibly leading to avoidance of the patient, which may worsen the patient's anxiety. Using a firm, matter-of-fact manner, set boundaries, such as asking the patient to save up requests for when checked on at regular intervals. It is important to follow through. Help the patient to make distinctions between what is controllable, partially controllable, or not controllable. Provide opportunity for decision making and choices within the boundaries to enhance sense of control (Badger, 1994).

Even when a patient cannot determine the cause of anxiety, it is possible to have a constructive means of controlling it. Decisions about timing interventions or scheduling the day or the visit provide patients with choices that are possible. Pain control is an essential part of promoting self-control (see Chapter 21). Sufficient analgesia reduces distress associated with procedures and prevents near-misses.

Reduce sensory deprivation and isolation. Sensory deprivation and isolation may heighten the patient's attention to various signals in the environment. Without the means to interpret these signals accurately and to be reassured and feel in control, the patient may allow signals to take on frightening meanings which make him or her feel abandoned and helpless. Feeling isolated and helpless increases the sense of vulnerability and danger.

Increase patient and family participation in care. Participation in care is a direct coping skill that can be taught to both the patient and family members. Consider first the question of how much participation, and by whom. With interested, attentive people and at a level that "fits," participation reduces helplessness and allows a sense of control. Participation may also help with the resolution of ineffective denial.

Build hope. Provide information about possible positive outcomes to reduce any tendency to avoidance behavior. Hope may be built around the ability to cope with the situation.

Treatment Strategies
(Leavitt & Minarik, 1989)

Presence of supportive persons. Supportive people, especially if they are familiar to the patient, can act as an "emotional anchor." The emotional anchor can be a staff member, a family member, or a friend. Family and friends may need coaching to handle a situation and prevent getting panicked themselves.

Expression of feelings, doubts, and fears. Such expressions provide an opportunity to correct or restructure unrealistically fearful appraisals. Do not aggressively encourage the expression of feelings. Cast doubt without direct confrontation and provide accurate information. Help the patient to identify any misconceptions, question automatic, anxiety-provoking thoughts, and substitute a more realistic view. Accurate information allows restructuring of perceptions and lends predictability to the situation. Zealous confrontation of unrealistic perceptions only serves to reinforce them.

Exploration of near-miss events. Exposure to near-misses in the immediate environment, such as another patient having a cardiac arrest, should be explored and realistically evaluated in view of the patient's situation.

Evaluation of antianxiety medications. When used, medications should be given concurrently with other interventions and monitored. Overuse can produce a delirium from intoxication, especially in the aged person.

Pain control. Medicate well in advance of painful or frightening procedures. Severe anxiety and attention focused on pain may increase the need.

Promotion of patient control. When a patient is very frightened of a particular procedure, wait, if possible, until the patient has regained enough composure to make the decision to proceed. Pushing ahead when the patient is panicked may save time in the immediate situation but it will increase the patient's sense of vulnerability and helplessness, possibly adding time over the long term.

Management of panic. When anxiety reaches panic, deal with the persistent thoughts by acknowledgment: "I know you are very frightened right now. I will stay with you." Use brief, simple statements. When a patient escalates or suddenly experiences severe to panic levels of anxiety, guide the patient to a smaller, quieter area, away from other people if possible, using quiet reassurance. Provide a calm, safe presence and reduce all environmental stimulation. Help the patient focus on a single object (see below) and guide the patient in recognizing the physical features of the object while breathing rhythmically. Consider the administration of prescribed anxiolytic medication.

Massage, touch, and physical exercise. Massage releases muscle tension and may also elicit emotional release. Physical exercise reduces muscle tension and other physiological effects of anxiety while providing a constructive way of releasing energy when direct problem solving is impossible or ineffective. Therapeutic touch is a treatment modality based on energy exchange between healer and patient that usually does not involve actual body contact (Macrae, 1988). It can provide both a soothing presence and reduce the physiological sequelae associated with anxiety. For further information, see Krieger (1981) and Quinn (1992), and Chapter 22.

Relaxation, Breathing, Focusing, and Imagery Techniques

1. *Relaxation techniques.* Relaxation techniques are usually effective for patients with mild to moderate anxiety who are able to concentrate and are interested in using them. Some relaxation techniques take time to learn and are more effective with regular practice. Relaxation techniques reduce awareness of the environment by focusing inward with deliberate concentration on breathing, a sound, or an image and suggestions of muscle relaxation. Progressive relaxation and autogenic relaxation are the most commonly used techniques and take approximately 15 minutes. It is helpful to start with the patient lying still in a quiet room with arms and legs uncrossed, the neck supported with a small pillow, the thighs supported above the knees with a pillow, and a light cover over the patient. Periodically during the technique, suggest that the patient can feel particular body parts supported softly but firmly by the pillow and mattress to promote a feeling of lightness or floating. The imagery script in Box 17-3 begins with a progressive relaxation technique.

2. *Deep breathing exercises.* Simple and easy to learn, breathing exercises provide slow, rhythmic, controlled breathing patterns that relax and distract the patient while slowing the heart rate, thus decreasing anxious feelings. Ask the pa-

tient to pay attention to his or her breathing while breathing normally. Then ask the patient to take a couple of slow, deep breaths all the way into the abdomen and say the word "relax" with each exhalation. Encourage practice throughout the day.

When teaching deep breathing, photographs and drawings may help patients visualize their actions. Show what lungs look like by using the images in a book such as *The Incredible Machine* (1986). Emphasize the size of the lungs filling the rib cage and demonstrate this by asking patients to place their hands on the lower ribs or waist. Ask patients to inhale deeply and direct the breath into their hands and feel the air move their diaphragm and ribs. Suggest imagining the lungs like an upside down cherry tree fully in bloom (Diane Scott, personal communication, 1990). Inhaling brings the air through the trunk, and out through the branches to the little air sacs that fluff up like a profusion of pink cherry blossoms gently blowing in the wind.

3. *Focusing on a single object and breathing techniques.* Useful for patients with severe to panic levels of anxiety, focusing repeatedly on one person or object in the room helps the patient to disengage from all other stimuli and promotes control. It is especially helpful when combined with demonstration and coaching of slow, rhythmic breathing by a nurse with a calm, low-pitched voice. These techniques give the patient a way of achieving self-control, which is desirable when the stress reaction is excessive and when the stressful event cannot be changed or avoided. Focusing and deep breathing techniques can be used without prior practice and during extreme stress.

4. *Listening to music or soothing nature sounds.* Soothing sounds reduce anxiety by providing a tranquil environment and promoting recall of pleasant memories. Music may serve to interrupt the stress response through distraction from stressful stimuli or direct action on the sympathetic nervous system (White, 1992). Mu-

sic recommended for relaxation is primarily of string composition, low-pitched, with a simple and direct musical rhythm and a tempo of approximately 60 beats per minute (White, 1992). Music with flute, *a cappella* voice, and synthesizer is also effective.

5. *Imagery or visualization.* Imagery inhibits anxiety by invoking an opposing, peaceful mental image, including memories, dreams, fantasies, and visions. Imagery is the deliberate, goal-directed use of the natural capacities of the imagination. Using all the senses, it serves as a bridge for connecting body, mind, and spirit (Dossey, 1988). Often combined with relaxation, imagery promotes coping with illness by anxiety reduction, enhanced self-control, feeling expression, symptom relief, healing promotion, and dealing with role changes (Stephens, 1993). Regular practice of imagery is essential to success over the long term. Guided imagery to decrease the intensity of pain or anxiety should not be attempted the first time in periods of extreme stress.

6. *Using imagery in conversation.* Use of imagery in conversation is subtle and spontaneous. We often are unaware that our questions and statements to patients include imagery. The deliberate use of imagery involves listening to the language, beliefs, and metaphors of the patient, and focusing on the positive aspects. Imagery in conversation is easily combined with routine activities.

The following are guidelines for developing the ability to use images in conversation (McCaffery & Beebe, 1989):

a. Identify a specific symptom relief measure. Explain how it relieves the symptom by using words that paint a mental picture, create sounds, or produce tactile-kinesthetic sensations. Create a positive expectation of relief. For example, when an analgesic is given, you could say, "It's as if the medicine is slowly floating through your body to find your pain and make it smaller, leaving feelings of comfort." Do not say, "If this doesn't help, there is another medica-
(text continues on p. 312)

BOX 17-3	**Imagery script**

Imagery is a fast way to connect body-mind-spirit by quieting the busy mind and allowing the mind to focus on a particular event. It is one way to learn to use your "wise self" to promote healing. . . I will start with a relaxation technique. . . You can communicate with me by raising your right index finger for yes and your left index finger for no. . . You are in complete control at all times during this session and you may stop the session at any time by simply opening your eyes. . . .

As you begin, pay attention to the patient's reactions—restlessness, agitation, breathing patterns, and facial expressions.

. . . I want to ask you, if you will, to allow yourself time to withdraw within. . . to take time for you. . . to rejuvenate and refresh yourself. . . And to begin I would like to ask you to count backwards with me from five to one. . . As I count backwards I would like to ask your subconscious mind to go back into comfort at the rate of one-fifth at a time. . . so that by the time we get to one, you can be as deeply relaxed as possible at this point in time. . . As you breathe in and out, ask your body to allow the relaxed feelings to flow all the way through. . . *five*

Speak slowly. Do not rush the session. Allow the person time to feel the gradual reduction in tension.

. . .As we go down (pause), ask your subconscious mind to release any unnecessary tensions in muscle groups like your eyes, eyelids, forehead, scalp . . . (pause) nostrils, lips and cheeks. . . releasing unnecessary tension that you don't wish to keep. . . It is not a requirement, simply an invitation that you are welcome to accept. . . Give up any tension around your cheeks, chin, and jaw. . . As you do this, you may find your mouth opening. . . It is a sign that your muscles are letting go. . . *four*. . . This is an internal exercise for your education, comfort. . .

Notice that the patient is given permission to have his or her own reactions to the treatment. There is no one right way to do this.

. . . Let go of any excess tensions across your neck and throat, down your biceps, triceps, past your elbow, forearm, wrist. . . breathing—calm, regular. . . even letting go of the tension of the little muscles between your ribs. . . Each time you let go of air, you might want to, if you wish, imagine blowing out tension with it, so that each and every breath becomes more relaxing. . . calm regular breathing. . . *three*. . . Just letting go of the tensions down your spine. . . each individual vertebra, each muscle in your vertebrae. . . almost as if warm water is being poured down the inside of the vertebrae and radiating warmth and comfort throughout your torso. . . all the way down. . . letting go of the tensions along your sides, abdomen, hips and seat. . . Very good. . . You're halfway there. . .

Remember to monitor facial expressions and bodily tension.

. . . Deeper and deeper into comfort you can go, at your own pace, in your own way. . . thighs, letting go. . . knees. . . letting go of tension along your calves and ankles. . . breathing and relaxing. . . *two* . . . heels letting go . . . And as you get down to your toes, you might want to continue letting your mind empty itself, much like that water, that warm water, going down your spine . . . releasing the cold tension . . . It's coming from your head and just emptying itself . . . cool forehead . . . *one* . . . as deep and comfortable as you wish, fully relaxed . . . That's right, nothing to do.

The pain reduction imagery begins here.

. . . Now let your imagination take you to a place that feels safe and comfortable.

It works best to have the patients choose a place where they have experienced pleasant memories.

BOX 17-3	**Imagery Script** (Continued)

Imagine a smooth white beach. . .

In this script we are using a beach scene.

. . . You walk through a garden filled with flowers to reach the beach . . . The air is filled with the gentle fragrance from the flowers
. . . As you reach the beach you see a hammock tied between two trees
. . . You go over to the hammock and lie down . . . The texture of the hammock is soft and nubby . . . You can feel the warm sun against your skin . . . You can feel a gentle breeze . . . Notice the sea gulls as they dip and glide on the wind currents . . . Hear the faint sounds of laughter in the background

Use all the senses to trigger imagic thought. Some patients work better with one sense than another. Speak slowly to allow time to create the scene.

. . . You have not been this comfortable for a long time . . . The hammock swings gently back and forth . . . back and forth . . .

Do not rush the patient. Time yourself if necessary so your own anxiety about using guided imagery does not make you speak too quickly.

. . . Nothing to do but relax and enjoy your special place . . . You look out over the crystal, clear, aquamarine waters and notice a sail boat slowly moving off in the distance . . .

Creating a background and a foreground adds to the imagery.

. . . Enjoy the differences in hues, as the light plays on the water . . . swinging, comfortably swinging in the hammock, with a breeze that keeps you at just the right temperature . . . Hear the water as it laps on the shore . . . and the wind as it ripples through the palm trees . . . And now, if you wish, get up and move to the water . . . Feel the cool water as it reaches your toes . . . Feel the sand on your feet as you slowly enter the water . . . As you swim through the water, each individual water molecule touching you, in its own way, finding a way to soothe and calm you . . . you are finding that new and ever emerging more comfortable you . . . It is nice to swim freely, comfortably through the water . . . Finally, you get out of the water and return to the hammock and lie down . . . You are relaxed and pleasantly tired . . . As the hammock moves slowly back and forth, you think back over the last few minutes . . . You enjoy your new-found freedom, your complete sense of comfort . . . You can retreat to this place of comfort whenever you wish . . . It is a place especially for you . . . You can change it . . .

Work toward adjusting the imagery to suit each patient.

. . . and enjoy it as much as you wish . . . Use this relaxation/imagery technique to escape the difficulties and pressures of daily life . . . and when you are ready to return from your special place, count slowly from one to five . . . Open your eyes and stretch your arms and legs . . . move around in your chair . . . You are awake and alert . . . feeling rested and comfortable.

Don't talk to the patient immediately after the session is over . . . Allow the patient to initiate the discussion . . . Your own anxiety over learning imagery may lead you to start conversation too quickly.

From Stephens, R.L. (1993). Imagery: A strategic intervention to empower clients. Part II—A practical guide. *Clinical Nurse Specialist* 7(5), p. 237–238. Copyright Williams & Wilkins. Adapted with permission.

tion I can give you." This can create an expectation of ineffectiveness.

b. Use words and phrases that convey relaxing, comforting, and healing images. Use such words as *softer, melting, dissolving, smooth, lighter, quieting, releasing, sinking into the soft support, healing, cooling* or *warming, letting go, soothing, less and less, loosening, powerful*, and *effective*. Notice your natural use of these words and practice using them more often.

c. Use permissive language—such as *may, can, might, should, let, allow*—that provides a direction, not a command.

d. When a patient is given an image of what causes a symptom, try also to give an image of how the symptom will subside or be relieved.

e. Use only those images or descriptors that are comfortable for you.

Be aware of the language used to describe the effects of medication or treatment, because descriptions can affect the patient's attitude and response. Nurses and physicians sometimes refer to amphotericin, the common antifungal drug, as "amphoterrible." One patient who heard this name said it frightened her, thinking something terrible, rather than something helpful, was going to happen when she took it.

Many people who are ill find their minds filled with fearful pictures of disaster with resultant feelings of helplessness, loss of control, and hopelessness. Providers can enhance hope, self-esteem, and a sense of control if they give empowering, healing messages, saying how they think treatment or medication will help (Minarik, 1993).

PHARMACOLOGIC MANAGEMENT OF ANXIETY

Anxiolytic medications are appropriate when the patient has moderate to severe anxiety or mild but persistent anxiety that is unresponsive to other interventions. Classes of drugs used for antianxiety effects include benzodiazepines, beta-blockers, antihistamine sedatives, sedatives with hypnotic effects, clonidine, and short-acting barbiturates. Use of nonbenzodiazepine antianxiety medications in

the physically ill is being studied (Badger, 1994; Wise & Taylor, 1990).

Benzodiazepines are the pharmacologic treatment of choice; they are effective at a standing dose, as necessary, or at night to aid sleep. The various benzodiazepines work equally well and the pharmacologic profile (such as fast to slow onset of action and sedative side effect) determines the choice in the physically ill. Those with a shorter half-life and accumulation of fewer active metabolites (such as lorazepam and oxazepam) are appropriate for the elderly and patients with liver disease. The most common side effect is sedation. Withdrawal symptoms may occur after chronic use.

A patient with depressive symptoms mixed with anxiety may be prescribed a tricyclic antidepressant or a selective serotonin reuptake inhibitor rather than a benzodiazepine. Patients with panic attacks also may be prescribed antidepressants. In patients with extreme fear or psychosis, such as those with delirium, low-dose neuroleptics are helpful. The most common neuroleptic prescribed for this purpose is haloperidol, as it is less potentially toxic to the physically ill person than other major tranquilizers. All pharmacologic treatments must be monitored for effectiveness and side effects.

EVALUATION

Evaluation of the effectiveness of interventions for anxiety includes observation of the anxiety level, self-control, sleep pattern, problem-solving ability, and ability to participate in care decisions. Look for a reduction in symptoms of severe anxiety and an increased sense of control and participation in care. The communicability of anxiety also provides a cue; the nurse's own sense of control is an indicator of whether the situation is being managed effectively.

THE PATIENT WITH POST-TRAUMA STRESS RESPONSE

The post-trauma response is defined as "the state in which an individual experiences a sustained, painful response to (an) overwhelming traumatic event(s)" (Kim, McFarland, & McLane, 1993). The response can be mild, moderate, or severe with symptoms falling on a continuum of post-trauma response to post-traumatic stress disorder (PTSD). Effects may be seen in a trauma victim, witnesses to an event, significant others, and health care workers who provide trauma care. Nurses as caregivers are in a position to assess and identify persons at risk. Not everyone exposed to a trauma will develop PTSD. Even without the full picture of PTSD symptoms, many people have significant readjustment issues following a trauma and benefit from nursing intervention. If a person uses adaptive coping skills and available support networks, the post-trauma response may not develop into PTSD (Ragaisis, 1994).

The defining feature of PTSD is the development of characteristic symptoms after exposure to an extreme traumatic stressor that is experienced with intense fear, helplessness, or horror (DSM-IV, 1994). It is experienced by normal people exposed to abnormally intense amounts of stress such as war, natural disasters, accidents, violent crime, or seeing a loved one killed or die suddenly (Ross & Wonders, 1993). Major symptoms include reexperiencing the traumatic event (intrusive memories, flashbacks, dreams); persistent avoidance of stimuli, thoughts, or feelings associated with the trauma; restricted responsiveness (general numbing, decreased affect, reduced interest, withdrawal from others); and persistent, increased arousal (difficulty sleeping, hypervigilance). Other symptoms include unpredictable episodes of explosive anger, exacerbations of substance abuse, thoughts of self-blame and guilt, anger at others, and interpersonal problems (Ross & Wonders, 1993). Persistent symptoms lasting 3 months or longer are considered to be chronic PTSD; symptoms of shorter duration may be thought of as an *adjustment disorder* or an *acute stress disorder* (*Diagnostic and Statistical Manual* [DSM-IV], 1994). In some patients, physical illness may precipitate PTSD (Hamner, 1994).

NURSING INTERVENTION

Social support interventions, including group and individual counseling, encourage verbal catharsis and identification of potential serious complications (Ross & Wonders, 1993). Most important are active listening to patients' detailed recollections and encouraging patients to identify specific aspects of the traumatic event that are most troubling. Ask patients to describe their feelings. One of the powerful effects of post-trauma response is that it conditions ongoing physiological sequelae, as if the body has frozen (Patricia Barry, personal communication). By talking about the traumatic event, patients gain some influence over their reactions to the memories.

Avoid judgmental statements that tell patients what to think, feel, and do. Assist patients in understanding their actual versus perceived roles in the traumatic event, and to separate areas where control is possible and those that are beyond control, to help them begin to let go of the sense of responsibility for the latter. Teach patients cognitive and behavioral strategies to manage anxiety and anger and encourage them to make their own choices about which ones are helpful.

Critical Incident Stress Debriefing (CISD) is a hybrid of crisis intervention that assists patients, families, and staff to normalize and master the stresses that result from being a witness to or a victim of violent acts. CISD is a facilitated, structured, formal process focused in the here-and-now. It consists of seven specific phases: an introduction phase, a fact phase, a thought phase, a reaction phase, a symptom phase, teaching about stress reactions and stress management skills, and a reentry phase to summarize and devise a future plan. Through encouragement of verbal expression and catharsis, the intervention helps to incorporate the thoughts and feelings associated with the traumatic experience into one's world view (Ragaisis, 1994).

EVALUATION

Outcome criteria include verbalization of awareness of symptoms of stress and anxiety, identification of events that trigger recollections, utilization of adaptive coping skills, a greater sense of self-control, identification of support systems, and identification of normal grief reactions.

THE PATIENT WHO IS DENYING

Denial minimizes fear and anxiety. In situations of permanent disability, denial may be called *hope*. In trauma or cancer, an aspect of denial is the belief that medical science will make a discovery that will change the outcome. Such denial does not hinder cooperation with care. Denial is a defense mechanism characterized by avoidance of disagreeable realities and unconscious refusal to face intolerable thoughts, feelings, needs, or desires. Denial may be functional, allowing time for emotional integration of overwhelming information or allowing a person to tolerate a chronic or progressive plight. During deterioration and decline, denial may be what helps the patient to face each day (Weisman, 1979).

Denial may be *adaptive* when it helps individuals get through a difficult, traumatic experience until they are better able to cope with reality (such as during the early stages of grief or when first diagnosed with a life-threatening illness). Denial can be *maladaptive* when a person persistently denies a serious problem (such as alcoholism, drug abuse, or the failure to seek medical attention for chest pain or a lump in the body that may be cancer). Negative repercussions of denial include refusal to submit to necessary or lifesaving treatments.

In studies of myocardial infarction and heart surgery patients, two types of denial have been reported: (1) *affective denial*, in which the patient denies anxiety or other painful symptoms or feelings, and (2) *cognitive denial*, in which the patient denies the nature and severity of the illness to various degrees. Studies have shown positive and negative outcomes associated with denial (Miller, 1989). Denial of illness during the acute hospital phase of MI is adaptive from a psychological and physiological standpoint, as it results in less anxiety and protects the patient from adverse effects of anxiety on the myocardium, leading to fewer days in intensive care, higher survival rates, and less cardiac dysfunction. Denial in the long run after discharge has been found to be maladaptive as the patient becomes less cooperative and compliant with recommendations and may deteriorate psychologically and physiologically (Billings, 1990).

Common situations in which ineffective denial occurs in the health care setting include learning about a catastrophic diagnosis such as cancer or AIDS, coping with a myocardial infarction or impending open-heart surgery, experiencing a traumatic injury, or dealing with a loved one's dying or death. In such circumstances, pervasive denial usually lasts a few days, gradually giving way to acknowledgment of the denied event and the feelings associated with it. When this does not occur, it is an indication that the threatening information or feelings continue to be too overwhelming to allow into conscious awareness.

NURSING INTERVENTION

The following analogy may be helpful in understanding how denial functions and in designing therapeutic intervention:

> If a person is very frightened, he might run into a room and barricade the doors and windows with anything available. He desperately needs to keep out the invader.
>
> Consider the invader seeking to enter the room. How might he be most successful, given these barricades and the state of the person taking refuge behind them? By battering in the door? By pounding on it and demanding to be let in? Or by talking gently so that the person inside is motivated to open the door?

The use of forceful confrontation in such a situation is unlikely to be successful; a gentle, indirect approach is usually more effective. Dealing with denial in the clinical situation is similar. The nurse can ask the patient and encourage the family to ask questions such as:

> "How are you (or your family) feeling about this illness?"
> "What have you been told about this illness?"
> "How do you think you will manage this illness when you go home?"

Similar questions can be asked of family members. Ask what they observe about their family member's condition. Their answers will indicate their grasp of the realistic aspects of the situation and their receptivity to more information. Provide objective observations of condition rather than comments on threatening implications. Encouraging the family to help provide care or be close to the patient during activities such as suctioning, turning, or intravenous line starts may also help them to begin to accept reality. Consistent information given repetitively over days is helpful.

A nonintrusive, questioning approach should yield a change in the denial in a few days. If the patient or family is unable to respond and continues to deny the illness beyond a few days or is unable to make important decisions about care, the denial is considered ineffective or maladaptive. At this point, consultation with liaison psychiatry should be considered. Continued ineffective denial may lead to difficulties with planning for future care, communication problems within the family, and so on.

Patients whose denial persists after the acute phase of illness may be less cooperative and compliant with treatment recommendations, may indulge in behavior threatening to health, and may deteriorate physically and psychologically. For example, a person recently diagnosed with arteriosclerotic heart disease may continue to smoke excessively. The nurse's intervention in this case should include the same nonintrusive questioning described above. In the example of the heart patient who continues to smoke heavily, the following questions can be used:

> "Mrs. Adams, what are the recommendations your health care provider has given you about smoking?"
> "How is your family reacting to your smoking?"
> "Tell me what you understand about how nicotine affects the blood vessels feeding your heart muscle."

If such questions result in continued ineffective denial by the patient, the nurse may consider a referral to counseling because of the self-destructive behavior, although this may not be a viable option because the denying person is not feeling any conscious emotional distress. The stress he or she is experiencing is more likely to be the result of the concerns of family, friends, and caregivers who are usually more distressed about the noncompliance. Family members may be more ready to benefit from counseling. If denial continues in spite of interventions, it may be necessary to recognize that ultimately, each person has responsibility for his or her own health.

THE PATIENT WHO IS DEMANDING, NONCOMPLIANT, AND/OR MANIPULATIVE

Some patients eventually tax the patience of caregivers because of their seemingly incessant demands for care, their dependency, and/or their manipulative behavior. Manipulative behavior, such as flattery, self-pity, helplessness, lying, playing staff against each other, hostility, intimidation, self-destructive threats, sexual innuendo and jokes, or use of vulgar language commonly occurs to gain attention, sympathy, dependence, or control (Keltner, Schwecke, & Bostrom, 1991; Sundeen et al., 1994). Many of these behaviors are characteristic of persons with personality disorders.

A *personality disorder* is defined as an "enduring pattern of inner experience and behavior that deviates markedly from the expectations of the individual's culture, is pervasive and inflexible, has an onset in adolescence or early adulthood, is stable over time, and leads to distress or impairment" (DSM-IV, 1994, p. 629). Such patients may also manifest behaviors called *entitlement* and *splitting*.

A person manifesting *entitlement* expects too much, views the world as owing him or her, and inevitably feels angry when staff fail to live up to the expectations. Manifestations of entitlement include frequent and excessive demands, angry affect, provocation of power struggles, easy feelings of rejection, rejection of care that is offered, and never feeling satisfied with received care because it is never enough (UCSF, 1995).

Splitting is a defense mechanism that prevents people from integrating positive and negative qualities of themselves or others into a cohesive image. When people use splitting, they view themselves or others as either all good or all bad at any given time, and behave correspondingly. Splitting behaviors include playing staff against one another with criticism or flattery, angry calls to those in authority, and manipulation (Sundeen et al., 1994; UCSF, 1995). Generally, people who use these coping mechanisms to relieve anxiety and tension lack insight and have no motivation to change because they feel no responsibility for their behavior (Daum, 1994). Because they are unlikely to want to change long-standing behavior patterns, nursing staff must develop approaches that minimize the negative impact.

Often these behaviors have the effect of staff anger, frustration, anxiety, helplessness, and embarrassment before they are recognized. Staff may not be conscious of their reactions to the patient. The patient care situation has the potential to deteriorate, with avoidance of assignment to the patient, avoidance of the patient's calls, negative comments about the patient among the staff, or polarized perceptions of the patient. These staff behaviors are signs that a systematic approach is needed. Avoidance of patients increases the avoided behavior due to the patient's anxiety and fear of abandonment.

NURSING INTERVENTION

The first interventions are to deal with staff reactions to the patient's behavior and maintain safety (Daum, 1994). If staff have an opportunity to share their negative reactions to the patient and attempts at behavioral intervention, they will learn that their responses are not unusual and they will be helped to develop effective interventions. The key intervention for splitting is continual communication among all the patient's care providers and consistent approaches to the patient's behavior. Safety is maintained by following appropriate policies and providing training regarding violence and the use of restraints (Daum, 1994).

Exploration of the cause of the patient's behavior (for example, delirium due to withdrawal or other factors, inadequate analgesia, staff avoidance resulting in increased anxiety) is essential for successful intervention with de-

manding and manipulative behavior. Communication must provide clarity, structure, and limit-setting. For example, confrontation directs attention to the patient's behavior and explores the consequences of it: "Jack, I've noticed that when you give me many compliments, you usually want something from me. When you do that, people are not likely to trust what you say." Power struggles and arguments are fruitless because they engage staff in giving attention to the patient, thereby actually rewarding the behavior.

It is important not to confront the patient about unrealistic demands by talking about the need to care for sicker patients; this will only increase anxiety and anger. To decrease excessive demands, use a proactive approach. Greet the patient early and talk about plans and sources of anxiety; acknowledge valid stressors in the situation. Explain any new procedures or treatments ahead of time. Provide opportunities for decision making and control. Give unsolicited attention when the patient has not called. Keep the patient well informed about changes in plans.

The intervention of limit-setting is a type of behavior modification best instituted early. Not a form of punishment, it should not be thought of only as a last resort when the patient is nearly out of control and the staff completely frustrated. It is a way of rewarding desirable behavior. Limit-setting involves directing attention to the behavior and its negative consequences, and suggesting alternate behavior with more positive consequences. Set limits on manipulative behaviors whenever they interfere with the patient's progress and the rights and safety of others (for example, yelling obscenities, breaking equipment, harming anyone). Signed contracts or agreements may be used. Limit-setting and contracting are most successful when the patient participates in the discussion and plan.

The steps in limit-setting begin with the nursing process as follows:

Assess the patient and diagnose the presenting problem. It is best to do this with others to ensure objectivity and decrease the impact of frustration.

Plan a limit-setting intervention designed to meet the patient's unique situation. It is helpful to schedule a formal meeting with an objective person from outside your unit, such as a psychiatric liaison nurse, who is specifically prepared to deal with this type of problem. In this meeting, develop a proposed plan to take to the patient. Interventions might include the nurse spending 5 minutes with the patient every 1½ hours, with the patient agreeing, in return, to call only in an emergency. The goal is to meet the patient's defined needs reasonably, so that the patient will eventually find it unnecessary to call indiscriminately.

Make an agreement with the patient about what he needs from the nursing staff and what the nursing staff needs from him. Tell the patient, in a low-key, nonthreatening manner, what it is that bothers the nursing staff. Emphasize the advantages the plan will have for him (e.g., knowing what to expect, more positive interactions). It is very important to allow the patient to discuss the plan. Revise the plan so it is acceptable to him. Contracting should not be done when a patient's emotional or intellectual functioning is so impaired that he is unable to understand or reason.

Implement the limit-setting approach. To ensure the success of limit-setting, outline the plan in appropriate written documentation to provide clear information to all staff who might be in contact with the patient. Unless everyone uses the approach, there will be no modification of the patient's behavior. Maintain consistency with all personnel.

Evaluate the effects of the limit-setting intervention. Modify the plan if indicated. Appraise the outcome of the intervention daily with the staff, and especially with the patient, and change the original expectations if necessary. When the patient is treated as a participating adult and given the opportunity to provide input, his behavior may become less child-like.

A limit-setting approach, especially if initiated early, will save time in the long run and can yield positive results for all concerned.

THE PATIENT WITH A COGNITIVE DISORDER OR "ICU SYNDROME"

Although cognitive disorders are organically based problems, the resultant behaviors are often viewed as problems in coping; therefore, they will be discussed in this chapter. The signs, symptoms, and causes for different types of cognitive disorders were presented in Chapter 11.

There are two main categories of cognitive disorders: delirium and dementia. *Delirium* manifests in different ways in different people, mimics other psychiatric disorders, develops over a short period of time, and fluctuates (waxes and wanes) during the course of a day, often with interspersed lucid intervals and is, therefore, often underdetected or misunderstood. It is often called "ICU syndrome." The essential feature of delirium is a disturbance of consciousness (DSM-IV, 1994). The altered consciousness may manifest as difficulties engaging the person in conversation due to impaired ability to focus, sustain, or shift attention. People who are delirious may experience memory impairment; disorientation; perceptual disturbances such as hallucinations; delusions; and language disturbances manifested by impaired ability to name objects, impaired ability to write, and/or rambling, irrelevant, or incoherent speech (DSM-IV, 1994).

"ICU syndrome" or "ICU psychosis" is generally not due to psychological stress or sensory overload alone, but develops due to altered brain function leading to a delirious state with psychotic features. Previously, it was believed to be due to stress felt by an individual in the foreboding ICU environment with little privacy, lack of sleep, and sensory overload. Current thinking is that delirium in the ICU is due to factors similar to those in other settings, the difference being that ICU patients react more severely because of their more severe illness. Stress and environmental factors play a contributory role (Eisendrath, 1994).

Dementia can be thought of as global intellectual decline with multiple cognitive deficits, especially in memory and the ability to learn new information. Memory impairment is common in both delirium and dementia; however, the person with a dementia only is alert and does not have the attention disturbance characteristic of a delirium. In dementia, symptoms are relatively stable rather than fluctuating (DSM-IV, 1994). Delirium can be superimposed on a dementia, as might occur when a person with memory impairment due to Alzheimer's disease is hospitalized for an orthopaedic procedure and receives anesthesia and analgesic agents.

For patients with cognitive disorders such as delirium and dementia, early recognition and intervention are essential to minimize patient morbidity and disability, prevent injury, maximize the use of intact functions, and minimize the necessity for impaired functions. Delirium may resolve quickly, except when a person has a coexisting dementia, in which case the symptoms are likely to persist for weeks. If the underlying etiological cause is promptly corrected or is self-limited, recovery is more likely to be complete (DSM-IV, 1994). It is unusual to be able to identify and correct just one single cause of delirium (Eisendrath, 1994).

Sensory deprivation may result in loss of reality testing and thought processing similar to that seen with cognitive impairment. This problem may occur in patients with impaired aural or visual acuity, decreased olfactory acuity, immobility due to extended bed rest, or confined to settings lacking in social or environmental stimuli.

NURSING INTERVENTION

Some general nursing care guidelines apply to both delirious and demented patients; other guidelines are more applicable to one or the other. Interventions adapted from Fortinash and Holoday-Worret (1995) and others will be described as they apply to particular symptoms or behavior.

GLOBAL COGNITIVE IMPAIRMENT (ATTENTION SPAN DISTURBANCE, DISORGANIZED THINKING, DISORIENTATION, OR MEMORY IMPAIRMENT)

• Assess patients on admission and every shift (unless cognitive impairment is stable) using a cognitive status examination. Particularly note any changes in attention span as this differentiates delirium from dementia. Elicit information from people familiar with the patient's usual behavior, especially regarding onset, pattern, and duration of any cognitive impairment, perceptual distortion, or abnormal thought content.

• For a delirious patient, identify all possible factors that may contribute to the patient's cognitive dysfunction and initiate treatments as necessary. Assist medical staff in determination of cause of delirium.

• Approach the patient in a gentle, calm, and friendly manner, using a clear, low-pitched voice. Patients will respond to the nurse's emotional tone. Address the patient by preferred name. Gain the patient's attention before speaking. Make eye contact and identify yourself each time you approach the patient.

• Eliminate or minimize competing and distracting background stimuli.

• Minimize changes of staff or placement. Establish predictable, familiar routines.

• Orient frequently to date, time, place, and activity. Convey the information in the context of routine conversation. Use visual memory aids such as a clock, calendar, and location signs.

• Speak in short, simple, concrete sentences; explain often what is being done and why. Avoid jargon and slang.

• Ask only one question, or make one statement at a time. Repeat the question, using the same words, if the patient does not seem to understand. After a few minutes, rephrase the question if the patient still doesn't understand. Use "yes" or "no" questions whenever possible, and avoid questions that require multiple choice or decision-making.

• Break down tasks into individual steps and ask the patient to do them one at a time. Enhance verbal communication with appropriate cues: "Do you want a blanket?" (while showing the patient the blanket).

• Refrain from agreeing with "made-up" stories that reflect memory impairment. Gently acknowledge the patient rather than try to convince them that they are wrong.

- Schedule rest periods and promote a normal day–night cycle.
- Attend to the patient's food, fluid, elimination, and hygiene needs.
- Safeguard the patient at all times, if possible using furniture rearrangement. Chemical or physical restraints may be necessary for patients with out-of-control behavior.

PERCEPTUAL DISTORTIONS (MISINTERPRETATIONS, ILLUSIONS, HALLUCINATIONS)

- Do not touch the patient or move towards the patient before gaining his/her attention.
- If you do not understand the patient, do not pretend that you do.
- Avoid contradicting or challenging the patient who is misinterpreting actual stimuli. Offer a simple, quiet explanation. Explain all unseen noises and activity simply and clearly.
- Avoid agreement, argument, or confrontation with a person experiencing a hallucination. Respond to the feeling in a noncommittal manner.

ABNORMAL THOUGHT CONTENT (DELUSIONS, PARANOIA)

- Avoid agreeing, confronting, or arguing with a suspicious, paranoid, or delusional patient about the "truth." Gently respond to the feelings instead. Redirect to a more concrete activity.
- Do not engage in laughter or whispering within view of the patient as the observation may confirm for the patient that the staff are against him or her.

COMBATIVENESS/AGITATION

- Remember that the patient is probably frightened and defensive, not actually trying to hurt you.
- Be alert to signals of increased restlessness, tension, rapid shifts in mental status, hallucinations, or delusions, indicative of escalating, out-of-control behavior that may be dangerous to the patient or others. Intervene early in the escalation of agitated behavior to maintain safety. The pre-

ferred drug in this situation is haloperidol (Ziehm, 1991). With some patients, benzodiazepines are used, either alone or in combination with haloperidol, to control behavior.

- Allow the patient adequate personal space. Use physical force as a last resort.
- Be alert to your own safety. Leave at least an arm's length between you and the patient. Do not let the patient get between you and the door. If you are frightened, leave the room to get help.
- Call security and use restraints if necessary to prevent injury.

SENSORY OVERLOAD

- Call the patient by name and introduce yourself by name and role.
- Taking the patient's point of view, explain the equipment, sounds, and other stimuli, including the therapeutic purpose.
- Provide *concrete, objective, preparatory information*.
- Reduce noise, especially at night. Staff conversation generally exceeds the noise from technology. Use of headphones and audiocassettes with the patient's favorite music will filter assaultive sounds.
- Modify lighting to simulate normal day-night cycles.
- Decrease vulnerability by ensuring privacy, modesty, and dignity and shielding from emergency events, such as cardiac resuscitation.

SENSORY DEPRIVATION

- Provide reality-orienting information in the context of routine conversation. Tell the patient about daily news, events, and weather. Involve other people in visiting and talking with the patient.
- Touch patients to show caring unless signs of suspiciousness, hallucinating, escalating anxiety, or agitation are present.
- Provide opportunities to use decision-making skills.
- Increase the meaningfulness of the environment by explaining the therapeutic purpose of all nursing actions and requests of the patient.
- If possible, use appropriate sensory aids.

USE OF PHYSICAL RESTRAINTS

Concerns about patient autonomy and safety by governmental and accrediting bodies have resulted in stringent standards of patient care when physical restraints are used (Weick, 1992; Joint Commission on Accreditation of Health Organizations [JCAHO], 1992a, 1992b). Restraints are to be used only when alternative strategies do not effectively control potentially harmful behavior, and then only as the last resort. JCAHO standards and Food and Drug Administration (FDA) guidelines require documentation of attempts to use alternatives (Food & Drug Administration, 1992, 1993). The use of restraints should trigger further identification and treatment of the problem causing the need for restraint, moving simultaneously to alternative measures to physical restraint when possible (Brower, 1991).

Restraints are most commonly used with patients with cognitive impairment and potentially dangerous, disturbed behavior (Evans & Strumpf, 1989; Berland et al., 1990). Alternatives to physical restraints are based on multidisciplinary assessment and individualized care (Minarik, 1994).

The FDA regulates as medical devices restraints that are defined as "a device, usually a wristlet, anklet, or other type of strap, that is intended for medical purposes and that limits a patient's movements to the extent necessary for treatment, examination, or protection of the patient" (Weick, 1992). Examples include, but are not limited to, safety vests, hand mitts, lap and wheelchair belts, body holders, straitjackets, protection nets, anklets, and wristlets.

> A medical device is not a substitute for nursing care. Like any other device, restraints must be monitored. A restraint is not an article of clothing.
> (Mary W. Brady, personal communication)

Federal regulations drafted in response to the Omnibus Budget Reconciliation Act (OBRA) of 1987, implemented in October 1990, state that nursing home residents have the right to be free from unnecessary physical and chemical restraints (Weick, 1992). Under the regulations, a resident's right to make choices, including the right to be free from restraints even when such freedom may pose possible risks, must be honored. OBRA states that restraints are allowed in these facilities only in restricted circumstances, that is, to ensure the physical safety of the resident or other residents, and only upon the written order of a physician that specifies the duration and circumstances under which the restraints are to be used (Weick, 1992). Evidence that restraints may actually be harmful, and recognition that the resident's dignity, mobility, and right to self-determination may be more important than perceived safety, provided the impetus to change practice (Rader et al., 1992).

Almost all types of restraints have been implicated in injuries and deaths reported to the FDA, but vest restraints caused most deaths. Most deaths occurred as the person tried to get out of or slid down within the restraint because caregivers tied the restraint incorrectly, the patient was not monitored or freed regularly, or personnel chose the wrong size or type for the patient.

Complications from use or misuse of restraints include immobility leading to bone resorption, pressure ulcers, skin tears, urinary retention or incontinence, fecal impaction, aspiration, restricted breathing, fractures and chafing, loss of self-esteem, confusion, forgetfulness, a sense of abandonment, depression, humiliation, fear, and anger.

According to the FDA, as long as an institution adheres to state and federal regulations and follows reasonable standards of care based on the patient's known mental and physical conditions, lawsuits are unsupportable. Generally, nurses are more likely to be held liable for failing to restrain a patient who should be restrained than for restraining a patient who should not be restrained (Weick, 1992).

Restraint differs from other interventions that limit a patient's movement, primarily on the basis of intent. Restraint is intended to limit movement as a means of protecting the patient or others from harm that might result from the patient's actions or behavior. The patient's behavior itself is the cause for limiting movement. When it is not customarily employed for a procedure, or when it is used with a cognitively impaired person, the intervention is considered a restraint.

No *pro re nata* (prn) orders for restraints are acceptable. It is important to follow applicable state and federal regulations and JCAHO requirements for the use of restraints. Documentation generally should contain at least the following:

- Physician time-limited order
- Events leading to restraint and rationale for use
- Documentation of attention to the needs of the patient
- Periodic observation of the patient
- Evidence that reapplication of restraints after a trial release is the result of the same condition that led to initial application; otherwise, each application requires a new order

The use of restraints is frightening to a patient. Always tell the patient what you are doing and why. Emphasize that restraints are a temporary measure to be applied with care. If necessary, use a team of staff, assigning each person to a limb and the head. Assign tasks in advance, including only one person to talk to the patient to reduce stimuli and prevent confusion that could result in injury to the patient or caregivers. Provide appropriate nursing care, including skin care and release from restraint at least every 2 hours (Fortinash & Holoday-Worret, 1991).

CONCLUSION

The stress of physical illness, injury, or disability, wherever it occurs, is a challenge for all people. People who cope effectively under normal circumstances may, if the stressors are severe enough, experience emotional complications. Family members and health care providers may also be affected. In this chapter, stress and the coping response to physical illness has been discussed with particular emphasis on anxiety-related responses considered ineffective. The responses described include anxiety; post-trauma stress response; denial, demanding, noncompliant and/or manipulative behavior; and cognitive disorders including "ICU syndrome." Nursing interventions for each response are recommended. When nurses recognize and understand the

response they are observing, individualized interventions can be more effectively designed to reduce the stress experienced by the patient, family members, and the nurses caring for them.

BIBLIOGRAPHY

Badger, J. M. (1994). Calming the anxious patient. *American Journal of Nursing, 94*(5), 46–50.

Berland, B., et al. (1990). Patient characteristics associated with the use of mechanical restraints. *Journal of General Internal Medicine, 5*(6), 485–486.

Billings, C. K. (1990). Anxiety and physical illness. *Psychiatric Medicine, 8*(3), 149–162.

Brower, H. T. (1991). The alternatives to restraints. *Journal of Gerontological Nursing, 17*(2), 18–22.

Christman, N. J., Kirchhoff, K. T., & Oakley, M. G. (1992). Concrete objective information. In G. M. Bulechek & J. C. McCloskey (Eds.), *Nursing interventions: Essential nursing treatments* (2nd ed.). Philadelphia: W. B. Saunders.

Daum, A. L. (1994). The disruptive antisocial patient: Management strategies. *Nursing Management, 25*(8), 46–51.

Diagnostic and statistical manual of mental disorders (4th ed.). (1994). Washington, DC: American Psychiatric Press.

Dossey, B. M. (1988). Imagery: Awakening the inner healer. In B. M. Dossey, L. Keegan, C. E. Guzzetta, & L. G. Kolkmeier, *Holistic nursing: A handbook for practice.* Rockville, MD: Aspen.

Eisendrath, S.J. (1994). Psychiatric problems. In F.S. Bongard & D. Y. Sue (Eds.), *Current critical care diagnosis and treatment.* Norwalk, CT: Appleton & Lange.

Evans, L. K. & Strumpf, N.E. (1989). Tying down the elderly: A review of the literature on physical restraint. *Journal of the American Geriatrics Society, 37*(1), 65.

FDA guidelines on physical restraint: Journal articles. (1993). IRD Report No. 930908. Rockville, MD: Food & Drug Administration.

FDA safety alert: Potential hazards with restraint devices. (1992). Rockville, MD: Food & Drug Administration.

Fortinash K. M., & Holoday-Worret, P. A. (1995). *Psychiatric nursing care plans* (2nd ed.). St. Louis: Mosby Year Book.

Hamner, M. B. (1994). Exacerbation of posttraumatic stress disorder symptoms with medical illness. *General Hospital Psychiatry 16*(2), 135–137.

The Incredible Machine. (1986). Washington, DC: National Geographic Society.

JCAHO. (1992a). Implementing restraint standards in hospitals. *Joint Commission Perspectives, 12*(6), 15, 17.

JCAHO. (1992b). Limitations on hospital patient movement that constitute restraint. *Joint Commission Perspectives, 12*(5), 11–12.

Keltner, N.L., Schwecke, L.H., & Bostrom, C. E. (1991). *Psychiatric nursing: A psychotherapeutic management approach.* St. Louis: Mosby Year-Book.

Kim, M. J., McFarland, G. K., & McLane, A. M. (Eds.), *Pocket guide to nursing diagnoses* (5th ed.). St. Louis: Mosby Year Book.

Krieger, D. (1981). *Foundations of holistic health nursing practices: The Renaissance nurse.* Philadelphia: J. B. Lippincott.

Lazarus, R. S., & Folkman, S. (1984). *Stress, appraisal and coping.* New York: Springer Publishing Co.

Leavitt, M., & Minarik, P.A. (1989). The agitated, hypervigilant response. In B. Riegel & D. Ehrenreich (Eds.), *Psychological aspects of critical care nursing.* Rockville, MD: Aspen.

Macrae, J. (1989). *Therapeutic touch: A practical guide.* New York: Alfred A. Knopf.

McCaffery, M., & Beebe, A. (1989). *Pain: Clinical manual for nursing practice.* St. Louis: C. V. Mosby.

McEnany, G. W., & Tescher, B. E. (1985). Contracting for care. *Journal of Psychosocial Nursing, 23*(4), 11–18.

Miller, N. (1989). Acute myocardial infarction. In B. Riegel & D. Ehrenreich (Eds.), *Psychological aspects of critical care nursing.* Rockville, MD: Aspen.

Minarik, P. A. (1994). Alternatives to physical restraints in acute care. *Clinical Nurse Specialist, 8*(3), 136, 162.

Minarik, P. A. (1993). Incorporating imagery in clinical practice. *Clinical Nurse Specialist, 7*(5), 234.

Minarik, P. A., & Leavitt, M. (1989). The angry, demanding hostile response. In B. Riegel & D. Ehrenreich (Eds.), *Psychological aspects of critical care nursing.* Rockville, MD: Aspen.

Quinn, J. (1992). Holding sacred space: The nurse as healing environment. *Holistic Nursing Practice, 6*(4), 26–35.

Rader, J., Semradek, J., McKenzie, D., & McMahon, M. (1992). Restraint strategies: Reducing restraints in Oregon's long-term care facilities. *Journal of Gerontological Nursing, 18*(11), 49–56.

Ragaisis, K. M. (1994). Critical incident stress debriefing: A family nursing intervention. *Archives of Psychiatric Nursing, 8*(1), 38–43.

Ross, M. C., & Wonders, J. (1993). An exploration of the characteristics of post-traumatic stress disorder in reserve forces deployed during Desert Storm. *Archives of Psychiatric Nursing, 7*(5), 265–269.

Runyon, N., Allen, C. L. M., & Ilnicki, S. H. (1988). The borderline patient on the med-surg unit. *American Journal of Nursing, 88*(12), 1644–1650.

Stephens, R. L. (1993). Imagery: A strategic intervention to empower clients. Part II—a practical guide. *Clinical Nurse Specialist, 7*(5), 235–240.

Sundeen, S. J., Stuart, G. W., Rankin, E. A. D., & Cohen, S.A. (1994). *Nurse-client interaction: Implementing the nursing process* (5th ed.). St. Louis: Mosby.

University of California, San Francisco (UCSF). Medical Center Department of Nursing. (1995). Patient/family with "difficult" behavior/communication. Intervention guidelines. Unpublished.

Weick, M.D. (1992). Physical restraints: An FDA update. *American Journal of Nursing, 92*(11), 74, 76–78, 80.

Weisman, A.D. (1979). *Coping with cancer.* New York: McGraw-Hill.

White, J. M. (1992). Music therapy: An intervention to reduce anxiety in the myocardial infarction patient. *Clinical Nurse Specialist, 6*(2), 58–63.

Wise, M. G., & Taylor, S. E. (1990). Anxiety and mood disorders in medically ill patients. *Journal of Clinical Psychiatry, 51*(1 Suppl), 27–32.

Ziehm, S. R. (1991). Intravenous haloperidol for tranquilization in critical care patients: A review and critique. *AACN Clinical Issues in Critical Care Nursing, 2*(4), 765777.

CHAPTER 18

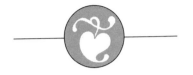

Psychosocial Intervention With Ineffective Coping Responses to Physical Illness: Depression-Related

Pamela Minarik

Anxiety and depression are common but distressing responses to the experience of illness. In the last chapter, anxiety-related coping responses were discussed. Depression-related responses are presented in this chapter.

The experience of illness is likely to be stressful or even provoke a crisis. The way people respond and cope depends upon their perception of the situation and the meaning of it for the person and family members involved.

DEPRESSION-RELATED COPING RESPONSE

As noted in Chapter 17, the nursing diagnosis of *ineffective individual coping* is defined as im-

pairment of adaptive behaviors and problem-solving abilities of a person in meeting life's demands and roles. When the psychological stress of illness is too great, patients manifest emotions and behaviors that present difficulties for care providers. Because a person may cope effectively in one context and not in another, it is useful to ask, "Coping with what? Ineffectively according to whom?"

Ineffective or maladaptive responses include unusual levels of depression and unmotivated behavior, suicidal thinking and behavior, and alcohol and psychoactive drug use. Depression, as well as delirium and anxiety, can

Patricia Barry: *Psychosocial Nursing: Care of Physically Ill Patients and Their Families,* 3rd ed.
© 1996 Lippincott–Raven Publishers

increase the severity of physical illness, prolong hospital stay, complicate the course of treatment, increase the utilization of health services, and increase patient disability. Because of their continuous contact with patients, nurses can recognize the more subtle signs of these disorders and obtain needed diagnosis and treatment, thereby decreasing morbidity and cost.

Each section of this chapter includes a description of the coping response and recommended interventions. In all instances, if symptoms persist despite interventions, or are severe, psychiatric or psychiatric nursing consultation should be requested to ensure the patient's safety, emotional comfort, and future adaptation, and/or to reduce the stress of care providers.

THE PATIENT WHO IS DEPRESSED OR UNMOTIVATED

Unmotivated behavior is often associated with depression and many of the interventions are similar; thus, depression and lack of motivation will be discussed together. Depression is found in men and women of all age groups and social classes. Depressive episodes occur twice as frequently in women as in men (*Diagnostic and Statistical Manual* [DSM-IV], 1994). Studies indicate that 12% to 36% of medical outpatients and approximately 33% of medical inpatients report depressive symptoms (Wise & Taylor, 1990). Major depression is found in 12% to 16% of elderly persons hospitalized with medical illness, with an additional 20% to 30% suffering appreciable depressive symptoms. Functional disability is strongly associated with depressive symptoms (Kurlowicz, 1994).

Depressive symptoms may result from the patient's psychological reaction to the illness, the medical disorder itself, or the medications used to treat the medical illness. Depressive symptoms in the physically ill may also predate the illness. Depression is associated with biological changes in neurotransmitter-receptor systems, the endocrine system, and the immune system (Eisendrath, 1994). Depression

and physical illness occurring together must both be treated. Causes of depression are not always known, but depression is probably due to combinations of family history and genetics, general medical illnesses, certain medications, drugs or alcohol abuse, stressful events, and personality traits (Stuart, 1994).

Depression in late life is due to a complex interaction of biological, psychological, and social events. Etiological factors include imbalance of neurotransmitters, structural brain changes, dysregulation of endocrine function, organ system disruption caused by physical illness, cognitive distortions, mourning and melancholia, sleep-wake cycle disruption, unsuccessful developmental task accomplishment, stressful life events, and chronic social stress (Kurlowicz, 1993). Older persons in particular may be misdiagnosed as demented when their slowed thinking and defects in memory, abstraction, and calculation are actually due to depression. Persons with this condition, called *pseudodementia*, may give up and no longer try to do anything.

RECOGNITION OF DEPRESSION

The recognition and diagnosis of depression in any health setting rely on the provider's awareness of risk factors associated with depression, and the provider's ability to elicit from the patient key signs, symptoms, and history of illness. Risk factors include prior episodes of depression, family history of depression, prior suicide attempts, female gender, age of onset under 40 years, postpartum period, medical comorbidity, lack of social support, stressful life events, personal history of sexual abuse, and current substance abuse (Stuart, 1994).

The situation of physical illness may increase dependency, helplessness, and uncertainty and generate a negative view of the world. Cognitive distortions can easily develop and the individual may make mistakes in judgment, interpreting benign events negatively or predicting catastrophe. Patients may feel themselves to be worthless and a burden to family and friends. Motivation to participate in care may be reduced. Family members may be immobilized, impatient, or angry with the patient's lack of communication, cooperation, or motivation (Minarik, 1989).

Generally, depressed patients present themselves as hopeless, helpless, clinging, dependent, guilty, obsessively ruminating, tearful, withdrawn, brooding, self-critical, and noncommunicative. Some patients who are depressed do not describe themselves as sad, however, but rather talk of feeling anxious, irritable, or worried about physical health or pain. Talking, moving, and eating are slowed. Decision making is hampered by slowed thinking, low self-esteem, and impaired concentration. Although some patients are slowed in their movements, others are agitated, unable to sit still, fidgeting and wringing their hands (DSM-IV, 1994; Minarik, 1989).

Culture can influence both the experience and communication of depressive symptoms. In some cultures, depression may be experienced mostly in somatic terms, rather than with guilt or sadness. Complaints of "nerves" and headaches (in Latino and Mediterranean cultures), of weakness, tiredness, or "imbalance" (in Chinese or Asian cultures), of problems of the "heart" (in Middle Eastern cultures), or of being "heartbroken" (among Hopi) may be expressions of depression. Cultures may differ in judgments about the seriousness of experiencing dysphoria; for example, irritability may be of more concern than sadness or withdrawal. Experiences distinctive to particular cultures, such as fear of being hexed, or vivid feelings of being visited by those who have died, must be distinguished from actual hallucinations or delusions that may be part of a major depressive episode with psychotic features. It is important not to dismiss a symptom because it is seen as the norm for a particular culture (DSM-IV, 1994).

DIFFERENTIATING DEPRESSIVE CONDITIONS IN THE MEDICALLY ILL

Because in most health care settings nurses have the most patient contact, they are in an ideal position to talk with individuals about their physical and emotional health problems and detect depression. Detection begins with knowing that the majority of the many people who experience depression seek treatment for related somatic complaints in general medical settings. Nurses should assess all patients for the risk factors related to depression and identify depressive conditions through the use of screening tools and by talking with the patient (Stuart, 1994). Although nurses are usually not making a differential diagnosis, it is helpful to know the diagnostic criteria for the major disorders.

Major Depressive Episode

According to the *Diagnostic and Statistical Manual of Mental Disorders* (1994), the essential feature of a *major depressive episode* is a period of at least 2 weeks during which there is either depressed mood or the loss of interest or pleasure in nearly all activities. For the diagnosis to be made, at least four additional symptoms from a list of nine (cognitive, affective, and somatic) must be present nearly every day during the same 2-week period and must represent a change from previous functioning (Box 18-1).

The physical symptoms caused by medical illnesses, such as fatigue, weight changes, anorexia, sleep disturbance, and psychomotor retardation, are difficult to distinguish from somatic symptoms of depression. Somatic symptoms, however, may be valid indicators of depression when they are severe or persistent despite treatment of the medical condition (Kurlowicz, 1994). Cognitive and affective symptoms such as persistent diminished interest, depressed or lowered mood, feelings of failure or punishment, feelings of guilt, hopelessness and helplessness, negative evaluation of the situation out of proportion to reality, withdrawal from friends and family, and thoughts of death may help to differentiate major depressive disorder in the presence of somatic symptoms.

Adjustment Disorder With Depressed Mood

Adjustment disorder is a maladaptive reaction to an identifiable psychosocial stressor, such as an acute illness, occurring within 3 months after the onset of the stressor. The essential feature is the development of clinically significant emotional or behavioral symptoms. The clinical significance of the reaction is indi-

BOX 18-1	Key Diagnostic Criteria for Major Depressive Disorder

1. Depressed mood most of the day, nearly every day, as indicated by either subjective report or observation by others
2. Markedly diminished interest or pleasure in all, or almost all, activities most of the day
3. Significant weight loss when not dieting, or weight gain, or decrease or increase in appetite
4. Insomnia or hypersomnia
5. Psychomotor agitation or retardation
6. Fatigue or loss of energy
7. Feelings of worthlessness or excessive or inappropriate guilt
8. Diminished ability to think or concentrate, or indecisiveness
9. Recurrent thoughts of death, recurrent suicidal ideation without a specific plan, or a suicide attempt or a specific plan for committing suicide

Five or more of nine symptoms must be present nearly every day during the same two-week period and represent a change from previous functioning; at least one of the symptoms is either #1 or #2.

Information adapted from DSM-IV, 1994.

cated either by marked distress in excess of what would be expected given the nature of the stressor or by significantly impaired social or occupational functioning. Typical symptoms are depressed mood, tearfulness, or feelings of hopelessness. This condition may be confused with major depressive disorder in the medically ill. The individual's culture should be considered when judging whether the response to the stressor is maladaptive or in excess of what would be expected. The meaning and experience of stressors and the evaluation of the response may vary across cultures (DSM-IV, 1994; Kurlowicz, 1994).

Reactions to Loss

Reactions to actual and symbolic losses are the most common depressive experiences of the physically ill and their significant others. Commonly called *reactive depressions*, these nonpathological reactions to stress arise in response to a specific, identifiable stressor. Even relatively minor illnesses may alter self-image of health, physical attractiveness, functional abilities, and invulnerability, and lead to a sense of loss. The stages of loss and grief are outlined in Chapter 9. In contrast to adjustment disorders, normal reactions to loss are adaptive and do not lead to marked distress in excess of what is expected and do not cause significant impairment in social or occupa-

tional functioning (DSM-IV, 1994). Uncomplicated grief reactions are time-limited, lasting less than 6 months.

Dysthymic Disorder

Dysthymic disorder and major depressive disorder are differentiated on the basis of severity, chronicity, and persistence. In *dysthymic disorder*, the depressed mood must be present more days than not, over a period of at least 2 years. The two disorders share similar symptoms; however, dysthymic disorder is characterized by chronic, less severe depressive symptoms that have been present for many years. Commonly encountered symptoms are feelings of inadequacy; generalized loss of interest or pleasure; social withdrawal; feelings of guilt, irritability, or anger; and decreased activity, effectiveness, or productivity (DSM-IV, 1994).

Depressive Symptoms Due to Medical Conditions or Substances

A variety of medical conditions, listed in Box 18-2, may cause mood symptoms. Mood symptoms may also be the direct physiological effect of a substance (i.e., a drug of abuse, a medication, other somatic treatment for depression, or toxin exposure). Onset may occur during intoxication or withdrawal. Drugs that may cause depression are listed in Box 18-3.

NURSING ASSESSMENT

Depressive conditions are found in the variety of settings where nurses engage in a range of nursing activities, including case-finding, counseling, enhancing self-care activities, administering somatic therapies, health teaching, case management, and health promotion (Stuart, 1994). The role of the nonpsychiatric nurse in the assessment of the depressed, physically ill person is to identify signs and symptoms of depression; distinguish between signs and symptoms in the normal range for the situation or those that require further assessment by a psychiatric professional; describe the signs and symptoms in an accurate, objective manner; and seek further evaluation for patients assessed as having a major depression or risk of suicide (Minarik, 1989). Because depression is often difficult to assess, the task of recognition, assessment, and diagnosis is likely to be ongoing. Thus, documentation and communication of observations, interventions, and outcomes are extremely important for all disciplines involved in the care of the patient.

The patient who has a major depression or is suicidal may benefit from somatic therapies, such as antidepressant medications. If medications are prescribed, the nurse must assess the response to the medication, watch for potential side effects, and educate the patient regarding the medication and management of common side effects.

General Observations and Questions

Specific screening instruments may be used, but if these are not available, direct questioning and clinical observation of mood, behavior, and thinking can be carried out concomitant with physical care. Observations of the patient's interactions with family members, friends, and staff members of various disciplines provide useful data. The following questions are adapted from Minarik (1989):

Questions on mood: How have your spirits been? How would you describe your mood? Have you felt sad or blue?

Questions relating to behavior (covering sleeping patterns, appetite, activity level, and

---

BOX 18-2	Medical Conditions Associated With Depression

Cardiovascular disease
cardiomyopathy, congestive heart failure, myocardial infarction

Collagen vascular disorders
rheumatoid arthritis, systemic lupus erythematosus, polyarteritis nodosa

Endocrine disorders
Addison's disease, diabetes mellitus, Cushing's syndrome, hyper- and hypoadrenalism, hyperaldosteronism, hyper- and hypo- parathyroidism, hyper- and hypothyroidism, hypopituitarism, premenstrual syndrome

Infections
Epstein-Barr virus, encephalitis, hepatitis, human immunodeficiency virus (HIV), mononucleosis, pneumonia, postinfluenza, syphilis

Neoplasms
central nervous system, lung, carcinoma of the pancreas

Neurologic disorders
cerebrovascular disease, dementia (e.g., Alzheimer's disease), epilepsy (particularly temporal lobe), Huntington's disease, hydrocephalus, multiple sclerosis, myasthenia gravis, narcolepsy, Parkinson's disease, postconcussion, progressive supranuclear palsy, stroke, subarachnoid hemorrhage

Vitamin deficiencies
vitamin B_1 deficiency, pellagra, pernicious anemia (vitamin B_{12} deficiency), Wernicke's encephalopathy

Others
alcoholism, anemia, electrolyte abnormalities, heavy metal poisoning, hemodialysis, hypertension, Kleinfelter's syndrome, porphyria, postoperative and postpartum affective disorders, uremia

Information adapted from DSM-IV, 1994; Valente, 1993; Wise & Taylor, 1990.

BOX 18-3	**Drugs Associated With Mood (Depression and/or Mania) Symptoms**

Associated with intoxication
alcohol
amphetamine and related
   substances
cocaine
hallucinogens
inhalants
opioids
phencyclidine and related substances
sedatives, hypnotics, and anxiolytics
other or unknown substances

Associated with withdrawal
alcohol
amphetamine and related
   substances
cocaine
sedatives, hypnotics, and anxiolytics
other or unknown substances

Medications reported to evoke mood symptoms
anesthetics
analgesics
anticholinergics
anticonvulsants
antihypertensives (especially high
   doses of reserpine)
antiparkinsonian medications
antiulcer medications
cardiac medications
oral contraceptives
psychotropic medications (e.g.,
   antidepressants, benzodiazepines, antipsychotics,
   disulfiram)
muscle relaxants
steroids (especially corticosteroids,
   anabolic steroids)
sulfonamides

Substances reported to evoke mood symptoms
heavy metals
toxins

Information adapted from DSM-IV, 1994.

changes in energy): How are you sleeping? How much energy do you have now compared with 1 month or 6 months ago? Has your appetite changed recently? Have you lost or gained weight? What do you usually do to cope with stress (e.g., talk to someone, go to a movie, work, exercise, drugs, alcohol)?

Questions related to cognition: How do you picture your future? What are the biggest problems facing you now? Are you as interested as usual in your work, hobbies, family, etc.? Have you felt satisfied with yourself and with your life? Can you concentrate as well as you usually can? Do you have family or close friends readily available to help you? Do you feel able to call on them?

All depressed patients should be asked directly about suicidal thinking, impulses, and past personal or family history of suicide attempts (Stuart, 1994). Severely depressed and/or potentially suicidal patients must be identified as soon as possible so that a safe environment can be assured and appropriate treatment can begin. Asking about suicide does not encourage suicidal behavior or thinking; rather, it opens up communication. Most patients are relieved to be asked. Assessment and interventions for the patient who is suicidal are discussed in a later section of this chapter.

NURSING INTERVENTION

Nurses sometimes plan care for the depressed patient with feeling better ("happier") as the goal. It may be more useful to think of the overall goal as maintenance of normal activity patterns. Specifically, the goals of nursing for the depressed patient are:

1. To ensure a safe environment.
2. To assist the patient to reduce symptoms and maladaptive coping responses.
3. To restore or increase the patient's level of functioning.
4. To improve quality of life, if possible.
5. To prevent future relapse and recurrence of depression (Minarik, 1989; Stuart, 1994).

Ensuring a safe environment will be discussed in the section about the suicidal patient.

The *self-care deficit theory of nursing* provides a useful framework for assessment of the patient's slow, dependent behaviors and/or lack of motivation, and intervention planning. The patient is assessed in terms of self-care ability (from severely limited to independent) and specific goals can be set in the following areas of functioning (Minarik, 1989; Underwood, 1980):

1. *Air, food, fluids*—breathing, smoking, fluid intake, food intake, behavior related to eating and drinking, alcohol and drug use
2. *Elimination*—bowel, bladder, elimination behavior, menstruation
3. *Personal hygiene*—clothing, activities of daily living
4. *Rest/activity balance*—sleep pattern, usual leisure time activities, usual work/school activities, usual physical activities, physical activity necessary for healing
5. *Solitude/social interaction balance*—suicide potential, mental status, ability to tolerate stimuli, interaction and communication patterns, sexuality, cultural factors

Crisis Intervention

Crisis intervention, described in Chapter 16, is appropriate when the patient is experiencing a grief and loss reaction. For grief and loss reactions and mild to moderate depression, useful strategies also include providing guidance on current problems, reinforcing patients' coping resources and strengths, and enhancing social supports (Stuart, 1994).

Cognitive Interventions

Cognitive approaches involve clarification of misconceptions and modification of faulty assumptions held by the patient by identifying and correcting the patient's distorted, negative, and catastrophic thinking. Cognitive approaches are useful with all of the depressive disorders.

Interpersonal Interventions

Interpersonal interventions assist with the balance of solitude and social interaction through clarification and potential resolution of interpersonal difficulties such as role disruptions, social isolation, delayed grief reaction, family conflict, or role enactment.

Behavioral Interventions

Behavioral interventions are based on a functional analysis of behavior and on social learning theory. The key to the behavioral approach is to stop reinforcing dependence. Instead, provide a contingency relationship between independent behavior and positive reinforcement, thereby altering behavior and subsequently influencing thoughts and feelings. It is helpful to organize this approach with the self-care areas previously identified (Minarik & Sparacino, 1990). The aim is to keep the patient active and moving.

Cognitive, interpersonal and behavioral interventions are summarized in Box 18-4.

PHARMACOLOGIC TREATMENT OF DEPRESSION

Antidepressant medications are easily administered and are an effective treatment strategy. Disadvantages include the need for repeated health care visits to monitor patient response and adjust the dosage, possible adverse side effects and medical reactions, potential use in suicide attempts, and the need for strict adherence to the schedule. Patients should be informed that most antidepressant medications must be taken for 3 to 4 weeks before a significant response is achieved. The nurse must be aware that suicidal patients become more energized with medications and appear to look better long before their depressive feelings and suicidal thoughts are relieved. *Careful monitoring of suicidal ideation should continue for weeks after the patient appears improved* (Stuart, 1994).

The major categories of antidepressant medications are the tricyclics (TCAs), heterocyclics/monocyclics, selective serotonin re-uptake inhibitors (SSRIs), and the monoamine oxidase inhibitors (MAOIs). No one medication is clearly more effective than another. The newer SSRIs are associated with fewer long-term side effects than the older TCAs, but are more expensive. MAOIs are usually not the

BOX 18-4	**Nursing Interventions for Treatment of Depression**

Cognitive Interventions
- Review and reinforce realistic ideas and expectations
- Help the patient examine the accuracy of self-defeating assumptions
- Review strengths and assets
- Set realistic goals
- Explain all actions and plans, seeking feedback and participation in decision making
- Provide choices, even if only about the timing of an activity
- Teach thought stopping or thought interruption
- Encourage the patient to explore feelings only for a specific purpose and only if the patient is not ruminating (constant repeating of failures, problems, etc.)
- Direct the patient to activities with gentle reminders to focus on that activity to discourage rumination
- Listen to physical complaints and take appropriate action, then redirect and assist the patient to accomplish activities
- Avoid telling the patient he or she is not sad or depressed or has no reason to be
- Avoid chastizing the patient for feeling sad

Interpersonal Interventions
- Enhance social skills through modeling, role playing, rehearsal, feedback, and reinforcement
- Build rapport with frequent, brief visits
- Engage in normal social conversation with the patient as often as possible
- Give consistent attention even when the patient is uncommunicative to show that the patient is worthwhile
- Direct comments and questions to the patient rather than to significant others
- Provide adequate time for the patient to formulate a response
- Mobilize family and social support systems
- Encourage the patient to maintain communication and share feelings with significant others
- Involve family and friends, providing them with support and suggestions about how to be helpful
- Avoid telling the patient about your personal reactions to the patient's dependent behavior
- Avoid medical jargon, giving advice, sharing personal experiences, or making value judgments
- Avoid false reassurance

Behavioral Interventions
- Provide directed activities
- Develop a hierarchy of behaviors with the patient
- Develop structured schedules
- Give homework assignments

(continued)

first choice because they require dietary restrictions and can have potentially fatal interactions with other medications. Side effects of antidepressant medications are usually dose-dependent and short-term (see Table 18-1). Effects on patient lifestyle can be minimized (see Table 18-2). Patient education is essential in this area

to decrease the possibility of nonadherence to the medication regimen.

In medically ill, depressed persons who have not used antidepressants previously, a psychostimulant such as dextroamphetamine or methylphenidate is often used if there is no medical contraindication such as tachyarrhy-

BOX 18-4	**NURSING INTERVENTIONS FOR TREATMENT OF DEPRESSION** (Continued)

- Use systematic application of reinforcement
- Encourage self-monitoring of predetermined behaviors, such as physical exercise
- Focus on goal attainment and preparation for adaptive coping in the future

Specific Behavioral Strategies

- Observe the patient's self-care patterns and routines and work with the patient to develop a structured, daily schedule
- Develop achievable, daily self-care goals with the patient to increase sense of control
- Upgrade the goals gradually to provide increased opportunity for positive reinforcement and goal attainment
- Utilize a chart for the patient and staff to monitor daily progress. Gold stars may be utilized as reinforcement and to secure more meaningful reinforcement, (i.e., the praise and positive attention of others). The chart also facilitates communication and consistency among caregivers.
- Provide sufficient time and repetitive reassurance ("You can do it") to help patients do self-care actions for themselves
- Positively reinforce even small achievements
- Assist the patient with activities, especially those related to appearance and hygiene, that the patient is unable to do
- Adjust assistance, verbal direction, reminders, and teaching to the actual needs/abilities of the patient. Do not overdo.
- Teach deep breathing techniques for management of anxiety generated by changing behavior

Information adapted from Stuart, 1994; Minarik & Sparacino, 1990; Minarik, 1989.

thmia. Dextroamphetamine is essentially free of side effects in most patients. Another advantage is the rapidity of response, 1 to 2 hours after the first or second dose, when it is successful. Different studies have shown a 48% to 80% improvement in depressive symptoms (Eisendrath, 1994).

Staff support. Staff members sometimes believe that depressed persons are only complainers and could be better if that was what they really wanted. Since this is rarely the case, the most important initial interventions for nurses to make are with themselves—increasing awareness of their attitudes toward depressed persons, their feeling reactions and their resultant behaviors toward the patient.

Dependency, helplessness, and a sense of futility are frustrating when nurses are trying to help the patient with physical and emotional care. If, in frustrated retaliation, they withdraw from the patient, the patient may become even more helpless and dependent in an attempt to regain the nurse's attention. Because physical care is needed when the patient is medically ill, a downward spiral may result: the patient becomes more dependent and the nurse takes over more and more of the patient's self-care, often out of concern and a desire to be helpful. The outcome of an apparently compassionate approach may be increased patient dependency and increased staff hopelessness. The time and encouragement necessary to promote self-care by depressed patients can be difficult to provide on a busy medical or surgical unit (Minarik, 1989; Minarik & Sparacino, 1990).

The constant need to push, encourage, and reassure can be fatiguing for the nursing staff. If several staff members share the assignment to depressed patients, they can validate each other's feelings and avoid directing anger or hopelessness to the patients. Patient care conferences help to maintain a therapeutic approach and provide for group problem-solving

TABLE 18-1 Antidepressant Medication Side Effect Profiles	
TCAs	**SSRIs**
• Dry mouth	• Nausea
• Blurred vision	• Nervousness
• Constipation	• Insomnia
• Sedation, drowsiness	• Sexual dysfunction
• Weight gain	• Headache
• Postural hypotension	
• Cardiac effects	
• Dizziness	

From Stuart, 1994.

and support. Few conditions require such a consistent approach, but the effort is likely to be gratifying as the depressed patient regains functional ability and independence (Minarik, 1989).

THE PATIENT WHO IS SUICIDAL

Suicide, defined as an *intentional, self-inflicted death*, is the eighth leading cause of death in the United States (Valente, 1983). Because suicide is underreported, statistics underestimate its magnitude; intentional overdoses by the terminally ill and intentional car accidents are rarely labeled as suicides. In primary care settings, high suicide rates are associated with cancer, acquired immune deficiency syndrome (AIDS), depression, substance abuse, and chronic illness. The suicide rate in people with AIDS is 66 times higher than the general population. Approximately 60% of depressed people have a high risk of suicide. In studies of people who committed suicide, most people consulted a health care provider about physical complaints, but their suicide risk was undetected (Valente, 1993).

For every patient who dies by suicide or attempts suicide, a large number of lives, including family members, friends, and health care professionals, are profoundly affected.

ASSESSMENT OF SUICIDE RISK

An important role of the nurse is to evaluate patients for potential suicidal behavior (Stuart, 1994). After recognizing the incidence of suicide, the basic steps in risk assessment are to evaluate risk factors, detect clues, and then estimate each individual's *lethality*, which is the potential to cause death. At the first hint of suicide, the health care provider should seriously evaluate suicidal warnings and despair and avoid the temptation to provide empty reassurance and cheerful reinforcement. Initial and periodic evaluation of suicidal potential is required for patients with history, thoughts, or risk factors of suicide (Valente, 1993).

Risk Factors

Groups at high risk for completed suicide are listed in Box 18-5. Other risk factors include hopelessness, physical illness, living alone, and psychosis, especially "command" hallucinations to commit suicide (Minarik, 1989; Stuart, 1994). Risk may also be increased by other factors such as pain, disability, recent loss of important relationships, or unexplained change

TABLE 18-2 Managing Antidepressant Medication Side Effects	
Symptom	**Remedy**
Nausea	Administer drugs with meals or at bedtime
Nervousness	Dose—slower escalation, temporary reduction
Insomnia	Dose as early in the day as possible
Sexual dysfunction	Dose after sexual intercourse
Headache	Mild analgesics: lower dose
Dry mouth	Adequate hydration: lozenges
Drowsiness	Dose at bedtime

From Stuart, 1994.

BOX 18-5	Risk Groups for Completed Suicide

Gender: Male

Age: Over 65

Ethnicity: White males higher than others. Suicide rates peak in young adulthood for African Americans, Hispanics, and some Native Americans.

Family history: Substance abuse or physical, sexual, mental, or emotional abuse

Psychiatric diagnoses: Depression, schizophrenia, substance abuse, phobia, post-trauma stress disorder, physical or sexual abuse, prior suicide attempt

Medical diagnoses: Cancer, AIDS, cardiorespiratory disorders, renal dialysis

Other: Gay men and lesbians (6–9 times higher rates of attempted suicide). Runaways and people recently detained in jail during the first 24 hours. Cult and gang members.

Adapted and reprinted by permission of the publisher. From Valente, S.M. (1993). Evaluating suicide risk in the medically ill patient. *Nurse Practitioner, 18,* 42. Copyright © 1993 by Elsevier Science Inc.

to careless or impulsive behavior (Minarik, 1989). Men complete suicide three to four times more often than women; the ratio is reversed for attempted suicide. Among the elderly, approximately one in four suicide attempts is fatal because of highly lethal methods. Chemical dependency, phobia, cognitive impairment, cancer, and alcoholism have been linked with elderly suicide (Valente, 1993).

Being in a high-risk group does not determine individual risk. Individual risk is based on the lethality of the suicide plan. Individual warning signs of suicide are listed in Box 18-6. In addition, a person who demonstrates a sudden feeling of happiness, peacefulness, and energy with no apparent reason after a long period of depression may have relieved the ambivalence about suicide by a decision to do it and therefore is at very high risk.

Recognition of Clues

Suicidal persons may give verbal and/or behavioral clues of their intent through their behavior, through writing in diaries or stories, through creative work such as art, and in their speech. Clues may be hidden, subtle, or obvious. Indicators include giving things away that

are usually needed or valued, making a will, unusual interest in settling personal affairs, asking questions about donating the body or body parts to science, making statements concerning thoughts of death (e.g., "How many of these pills would it take to kill someone?") or statements indicating hopelessness or helplessness. Any jokes about suicide or suicide messages must be taken seriously and investigated. Social withdrawal, self-mutilation, running away, aggressive acting out, anorexia, changes in sleeping pattern, slowed psychomotor activity, and resistance or refusal of treatments, food, or fluids may indicate suicidal ideation or intent and require further assessment (Valente, 1993).

Ascertaining Lethality

The important factors in determining lethality are suicide plan, method, intended outcome (e.g., death or rescue), and availability of resources and ability to communicate (Minarik, 1989; Valente, 1993). Verbal and nonverbal behavior with a theme of ending or giving up should be clarified with direct questions. Presence of suicidal thinking can be assessed by asking questions such as:

"You sound discouraged. Have you wanted to stop living?"

BOX 18-6	Individual Warning Signs of Suicide	
Historical	Previous suicide attempts	
Behavioral	• Verbal statements of suicidal thoughts	
	• Behavioral changes	
	• Saying goodbye (e.g., writing a will,[1] giving away prized belongings)	
Mood	• Depressed, hopeless, helpless, ambivalent	
Social	• Isolated, withdrawn	
Death wishes or death themes	• In art, writing, play, conversation	

[1] This may be a normal task of aging or terminal illness. Evaluate whether individual has any intent or wish to actively hasten death.

Adapted and reprinted by permission of the publisher. From Valente, S.M. 1993. Evaluating suicide risk in the medically ill patient. *Nurse Practitioner, 18,* 43. Copyright © 1993 by Elsevier Science Inc.

"Have you thought about harming yourself or about suicide?"

"When people are feeling down, they sometimes think of taking their own lives. I am concerned that you seem sad. I wonder if you have thought of suicide?"

Ask the patient about a suicide plan and, if present, ask about the method and determine its lethality and accessibility:

"Do you have a suicide plan?"
"How would you kill yourself?"
"Is that method available to you?"
"Have you rehearsed your plan?"
"What do you hope will happen?"
"Do you have plans for rescue?"
"When are you planning on killing yourself?"
"Are you planning on killing yourself now?"
"Have you felt able to control your suicidal impulses?"

Lethal methods include guns, knives, jumping from heights, drowning, and carbon monoxide. Other *potentially lethal methods* include hanging or strangulation (using strong pieces of twine, rope, electric cords, sheets), taking high doses of aspirin or Tylenol, being in a car crash, or undergoing exposure to extreme cold. Wrist cutting and mild aspirin overdose are considered low and barbiturates are moderate in lethality (Valente, 1993). Ask if the patient has a history of suicide attempts. If yes, what was the method? What was the outcome? Was the patient rescued accidentally or did he or she call for help?

Ask the patient about factors favoring and disfavoring suicide and about available internal and external resources (Stuart, 1994):

"What has kept you from suicide (for example, significant others, religious or spiritual values, unfinished business)?"
"Is there anything keeping you from going ahead with your plan?"
"Who can you turn to when you are upset?"
"Who is available to stay with you or help you?"

NURSING INTERVENTION

A patient with an immediate, lethal, and precise suicide plan needs strict safety precautions such as hospitalization or continuous or close supervision. Inform the patient's primary health care provider immediately. Psychiatric consultation is recommended to confirm lethality and plan for safety and therapeutic intervention. The patient in the hospital or outpatient setting should be observed constantly, one-to-one, with eye contact, and not allowed to leave until the consultant arrives. The low-risk patient should not be underestimated. If circumstances change, risk could change. In all cases notify the primary provider, and document the patient's behavior and verbatim statements as well as the time and date the provider was notified. If the provider is not responsive to the nurse's report of the patient's suicidal ideation, it is important to maintain observation and continue to pursue psychiatric consultation. The legal responsibility for an attempted or completed suicide will, at least partially, belong to the nurses on duty at the time (Valente, 1993).

Suicide risk can be reduced by using a written and signed no-suicide contract, ensuring a safe environment, reducing symptoms, increasing social support, encouraging a plan for living, and providing referrals. A no-suicide (or no-harm) contract is a promise not to do anything self-destructive without calling the nurse or other health care provider. It may be ineffective with impulsive people or manipulative and/or angry patients who lack a caring relationship with the provider (Valente, 1993).

Members of some cultural groups may be uncomfortable with the formality of signing a contract with a health care provider.

For an actively suicidal patient, safety can be best ensured by transfer to a psychiatric unit. If the patient must remain on a medical or surgical unit, specific nursing care recommendations can be obtained from the psychiatric or psychiatric nursing consultant. It will be necessary to assess suicide potential continuously by observing impulse control, suicidal ideation and intent, behavior changes, emotional state, physical complaints, the patient's response to observation, and safety needs. Let the consultant know that the nurses are not experienced with suicidal patients, may be anxious and uncertain, and require help in developing a nursing care plan.

BOX 18-7	Alcohol and Psychoactive Substances: Commonly Used Terms	
	substance	drug of abuse (including alcohol), a medication, or a toxin
	misuse	used for other than intended purposes, or used incorrectly
	abuse	excessive use differing from accepted social practices; maladaptive pattern of substance use with resulting social, work, or personal problems or use in physically dangerous situations
	craving	persistent psychological or physical need
	dependence (also called addiction)	impaired control and continued use of a substance on a continual or periodic basis despite significant substance-related problems resulting in cognitive, behavioral, and physiological symptoms and resulting in withdrawal symptoms with abstinence
	tolerance	need for greatly increased amount of the substance to achieve intoxication (or the desired effect) because of metabolic changes and alterations in cell functions that diminish the tissue reaction to a drug
	intoxication	recent ingestion of a substance with development of a reversible syndrome of clinically significant maladaptive behavioral or psychological changes
	withdrawal	substance-specific physiological signs that occur when the addictive substance is reduced or stopped; sometimes called abstinence syndrome
	cross dependence	condition in which a substance prevents withdrawal symptoms caused by abstinence from a substance in the same pharmacological class
	cross tolerance	condition in which tolerance to one substance results in tolerance to another
	dual diagnosis	substance dependence occurring concurrently with mental illness
	polyaddiction	dependence on a number of substances
	relapse	addiction reoccuring after a period of abstinence
	codependency	stress-induced preoccupation, dependence, and excessive concern with the addicted person's life

Information adapted from DSM-IV, 1994; Naegle, 1992; Gerace, 1993.

THE PATIENT WHO ABUSES ALCOHOL AND/OR PSYCHOACTIVE DRUGS

In the United States, substance abuse is a major public health problem (Frances, 1994). Terms commonly used in describing this problem are listed in Box 18-7.

Approximately 9.3 to 10 million persons, or about 7% of the U. S. adult population, are alcoholics. Families of alcoholics experience increased stress-related health problems. Other drugs that are abused are tobacco, caffeine, amphetamines, barbiturates, benzodiazepines, marijuana (cannabinoids), cocaine, hallucinogens, and opiates. Patients with alcohol, tobacco, and other substance abuse problems commonly present in general hospital services, such as gastroenterology (due to liver disease); heart and lung units; burn units (due to smoking and alcoholism); chronic pain programs; trauma services; cancer treatment programs; infectious disease (due to tuberculosis and HIV infection); and pediatrics, obstetrics, and gynecology (Frances, 1994). The effects of most of the drugs of abuse are summarized in Table 18-3.

TABLE 18-3
Effects of Psychoactive Substances

Substance	Physical Dependence	Psychological Dependence	Tolerance	Possible Effects
alcohol	yes	yes	yes	relaxation, euphoria, sedation, release of inhibitions, depression, impaired judgment, incoordination, slurred speech, nausea and vomiting
amphetamines	possible	high	yes	increased alertness, euphoria, insomnia, hyperactivity, anorexia, anxiety, tachycardia, hypertension
barbiturates	high-moderate	high-moderate	yes	slurred speech, disorientation, drunken behavior without odor of alcohol, sedation, emotional lability, decreased inhibitions
benzodiazepines	low	low variable	yes	anxiety relief, increased self-confidence, ataxia, drowsiness, slurred speech, hypotension
cannabinoids	degree unknown	moderate	yes	euphoria, relaxed inhibitions, increased appetite, disoriented behavior, failure in judgment, reddened eyes, dry mouth, incoordination
cocaine	possible	high	possible	increased alertness, excitation, euphoria, irritability, pressured speech, tachycardia, hypertension, anorexia, diaphoresis, insomnia
hallucinogens	no or unknown	no except phencyclidine	yes	distorted perception, heightened sense of awareness, illusions, hallucinations, distortions of time and space, depersonalization, dilated pupils, increased blood pressure, increased salivation
opiates	moderate to high	moderate to high	yes	euphoria, drowsiness, pain relief, lack of concern, respiratory depression, constricted pupils, nausea, impaired judgment

Information adapted from Naegle, 1992; Gerace, 1993; Stuart & Sundeen, 1991.

Attitudes toward substance abuse vary depending on the substance being abused, the person who is abusing it, and the setting in which abuse occurs. Nurses must be aware of different cultural attitudes and their own attitudes toward substance abuse to care for these individuals effectively. Addictive behavior is considered a biopsychosocial problem, with the key feature being the loss of control over, and preoccupation with, substance use (Gerace, 1993). Dysfunctional behavior patterns seen include manipulation, impulsiveness, dysfunctional anger, avoidance, grandiosity and entitlement, denial, and codependence (Naegle, 1992). Only 25% of those needing alcohol and drug treatment receive it (Frances, 1994).

NURSING INTERVENTION

The immediate concern of the nurse caring for a substance-abusing patient is recognizing and monitoring dangerous symptoms of withdrawal, particularly from alcohol, barbiturates, and benzodiazepines, as these are potentially fatal. Because a high level of denial is common in substance abusers, the patient may not identify substance dependence. First symptoms of withdrawal can proceed to more severe symptoms if the warning signs are missed. Table 18-4 presents the time periods and symptoms of alcohol withdrawal. Treatment of withdrawal commonly includes close monitoring of vital and other signs, gradually

TABLE 18-3
Effects of Psychoactive Substances (Continued)

Onset of Effect	Duration of Effect	Effects of Overdose	Withdrawal Syndrome
20 min–1 hr	dose-related	unconsciousness, coma, respiratory depression, death	tremors, hallucinosis, seizure disorder, delirium tremens (alcohol withdrawal delirium)
route-related, 10–30 min	drug-related, 2–4 hr	agitation, increased body temperature, hallucinations, convulsions, possible death	apathy, long periods of sleep, irritability, depression, disorientation
30–40 min	1–16 hr	shallow respiration, cold and clammy skin, dilated pupils, weak and rapid pulse, coma, possible death	anxiety, insomnia, tremors, delirium, convulsions, possible death
30–40 min	4–8 hr	shallow respiration, cold and clammy skin, dilated pupils, weak and rapid pulse, coma, possible death	anxiety, insomnia, tremors, delirium, convulsions, possible death
route and dose dependent, 20–30 min	route- and dose-dependent, 2–4 hr	fatigue, paranoia, possible psychosis	insomnia, hyperactivity, decreased appetite occasionally reported
route-related, 10–30 min	1–2 hr	agitation, increase in body temperature, hallucinations, convulsions, possible death	apathy, long periods of sleep, irritability, depression, disorientation
40–60 min	6–12 hr or variable	longer, more intense "trip" episodes, psychosis, possible death	withdrawal syndrome not reported
20–30 min	3–8 hr	slow and shallow breathing, clammy skin, convulsions, coma, possible death	watery eyes, runny nose, yawning, loss of appetite, irritability, tremors, panic, chills and sweating, cramps, nausea

TABLE 18-4 Timetable of Alcohol Withdrawal		
Stage	**Timing and Duration**	**Withdrawal Behaviors**
Stage 1	Begins shortly after drinking has ended; lasts 2–7 days (may be self-limiting or may progress to a more severe stage)	Tremors (hand, eye, and tongue), anxiety, hyperalertness, psychomotor agitation, nausea and vomiting, autonomic hyperactivity (hypertension, tachycardia, diaphoresis), anorexia, insomnia, irritability, headache, illusions
Stage 2	Begins within 12–24 hours; lasts for a few hours or days; alcoholic hallucinosis may, on rare occasions, become chronic	Stage 1 symptoms plus hallucinations: auditory, visual, tactile, and olfactory (rare), and paranoid ideation and behavior. Hallucinations may be transient and intermittent. Alcoholic hallucinosis is characterized by auditory hallucinations in a patient with no other psychotic behavior.
Stage 3	Usually occurs on the 2nd or 3rd day after the last drink; usually over within 48–72 hours after onset	Alcohol withdrawal delirium or delirium tremens (DTs) is a medical emergency. Stage 1 and stage 2 symptoms with marked autonomic hyperactivity, disorientation, delusions, delirium, severe agitation. May be seizure activity. Increased incidence of death.

Information adapted from Naegle, 1992; Gerace, 1993; Stuart & Sundeen, 1991.

reduced benzodiazepine or nonbenzodiazepine sedatives, patient safety using restraints for short periods if necessary, a low stimulation environment, and attention to nutrition.

Education, counseling, and referral to alcohol or drug treatment is an important but often neglected aspect of care. The crisis of hospitalization may create more patient receptivity to these ideas (Fuller & Jordan, 1994). Self-help groups include Alcoholics Anonymous (AA), Narcotics Anonymous (NA), Al-Anon, Nar-Anon, Ala-Teen, Adult Children of Alcoholics (ACOA), and Families Anonymous (Naegle, 1992).

Many treatment programs emphasize abstinence from mood-altering drugs and the need for ongoing treatment (Naegle, 1992). A challenge to current practices is presented by the field of harm reduction in public health. Harm reduction takes a wide view of the variety of harms associated with drug use and ways to reduce harm. Attention is focused on reducing the harmful consequences of use rather than reducing or attempting to eliminate use per se. This approach normalizes rather than marginalizes substance users and places substance abuse on a continuum relating use to problem severity for each individual (Somers, Tapert, & Marlatt, 1992).

CONCLUSION

The stress of physical illness challenges the coping abilities of patients and their families. Depression-related coping responses occur along a continuum from normal but distressing responses to maladaptive responses that present challenges to health care providers. In this chapter, coping responses to physical illness have been discussed with particular emphasis on depression-related responses considered ineffective. The responses described include depression and unmotivated behavior, suicidal thinking and behavior, and alcohol and psychoactive drug use. Interventions are recommended. As with all coping responses, when nurses understand and recognize the responses they observe, they can plan and implement effective, individualized interventions to reduce the stress experienced by patients, family members, and the health care providers caring for them.

BIBLIOGRAPHY

Billings, C.K. (1990). Anxiety and physical illness. *Psychiatric Medicine 8* (3), 149-162.

Diagnostic and statistical manual of mental disorders (4th ed.). (1994). Washington, DC: American Psychiatric Press.

Eisendrath, S. J. (1994). Psychiatric problems. In F. S. Bongard & D. Y. Sue (Eds.), *Current critical care diagnosis & treatment.* Norwalk, CT: Appleton & Lange.

Frances, R. J. (1994). Substance abuse in the general hospital: A priority area for evaluation and treatment. *General Hospital Psychiatry, 16,* 71.

Fuller, M. G., & Jordan, M. L. (1994). The substance abuse consultation team: Addressing the problem of hospitalized substance abusers. *General Hospital Psychiatry, 16(2),* 73–77.

Gerace, L. M. (1993). Addictive behavior. In R. P. Rawlins, S. R. Williams, & C. K. Beck (Eds.), *Mental health-psychiatric nursing: A holistic life-cycle approach* (3rd ed). St. Louis: Mosby Year Book.

Kurlowicz, L. H. (1993). Social factors and depression in late life. *Archives of Psychiatric Nursing, 7*(1), 30–36.

Kurlowicz, L. H. (1994). Depression in medically ill elders. *Archives of Psychiatric Nursing, 8*(2), 124–136.

Minarik, P. A. (1989). *The depressed patient: Nursing in the acute care setting* (syllabus and video). New York: Hospital Satellite Network and AJN Company.

Minarik, P. A., & Sparacino, P. S. A. (1990). Clinical nurse specialist collaboration in a university medical center. In P. S. A. Sparacino, D. M. Cooper, & P. A. Minarik (Eds.), *The clinical nurse specialist: Implementation and impact.* Norwalk, CT: Appleton & Lange.

Naegle, M. A. (1992). Management of chemical dependence. In J. Haber, A. L. McMahon, P. Price-Hoskins, & B. F. Sideleau, *Comprehensive psychiatric nursing* (4th ed.). St. Louis: Mosby Year Book.

Somers, J., Tapert, S. S., & Marlatt, G. A. (1992). Bringing harm reduction home. Harm reduction: Principles, applications and possibilities. In A. S. Trebach & K. B. Zeese (Eds.), *Strategies for change: New directions in drug policy.* Washington, DC: Drug Policy Foundation.

Stuart, G. W. (1994). *Detection and treatment of depression: The nursing perspective.* Washington, DC: American Nurses Association.

Stuart, G. W., & Sundeen, S. J. (1991). *Principles and practice of psychiatric nursing* (4th ed). St. Louis: Mosby Year Book.

Underwood, P. R. (1980). Facilitating self-care. In P. C. Pothier (Ed.), *Psychiatric nursing: A basic text.* Boston: Little, Brown & Co.

Valente, S. M. (1993). Evaluating suicide risk in the medically ill patient. *Nurse Practitioner, 18*(9), 41–50.

Wise, M. G., & Taylor, S. E. (1990). Anxiety and mood disorders in medically ill patients. *Journal of Clinical Psychiatry, 51*(1 Suppl), 27–32.

CHAPTER 19

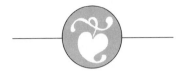

Psychosocial Aspects of Specific Physical Conditions

Patricia Barry
Pamela Minarik

Living with a condition that makes a person look or feel "different" can be a major adaptive challenge. The conditions selected for discussion in this chapter are infertility; menopause and hysterectomy, including sexual dysfunction due to physical conditions; the disfiguring conditions of mastectomy, ostomy, and amputation; and obesity and morbid obesity. The issues of trust, self-esteem, control, loss, guilt, and intimacy described in Chapter 9 will be applied to the challenge of adaptive coping with each condition. The purpose of this chapter is to serve as a resource to nurses in providing care and enhancing adaptive coping. Recommendations for specific nursing approaches that can reduce the risk of maladaptive responses will be included.

INFERTILITY

For couples who desire a child but are unable to conceive, the lack of a child can become a crisis that touches every aspect of their relationship, including feelings about self and each other, and relationships with family members and friends. Inability to conceive can result in frustration, depression, tension, anxiety, anger, obsession, guilt, isolation, a decrease in self-esteem in one or both partners, and ultimately grief (Berg & Wilson, 1992; Hirsch & Hirsch, 1989).

Considered a transitional phenomenon, infertility is usually experienced as an unexpected, unpleasant, undesired, and negative life event (Sandelowski, 1995). In a study of gender differences in coping with infertility, Draye, Woods, and Mitchell (1988) found that women were more vulnerable to the infertility crisis as manifested in lower self-esteem, higher rates of depression, and greater problems in personal life and with the health care system. Women were more likely than men to attribute the cause of the infertility to themselves. Both women and men used similar problem-focused coping strategies; women used more emotion-focused strategies.

Patricia Barry: *Psychosocial Nursing:*
Care of Physically Ill Patients and Their Families, 3rd ed.
© 1996 Lippincott–Raven Publishers

Causes of infertility include but are not limited to anovulation, tubal disease, and endometriosis in women, and varicocele and hypospermia in men. The contribution of psychosocial factors to infertility has interested investigators for many years; in the past, the trend was to focus on psychosocial antecedents or causes of infertility (Olshansky, 1987; Wright et al., 1989). A review of controlled research on the relationship of psychosocial distress and infertility found no evidence to support the often-cited hypothesis that psychosocial distress was more frequently an etiologic factor for women than men (Wright et al., 1989). These findings suggest that women tend to be more distressed by the entire experience of infertility and its medical management, but more likely this is a result, rather than a cause, of the fertility problem in the majority of cases. Parenthood may be more significant to adult role fulfillment for women.

New treatment approaches to infertility include microsurgery, sometimes with lasers, to open destroyed or blocked egg or sperm ducts; new hormone preparations to induce ovulation; and ultrasound to monitor ovulation. Other successful but potentially controversial techniques include in vitro fertilization (IVF), gamete intrafallopian transfer (GIFT), embryo transfer, host uterus, and surrogacy (Alexander and LaRosa, 1994).

PSYCHOSOCIAL ISSUES

Trust

The couple who desires a child and is unable to conceive can have many issues related to trust. Trust in normal body functioning is something that most persons take for granted. Trust in one another can also be affected, particularly if the cause of the infertility is identified. Even when the cause is unknown, women and men experience infertility differently (Draye, Woods, & Mitchell, 1988). Because of differences in experience or differences in coping, couples may experience difficulty in communicating and in supporting each other, especially if there was a prior lack of communication (Hirsch & Hirsch, 1989).

Another aspect of trust that becomes important for the couple is their belief in the health care provider. The care of infertile couples requires that the provider be knowledgeable about many intimate aspects of a couple's life. Care can be felt as intrusive and often includes direction about timing intercourse. Specialists in infertility are advised to pay particular attention to the patients' emotional needs, to the patients' understanding of procedures explained to them, to discussion of adoption, to greater involvement of the spouse in treatment, and to assisting the patient to have more control over the treatment course (Halman, Abbey, & Andrews, 1993).

Self-esteem

Infertility can present a developmental crisis depending upon the importance of parenthood to the individual, the couple, their families, and their social and cultural group (Draye, Woods, & Mitchell, 1988). When infertility occurs, and especially if it continues despite treatment, self-esteem, particularly of the infertile individual, can be seriously undermined. The maintenance of self-esteem is partially due to a person's being able to fulfill adult role expectations. When this ability is lost or hope of fulfilling it is lost, self-esteem decreases. The resulting sense of failure may lead to withdrawal from social contacts, possibly further eroding self-esteem.

Control

Infertility can result in a sense of loss of control, and participation in infertility treatment may be one way to seek control. Infertility treatment itself involves other issues of control. A couple's sexual technique, frequency, and bodies are subject to the control of the treating health care provider. Infertility and the drive to achieve their goal to conceive takes precedence over all other aspects of life (Mahlstedt, 1985; Olshansky, 1987). Making decisions about treatment, "taking medication, recuperating from surgery, dealing with the emotional consequences of infertility, and hoping *daily* that the process will end soon" take control (Mahlstedt, 1985).

Loss

The experience of infertility may involve a sense of profound loss for couples as they accept the reality of never conceiving a child. It is difficult to accept this loss because of the uncertain state in which infertile couples live as they continue in treatment. Ambivalence and mood swings may result from this uncertainty. Other simultaneous and complex feelings of loss may be involved (Mahlstedt, 1985). These include:

1. Loss of relationship
2. Loss of health, important body functions, or attractiveness
3. Loss of status or prestige
4. Loss of self-esteem
5. Loss of self-confidence, competence, or control
6. Loss of security
7. Loss of hope of fulfilling an important fantasy
8. Loss of something or someone of great symbolic value

Guilt

Infertile couples may experience guilt related to past sexual activities, sexually related diseases, or abortions (Rosenthal, 1992). The presence of guilt may be influenced by which member of the couple is infertile. Sexual activity may become associated with failure rather than pleasure (Hirsch & Hirsch, 1989). Guilt also may be an attempt to gain control of the answer to the question "why" (Mahlstedt, 1985).

Intimacy

Intimacy in a relationship is the degree of openness, honesty, and trust experienced together. Problems in communication that result from infertility or the treatment process can develop or serve to further undermine an already conflicted relationship. The level of intimacy that each partner experiences in all aspects of the relationship—emotional, intellectual, and physical—can deteriorate as the infertility treatment period progresses without positive results. Couples with good communication and mutual support may find their relationship strengthened by working together on the problem of infertility (Hirsch & Hirsch, 1989).

NURSING APPROACHES

The issues and outcomes outlined above are not necessarily permanent or as crisis-producing as they may initially sound. Infertile couples may experience some or all of the normal but distressing psychosocial effects described above as the process of infertility awareness and treatment unfolds. Because of the shame that many infertile couples experience about their condition, they rarely discuss it with others. Their communication with each other may be affected as each member tries to protect the other. This caring behavior, however, can result ultimately in a shutdown of their communication.

Counseling

Nurses can be very helpful by providing education, counseling, and empathic listening and support. Draye, Woods, & Mitchell (1988), Hirsch & Hirsch (1989), and Rosenthal (1992) make the following suggestions:

- Develop therapeutic and empathic relationships to help decrease feelings of isolation and loneliness.
- Allow patients to express and work through their feelings about infertility.
- Provide anticipatory guidance about what to expect in infertility and infertility treatment.
- Educate and clarify, providing information about options, and help patients in problem solving and decision making.
- Encourage verbalization of feelings between spouses, especially in noncommunicating couples. Emphasize the importance of open communication and mutual support to a healthy marital relationship.
- Help the couple recognize the differences in the way they are coping and how that may result in perceptions of underconcern or overconcern.
- Help men understand how encompassing the infertility identity can be for a woman.
- Pay particular attention to the needs of women because of the likelihood of greater distress in women.
- Normalize feelings and behavior.
- Refer to therapists knowledgeable about the psychological issues of infertility.

Couple Support Group

One approach to the psychosocial stress of infertility can be participation by couples in a group experience with other infertile couples. Rather than offering the group on an "as needed" basis, include the group as a part of the overall treatment. Frequently, if people must acknowledge that they "need" a group, their typical response is to deny that they are having any difficulty.

The advantages of a peer support group are that feelings of uniqueness, inadequacy, and isolation are decreased. Since all members are experiencing many similar emotions, they find support and approval. One of the advantages of a couples' group is that feelings and thoughts that a husband or wife may be afraid to express to the spouse may be identified, discussed, and defused in a group environment. Frequently, the members find great relief when they realize that they and their spouses are similar to other members of the group. Self-acceptance can be promoted by an awareness that one's feelings are normal.

MENOPAUSE AND HYSTERECTOMY

In Western societies there are many myths and misconceptions about the consequences of hysterectomy leading to surgically induced menopause, as well as natural menopause. These myths and misconceptions may cause women to approach these events negatively. In this section, information on menopause and hysterectomy, psychological effects, and issues of midlife, when natural menopause usually occurs, will be presented so that caregivers can form a conceptual base to use with patients in clinical practice.

DEVELOPMENT OF A FEMININE BODY IMAGE

During early and middle childhood, there is a heightened curiosity about sexual functioning in children of both sexes. Young girls incorporate their mother's and other important females' expressed opinions and nonverbal responses to sexual matters. The curiosity about their own and others' sexual functioning remains high in young girls during the latency stage of psychosexual development. By the time a female adolescent begins sexual development, many of her concepts about her own immature breasts and uterus, as well as her own potential sexuality, are formed. These are primarily the result of socialization within the family and social group.

The presence and functions of the breasts and uterus become integrated into the self-concept of the adolescent female. Depending on her socialization, a young girl's emotional investment in her uterus's child-bearing potential can be great or small. If a woman has little interest in raising a family, she will adapt to the effects of natural menopause or artificially induced menopause due to drug treatment or hysterectomy, similarly to any other change in her life. If however, there is or was great emotional investment in child-bearing ability, hysterectomy or artificially induced menopause at any age can be psychologically threatening (Hordern, 1994). On the other hand, the freedom to be unconcerned about pregnancy may be a relief for some women.

Unlike most body system functioning, which occurs outside of one's awareness, the menstrual cycle is part of a woman's conscious life. Some women describe their periods as being a nuisance or worse, being physiologically or emotionally symptomatic. On the other hand, the menstrual cycle is an affirmation of womanliness. Although rarely acknowledged, the ongoing rhythm of the menstrual cycle is psychologically comforting to some women. The loss of this cycle, which has been a conscious part of normal body functioning, body image, and self-image for 30 or more years, may normally be accompanied by feelings of sadness or, sometimes, of relief.

PSYCHOSOCIAL RESPONSE TO MENOPAUSE

Menopause, the cessation of menses, occurs gradually and naturally in midlife as an important physical and emotional life transition (Boston Women's Health Book Collective,

1984; Schover, 1988). Menopause lasts from a few months to 2 to 3 years and occurs when the ovaries begin to fail to produce estrogen and progesterone. Artificially induced menopause may occur as a result of surgery or treatments such as chemotherapy or radiation (Alexander & LaRosa, 1994). Premature menopause is more abrupt than natural menopause and the physical symptoms may be more severe. The occurrence of menopause is but one aspect of the adaptive and developmental challenges of women in midlife.

Frequently, menopause is used to explain any kind of psychological distress a woman experiences during this time. Actually, the hormonal changes of menopause are seldom the actual reason for emotional distress or depression. Rather, it is the *meaning* of menopause to the woman and her significant others, and her overall health coupled with the shifts and stresses of midlife, that influence her reaction (Johnson, 1991; Kaufert, Gilbert, & Tate, 1992). The multiple potential events of midlife that may be attributed to menopause include:

1. Changes in body image and youthful appearance.
2. Changes in health status, with increased incidence of major diseases.
3. Loss of menses and fertility.
4. Increasing awareness of mortality.
5. Loss of a daily relationship with children as they leave home.
6. Loss of active mothering role as result of above. If children return home due to financial pressures or develop drug or alcohol problems, a reluctant resumption of the parental role may occur.
7. Changes in the marital relationship may become evident as husband and wife are alone for the first time since they were newly married, or widowhood or divorce may occur.
8. Change in relationship to parents. Physical illness or a senile dementia in the parent(s) results in role reversal. The adult child becomes the caretaker of the parent.
9. Death of parents or loved relatives.
10. Awareness of lost opportunities with the passing of youth.
11. Job advancement opportunities may be given to younger people.

(Johnson, 1991; Kaufert, Gilbert, & Tate, 1992)

The loss of menses, in the context of the other changes a woman is experiencing, is only one of many factors that can contribute to psychological distress. Stereotypical thinking about menopausal women contains many fallacies and myths: "partial death," "a living decay," "raging hormones...incapable of rational thought and behavior," "fear of going crazy at menopause," the menopausal woman as "not really a man but no longer a functional woman" (Boston Women's Health Book Collective, 1984). In contrast to the stereotypes, women in their early 40s to early 50s have been found to increase in confidence, decisiveness, comfort and stability, and coping (Helson & Wink, 1992). The combination of events in midlife can be invigorating for women seeking new forms of activity and self-expression (Alexander & LaRosa, 1994).

Three physical signs are directly attributable to changes in estrogen production: 1) changes in the menstrual cycle; 2) hot flashes and sweats (vasomotor instability); and 3) decrease of moisture and elasticity in the vagina (vaginal atrophy). Because of the decreased moisture and elasticity in the vagina, intercourse can be painful, leading to fear of pain and intercourse. Other reported changes include decreased libido, decreased frequency of coitus, and reduced pleasure from coitus (Nathorst-Boos & von Schoultz, 1992; Nathorst-Boos, von Schoultz, & Carlstrom, 1993; Williamson, 1992). Some women report crying more readily, feeling more irritable, having less tolerance for others, and feeling more disorganized. Most women have few if any psychological symptoms and feel that the symptoms are manageable (Alexander & LaRosa, 1994).

Confusion and controversy surrounds the question of appropriate treatment for menopausal symptoms and the prevention of long-term health outcomes associated with postmenopausal women. Many medications are available for hormone replacement therapy, but not all women should take them. Estrogen has demonstrated clinical value in the treatment of postmenopausal conditions. It alleviates menopausal symptoms such as vasomotor instability (hot flashes) and vaginal dryness, and helps to prevent cardiovascular disease and osteoporosis, but it increases the risk of certain cancers and in some women raises triglyceride levels which contribute to heart disease (Alexander & LaRosa, 1994; Cadelago, 1994). Determining whether to use hormone replacement therapy for a given woman requires that the woman and her primary care provider work closely in partnership to evaluate dosage, effects, side effects, duration of treatment, and the use of other alternatives. Alexander and LaRosa (1994) point out that prevention of cardiovascular disease and osteoporosis by lifestyle modification—quitting cigarettes, eating a diet low in fat with adequate levels of calcium, and regular physical exercise—is the best strategy.

Factors in the Psychological Outcome of Hysterectomy

Hysterectomy is one of the most common major surgical procedures in the United States. Approximately 665,000 women undergo a hysterectomy each year; half of these women are still in their reproductive years (Williamson, 1992). Indications for hysterectomy include cervical or endometrial cancer, although the majority of hysterectomies are performed for nononcologic reasons (Cohen, Hollingsworth, & Rubin, 1989). If the ovaries are also removed, premature or artificial menopause will result. Although they are concerned about the surgical procedure itself and how soon they can return to normal routines, women are most concerned about their sexuality after hysterectomy (Williamson, 1992). The removal of the uterus has potential implications for altered body image ("empty shell"), altered self-perception of sexual functioning, and altered gender identity ("less feminine") if the latter was based on the uterus and childbearing ability (Schover, 1988; Williamson, 1992). Education and counseling before and after hysterectomy are an important part of recovery (Dulaney, Crawford, & Turner, 1990; Williamson, 1992).

Dispelling myths and misconceptions about the effects of hysterectomy is important in the adjustment of women posthysterectomy. Women may not know that they will no longer menstruate. They may erroneously believe that the vagina will be removed or sewn shut, rendering intercourse impossible, or they may believe that a uterus is necessary for orgasm or strength. Some women believe that the uterus is essential as an organ of excretion and that menstruation is important to good health. Women having a hysterectomy for cancer may believe that their disease was punishment for previous sexual behaviors or that cancer itself is contagious through sexual contact (Lamb, 1990; Schover, 1988; Williamson, 1992).

Influential early research on psychological complications posthysterectomy cited depression, anxiety, lowered self-esteem, altered sexual functioning, and posthysterectomy syndrome (severe depression and physical symptoms), the latter attributed to endocrine imbalance (Cohen, Hollingsworth, & Rubin, 1989; Richards, 1974). Later research does not support earlier findings about the incidence of posthysterectomy depression; part of the difference in the findings may be due to the different perceptions of women by themselves and others in the time periods (1940s to 1980s) in which the studies were done (Cohen, Hollingsworth, & Rubin, 1989; Kalisch & Kalisch, 1987). However, as with other surgical procedures, sadness and anxiety are common pre- and posthysterectomy. Women may grieve the loss of menstrual rhythmicity and reproductive ability even when the hysterectomy brings welcome symptom relief (Williamson, 1992). In a minority of women, usually those with prior history of depression, depression requiring professional intervention may develop after hysterectomy.

In a study of men's views about hysterectomies and the women who have them, Bernhard (1992) found that men, although not knowledgeable about hysterectomy, perceived negative psychological, social, and sexual effects of hysterectomy on women, but their relationships with women were not affected by hysterectomy. The findings could confirm fears of some women about men's beliefs about hysterectomy.

After hysterectomy, the vagina is shallower and orgasm will not include rhythmic uterine contractions as before, but these effects will not prevent orgasm (Schover, 1988; Williamson, 1992). Williamson (1992) also reported paresthesia and altered genital and pelvic sensations.

Lamb (1990), Schover (1988), and Williamson (1992) provide detailed information and suggestions for adjusting to these changes and enhancing sexuality, such as using lubricating gel on genitals and thighs and pressing thighs together during intercourse. Recent studies show that women do not experience significant changes in sexual functioning after surgical recovery from hysterectomy and may experience marked improvement in quality of life (Carlson, Miller, & Fowler, 1994; Cohen, Hollingsworth, & Rubin, 1989).

In spite of the myths about responses to hysterectomy, a relatively small number of women experience psychological maladaptation after hysterectomy. Women at high risk for emotional problems following a hysterectomy include those who have a history of depression, who are under 40, who have marital or sexual problems, who have conflicts about childbearing, and who have lower educational levels (Dulaney, Crawford, & Turner, 1990; Hallstrom & Samuelsson, 1985; Williamson, 1992). Adequate preoperative and postoperative information and social support are crucial in coping after hysterectomy (Cohen, Hollingsworth, & Rubin, 1989; Dulaney, Crawford, & Turner, 1990; Hallstrom & Samuelsson, 1985).

PSYCHOSOCIAL ISSUES

Trust

Trust in self and others relating to acceptance, and lack of rejection relating to age or loss of reproductive capacity can be major issues. For a woman having a hysterectomy, trust in the surgeon and other care providers may be an issue.

Self-esteem

Self-esteem can be threatened during midlife or after artificially induced menopause because of the sociocultural messages about aging and women, and the life events described above. However, women have been shown to increase in confidence (Helson & Wink, 1992) and be invigorated by new opportunities. When troubling symptoms are ended by hysterectomy, quality of life may improve.

Control

Many of the events of midlife can cause a woman to feel that she has little control over what is happening to her. The period of middle age for people with families has been called "the sandwiched generation." The needs of children and elderly parents can cause a woman to feel that her own needs are unimportant or nonexistent. On the other hand, women may find themselves with a greater sense of control, confidence, and freedom to pursue new interests. For women having surgery, lack of information and lack of control can be an issue.

Loss

The losses potentially experienced by a woman postmenopause or at midlife are listed above.

Guilt

Midlife may be a time of conflict in some women, particularly those who heavily invested their time and emotional energy in meeting the needs of others during previous years. Guilt may relate to anger about choices made earlier in life.

Intimacy

Intimacy in the marital relationship and in friendships can be especially meaningful during midlife. Sexuality may or may not be affected by natural or artificially induced menopause depending upon many factors such as quality of previous sex life, openness of communication within the relationship, and attitudes about menopause.

NURSING APPROACHES

Nurses caring for hysterectomy patients can encourage patients to discuss their concerns about themselves and their emotional, intellectual, and sexual relationships with their partners. Caregivers can help by correcting misconceptions and myths; educating patients about what will and will not be removed by the surgery; the physical and emotional changes, including grief, that may occur; and exploring practical ways to adjust sexually (Dulaney, Crawford, & Turner, 1990; Schover, 1988; Williamson, 1992). Many women are helped by participating in support groups with other women undergoing similar transitions.

After vaginal hysterectomy, the majority of women experience a loss of vaginal sensation for up to 6 months as a result of nerve trauma caused by the surgery. Eventually, sensation should return to normal (Williamson, 1992). If she is not informed that this is a common outcome of the surgery, a woman can become distraught that her normal sexual functioning may be permanently impaired. She should be encouraged to talk to her surgeon about her concerns.

After abdominal hysterectomy, most women do not experience a change in sexual desire and functioning, although they may be afraid of breaking or hurting something. Gradually following postoperative healing, a normal sexual activity pattern is likely to return. Women may have questions and concerns that they may be hesitant to bring up. It is often comfortable for a patient to discuss her sexuality with a knowledgeable nurse who can provide verbal and written information. She should be encouraged to discuss her concerns with her partner if she is experiencing increased anxiety. Lamb (1990), Schover (1988), and Williamson (1992) provide practical suggestions for enhancing sexuality, such as experimenting with positions, sexual fantasy, and the use of water-soluble jellies intravaginally to reduce initial discomfort during intercourse. Generally, the post-hysterectomy woman can look forward to unchanged and possibly increased sexual pleasure after her surgery. If nurses observe signs of significant depression or anxiety, they should talk with the patient about a referral for psychotherapy or counseling.

DISFIGURING CONDITIONS

A disease process can be cured by surgery that removes the diseased tissue. At times it is necessary to remove more than the exact site of pathology. Whenever the result is visible to the patient and others and results in a changed body image, it can be classified as disfiguring surgery.

MASTECTOMY

Breast cancer is the most common cancer and the leading cause of death among American women between the ages of 35 to 54 years (Knobf, 1991). Approximately 182,000 new cases of breast cancer were diagnosed in 1993 (Wyatt, Kurtz, & Liken, 1993). However, of the more than 900,000 breast biopsies performed in a year, 8 of every 10 will not identify malignancies, according to the American Cancer Society (Wilcox, 1994). Among African American women, the incidence of breast cancer is lower than among Caucasian women, although African American women have more advanced stages at diagnosis and lower survival rates (Lauver, 1992). This difference could be due to differences in prompt care-seeking, since earlier stage at diagnosis is related to improved survival (Knobf, 1991; Lauver, 1992).

Recognized risk factors for breast cancer include history of previous breast cancer, age older than 40 years, late menopause, no children or first pregnancy after age 30, and family history of breast cancer. Potential risk factors still being studied are diet, obesity, benign breast disease, oral contraceptive use, radiation exposure, and replacement estrogen use. Basic choices for treatment of breast cancer include lumpectomy plus irradiation and/or chemotherapy, modified radical mastectomy, and radical mastectomy. The modified radical mastectomy, which includes removal of the breast and axillary lymph nodes and preservation of the pectoralis muscle, with or without preservation of the pectoralis minor muscle, has been the standard of care since the 1970s. It involves considerable alteration in body image, function, and adjustment. When possible, breast reconstruction is an alternative that achieves symmetry and preserves body image (Knobf, 1991).

For some women, breast-preserving surgery combined with radiation is a choice. In some comparisons with mastectomy patients, these women have fewer negative feelings about themselves nude, resume sexual relations earlier, and experience less change in body satisfaction (Knobf, 1991). In other studies, findings have shown no relationship between type of treatment chosen and psychological and functional status, or that lumpectomy and mastectomy patients had similar emotional reactions and functional status. Possible explanations for this finding are that radiation therapy leads to more functional impairment than usually assumed due to fatigue and schedule disruption, or that lumpectomy patients receive less emotional support because others minimize the seriousness of breast-conserving surgery relative to the mastectomy (Hughes, 1993).

Following a breast cancer diagnosis, the decision-making process is complex, with many variables—the actual choices, information, relationships with providers, health behavior, attitudes and beliefs, coping style, personality, time, and significant others. Patients and their families need adequate time to process information, review treatment options, and seek a second opinion (Knobf, 1991; Long, 1993). Resources are available to help women decide which questions to ask and how to evaluate alternatives (Kelly, 1991; National Cancer Institute, 1991).

Mastectomy involves dealing both with a diagnosis of cancer and with the loss of a body part that is significant to womanliness. Breasts are viewed as an essential part of feminine beauty. After diagnosis it is common to experience fear, sadness, anger, perhaps guilt, and uncertainty, but this will happen on each person's individual timetable (Hughes, 1993; McGinn & Haylock, 1993). After surgery, frequently reported psychological problems include worry about recurrence, anxiety, depressed mood, feeling overwhelmed by emotions, worries about family, angry mood, and worries about self (Knobf, 1991). Studies of quality of life of long-term survivors have been limited, but generally have shown that women with treated breast cancer manifest nearly the same quality of life as asymptomatic women (Wyatt, Kurtz, & Liken, 1993).

In a review of the literature covering the period from 1989 to 1992, Carlsson and Hamrin (1994) reviewed studies and grouped them according to studies that examined 1) the relationship between psychological characteristics and breast cancer; 2) the relation-

ship between psychosocial interventions and breast cancer; 3) quality of life after breast cancer surgery and treatment; and 4) the relationship between social support and breast cancer. The authors made the following conclusions:

- In the studies of the relationship between psychological characteristics and breast cancer, most showed that the psychological adjustment (ways of coping) before the onset of cancer is one of the most important factors for understanding the psychological responses to breast cancer.
- Studies of the relationship between psychosocial interventions and breast cancer showed that psychosocial intervention, such as group and family treatment, had positive outcomes for participating women in regard to feelings of well-being and cancer regression.
- Studies of quality of life after breast cancer surgery and treatment indicated that the differences in outcome between mastectomy and breast-conserving surgery were small and insignificant, but most showed a nonsignificant trend toward an overall better quality of life in the breast-conserving group.
- Studies of the relationship between social support and breast cancer showed that social support (from partner, family, friends, relatives, and medical professionals) is an important factor in psychosocial adjustment and survival.

According to Carlsson and Hamrin, the question of the impact of psychological characteristics is difficult to answer unambiguously. Based on their review of the literature, they concluded:

- Fighting spirit and denial are better coping behaviors than stoic acceptance, anxiousness, or helplessness.
- Women react to the diagnosis of breast cancer with grief, anger, and intense fear, but the majority do not experience long-term emotional distress.
- Psychiatric morbidity, specifically depression and anxiety, was more likely in people with previous psychiatric illness who lacked a confiding relationship,

and greater in women with malignant disease.

- Risk factors for psychological distress included many medical symptoms, little or no social support from family and significant others, little or no hope of a recovery, a desire to give up, and great concern about death.
- Psychological state before cancer was one of the best predictors for postcancer adjustment. Sexual satisfaction seemed to be predicted by overall psychological health, relationship satisfaction, and premorbid sexual life.

Psychosocial Issues

Trust

Multiple issues of trust occur for a woman with breast cancer. Assembling a cancer care team she trusts and educating herself to be a participating member are important (McGinn & Haylock, 1993). Another issue is trusting herself to make good decisions and cope with multiple intense and difficult feelings. A major issue is trusting her partner, family, and friends to support her and accept her as a woman.

Self-esteem

As a result of cancer or surgical treatment for cancer, women may see themselves as *"unhealthy, not in control, unfeminine, asexual"* (McGinn & Haylock, 1993). Losing one or both breasts can be traumatic, damaging a woman's feelings of attractiveness. The impact on body image is significant. The effort to manage powerful feelings such as anger may leave a person feeling immobilized or "unladylike" (McGinn & Haylock, 1993). Sense of self-worth and value may be damaged and may affect relationships negatively.

Control

Women may feel helpless, out of control, and suddenly dependent on a new set of advisors and health care providers (McGinn & Haylock, 1993). Uncertainty about the future as well as strong and frightening feelings may lead to feeling out-of-control. Women with cancer may be afraid to feel or talk about fear or other negative feelings because they believe it means they do not have a positive attitude. Lack of in-

formation may exacerbate feelings of being out-of-control.

Loss

Removal of the breast is a significant loss (Knobf, 1991). Other potentially devastating losses include the loss of former body concept, sense of femininity, sources of sexual pleasure, attractiveness to her partner, and potential loss of full arm function if lymphedema continues (Granda, 1994; McGinn & Haylock, 1993). Radiation or chemotherapy treatment may also cause other losses—hair and figure—that may be temporary but still are difficult to cope with. Grief is a normal response to loss, but because mastectomy is a treatment for breast cancer, a more prominent feeling may be relief at being cured of cancer.

Guilt

Women can experience guilt about causing or being responsible for cancer. They can also feel guilty if they delayed before seeking a medical opinion about a breast lump or about not meeting their expectations for performance and positive attitude during treatment (McGinn & Haylock, 1993). Women may feel guilty if they believe they are no longer physically or sexually attractive to their partners and their partners "are stuck" with them.

Intimacy

Changes in self-esteem, feelings of vulnerability, and physical changes may disrupt intimacy, in terms of both openness and sexuality. A woman may feel insecure about whether her partner will accept her and find her attractive and pleasing. Sensations may be different, especially in the beginning. Loss of the breast and nipple obviously interferes with pleasure from breast caressing, or skin may be tender during radiation. Self-consciousness about the scar and chest or shoulder pain may interfere with touching or intercourse (Schover, 1988).

Nursing Approaches

Education and emotional support are important psychosocial interventions. Encourage women to take a family member or trusted friend when they see the surgeon and take the time to give careful consideration to the alternatives as indicated earlier. Provide educational materials and information about procedures, side effects, and follow-up care at the level of the woman's ability to hear and understand.

Emotional support includes exploring with the patient her feelings and responses to the losses, her thoughts about the alternatives available to her, how she thinks mastectomy will affect her life and her relationships, and other psychosocial support resources available to her and her family (Knobf, 1991). Many patients benefit from support groups and interventions such as guided imagery and relaxation described by Siegel (1989) that enhance coping and increase sense of control. Information about adapting to changes and enhancing sexual functioning should be included in nursing care. Patients are often embarrassed to bring up questions about sexuality to their health care providers. Unfortunately, providers may be uninformed, embarrassed, or set other priorities. At the minimum, written materials such as *Sexuality & Cancer* (Schover, 1988) or other booklets by the American Cancer Society should be provided.

OSTOMY

Over the last few decades, an increase in the number of intestinal and genitourinary diseases diagnosed in North America has resulted in a higher incidence of ostomy surgery (Rheaume & Gooding, 1991). Surgical treatment of gynecological cancer may also result in ostomy creation (Lamb, 1990). The word *ostomy* is used here to define an abdominal stoma that is the result of a temporary or permanent diversion of the intestinal or urinary tract to the outside of the body. People with ostomies report many problems after the surgery, including shock, rage, and depression during hospitalization and immediately after; fear of rejection, shame, and low self-esteem, resulting in withdrawal and increased difficulty forming interpersonal relationships; and a dramatic change in body image that may cause sexual dysfunction (Grosso-Hacker, 1991; Ramer, 1992). Psychological factors also influence the patient's ability to learn stoma care (Deeny & McCrea, 1991; Model, 1990).

Many variables influence adjustment to ostomy surgery. One of the major factors that can cause difficulty in a patient's ability to accept an ostomy is the emphasis in U. S. culture on cleanliness, grooming, and the normal privacy of the process of elimination. These values evolve from early childhood experience and are deeply embedded in the personality. Youngsters of 2 and 3 years are socialized to conform to society's expectations regarding toileting. Self-esteem, body image, and many personality traits are developed in the youngster when he or she is acquiring beliefs about elimination. As a result, when an ostomy is necessary, it can be a major adaptive challenge.

The circumstances surrounding the ostomy surgery impact the patient's response. Is this a sudden, unexpected ostomy (as a result of trauma) that left the patient no time for psychological preparation? Is this a temporary ostomy being performed to give the bowel a rest from diverticulitis or another type of bowel disease? Is there a possibility that there is a malignant tumor? In the latter case, the patient's concern about the ostomy will usually be secondary to major concerns for life.

Psychosocial Issues

Trust
The patient with an ostomy is in an unfamiliar, possibly frightening situation, feeling total dependence on the nurse for the care of the stoma, removal of waste products, and teaching self-care. Initially, the patient will watch the nurse closely for a reaction to the appearance of the stoma, the odor, or the feces or urine. The patient may expect rejection from the nurse, from family and friends, and from strangers.

Self-esteem
Because an ostomy, like many surgical procedures, returns a patient to a dependent status and causes a major shift in body perception, the patient is subject to shame and feelings of self-rejection. Body image has the potential to change markedly. A drop in self-esteem may be seen initially as the person adapts to the new circumstances.

Control

There are two major factors that can further add to the sense of loss of control that is common for ostomy patients.

1. What is the person's normal personality style? Is he or she fastidious? Does he or she have a controlling personality type? (See Chapter 15.) If so, this patient will be even more threatened by this condition than someone whose approach to life and to new situations is more relaxed and easygoing.

2. Where was the ostomy performed? Was it high in the bowel, in the jejunum, in the lower part of the colon, or in the ureter? Jejunostomies or ureterostomies can be more threatening to people because the contents are watery and unformed, leading to greater fear of leakage or "accidents," especially in public places. On the other hand, if the ostomy is performed near the end of the bowel, the feces are usually well formed. Once the ostomy is healed, it is usually possible to obtain a degree of control of the timing of bowel movements.

Loss

As mentioned above, the ostomy patient initially loses control over bowel function. In addition, if surgery involved the removal of a section of bowel, rectum, ureter, or bladder, this represents the loss of a body part. Initially the patient may anticipate lifestyle changes—ability to travel, to sit in a theater near other people, to make love or be intimate in other ways, and so on. Usually these expected limitations can be resolved and the patient is able to resume normal activities. Resolution usually depends far more on psychosocial adaptation than on physiological adaptation to the surgery.

Guilt

If the patient's ostomy is the result of bowel disease that was aggravated by poor adherence to a prescribed diet, guilt may result. Guilt may be expressed during the nurse's care of the stoma and feces or urine. The patient may apologize for the inconvenience, messiness, and so on. The patient is actually looking for reassurance when making such comments that

he or she (as a person) is still accepted by the nurse.

Intimacy

One of the major concerns of ostomy patients who have sexual partners is *whether* they can function sexually, *how* they will function sexually, and *how* their partner will react to them. One study of 250 ostomy patients found that single and widowed males enjoyed better emotional health than married men and than women, leading to the conclusion that intimacy may be less important in that group (Wade, 1990). Women who have undergone ostomy creation as a result of tumor debulking for ovarian cancer or pelvic exenteration for recurrent cancer of the cervix commonly report sexual dysfunction (Lamb, 1990). Sexual dysfunction results not only from drastic changes in body image and fears associated with stomal/pouch appearance, noise, leakage, odor, and rejection by partner, but also from disruption in the innervation within the pelvis that may result in orgasmic problems. During pelvic exenteration, urinary and/or bowel ostomies are created and the vaginal canal is removed. Sexual disruption after this surgery includes a decrease in the frequency of sexual activity, low sexual satisfaction and arousal, and changes in sexual confidence and body image; the degree of distress depends on past sexual habits and desire to continue (Lamb, 1990).

Patients can become fearful of developing any intimate relationship with a member of the opposite sex. When these concerns are not addressed in the hospital before discharge, the uncertainty that the patient feels can contribute to an overall reduction of interpersonal communication. This can create stress in a relationship, which, if prolonged, can be more difficult to resolve. It is wise to wait to discuss these issues until the patient has made progress in coping with the diagnosis that led to the surgery and dealt with concerns about survival right after the surgery (Gloeckner, 1991).

Nursing Approaches

An essential aspect of nursing care of the ostomy patient is the nurse's response to the patient. The patient will be watching the nurse for the slightest negative clue. If the nurse demonstrates acceptance of the patient, first as a human being with worth and dignity and second as a person with an ostomy who is acceptable, the patient will be more able to incorporate this acceptance into his or her own self-image; the nurse's acceptance can form the basis of the patient's self-acceptance. The nurse can also serve as a role model to the patient's partner, family members, and friends. Family members may need support in dealing not only with stoma care but also with psychological and social issues that may be stressful (Malett, 1993).

The importance of talking with an ostomy patient cannot be overemphasized. By asking open-ended questions (see Chapter 2), the nurse can encourage the patient to talk about feelings and thoughts. Verbal exploration of important psychological issues enhances adaptation. On occasion, the spouse or other important support person should be included. Many problems with adaptation can be easily avoided by perceptive nursing care. For example, if the nurse notices that the patient is unwilling to look at the ostomy after a few days of care, talking about feelings is very important. If the patient's behavior is unchanged despite these efforts, the nurse may recommend counseling from an enterostomal and/or psychiatric liaison nurse specialist. Nursing assessment and intervention also should include talking about sexual function and concerns (Lamb, 1990).

Support from family, friends, health professionals, or self-help groups is beneficial to adjustment (Grosso-Hacker, 1991; Rheaume & Gooding, 1991). Whenever patients express major concerns about whether they will be able to resume a normal lifestyle, it can be very helpful for them to talk with someone who has an ostomy and is fully active. If the hospital has an enterostomal therapist or clinical nurse specialist, he or she can help to arrange an ostomy visitor before the patient goes home. If there is not an ostomy specialist, contact the local chapter of the United Ostomy Association or the American Cancer Society for information about how to arrange for an ostomy visitor. Meeting, listening, and talking to another person with an ostomy, especially someone well-

adjusted to it, helps decrease feelings of being the only one with an ostomy and increase feelings of self-acceptance (Grosso-Hacker, 1991). If, despite these interventions, the nurse continues to be concerned about actual or potential psychosocial maladaptation, formal psychiatric consultation or outpatient counseling should be requested.

AMPUTATION

More than 90 percent of the approximately 600,000 amputations performed annually are due to complications of chronic disease (Butler, Turkal, & Seidl, 1992). Most surgical amputations involve the lower limbs (Rybarezyk et al., 1992). The present-day amputee population is likely to be older, chronically ill, male with limited social support, and suffering the complications of peripheral vascular disease or diabetes mellitus (Butler, Turkal, & Seidl, 1992).

Amputation is a surgical procedure that results in psychological trauma for the patient. It poses serious physiological and psychological problems, both short- and long-term (Medhat, Huber, & Medhat, 1992). The patient's reaction to amputation is complex and influenced by many factors including age, sex, type of amputation, expectations for rehabilitation, the perceived or functional value of the lost body part, and the reason the amputation is done (Butler, Turkal, & Seidl, 1992; Pierce, Kernek, & Ambrose, 1993). If the surgery is planned, there will be more time to prepare emotionally and grieve for the loss of a limb or part of a limb. Traumatic amputation, however, may be more likely to precipitate psychosocial crisis (Raven & Brugger, 1992). If the amputation is preceded by extended suffering due to chronic disease, it may be perceived as a relief, resulting in less severe body image conflicts (Butler, Turkal, & Seidl, 1992).

Psychological challenges facing amputees and their families include grief reactions, anger, anxiety, phantom limb sensation or pain, and preoccupation with body image. Potential consequences include social withdrawal, isolation, and long-term difficulties with social adjustment, occupational rehabilitation, and loss of income (Butler, Turkal, & Seidl, 1992; Heafy, Golden-Baker, & Mahoney, 1994).

Psychosocial Issues

Trust

The initial surgical recommendation that the limb should be removed results in many doubts for the patient. The ability to trust a surgeon and the validity of the recommendation can be a major challenge (Butler, Turkal, & Seidl, 1992). If a patient is highly suspicious, reluctant, or anxious about such a recommendation, and his or her overall physical condition is deteriorating, it is advisable to do the following:

1. Seek immediate psychiatric liaison consultation to determine the patient's reasons for refusing surgery.
2. Avoid doing the surgery, unless the patient's life is jeopardized, until some resolution of the patient's psychic distress is achieved. Without such resolution the patient's adaptation following surgery can be severely compromised, resulting in a paranoid psychotic reaction, marked anxiety, severe depression, and/or concomitant physical complications as the result of severe mental stress. Another outcome of a patient's being coerced into an unwanted amputation is a complex rehabilitation process.

The patient must trust in the recommendations and plans of rehabilitation physicians (physiatrists) and physical therapists to work in rehabilitation. Rehabilitation may be a painful process because of the use of stumps that have not yet fully healed or give the patient phantom limb pain. One of the most difficult adjustments of the person who has had lower limb amputation is to develop trust in caregivers that they will hold securely and not allow falling.

Self-esteem

The amputee, whether he or she has lost part of a hand, arm, foot, or leg, may experience a marked drop in self-esteem. The amputee may expect rejection by others and doubt the ability to return to full functioning, even with a prosthetic device. These ideas, accurate or not, diminish self-esteem. In addition, the gradual awareness of lost former abilities may also have an effect on a person's sense of worth and self-image.

Control

Feelings of powerlessness are common and necessitate a major adaptive effort in order to overcome them. When the patient thinks about future functioning, he or she frequently believes that previously normal circumstances will be difficult to manage and control. As with many postoperative patients, the initial enforced dependency is one of the most difficult aspects of the recovery period.

Feelings of anger and frustration in amputees are common as the slow rehabilitation process is underway. Many male amputees fear that they may cry uncontrollably. They may have been socialized into feeling that crying is not acceptable in men. Permission by caregivers that such feelings are normal and acceptable to them can allow amputees to grieve their loss adaptively both in the hospital and after discharge, as the grief process continues. Excessive control of emotions disrupts the normal grief response.

Loss

The amputee faces many types of loss, including actual loss of the physical part and loss of function of the limb. Depending on the limb affected, the availability of a prosthesis, and adaptation to the prosthesis, the patient may no longer be able to walk, run, write, play sports, drive, or operate complex machinery. The patient also loses previous self-image, body image, and role function if no longer able to work in his or her former occupation. Commonly, patients fearfully anticipate subsequent amputations that may be necessitated by their chronic medical problems.

Guilt

Guilt feelings in amputees whose surgeries were necessitated by traumatic injury may occur if their accidents were due to their own carelessness. Guilt may also be experienced by people with circulatory problems whose poor personal hygiene or carelessness may have contributed to the deterioration of the affected limb.

Intimacy

One of the common fears of an amputee is rejection by his or her sexual partner or unattractiveness to a future partner because of the missing part and changed appearance. This subject, often avoided by patients, is of intense concern for many. The patient frequently is too embarrassed to discuss concerns about his or her own sexuality, but caregivers should initiate discussion and encourage the patient to talk about these fears, as part of the rehabilitative effort. The patient's ability to share feelings may be decreased as he or she tries to resolve many concerns privately. The intimacy and closeness of nonsexual relationships also may be affected. Sharing feelings with another person, even a normally trusted person, may initially be too risky because of a feeling of vulnerability.

Nursing Approaches

An important role of the nurse in caring for the amputee is to discuss the amputation supportively, allowing the patient to talk about feelings. Patients can be encouraged to talk about their emotions and thoughts on their changed body and how they think others may react to them. Discussion about intimacy and sexuality is also important. As described above, amputees often are concerned about rejection by their partner. The counseling techniques described in Chapter 2, specifically the section on leading skills, can be helpful. Include information on the normal emotional responses to loss. When uncontrollable emotion is expressed, the nurse can sit quietly with the patient and listen attentively.

One of the most important themes of intervention is to maintain a focus on the enduring qualities of the person and to reinforce the person's ability to cope with past crises (Butler, Turkal, & Seidl, 1992). Keep the family informed and involved, providing opportunities for them also to share their feelings and fears. Another helpful intervention is to arrange a visit from an amputee who has had a similar surgery and made a positive adjustment. The setting of realistic, short-term goals is an important therapeutic approach. Avoid falsely optimistic predictions or platitudes which usually result in patient anger, resentment, and or withdrawal. Honest, encouraging feedback can provide much-needed support and reassurance.

OBESITY AND MORBID OBESITY

Obesity is a complex and multifaceted problem needing multifaceted treatment programs (Brink, 1992; McBride, 1988; Vickers, 1993). One in three Americans is overweight, according to researchers ("America's Getting Fatter," 1994; "Failing in Our *Healthy People 2000* Objectives," 1994). The prevalence of overweight, defined as body mass index values correlating with approximately 120% or more of desirable weight, soared between the late 1970s and the early 1990s. Although the increase in overweight cut across gender and racial lines, not all groups are equally prone to overweight. Less than a third of white women and non-Hispanic white or black men were overweight but nearly half of Hispanic or black women were. The researchers urged early intervention in childhood to prevent overweight and resultant health problems. However, there is controversy about the relationship of overweight to health problems, especially in regard to the dismal record of treatment for obesity (Ciliska, 1990; Popkess-Vawter, 1989). An additional problem is the cultural context of stigma and discrimination against the obese (Brink, 1992, 1994; McBride, 1988; Rossi, 1988).

The relationship of health to overweight is not completely clear. Excess body weight has been associated with hypertension, hyperlipidemia, diabetes mellitus, carbohydrate intolerance, increased surgical and anesthesia risk, osteoarthritis, higher mortality risk, pulmonary and renal problems, and complications during pregnancy ("Failing in Our *Healthy People 2000* Objectives," 1994; Vickers, 1993). Research has not, however, demonstrated a causal relationship between obesity and these diseases (Brink, 1992). There is evidence to support the idea that total body mass is not predictive of diabetes or heart disease but that placement of fat on the belly region (truncal or android adiposity) rather than in the hip region (gynecoid adiposity) or all over, is predictive (Brink, 1992). Significant for health of the overweight person are family history of high-risk diseases and prior history of dieting and exercise (Brink, 1992). "Yo-yo" dieting almost inevitably leads to failure and results in a tendency toward android adiposity (Brink, 1992; McBride, 1988). The latter, fortunately, is responsive to exercise.

Rather than a single, standardized, valid measure for estimating healthy or unhealthy weights, a number of methods are used. The preferred method is the body mass index (BMI), a simple calculation of height and weight in which an individual's weight in kilograms (k) is divided by height in meters (m) squared (k/m^2). A BMI between 20 and 25 is considered healthy for both men and women. A further rating scale discriminates levels of obesity, with individuals whose BMI exceeds 45 considered morbidly obese (Brink, 1992). Other definitions of morbid obesity are excess weight (for height) of 100 pounds or more above the life insurance standards, or weight more than twice ideal body weight (Black & Mangan, 1991; Brentin & Sieh, 1991).

However obesity is defined, many nurses find caring for obese patients frustrating, offensive, and potentially hazardous (Brentin & Sieh, 1991; Vickers, 1993). Nurses are prey to the same cultural prejudice against fat that currently characterizes Western society (Brink, 1992; Fontaine, 1991a; Rossi, 1988). Trends in ideal body shape and size reflect society's expectations of women at the time; there is a wider range of acceptable body types for men than for women (McBride, 1988; Rossi, 1988). Men are less dependent on body shape and size as a primary definition of masculinity (Fontaine, 1991a).

Body-image disturbances such as body-image distortion, body-image dissatisfaction, and obsession with weight loss are seen in anorexia nervosa, bulimia nervosa, and compulsive overeating, as well as in obesity (Kiszka, 1994; Miller, 1991). Women are particularly susceptible to social pressure to be thin (Brink, 1994; Popkess-Vawter & Banks, 1992). The obese are seen as physically deformed, lacking character and self-control, stupid, lazy, gluttonous, morally defective, less likable, and ugly; the assumption is that they like being fat or they would do something about it. Discrimination occurs in lower college acceptance rates, reduced likelihood of being hired, lower salaries, and problems in education, seating in public transportation, and in social relationships (Brink, 1994; Ciliska, 1990; Weiler & Helms, 1993).

PSYCHOSOCIAL ISSUES

The following issues are closely tied to the sociocultural context and the transmission of cultural ideals related to shape and size. In some cultures and subgroups, these may not apply.

Trust

Social influences on body image begin in infancy and continue throughout life, with the possibility that obese people will internalize society's negativity and rejection (Brink, 1994; Fontaine, 1991a).

Self-esteem

Much has been written about the negative impact of culture on the self-esteem of obese people and the psychological trauma of being stigmatized (Brink, 1994; Ciliska, 1990; Fontaine, 1991a; Rossi, 1988; Popkess-Vawter & Banks, 1992) although the obese show no greater psychopathology than the nonobese (Ciliska, 1990). Negative body image, body distortion, and body dissatisfaction are far more common among women than men (Ciliska, 1990; Miller, 1991). Relatively few people who lose weight through dieting are able to maintain their losses, leading then to a greater sense of failure (Ciliska, 1990; McBride, 1988).

Control

According to Fontaine (1991a), in the American value system, thinness is equated with power, control, independence, and achievement, and fatness with helplessness, lack of self-control, and nonachievement. Efforts to control weight include the use of drugs, surgery, diet and exercise plans, behavior modification, self-help programs, and individual and group support (Ciliska, 1990). The surgical procedure gastric stapling is effective but usually is reserved for morbid obesity (Black & Mangan, 1991; NIH Conference, 1991).

Loss

The sense of not fitting in can leave the obese person socially isolated, with resultant loss of social supports (McBride, 1988).

Guilt

According to Fontaine (1991a), a cultural assumption is that obese people could be thin and happy if they were not so lazy; they have only themselves to blame for their size, shape, and unhappiness.

Intimacy

Some people are hostile or ridiculing toward fat people. For the obese or self-perceived obese person, body dissatisfaction may impair social functioning and limit openness to intimacy and sexuality (Fontaine, 1991b; Miller, 1991). Eating-disordered patients may suffer from concurrent sexual problems that are the result of a complex interaction of biological, intrapersonal, and interpersonal factors (Fontaine, 1991b).

NURSING APPROACHES

The first task of caring for the obese or morbidly obese patient is to examine one's own beliefs about body shape and size and to rethink internalized cultural values. It is important to avoid feeding into the stereotype that anyone can be thin and a thin body is a magical solution to life's problems. This means consciously defining identity broadly to include characteristics other than body shape and size (Fontaine, 1991a).

Morbidly obese people who are hospitalized either for gastric stapling to control weight or for other comorbid conditions require individualized assessment, care planning, and intervention, as well as good teamwork (Black & Mangan, 1991; Brentin & Sieh, 1991). This is likely to involve changes in usual methods of assessment and usual equipment, adjustments of drug and IV therapy, and aggressive skin care and respiratory support, as well as encouragement of self-care and mobility. Safety of staff and patient is a major concern. The patient will likely be afraid of falling and not being able to get up and the staff is likely to be afraid of being injured when lifting or turning the patient.

Health professionals must also avoid assuming that all overweight people desire primarily to lose weight. McBride (1988) recommends the development of multiple criteria for treatment success; do not equate success only with losing weight. Promote and provide psychoeducational interventions that deemphasize the importance of body size in determining self-worth, increase self-esteem, decrease body dissatisfaction, and normalize eating, such as Ciliska's (1990) *Beyond Dieting: The Weekly Program* and Miller's (1991) body-image therapy using cognitive, mind-body, and kinesthetic strategies. Nursing care should also include sexual assessment, education about anatomy and physiology of sexual response and the effect of eating disorders, and counseling, depending on the nurse's level of preparation (Fontaine, 1991b).

CONCLUSION

Living with a condition that makes a person look or feel "different" can be a major challenge. Nurses can help patients work through their psychological, emotional, and behavioral responses to their condition and experience life more fully. Adaptation to such a condition can enrich family relationships and promote quality of life in which a person is able to accept and appreciate a variety of life's invitations.

Because of the many types of clinical settings in which nurses work—acute care, ambulatory clinics and offices, rehabilitation, home care, occupational health, schools—they have continuous opportunities to assess and intervene to enhance the psychosocial adaptation of people and their families living with various types of physical conditions.

BIBLIOGRAPHY

Alexander, L. L., & LaRosa, J. H. (1994). *New dimensions in women's health.* Boston: James and Bartlett Publishers.

America's getting fatter. (1994). *American Journal of Nursing, 94*(9), 9.

Berg, B. J., & Wilson, J. F. (1990). Psychiatric morbidity in the infertile population: A reconceptualization. *Fertility and Sterility, 53*(4), 654–661.

Bernhard, L. A. (1992). Men's views about hysterectomies and women who have them. *Image: The Journal of Nursing Scholarship, 24*(3), 177–181.

Black, J., & Mangan, M. (1991). Body contouring and weight loss surgery for obesity. *Nursing Clinics of North America, 26*(3), 777–788.

Blenner, J. (1990). Passage through infertility treatment: A stage theory. *Image: Journal of Nursing Scholarship, 22* (3): 153–158.

Boston Women's Health Book Collective. (1984). *The New Our Bodies, Ourselves.* New York: Simon & Schuster.

Brentin, L., & Sieh, A. (1991). Caring for the morbidly obese. *American Journal of Nursing, 91*(8), 40–43.

Brink, P. J. (1992). Challenging commonly held beliefs about obesity. *Clinical Nursing Research, 1*(4), 418–429.

Brink, P. J. (1994). Stigma and obesity. *Clinical Nursing Research, 3*(4), 291–293.

Butler, D. J., Turkal, N. W., & Seidl, J. J. (1992). Amputation: Preoperative psychological preparation. *Journal of the American Board of Family Practice, 5*(1), 69–73.

Cadelago, L. G. (1994). Coronary artery disease: Are there differences between women and men? *Clinician Reviews, 4*(10), 57–58, 60–62, 65, 68–70, 72, 75–76, 78.

Carlson, K. J., Miller, B. A., & Fowler, F. J. Jr. (1994). The Maine women's health study: I. Outcomes of hysterectomy. *Obstetrics and Gynecology, 83*(4), 556–565.

Carlsson, M., & Hamrin, E. (1994). Psychological and psychosocial aspects of breast cancer and breast cancer treatment: A literature review. *Cancer Nursing, 17*(5), 418–428.

Chandarana, P. C., Conlon, P., Holliday, R. L., Deslippe, T., & Field, V. A. (1990). A prospective study of psychosocial aspects of gastric stapling surgery. *Psychiatric Journal of the University of Ottawa, 15*(1), 32–35.

Ciliska, D. (1990). *Beyond dieting: The weekly program.* New York: Brunner/Mazel.

Cohen, S. M., Hollingsworth, A. O., & Rubin, M. (1989). Another look at psychologic complications of hysterectomy. *Image: The Journal of Nursing Scholarship, 21*(1), 177–181.

Deeny, P., & McCrea, H. (1991). Stoma care: The patient's perspective. *Journal of Advanced Nursing, 16*(1), 39–46.

Downey, J., & McKinney, M. (1992). The psychiatric status of women presenting for infertility evaluation. *American Journal of Orthopsychiatry, 62*(2), 196–205.

Draye, M. A., Woods, N. F., & Mitchell, E. (1988). Coping with infertility in couples: Gender differences. *Health Care for Women International 9*(3), 163–175.

Dulaney, P. E., Crawford, V. C., & Turner, G. (1990). A comprehensive education and support program for women experiencing hysterectomies. *Journal of Obstetric, Gynecologic, and Neonatal Nursing, 19*(4), 319–325.

Erikson, E. (1963). *Childhood and society* (2nd ed.). New York: Norton.

Failing in our *Healthy People 2000* objectives. (1994). *Clinician Reviews, 4*(10), 31–32, 35.

Fiorentini, A. (1990). Acute meningococcaemia: A case study. *Intensive Care Nursing, 6*(1), 17–24.

Fontaine, K. L. (1991a). The conspiracy of culture. *Nursing Clinics of North America, 26*(3), 669–676.

Fontaine, K. L. (1991b). Unlocking sexual issues. *Nursing Clinics of North America, 26*(3), 737–743.

Gloeckner, M.(1991). Perceptions of sexuality after ostomy surgery. *Journal of Enterostomal Therapy, 18*(1), 36–38.

Granda, C. (1994). Nursing management of patients with lymphedema associated with breast cancer therapy. *Cancer Nursing, 17*(3), 229–235.

Grosso-Haacker, M. (1991). Coping with an ostomy. *Ostomy/Wound Management 33*: 43–46.

Hallstrom, T., & Samuelsson, S. (1985). Mental health in the climacteric: The longitudinal study of women in Gothenburg. *Acta Obstetricia et Gynecologica Scandinavica. Supplement,* 130, 13–18.

Halman, L. J., Abbey, A., & Andrews, F. M. (1993). Why are couples satisfied with infertility treatment? *Fertility and Sterility 59*(5), 1046–1054.

Heafey, M. L., Golden-Baker, S. B., & Mahoney, D. W. (1994). Using nursing diagnoses and intervention in an inpatient amputee program. *Rehabilitation Nursing, 19*(3), 163–168.

Helson, R., & Wink, P. (1992). Personality change in women from the early 40's to the early 50's. *Psychology and Aging, 7*(1), 46–55.

Hirsch, A. M., & Hirsch, S. M. (1989). The effect of infertility on marriage and self-concept. *Journal of Obstetric, Gynecologic, and Neonatal Nursing, 18*(1), 13–20.

Hordern, B. B. (1994). Hysterectomy before 40: One woman's story. *Seasons* (Wyeth-Ayerst Laboratories), *4*(1), 3–6.

Hughes, K. K. (1993). Psychosocial and functional status of breast cancer patients: The influence of diagnosis and treatment choice. *Cancer Nursing, 16*(3), 222–229.

Hunt, K., Vessey, M., & McPherson, K. (1990). Mortality in a cohort of long-term users of hormone replacement therapy: An updated analysis. *British Journal of Obstetrics and Gynaecology, 97*(12), 1080–1086.

Johnson, K. (1991). *Trusting ourselves: The complete guide to emotional well-being for women.* New York: Atlantic Monthly Press.

Kalisch, P. A., & Kalisch, B. J. (1987). *The changing image of the nurse.* Menlo Park, CA: Addison-Wesley.

Kaufert, P. A., Gilbert, P., & Tate, R. (1992). The Manitoba Project: A re-examination of the link between menopause and depression. *Maturitas, 14*(2), 143–155.

Kelly, P. T. (1991). *Understanding breast cancer risk.* Philadelphia: Temple University Press.

Kiszka, S. A. (1994). Dieting to death. *Advance for Nurse Practitioners, 2*(9), 8–10, 42.

Knobf, M. T. (1991). Breast cancer. In S. B. Baird, R. McCorkle, & M. Grant (Eds.), *Cancer nursing: A comprehensive textbook.* Philadelphia, W. B. Saunders.

Lamb, M. A. (1990). Psychosexual issues: The woman with gynecologic cancer. *Seminars in Oncology Nursing, 6*(3), 237–243.

Lauver, D. (1992). Psychosocial variables, race, and intention to seek care for breast cancer symptoms. *Nursing Research, 41*(4), 236–240.

Long, D.S. (1993). How breast cancer patients choose a treatment method. *Radiologic Technology 65*(1), 30–33.

Mahlstedt, P. P. (1985). The psychological component of infertility. *Fertility and Sterility, 43*(3), 335–346.

Malett, J. (1993). Caring for the caretakers: The patient's family. *Journal of ET Nursing, 20*(2), 78.

Marshall, M., Helmes, E., & Deathe, A. B. (1992). A comparison of psychosocial functioning and personality in amputee and chronic pain populations. *The Clinical Journal of Pain 8*(4), 351–357.

McBride, A. B. (1988). Fat: A women's issue in search of a holistic approach to treatment. *Holistic Nursing Practice, 3*(1), 9–15.

McGinn, K. A., & Haylock, P. J. (1993). *Women's cancers: How to prevent them, how to treat them, how to beat them.* Alameda, CA: Hunter House, Inc.

Medhat, A., Huber, P., & Medhat, M. (1992). Factors that influence the level of activities in persons with lower extremity amputation (or ambulation?). *Rehabilitation Nursing, 15*(1), 13–18.

Miller, K. D. (1991). Body-image therapy. *Nursing Clinics of North America, 26*(3), 727–736.

Model, G. (1990). A new image to accept: Psychological aspects of stoma care. *Professional Nurse, 5*(6), 310–316.

National Cancer Institute. (1991). *Questions to ask your doctor about breast cancer.* Bethesda, MD.

Nathorst-Boos, J., & von Schoultz, B. (1992). Psychological reactions and sexual life after hysterectomy with and without oophorectomy. *Gynecologic and Obstetric Investigation, 34*(2), 97–101.

Nathorst-Boos, J., von Schoultz, B., & Carlstrom, K. (1993). Elective ovarian removal and estrogen replacement therapy—Effects on sexual life, psychological well-being and androgen status. *Journal of Psychosomatic Obstetrics and Gynaecology, 14*(4), 283–293.

NIH Conference. (1991), Gastrointestinal surgery for severe obesity. Consensus Development Conference Panel. *Annals of Internal Medicine 115*(12), 956–961.

Olshansky, E. F. (1987). Infertility and its influence on women's career identities. *Health Care for Women International, 8*(2–3), 185–196.

Pierce, R. O., Kernek, C. B., & Ambrose, T. A. (1993). The plight of the traumatic amputee. *Orthopedics, 16*(7), 793–797.

Popkess-Vawter, S., & Banks, N. (1992). Body image measurement in overweight females. *Clinical Nursing Research, 1*(4), 402–417.

Popkess-Vawter, S. (1989). Assessment of positive and negative body image in normal weight and overweight females. In R.M. Carroll-Johnson (Ed). *Classification of nursing diagnoses: Proceedings of the Eighth Conference, North American Nursing Diagnosis Association.* Philadelphia: J.B. Lippincott Co.

Ramer, L. (1992). Self-image changes with time in the cancer patient with a colostomy after operation. *Journal of ET Nursing, 19*(6), 195.

Raven, K. A., & Brugger, C. A. (1992). Hemicorporectomy: A nursing challenge. *Orthopeaedic Nursing, 11*(2), 73–78.

Rheaume, A., & Gooding, B. A. (1991). Social support, coping strategies, and long-term adaptation to ostomy among self-help group members. *Journal of Enterostomal Therapy, 18*(1), 11–15.

Richards, D. H. (1974). A post-hysterectomy syndrome. *Lancet, 2*(7887), 983–985.

Rosenthal, M. B. (1992). Infertility: Psychotherapeutic issues. *New Directions for Mental Health Services, 55,* 61–71.

Rossi, L. R. (1988). Feminine beauty: The impact of culture and nutritional trends on emerging images. *Holistic Nursing Practice, 3*(1), 1–8.

Rybarezyk, B. D., Nyenhuis, D. L., Nicholas, J. J., Schulz, R., Alioto, R. J., & Blair, C. (1992). Social discomfort and depression in a sample of adults with leg amputations. *Archives of Physical Medicine and Rehabilitation, 73*(12), 1169–1173.

Sandelowski, M. (1995). A theory of the transition to parenthood of infertile couples. *Research in Nursing and Health, 18* (2), 123–132.

Schain, W. S. (1991). Sexual rehabilitation: Whose responsibility is it anyhow? Oncology Nursing Conference, Contemporary Forums. San Francisco, September 27.

Schover, L. R. (1988). *Sexuality & cancer: For the woman who has cancer, and her partner.* New York: American Cancer Society, Inc.

Siegel, B. S. (1989). *Peace, love & healing.* New York: Harper & Row.

Turner, C. (1994). Pharmacologic highlights. Hormone replacement therapy: Its use in the management of acute menopausal symptoms. *Journal of the American Academy of Nurse Practitioners, 6*(7), 318–320.

Vickers, M. J. (1993). Understanding obesity in women. *Journal of Obstetric, Gynecologic, and Neonatal Nursing, 22*(1), 17–23.

Wade, B. E. (1990). Colostomy patients: Psychological adjustment at 10 weeks and 1 year after surgery in districts which employed stoma-care nurses and districts which did not. *Journal of Advanced Nursing, 15*(11), 1297–1304.

Weiler, K., & Helms, L. B. (1993). Responsibilities of nursing education: The lessons of Russell v Salve Regina. *Journal of Professional Nursing, 9*(3), 131–138.

Wilcox, P. M. (1994). Recognizing breast problems and promoting breast health. *Advance for Nurse Practitioners, 2*(5), 12–15, 39.

Williamson, M. L. (1992). Sexual adjustment after hysterectomy. *Journal of Obstetric, Gynecologic, and Neonatal Nursing, 21*(1), 42–47.

Wright, J., Allard, M., Lecours, A., & Sabourin, S. (1989). Psychosocial distress and infertility: A review of controlled research. *International Journal of Fertility, 34*(2), 126–142.

Wyatt, G., Kurtz, M. E., & Liken, M. (1993). Breast cancer survivors: An exploration of quality of life issues. *Cancer Nursing, 16*(6), 440–448.

CHAPTER 20

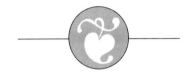

Psychosocial Aspects of Chronic Illness*

Karen Inaba

Chronic illness is a primary health care problem, and refers to a trajectory of enduring alterations in health status leading to incurable, recurrent symptoms; impaired functioning; ongoing, illness-related demands; and challenges to adaptation (Corbin & Strauss, 1991; Miller, 1992a). Chronic illness differs from acute illness in that it does not usually end in recovery and is not self-limited in course. Examples of chronic conditions include AIDS, alcohol abuse, chronic obstructive pulmonary disease, chronic renal failure, coronary artery disease, diabetes mellitus, paralytic conditions secondary to spinal cord injury or stroke, and rheumatoid arthritis.

Chronic illness occurs in many configurations. For some individuals, the experience of chronic illness is merely a fluctuating course with exacerbation of symptoms and periods of remission. For others, symptoms are continuous with a steady, deteriorating course until death. A compromised person may experience acute episodes of other illnesses superimposed onto the existing, primary, chronic condition, complicating recovery from the secondary illness. Also, multiple, interrelated chronic conditions may exist concurrently over the course of an individual's life span as vulnerability increases. In some situations, for example, one chronic illness may precipitate another chronic condition, as in the case of chronic renal failure related to diabetes mellitus.

Within this context, and with the increased life span of the chronically ill, nurses in a variety of care settings face numerous challenges in supporting adaptation to disability, enhancing quality of life, and supporting individual and family decision-making about aggressiveness of medical treatment in advanced disease. Nursing models of the illness experience are now focusing on individual and family perspectives, self-help and self-care, behavioral responses to illness, developmental and systems perspectives, the context of illness, and stress adaptation, instead of merely the disease and diagnostic categories.

The individual with chronic illness accesses the healthcare system for symptom management or treatment of concurrent acute illness,

---

*Note: The opinions expressed by the author do not necessarily reflect those of the Department of Veterans Affairs.

Patricia Barry: *Psychosocial Nursing: Care of Physically Ill Patients and Their Families,* 3rd ed. © 1996 Lippincott–Raven Publishers

and may repeatedly enter a variety of health care settings depending upon the phase and severity of illness. Relationships with health care providers, access to care, and new systems of care influence patient outcomes and health care delivery for the chronically ill individual. Case management, advanced practice nursing providers, shorter hospital stays, and greater collaboration with home health care agencies and community resources are now paradigm shifts for chronic care (Hinton-Walker, 1993). Numerous strategies to assess and support coping skills in the chronically ill, such as self-regulation and cognitive control strategies, are also being utilized (Miller, 1992a).

CHARACTERISTICS AND STAGES OF CHRONIC ILLNESS

Characteristics and stages of chronic illness can be described by a trajectory framework that takes into consideration the illness course and impact on the individual within the context of his or her life situation. The trajectory model refers to the clinical progression of the disease over time, with various coping tasks required at each stage (Corbin & Strauss, 1991; Hawthorne, 1991). Some individuals remain fixated at initial stages due to new illness events or other complications.

Corbin and Strauss (1991) described eight phases representing changes in health status in chronic illness. These stages were described as pretrajectory (preillness); trajectory onset (signs and symptoms appear); crisis; acute (active illness or complications); stable (symptoms controlled); unstable; downward (progressive deterioration); and dying.

Morse and Johnson (1991) presented a four-stage illness constellation model describing coping responses of individuals and families based on the stage of illness. These stages included uncertainty when illness is first suspected; disruption and crisis when medical care is sought; striving to regain self or attempts to continue usual responsibilities; and regaining health or accepting limitations imposed by the disease.

COPING IN CHRONIC ILLNESS

Factors influencing patient and family coping in chronic illness include cognitive appraisal of threat and stress; the meaning of the illness to the person; attribution or beliefs about causation of illness; hope; personal factors such as age, sex, roles, cognitive capacity, and premorbid personality; disease-related factors such as type of illness, rate of onset and progression of illness, level of disability or alterations in body image, prognosis, and demands of illness; and interpersonal factors such as available family and social support systems, developmental level, cultural beliefs and values; and concurrent life crises (Seaburn, Lorenz, & Kaplan, 1992; Woods, Haberman, & Packard, 1993).

Coping with a chronic disease and adjusting to an illness role are also influenced by the individual's past family relationships, developmental history, and life experiences affecting trust, relatedness to others, intimacy, self-esteem, and coping with loss. For example, a person who has been unable to form healthy attachments to others may feel anxious and threatened by multiple caregivers in a hospital setting, loss of autonomy, and intrusions into personal space. Likewise, an individual with a body-image disturbance may adjust poorly to a changed appearance brought about by a chronic disease.

Chronic illness and disability may further threaten an individual with a fragile self-concept and limited emotional reserves related to a history of major physical and emotional trauma, catastrophic losses, repeated shaming, and situations of powerlessness. Loss of personal worth, weakened defense mechanisms, fear of abandonment, and guilt may impair adjustment to the chronic disease. Also, changes in prior family roles and role expectations, loss of control, and the type and magnitude of the illness disability experienced may contribute to ineffective individual or family coping and other nursing diagnoses.

COPING STYLES IN CHRONIC ILLNESS

Coping in the chronically ill individual has been described as a process of appraisal and adaptation to multiple stressors in the context of the person's experience. In chronic illness, stressors such as role changes, loss of functioning, and other sources of threat often overwhelm the individual, disrupting equilibrium and precipitating a crisis. In the more resilient, hardy person, on the other hand, adjustment to chronic health problems occurs more rapidly.

Lipowski (1970) described two cognitive coping styles in adjustment to illness. These styles included minimization responses such as ignoring, denying, or rationalizing; and vigilant focusing or obsessional, anxious, intellectualized hypervigilance. He also described behavioral coping styles in illness as *tackling*, or approach behaviors; *capitulating*, or passivity and dependent clinging; and avoiding stressors, or *flight*.

Lipowski also asserted that the individual's coping capacity was influenced by meanings and attitudes held toward the illness and disability. These meanings include illness as challenge; illness as enemy; illness as punishment; illness as weakness; illness as relief; illness as strategy; illness as irreparable loss or damage; and illness as value. Schussler (1992) later tested these concepts on chronically ill individuals and confirmed Lipowski's formulations.

Lazarus and Folkman (1984; Lazarus, 1993) described two coping styles used in stressful situations that can apply to the chronically ill individual. These include *emotion-focused* or *emotion-regulating* coping, such as venting feelings, vigilance, distraction, and distancing behaviors. *Problem-focused* coping occurred when the stressor could be modified through problem-solving, acting on the environment or oneself, or new learning.

Expanding on Lazarus' work, Burckhardt (1987) summarized coping strategies of the chronically ill as information-seeking, direct action, inhibition of action, intrapsychic processes, and turning to others for support.

COPING TASKS IN CHRONIC ILLNESS

Demands of illness refer to illness-related stressors and events experienced by individuals and families facing chronic illness. Some of these major tasks include managing everyday life activities, monitoring a chronic course of symptoms,

adapting to disability and changes in family, social, and vocational roles, negotiating through the complex systems and settings of health care, preventing and managing medical crises, managing care regimens, establishing relationships with caregivers, preserving self-esteem, and maintaining meaning and quality of life in the face of uncertainty. Table 20-1 summarizes common coping tasks of chronically ill adults (Miller, 1992a).

PSYCHOSOCIAL RESPONSES TO CHRONIC ILLNESS

There are many diverse psychosocial responses to the chronic illness experience and the crisis of coping with chronic alterations in health status. Individuals and families respond to chronic illness from unique personal and group contexts; society reacts to issues surrounding chronicity caregiving; and health care providers face ongoing challenges of helping the chronically ill and their families adjust to disability and maintain quality of life.

INDIVIDUAL RESPONSES

In the initial stages of chronic illness, many individuals face uncertainty about the impact of their newly diagnosed disease and outcomes, especially when a deteriorating course is predicted. Anxiety, fears about disability and ongoing medical treatment, and feelings of hopelessness, helplessness, and powerlessness are frequently experienced. Common responses to chronic disease and disability include acute and dysfunctional grieving for continuing losses, decrease in functioning and ability to live independently; self-esteem disturbance; body-image disturbance; altered role performance; ineffective individual coping; defensive coping; and impaired adjustment (Conwill, 1993; Lindgren et al., 1992). Common nursing diagnoses and behavioral manifestations are summarized in Table 20-2.

In addition to emotional adjustment, chronically ill individuals must also establish and maintain trusting relationships with multiple health care providers in a number of settings.

TABLE 20-1
Typology of Coping Tasks of Chronically Ill Adults

Broad Task Category	Subconcepts in the Category
1. Maintaining a sense of normalcy.	Hiding, minimizing illness and/or responding to curious inquiries of others. Living as normally as possible despite daily therapy and obvious symptoms.
2. Modifying daily routine; adjusting lifestyle.	Including therapy and symptom control in daily routine. Providing for safety.
3. Obtaining knowledge and skill for continuing self-care.	Having internal awareness. Monitoring effects of therapy.
4. Maintaining a positive self-concept.	Integrating illness into self-concept. Maintaining or enhancing self-esteem.
5. Adjusting to altered social relationships.	Experiencing loneliness or social isolation. Undergoing patient- or other-initiated disengagement. Preserving relationships with friends and family who satisfy dependency needs. Maintaining family solidarity.
6. Grieving over losses concomitant with chronic illness.	Losing physical abilities, function. Losing status. Losing income and social relationships. Losing roles and dignity. Dealing with financial losses.
7. Dealing with role change.	Losing roles—social, work, family. Gaining roles—dependent help seeker, self-care agent, chronically ill patient.
8. Handling physical discomfort.	Handling illness-induced discomfort. Handling pain caused by therapy.
9. Complying with prescribed regimen.	
10. Confronting the inevitability of one's own death.	
11. Dealing with social stigma of illness or disability.	
12. Maintaining a feeling of being in control.	Exerting cognitive control. Exerting behavioral control. Exerting decisional control.
13. Maintaining hope despite uncertain or downward course of health.	Experiencing effects of hope. Finding meaning in physical changes.

Miller, J. F. (1992). Analysis of coping with illness. In J. F. Miller (Ed.), *Coping with chronic illness: Overcoming powerlessness*. Philadelphia: F. A. Davis Co. Used with permission.

Adjusting to treatment regimens, handling medical crises, dealing with uncomfortable symptoms, and coping with hospitalization or other unfamiliar systems of care may overwhelm vulnerable individuals. Difficult, reactive behaviors may occur, and should be acknowledged and understood within the context of the person's multiple physical and emotional stressors.

In the elderly, self-care deficits, social isolation, diminished support resources, and coping with developmental crises such as retirement and death of a spouse frequently impact quality of life and adjustment to chronic illness. Often, the elderly must adjust to a constellation of several chronic, interrelated conditions, as illness sequelae progress. Repeated hospitalizations, relocation, adjusting to family caregiving or institutionalization, and preparing for one's death are often a part of the chronic illness trajectory for many elderly.

SOCIETAL RESPONSES

Another psychosocial response to the condition of chronic illness lies in society's stigmatization, or devaluing, of the chronically ill, disabled individual who is unable to meet societal expectations for functioning and assumes the sick role as a lifestyle (Saylor, 1990). Some chronic diseases, for example, alcoholism and AIDS, carry greater stigma than others, due to negative appraisals of behavior or lifestyles assumed to be associated with the illness condition. For some individuals, their chronic illness is not obvious, so they are more easily misjudged or stigmatized than others with more apparent disabilities or advanced age. Isolation, withdrawal, and a sense of rejection by caregivers are common reactions of stigmatized groups.

Another societal response to chronicity involves an increase in ethical dilemmas in health care of the chronically ill (Johnson, 1991). As the population ages, chronic illnesses increase, as do questions about distribution of scarce health care resources, end-of-life decision making, aggressiveness of care in progressive diseases, who will provide care and in what setting, and who will finance treatment. New models of holistic care for incurable,

chronic conditions will be needed in the future (Hinton-Walker, 1993).

FAMILY RESPONSES

The many demands of chronic illness and illness-related events create ongoing crises and continually challenge the coping skills of families and partners. Chronic illness taxes personal and social resources; creates stress and disequilibrium within the family system; and often leads to responses such as altered family processes, ineffective family coping, altered role performance, altered sexuality patterns, caregiver role strain, and decreased social support and isolation for the well partner (Archbold et al., 1990; DesRosier, Catanzaro, & Piller, 1992). Guilt reactions may also appear in family members impacted by sudden catastrophic events that later result in chronic disability, or may simply result from cumulative frustration, anger, and physical and emotional strain associated with caring for the chronically ill family member in the home (Flannery, 1990; Lubkin, 1992).

How well a family copes may depend upon the meanings attributed to the illness and family members' perceptions of the illness; disability and accompanying demands, as well as the nature and stage of the illness; illness course; family characteristics; resources and support network; coping skills; family rules and roles; and perception of health care (Seaburn, Lorenz, & Kaplan, 1992; Youngblood & Hines, 1992). Periodic crises may also occur as chronic illness demands overwhelm family resources and coping with usual stresses of daily living. Developmental demands impacting the family are also important to assess (Shaw & Halliday, 1992).

Family involvement in care of the chronically ill member is now increasing as resources for chronic care shift away from the acute hospital. Because of this trend, the chronically ill individual and family or partner caregivers, together with professional caregivers or care managers, must collaborate early in all phases of teaching, treatment planning, and decision making. Identifying community resources; increasing availability of relevant information, support, and respite care for caregivers; and improving access to systems of care are essen-

<table>
<tr><td colspan="2" align="center">**TABLE 20-2**
Examples of Nursing Diagnoses for Chronic Illness</td></tr>
</table>

Nursing Diagnosis	Behavioral Manifestation
Impaired adjustment related to lifestyle and behavioral changes or inadequate support systems.	Job loss and career disruptions result from physical disabilities.
Impaired social interaction related to self-concept disturbance.	Dramatic physical changes as well as psychological disturbances diminish self-confidence and affect interpersonal relationships.
Hopelessness related to deteriorating physical condition.	Prolonged confirmation of diagnosis or unsuccessful treatment may cause patients to lose faith or decrease perseverance.
Knowledge deficit related to limited exposure to information and anxiety.	Patients and families may be overwhelmed by illness-related tasks and unable to process new information.
Fear related to powerlessness.	Expressions of "loss of control" are made when chronic illnesses affect activities of daily living.
Body-image disturbance related to chronic disease and debilitation.	Significantly altered physical appearance or need for adaptive devices affect identity and self-concept.
Altered sexuality patterns related to body-image disturbance, loss of body function, and psychological stress.	Changes in sexual behavior and sexual dysfunction are associated with fatigue, chronic pain, impaired physical mobility, and illness-related anxiety.

Adapted from Piringer, P., Agana-Defensor, R., Mullen, N. M., & Lee, L. (1993). A model for development and implementation of a patient support group in a medical-surgical setting. *Holistic Nursing Practice, 8* (1), 16–26, with permission of Aspen Publishers, Inc.

tial strategies that will empower families caring for the chronically ill.

RESPONSE OF THE NURSE

Caring for a chronically ill individual presents many clinical as well as emotional challenges to nurses working in acute care settings, rehabilitation centers, nursing homes, outpatient clinics, or the person's residence. Goals of nursing care focus on improving the quality of life; minimizing symptoms and further disability; teaching symptom management; facilitating self-care and self-help competence; decreasing a sense of powerlessness; providing acknowledgement, support, and encouragement; advocating for the chronically ill person and family by assisting them in identifying and utilizing appropriate resources; and developing effective strate-

gies to help the individual become an empowered, effective partner in care.

Nurses can provide several types of support for the chronically ill and their families. Woods and colleagues (1989) studied nursing support and noted three types of support that are helpful in relieving troublesome symptoms: emotional, informational, or instrumental. They suggested that support is most effective in the following situations:

The type of support given matches the specific illness demands and patient problems (e.g., instrumental support to relieve physical symptoms versus emotional and informational support to decrease emotional distress).

The nature and source of support are appropriate to the individual's stage of illness and situation.

The nature and timing of support are appropriate (e.g., informational support during the early and transitional stages of illness). The nature of support matches the desired outcomes.

Caring for the chronically ill individual and family involves therapeutic use of self in providing support throughout the various stages of the illness trajectory. Some problematic areas for nurses include overinvolvement, overidentification, and lack of emotional boundaries with the chronically ill individual and family; rescuing behaviors and relating to the person in paternalistic ways that increase dependency and helplessness; anger and frustration at difficult behaviors, such as noncompliance with the treatment regimen and rejection of help or goals; and grieving as the chronically ill individual becomes progressively more disabled and eventually dies. Consulting with colleagues who are part of the caregiving team is another effective method of decreasing stress following the death of a chronically ill individual.

PSYCHOSOCIAL ISSUES WITH SPECIFIC CHRONIC ILLNESSES

Psychosocial issues associated with many common chronic illnesses are frequently identical or interrelated, and are affected by the stage and duration of the condition; personal and family factors, including age, premorbid personality, and family and social support; cultural beliefs and practices; and availability of other coping resources. While shared patterns of disability or common concerns exist in each disease category, it is important to acknowledge personal responses and individualize care as much as possible.

THE INDIVIDUAL WITH AIDS

The individual diagnosed with AIDS faces an uncertain future with an ominous course, as AIDS is a terminal, multisystem illness. While a cure is not available, advances in medical science have prolonged the lives of many affected with AIDS, and changed its course into a chronic as well as terminal illness.

The initial stage of AIDS involves diagnosis with a positive HIV antibody serostatus. The second stage involves development of AIDS-indicating symptoms or AIDS-related complex (ARC) of symptoms. The third, or terminal, stage is a period characterized by multiple opportunistic infections, neoplasms, and organic mental disorders such as AIDS dementia (Flaskerud, 1992; Oechsner, Moller, & Zaudig, 1993).

Common psychosocial issues faced by the individual with AIDS may include living with stigmatization and others' fears of contagion; adjusting to multiple losses and uncertainty; maintaining quality of life with increasing debilitation; coping with body-image changes; confronting end-of-life decision-making in the terminal stages of illness; and maximizing functioning in spite of cognitive impairments (Gaskins & Brown, 1992; Hall, 1992).

Nursing Diagnoses

The individual diagnosed with AIDS faces a shortened life span with many demands on coping. Anxiety often develops while waiting for confirmation of seropositivity and experiencing an often vague onset of early symptoms of the disease. Anger, guilt, and anticipatory grieving related to loss of comfort and body functioning, body-image disturbance, loss of relationships, loss of autonomy, and altered role performance related to job loss and changed financial status may lead to profound states of hopelessness. As the disease restricts functioning, powerlessness related to loss of control may increase. Altered sexuality patterns or sexual dysfunction related to changes in close personal relationships and partner's fears of contagion, may also occur. Dysfunctional grieving responses may also occur throughout the illness or escalate in the terminal stages of the disease as patients confront quality-of-life and other existential issues.

Since AIDS also attacks the central nervous system, chronic mental status changes may occur and progress into chronic conditions such as AIDS-related dementia complex. Alterations in thought processes, acute confusion and sensory/perceptual alterations related to brain infections, or side effects of medications may impair decision making and coping and create crises for caregivers. Potential for injury related to cognitive impairment, mood lability, and impulsivity may also increase as the AIDS patient enters terminal stages of the illness.

Nursing Interventions

The individual diagnosed with AIDS must often share stigmatizing information about lifestyle risk factors that may compromise privacy and a sense of safety. Disclosure that one is homosexual, bisexual, and/or an intravenous drug user is difficult, especially if the individual has not shared this information openly. Conveying nonjudgmental acceptance is essential in relationship-building with the individual with AIDS, since many are often blamed for their condition and may experience discrimination and rejection from family and usual support systems. Allowing proximity and focusing on the person's strengths and uniqueness will also bolster self-esteem and decrease withdrawal and fears of rejection by caregivers.

Encouraging the individual with AIDS to verbalize feelings about the diagnostic process and outcomes, responding to questions and concerns about symptoms, providing information, and acknowledging versus minimizing concerns related to symptoms, decreases anxiety and increases a sense of control.

Consistent care providers, whenever possible, will decrease the individual's fear of abandonment as the disease progresses and the person becomes more dependent on others for care. Social isolation may be reduced by helping the individual with AIDS network with an appropriate support group of others affected by the same disease or accessing community resources for AIDS support.

Individuals with AIDS benefit from extra support during crisis periods in the illness, such as initial confirmation of seropositivity and initial appearance of opportunistic diseases. Assessment for suicidal tendencies should occur during these crisis periods, especially when other major losses also impact the patient. High-risk factors include a history of affective disorder and drug use, family history

of suicide, recent catastrophic losses, and an inadequate social support network.

In the later stages of AIDS, organic mental disorders may develop. Ensuring safety, decreasing overstimulation, providing a familiar environment, arranging for consistent caregivers, and assessing medical causes for confusion and agitation are essential. Administering antipsychotic medication (e.g., haloperidol) and restraints may also be indicated.

THE INDIVIDUAL WITH ALCOHOL DEPENDENCE

The individual with alcohol dependence has persistent patterns of excessive drinking, behaviors that are maladaptive, preoccupation with obtaining the substance, marked tolerance for achieving intoxication, and withdrawal reactions in the absence of the drug. Since it is a chronic mental disorder, alcohol dependence has periods of remission following treatment and relapses or acute exacerbations throughout the course of the disease. Alcohol dependence in the elderly population is also of increasing concern (Liberto, Oslin, & Ruskin, 1992).

The individual with alcohol dependence may develop a spectrum of chronic physical complications that require acute or repeated hospitalization. Alcohol-induced hepatic disorders such as fatty liver disease, hepatitis, and cirrhosis are common complications of heavy alcohol consumption. Other conditions associated with chronic alcohol use include recurrent gastrointestinal hemorrhages, esophageal inflammation, malnutrition, vitamin deficiencies, anemia, chronic pancreatitis, cardiomyopathy, cardiac arrhythmias, and dementia. The alcohol-dependent person is also at high risk for developing alcohol withdrawal delirium, seizures, and traumatic injuries that may result in chronic disability (Auerhahn, 1992; U. S. Department of Health and Human Services, 1990).

Many alcoholics mismanage other chronic health problems and are hospitalized for acute exacerbations related to noncompliance with treatment regimens. For example, mental illness and alcohol dependence often occur together and must be treated concurrently. These dual-diagnosis patients often present with primary mental illness with substance abuse sequelae, or primary substance abuse with psychiatric sequelae (Lehman, Myers, & Corty, 1989). With advanced age and the debilitating course of alcohol dependence, individuals with dual diagnoses may often experience several chronic physical conditions that are ineffectively managed.

Nursing Diagnoses

The individual with chronic alcohol dependence focuses activities around obtaining the substance and maintaining a state of intoxication. Besides physical complications, psychosocial responses to this disease include self-care deficit related to constant inebriation; high risk for injury related to loss of judgment and coordination; altered role performance related to frequent neglect of obligations and preoccupation with drinking; ineffective individual coping related to decreased ability to problem-solve; defensive coping related to denial of the problem; self-esteem disturbance related to loss of control; noncompliance related to self-care difficulties; and altered thought processes related to intoxication.

Nursing Interventions

Nursing interventions with the individual with alcohol dependence often focus on detoxification and stabilization after acute exacerbations of the illness. Discharge care involves outpatient follow-up for case management, group therapy, or other activities to promote maintenance of sobriety and management of other chronic problems associated with the disease. Assessing patterns of abuse, patient use of other illicit substances, degree of motivation for treatment, available social support networks, and history of previous treatment for alcoholism are essential. Assessing and treating acute episodes of mental illness, if present, and making appropriate referrals for psychiatric or substance abuse treatment and evaluation of competency may be indicated, especially if life-threatening physical conditions develop. Collaboration with community agencies in developing aftercare goals for management of both physical and mental illness is essential.

THE INDIVIDUAL WITH CHRONIC OBSTRUCTIVE PULMONARY DISEASE

The individual with chronic obstructive pulmonary disease (COPD), such as asthma, bronchitis, and emphysema, faces progressive debilitation and daily struggles with breathing and adequate airway exchange. Loss of control over one's ability to breathe creates a constant sense of threat and feelings of helplessness. Dyspnea, a core symptom, is associated with increased expenditure of energy from rapid, shallow breathing patterns, and often leads to a profound sense of fatigue and chronic debilitation. Symptoms may be exacerbated by smoking, allergens, exercise, and intense emotional states. Hypoxemia frequently creates tachycardia, weakness, and changes in mental status.

The individual with chronic obstructive pulmonary disease must also cope with restrictions in activities, increased dependency on others as the disease progresses, and loss of control. In advanced stages, the individual may be dependent on oxygen in order to survive, further decreasing quality of life and increasing negative mood (McBride, 1993; Small & Graydon, 1992).

Nursing Diagnoses

The individual with chronic obstructive pulmonary disease must often cope with activity intolerance and fatigue related to dyspnea and altered breathing patterns; anxiety related to the subjective experience of breathlessness, airflow obstruction, and a fear of suffocation; powerlessnesss related to inability to control breathing, a basic physiologic function; body-image disturbance related to side effects of medications, noisy respirations, frequent coughing, and chronic debilitation; self-esteem disturbance related to loss of control and feelings of helplessness; altered role performance related to fatigue and restrictions in activity levels; sleep pattern disturbance related to dyspnea and the discomforts of breathlessness; and activity intolerance related to dyspnea and fatigue. Alterations in thought processes, sensory/perceptual alterations, and other cognitive changes may also occur in advanced stages of illness due to hypoxemia (DeVito, 1990; McMahon, 1992).

Nursing Interventions

Since dyspnea and fatigue are often the most disruptive symptoms to the individual with chronic obstructive pulmonary disease, many nursing interventions focus on energy conservation and fatigue reduction by pacing activities, regulating breathing through controlled breathing exercises; using conditioning exercises to increase endurance and decrease fatigue; and practicing relaxation techniques. Many of these strategies are taught in pulmonary rehabilitation programs.

Decreasing emotional stressors and modulating emotional responses are also helpful strategies in decreasing dyspnea. For example, one study by Gift (1991) showed that anxiety, depression, somatization, and hostility were higher during periods of high dyspnea. DeVito (1990) also discussed the importance of timely responses by caregivers to a person's complaints of dyspnea, comparing the condition to the subjective experience of pain.

It is also important to assess for mood disturbances such as dysfunctional grieving responses and chronic anxiety in the individual with chronic obstructive pulmonary disease. Loss of control, fatigue, social isolation, altered body image, and side effects of corticosteroid medication may contribute to depression and hopelessness. Dyspnea may also contribute to severe anxiety or panic reactions. Side effects of bronchodilator medication may lead to anxiety and sleep pattern disturbance. Educating individuals and families about the side effects of medications for COPD is essential.

THE INDIVIDUAL WITH CHRONIC RENAL FAILURE

The individual with chronic renal failure or end-stage renal disease (ESRD) faces many physiological and cognitive problems due to metabolic abnormalities, toxic conditions from organ failure, and major lifestyle changes brought about by ongoing hemodialysis treatment and related complications. Many patients with chronic renal failure develop this condition secondarily from other chronic conditions such as diabetes mellitus, and must cope with debilitating problems and management of both diseases (Hampton, 1992; Kopp, 1992).

Maintaining quality of life, adjusting to chronic hemodialysis, and coping with chronic depression and hopelessness are common concerns of the individual with chronic renal failure (Kopp, 1992; O'Brien, 1992). The treatment regimen demands may be overwhelming for a debilitated patient, and further reduce role functioning within the family. Also, severe fluid and dietary restrictions further increase discomfort and frustration with the disease.

Nursing Diagnoses

The individual with chronic renal failure or ESRD must face continual powerlessness from dependency on hemodialysis machines and rigid, long-term maintenance regimens including dietary and fluid restrictions; alterations in comfort related to thirst and itching; anxiety related to the uncertainty of waiting for a cadaveric kidney transplantation, if indicated; body-image disturbance related to shunts or fistulas and skin discoloration; fatigue related to chronic toxicity and organ failure; fear of death and failure of hemodialysis equipment; altered role performance related to the weekly time demands of hemodialysis treatment; and hopelessness related to catastrophic illness and lowered quality of life (Frank, 1988; Gurklis & Menke, 1988).

Nursing Interventions

Nursing interventions to assist coping in the individual with chronic renal failure include individualizing care as much as possible (e.g., diet) and goal-setting to increase compliance and self-management; acknowledging emotional responses to restrictions in diet and fluid intake; decreasing powerlessness by involving the person in decision-making about care whenever possible; and supporting the family or partner's adjustment to altered role performance. Assessing for mood disorders and changes in mental status is also indicated, as many individuals with chronic renal failure appear lethargic, depressed, and delirious due to metabolic and toxic factors.

THE INDIVIDUAL WITH CORONARY ARTERY DISEASE

The individual with coronary artery disease may suffer from chronic angina pectoris, valvular disease, or myocardial infarctions and may require coronary artery bypass surgery as part of treatment. These diseases are often associated with early death and activity restrictions following the acute coronary event, and often impact individuals in their middle and most productive years. While once thought to affect predominantly males, coronary artery disease is now a leading problem in older women (Wenger, 1990).

The role of personality risk factors in the development of coronary artery disease is widely accepted. Individuals with coronary artery disease are often characterized as having Type A behavior or a personality style with high needs to maintain control, competitiveness, repression of emotions, and hyperactivity (Drory & Florian, 1991; Pancheri et al., 1978). Prolonged stress or stressful life changes and a lifestyle with other high-risk factors such as obesity, smoking, hypertension, and a fatty diet also contribute to development of this disease.

While coronary artery disease is one of the leading causes of premature death, advances in treatment modalities have prolonged life and increased chronicity. Invasive procedures and surgery have resulted in increased survival of many cardiac patients who are now sicker and need repeated hospitalization. The "chronically critically ill" elderly individual is an example of a health care recipient reflecting this trend in medical care (Hawthorne, 1991).

Nursing Diagnoses

The individual with coronary artery disease often experiences powerlessness related to the unpredictability and lethality of the illness; ineffective coping related to a typical pattern of denial and repressing emotions; impaired adjustment related to difficulties complying with cardiac rehabilitation regimens and lifestyle changes; ineffective denial related to sense of threat; high anxiety related to the high acuity of the illness and unpredictable course; self-esteem disturbance related to restrictions in activities that provide self-worth (e.g., a career); altered role performance associated with role loss, fatigue, and role reversals within the marital and family unit; ineffective family coping related to alteration in family roles and increased responsibilities on the spouse or partner; and altered sexuality patterns related to fears about sexual dysfunction, overexertion, or further cardiac damage. In some patients with end-stage cardiac illness, alterations in thought processes and sensory/perceptual alterations may occur due to hypoxemia and organ failure.

Nursing Interventions

Nursing interventions most helpful to the individual with coronary artery disease include strategies to reduce anxiety and hypervigilance, and interventions to increase a sense of control. Relaxation exercises, providing information, adequate pain management, and assessing and addressing unexpressed emotional distress is essential. Including the individual in all stages of cardiac rehabilitation treatment and collaborating in decision making about care decreases powerlessness and promotes a sense of mastery over an overwhelming situation. Determining a person's expectations and health beliefs may help identify individuals who may abandon medical recommendations after discharge and need further support with cardiac rehabilitation activities (Robertson & Keller, 1992).

Referrals to support groups and including spouses and partners in discussion of realistic expectations, losses, and lifestyle changes are also helpful in facilitating family system adjustment and resumption of intimacy following acute cardiac events or cardiac surgery (Miller et al., 1990; Nymathi et al., 1992).

THE INDIVIDUAL WITH DIABETES MELLITUS

The individual with diabetes mellitus must learn and perform ongoing self-care tasks throughout his or her lifetime to manage the disease and prevent catastrophic complications that can further restrict independence and quality of life. Whether the person is diagnosed with Type I (insulin-dependent) or Type II (non–insulin-dependent) diabetes, daily self-management activities often create restrictions that may lead to a sense of frustration. Restricting one's diet, regulating meal times, monitoring blood sugar throughout the day, administering and/or injecting self with insulin, preventing and managing insulin reactions, and other aspects of the diabetic regimen must be incorporated into the person's lifestyle and personal identity.

Adequate metabolic control of diabetes is essential in preventing long-term complications such as visual impairment related to proliferative retinopathy, glaucoma, or cataracts; macroangiopathy or hardening and degeneration of blood vessels; cardiac disease; cerebrovascular disease, peripheral vascular disease; focal, sensory, peripheral, and autonomic neuropathies; end-stage renal disease; and foot ulcers, gangrene, and injuries caused by lack of sensation and other problems (Haas, 1992; Nyhlin, 1990). Multiple complications often coincide with each other, resulting in a sense of failure and powerlessness, especially if a patient has attempted to manage the disease independently and has been compliant with a recommended self-care regimen.

In order to manage diabetes mellitus successfully, the individual must learn principles of managing blood sugar and medication administration techniques that may be painful, threatening, and invasive. The insulin-dependent diabetic must cope with repeated, daily injections in order to survive, as well as multiple finger pricks to monitor blood sugar. Commitment to self-care practices and level of motivation are often influenced by the life stage of the person at the time of diagnosis. In adolescent diabetics, for example, self-care tasks are often affected by self-concept, body image, and peer relationship issues. In older adults, major changes in lifestyle required by the disease may be difficult (Nelson, 1992).

Nursing Diagnoses

Individual responses to diabetes often depend upon the type and stage of the illness, degree of metabolic control, and readiness for learning self-management behaviors. These responses may include grieving related to loss of independence and changed health status; powerlessness related to difficulties in daily management of the disease or complications; anxiety related to learning new regimens of care and uncertainty about the future; noncompliance related to lack of readiness to learn self-care tasks; impaired adjustment related to lack of acceptance of the disease and unwillingness to modify lifestyle; ineffective coping related to anger about lifestyle changes and restrictions imposed by the illness; altered role performance related to physical disability and role changes; and altered thought processes related to metabolic abnormalities affecting the brain (LeMone, 1993; Nelson, 1992).

Nursing Interventions

Nursing interventions in the care of the individual with diabetes mellitus should focus on empowering the person in self-management of the disease; assisting with adaptation to self-care tasks; respecting autonomy and encouraging choices whenever possible; promoting independence and mastery in self-care regimens to increase self-esteem; tailoring information and teaching to the stage of acceptance of the disease and readiness to learn new behaviors; and using problem-solving and empowerment strategies in diabetes education programs (Curry, 1993; Hurley & Shea, 1992). Helping the diabetic manage stressors and psychological factors that may affect glucose regulation is also beneficial (Helz & Templeton, 1990). In the early stages of the disease, effective self-care strategies can prevent debilitating complications that further decrease quality of life, as well as help the individual achieve some degree of control over the disease.

THE INDIVIDUAL WITH A PARALYTIC CONDITION

Paralysis is a chronic condition resulting from traumatic spinal cord injury (SCI) or cerebral vascular accident (CVA). While the cause, onset of illness, and degree of disability may differ, the individual with a paralytic condition experiences many similar emotional and physical adjustments during rehabilitation. Sudden loss of mobility and independence are common problems that create a sense of powerlessness and quality-of-life concerns for the individual and family members. While paralysis may decrease in some situations, extended rehabilitation and treatment is often needed to maximize remaining functioning in most individuals, and the condition remains largely permanent. Managing physical disabilities such as loss of bowel and bladder function, mobility and position restrictions, and decreased capacity for self-care require major lifestyle changes for both the paralyzed individual and family members.

In the acute phase, the paralyzed individual who is paraplegic or quadriplegic must often recover from other traumatic physical injuries as well and cope with sudden, permanent loss of body functioning and increased dependency on others. Control of one's life may be completely or partially relinquished to others. The occurrence of powerlessness is pervasive throughout hospitalization, increasing in quadriplegics and older individuals (Richmond et al., 1992).

Many individuals with spinal cord injuries are young, healthy males who sustain injuries resulting from motor vehicle or motorcycle accidents, athletic injuries, gunshot wounds, or industrial accidents. Because of the catastrophic nature of these injuries, normal adult development is often disrupted (Bozzacco, 1993). Vocational status is also disrupted, although adjustment tends to improve significantly with time (Krause, 1992; Nieves, Charter, & Aspinall, 1991).

The individual who is paralyzed from a cerebral vascular accident is frequently coping with other preexisting chronic illnesses such as atherosclerosis, diabetes mellitus, or hypertension that preceded the stroke. The person may suffer from a single, disabling event or from multiple infarcts that lead to gradual, increasing disability. Advanced age and debilitation from other conditions may overwhelm coping resources of family or partner caregivers. Furthermore, since infarcts decrease blood supply to the brain, mental status changes such as acute confusion, memory loss, and dementia may occur as well as mood disorders such as

depression (Robinson & Starkstein, 1990; Tatemichi et al., 1992). Loss of mobility, with paralysis generally occurring on the side opposite from the brain lesion; speech and language deficits; and other neurocognitive changes, are common (Bronstein, 1991; Ragsdale, Yarbrough, & Lasher, 1993).

Nursing Diagnoses

The individual with a paralytic condition secondary to spinal cord injury or cerebral vascular accident often responds with powerlessness related to immobility and loss of control over self-care; grieving related to loss of independence and loss of body functioning; body-image disturbance related to loss of uprightness and use of adaptive equipment; self-esteem disturbance related to negative changes in self-perception; self-care deficit related to loss of functional capacity; altered sexuality patterns related to limitations in sexual performance; altered family processes related to lifestyle adjustments and role changes; and altered role performance related to physical disability (Bozzacco, 1993; Richmond et al., 1992).

Nursing Interventions

Nursing interventions helpful to the paralyzed patient include supporting the grief process by allowing for periods of withdrawal and emotional shock; encouraging verbalization about the injury and changes in health status; including the person in decision making about daily care to decrease a sense of powerlessness; facilitating opportunities for the patient to participate in support groups or other peer activities; involving family members or partners in support groups; using crisis intervention strategies to reinforce healthy coping; and providing sexual counseling and education with the individual and his or her partner.

As the rehabilitation process is difficult for both the paralyzed individual and family members, assessment for dysfunctional grieving responses, hopelessness, and ineffective coping should be ongoing. Providing encouragement and arranging respite care for family caregivers may also be helpful. Making early referrals for psychiatric treatment, if indicated, and encouraging participation in community groups will support adjustment and decrease social isolation associated with this devastating condition.

THE INDIVIDUAL WITH RHEUMATOID ARTHRITIS

The individual with rheumatoid arthritis must cope with a systemic, connective-tissue, inflammatory disorder that has a fluctuating, uncertain course. Localized chronic joint pain and swelling, morning stiffness, progressive deformities, muscle atrophy, weakness, fever, fatigue, and progressive disability are characteristics of this disease that affects women in greater numbers than men (Lambert & Lambert, Young, 1992). Fatigue is also a significant problem and is often associated with pain and depression (Tack, 1990).

Acute flare-ups of rheumatoid arthritis lead to progressive disability, with activities of daily living becoming progressively more difficult. Frequently, the individual requires assistance with ambulation and may need other modifications in the living environment to maintain activities of daily living. Often, the person must also cope with side effects of antiinflammatory medications that may affect mood and increase discomfort. Smith and Wallston (1992) described the emotional experience of the individual with rheumatoid arthritis as a vicious cycle of helplessness appraisals, passive coping with pain, and psychological impairment leading to maladaptive coping.

Depression or dysfunctional grieving is a common psychological disturbance in many individuals with rheumatoid arthritis, as they face chronic pain and disability (Blalock & De-Vellis, 1992; Young, 1992). In several studies, social factors influenced patient coping and quality of life. These factors included degree of spousal support (Manne & Zautra, 1990) and use of social resources within and outside of the marriage (Revenson & Majerovitz, 1991).

Nursing Diagnoses

The individual with rheumatoid arthritis often experiences chronic pain related to joint inflammation; self-care deficits related to pain and stiffness; body-image disturbance related to swollen joints, disfigurement, and need for assistive devices in activities of daily living; self-esteem disturbance related to perception of self as disabled; fatigue related to high energy expenditures needed for ambulation and other activities of daily living, pain, anemia, or fever; activity intolerance related to pain and self-protection of painful joints; grieving related to loss of functioning and leaving the workplace; powerlessness related to progression of the disease, uncertainty, relapsing course, and loss of control over one's mobility; social isolation related to changes in social and leisure activities brought on by the disease; and altered role performance related to changes in usual functioning and increased dependency.

Nursing Interventions

Nursing interventions in care of the individual with rheumatoid arthritis include strategies to conserve energy, decrease pain and stress, and prevent further disability in affected joints; strategies to help the person adjust to mobility and dexterity problems; strategies to assist coping with disfigurement, chronic resting and movement pain, and body-image changes; and strategies to maintain the social and family support networks (Miller, 1992b; Mirabelli, 1990). Pacing of activities, especially in morning hours; regular exercise; the use of cognitive-behavioral techniques to decrease discomfort and stress; facilitating social interaction with others; and helping the patient participate in new recreational outlets realistic for level of functioning may also prove helpful.

CONCLUSION

Living with a chronic illness presents many coping challenges to individuals and their families. Maintaining quality of life in spite of decreased body functioning, managing physical and emotional discomfort, and adjusting one's lifestyle to limitations imposed by the disease are major tasks in the adjustment process. The nurse's role in supporting the chronically ill individual and family includes fostering hope, maximizing comfort, acknowledging concerns, and empowering patients to achieve appropriate self-management of their disease.

BIBLIOGRAPHY

Archbold, P. G., Stewart, B. J., Greenlick, M. R., & Harvath, T. (1990). Mutuality and preparedness as predictors of caregiver role strain. *Research in Nursing and Health, 13*, 375–384.

Auerhahn, C. (1990). Recognition and management of alcohol-related nutritional deficiencies. *Nurse Practitioner, 17*(12), 40, 43–44, 49.

Blalock, S. J., & DeVellis, R. F. (1992). Rheumatoid arthritis and depression: An overview. *Bulletin on the Rheumatic Diseases, 41*(1), 6–8.

Bozzacco, V. (1993). Long-term psychosocial effects of spinal cord injury. *Rehabilitation Nursing, 18*(2), 82–87.

Braden, C. J. (1993). Research program on learned response to chronic illness experience: Self-help model. *Holistic Nursing Practice, 8*(1), 38–44.

Bronstein, K. S. (1991). Psychosocial components in stroke: Implications for adaptation. *Nursing Clinics of North America, 26*(4), 1007–1017.

Burckhardt, C. S. (1987). Coping strategies of the chronically ill. *Nursing Clinics of North America, 22*(3), 543–549.

Connelly, C. E. (1993). An empirical study of a model of self-care in chronic illness. *Clinical Nurse Specialist, 7*(5), 247–253.

Conwill, J. (1993). Understanding and combating helplessness. *Rehabilitation Nursing, 18*(6), 388–394, 399.

Corbin, J. M., & Strauss, A. (1991). A nursing model for chronic illness management based upon the trajectory framework. *Scholarly Inquiry for Nursing Practice, 5*(3), 155–174.

Curry, S. J. (1993). Commentary. *Diabetes Spectrum, 6*(1), 34.

DesRosier, M. B., Catanzaro, M., & Piller, J. (1992). Living with chronic illness: Social support and the well spouse perspective. *Rehabilitation Nursing, 17*(2), 87–91.

DeVito, A. J. (1990). Dyspnea during hospitalizations for acute phase of illness as recalled by patients with chronic obstructive pulmonary disease. *Heart and Lung, 19*(2), 186–191.

Drory, Y., & Florian, V. (1991). Long-term psychosocial adjustment to coronary artery disease. *Archives of Physical Medicine and Rehabilitation, 72*, 326–331.

Flannery, J. (1990). Guilt: A crisis within a crisis. *Journal of Neuroscience Nursing, 22*(2), 92–99.

Flaskerud, J. H. (1992). Psychosocial and neuropsychiatric care. *Critical Care Nursing Clinics of North America, 4*(3), 411–420.

Frank, D. (1988). Psychosocial assessment of renal dialysis patients. *American Nephrology Nurses Association Journal, 15*, 207–210, 232.

French, J. K., & Phillips, J. A. (1991). Shattered images: Recovery for the SCI client. *Rehabilitation Nursing, 16*(3), 134–136.

Funnell, M. M., Arnold, M. S., Donnelly, M., & Taylor-Moon, D. T. (1991). Empowerment: An idea whose time has come in diabetes education. *The Diabetes Educator, 17*(1), 37–41.

Gaskins, S., & Brown, K. (1992). Psychosocial responses among individuals with human immunodeficiency viral infection. *Applied Nursing Research, 5*(3), 111–121.

Gift, A. G. (1991). Psychologic and physiologic aspects of acute dyspnea in asthmatics. *Nursing Research, 40*(4), 196–199.

Gurklis, J., & Menke, E. (1988). Identification of stressors and use of coping methods in chronic hemodialysis patients. *Nursing Research, 37*(4), 236–239.

Haas, L. B. (1992). Chronic complications of diabetes mellitus: Peritoneal dialysis. *American Nephrology Nurses Association Journal, 19*(5), 439–446.

Haberman, M. R., Woods, N. F., & Packard, N. J. (1990). Demands of chronic illness: Reliability and validity assessment of a demands-of-illness inventory. *Holistic Nursing Practice, 5*(1), 25–35.

Hall, B. A. (1992). Overcoming stigmatization: Social and personal implications of the human immunodeficiency virus diagnosis. *Archives of Psychiatric Nursing, 6*(3), 189–194.

Hampton, J. K. (1992). Long-term effects of hemodialysis in diabetic patients with end stage renal disease. *American Nephrology Nurses Association Journal, 19*(5), 455–456.

Hawthorne, M. H. (1991). Using the trajectory framework: Reconceptualizing cardiac illness. *Scholarly Inquiry for Nursing Practice, 5*(3), 185–195.

Helz, J. W., & Templeton, B. (1990). Evidence of the role of psychosocial factors in diabetes mellitus: A review. *American Journal of Psychiatry, 147*(10), 1275–1282.

Hinton-Walker, P. (1993). Care of the chronically ill: Paradigm shifts and directions for the future. *Holistic Nursing Practice, 8*(1), 56–66.

Hurley, C. C., & Shea, C. A. (1992). Self-efficacy: Strategy for enhancing diabetes self-care. *The Diabetes Educator, 18*(2), 146–150.

Johnson, S. H. (1991). Ethics: Focus for the 90s. *Dimensions in Critical Care Nursing, 10*(1), 3.

Kopp, J. (1992). Psychosocial correlates of diabetes and renal dysfunction. *American Nephrology Nurses Association Journal, 19*(5), 432–437.

Krause, J. S. (1992). Longitudinal changes in adjustment after spinal cord injury: A 15-year study. *Archives of Physical Medicine and Rehabilitation, 73*, 564–568.

Kvam, S. H., & Lyons, J. S. (1991). Assessment of coping strategies, social support, and general health status in individuals with diabetes mellitus. *Psychological Reports, 68*, 623–632.

Lambert, C. E., & Lambert, V. A. (1987a). Psychosocial impacts created by chronic illness. *Nursing Clinics of North America, 22*(3), 527–533.

Lambert, V. A., & Lambert, C. E. (1987b). Coping with rheumatoid arthritis. *Nursing Clinics of North America, 22*(3), 551–558.

Lazarus, R., & Folkman, S. (1984). *Stress appraisal and the coping process.* New York: McGraw-Hill.

Lazarus, R. S. (1993). Coping theory and research: Past, present, and future. *Psychosomatic Medicine, 55*, 234–247.

Lehman, A. F., Myers, C. P., & Corty, E. (1989). Assessment and classification of patients with psychiatric and substance abuse disorders. *Hospital and Community Psychiatry, 40*(10), 1019–1025.

LeMone, P. (1993). Human sexuality in adults with insulin-dependent diabetes. *Image: Journal of Nursing Scholarship, 25*(2), 101–105.

Liberto, J. G., Oslin, D. W., & Ruskin, P. E. (1992). Alcoholism in older adults: A review of the literature. *Hospital and Community Psychiatry, 43*(10), 975–984.

Lieber, C. S., & Guadagnini, K. S. (1990). The spectrum of alcoholic liver disease. *Hospital Practice, 25*(2A), 51–69.

Lindgren, C. L., Burke, M. L., Hainsworth, M. A., & Eakes, G. G. (1992). Chronic sorrow: A lifespan concept. *Scholarly Inquiry for Nursing Practice*, 6(1), 27–43.

Lipowski, Z. W. (1970). Physical illness, the individual and the coping processes. *Psychiatry in Medicine*, 1(2), 91–101.

Lubkin, I. M. (Ed.). (1992). The family caregiver. In I. M. Lubkin (Ed.), *Chronic illness: Impact and interventions* (2nd ed.). Boston: Jones and Bartlett Publishers.

Manne, S. L., & Zautra, A. J. (1990). Couples coping with chronic illness: Women with rheumatoid arthritis and their healthy husbands. *Journal of Behavioral Medicine*, 14(4), 327–342.

McBride, S. (1993). Perceived control in patients with chronic obstructive pulmonary disease. *Western Journal of Nursing Research*, 15(4), 456–464.

McMahon, A. (1992). Coping with chronic lung disease: Maintaining quality of life. In J. F. Miller (Ed.), *Coping with chronic illness: Overcoming powerlessness* (2nd ed.). Philadelphia: F. A. Davis Company.

Miller, J. F. (1992a). Analysis of coping with illness. In J. F. Miller (Ed.). *Coping with chronic illness: Overcoming powerlessness* (2nd ed.). Philadelphia: F. A. Davis Company.

Miller, J. F. (1992b). Energy deficits in chronically ill persons with arthritis. In J. F. Miller (Ed.), *Coping with chronic illness: Overcoming powerlessness* (2nd ed.). Philadelphia: F. A. Davis Company.

Miller, P. M., Wikoff, R., McMahon, M., Garett, M. J., & Ringel, K. (1990). Marital functioning after cardiac surgery. *Heart & Lung*, 19(1), 55–61.

Mirabelli, L. (1990). Caring for patients with rheumatoid arthritis. *Nursing 90*, 20(9), 67–72.

Morse, J. M., & Johnson, J. L. (1991). Toward a theory of illness: The illness constellation model. In J. M. Morse & J. L. Johnson (Eds.), *The illness experience*. Newbury Park, CA: Sage.

Nelson, J. B. (1992). Psychosocial aspects of diabetes. *Journal of Home Health Care Practice*, 4(3), 72–90.

Nieves, C. C., Charter, R. A., & Aspinall, M. J. (1991). Relationship between effective coping and perceived quality of life in spinal cord injured patients. *Rehabilitation Nursing*, 16(3), 129–132.

Nyhlin, K. T. (1990). Diabetic patients facing long-term complications: Coping with uncertainty. *Journal of Advanced Nursing*, 15(9), 1021–1029.

Nymathi, A., Jacoby, A., Constancia, P., & Ruvevich, S. (1992). Coping and adjustment of spouses of critically ill patients with cardiac disease. *Heart & Lung*, 21(2), 160–166.

O'Brien, M. E. (1992). Compliance behavior and long-term maintenance dialysis. *American Journal of Kidney Diseases*, 15(3), 209–214.

Oechsner, M., Moller, A. A., & Zaudig, M. (1993). Cognitive impairment, dementia, and psychosocial functioning in human immunodeficiency virus infection. *Acta Psychiatrica Scandinavia*, 87, 13–17.

Pancheri, R., et al. (1978). Infarct as a stress agent: Life history and personality characteristics in improved vs. not-improved patients after severe heart attacks. *Journal of Human Stress*, 4, 16.

Piringer, P., Agana-Defensor, R., Mullen, N. M., & Lee, L. (1993). A model for the development and implementation of a patient support group in a medical-surgical setting. *Holistic Nursing Practice*, 8(1), 16–26.

Ragsdale, D., Yarbrough, S., & Lasher, A. T. (1993). Using social support theory to care for CVA patients. *Rehabilitation Nursing*, 18(3), 154–172.

Revenson, T. A., & Majerovitz, S. D. (1991). The effects of chronic illness on the spouse: Social resources as stress buffers. *Arthritis Care and Research*, 4(2), 63–72.

Richmond, T. S., Metcalf, J., Daly, M., & Kish, J. R. (1992). Powerlessness in acute spinal cord injury patients: A descriptive study. *Journal of Neuroscience Nursing*, 24(3), 146–152.

Robertson, D., & Keller, C. (1992). Relationships among health beliefs, self-efficacy, and exercise adherence in patients with coronary artery disease. *Heart & Lung*, 21(1), 56–63.

Robinson, R. G., & Starkstein, S. E. (1990). Current research in affective disorders following stroke. *Journal of Neuropsychiatry*, 2(1), 1–14.

Saylor, C. R. (1990). The management of stigma: Redefinition and representation. *Holistic Nursing Practice*, 5(1), 45–53.

Schussler, G. (1992). Coping strategies and individual meanings of illness. *Social Science and Medicine*, 34(4), 427–432.

Seaburn, D. B., Lorenz, A., & Kaplan, D. (1992). The transgenerational development of chronic illness meanings. *Family Systems Medicine*, 10(4), 385–394.

Shaw, M. C., & Halliday, P. H. (1992). The family, crisis, and chronic illness: An evolutionary model. *Journal of Advanced Nursing*, 17, 537–543.

Shekleton, M. E. (1987). Coping with chronic respiratory difficulty. *Nursing Clinics of North America*, 22(3), 569–581.

Simmons, R. G., & Abress, L. (1990). Quality-of-life issues for end-stage renal disease patients. *American Journal of Kidney Diseases*, 15(3), 201–208.

Small, S. P., & Graydon, J. E. (1992). Perceived uncertainty, physical symptoms, and negative mood in hospitalized patients with chronic obstructive pulmonary disease. *Heart & Lung*, 21(6), 568–574.

Smith, C. A., & Wallston, K. A. (1992). Adaptation in patients with chronic rheumatoid arthritis: Application of a general model. *Health Psychology*, 11(3), 151–162.

Tack, B. B. (1990). Self-reported fatigue in rheumatoid arthritis. *Arthritis Care & Research*, 3(3), 154–157.

U. S. Department of Health and Human Services. (1990). *Seventh special report to the U. S. Congress on Alcohol and Health* (DHSS Publication No. ADM 90-1656). Washington, DC: U. S. Government Printing Office.

Wenger, N. K. (1990). Gender, coronary artery disease, and coronary bypass surgery. *Annals of Internal Medicine*, 112, 557–558.

White, N. E., Richter, J. M., & Fry, C. (1992). Coping, social support, and adaptation to chronic illness. *Western Journal of Nursing Research*, 14(2), 211–224.

Woods, N. F., Haberman, M. R., & Packard, N. J. (1993). Demands of illness and individual, dyadic, and family adaptation in chronic illness. *Western Journal of Nursing Research*, 15(1), 10–30.

Young, L. D. (1992). Psychological factors in rheumatoid arthritis. *Journal of Counseling and Clinical Psychology*, 60(4), 619–627.

Youngblood, N. M., & Hines, J. (1992). The influence of the family's perception of disability on rehabilitation outcomes. *Rehabilitation Nursing*, 17(6), 323–326.

CHAPTER 21

Pain Management in Acute Care and Home Care Settings

Mary Beth Singer

Pain is a common human response to illness. As such, it has been identified as a high-frequency nursing diagnosis and a nursing research priority (Cancer Consortium, 1987; Ferrell, Rhiner, & Grant, 1991). While pain is ubiquitous, it remains a decidedly subjective experience, with unique individual expression. Both the subjective nature of pain and the many barriers to effective pain management present challenges to clinicians caring for patients and their families across care settings.

This chapter will present a cohesive summary of state-of-the-art pain management. It will present a general overview and definition of the problem, followed by general assessment and treatment guidelines. The remainder of the chapter will address specific types of pain problems: acute pain; chronic, nonmalignant pain; and cancer-related pain. Prototypes will be used to illustrate specific assessment and treatment strategies for each type of pain. The psychosocial impact of ineffective pain management on the individual and family will be integrated throughout the text. The role of the

nurse generalist and advanced practice nurse in managing pain will be delineated. The reader is reminded that several excellent guidelines and manuals are available that provide extensive review of the clinical management of pain (see Table 21-1).

Pain is the most common reason that individuals seek health care. In 1989, over 23 million operative procedures were performed (AHCPR, 1992). Chronic, nonmalignant pain affects approximately 80 million Americans (Christenson, 1993) at an annual estimated cost of from $60 to $85 billion (Hazard, 1994; Mooney, 1991). Annually, over 1 million Americans are diagnosed with cancer. Cancer is responsible for the deaths of one in five Americans, approximately 1400 deaths per day (*Cancer Facts and Figures,* 1994). In advanced cancer, pain is a prevalent symptom, occurring in 60% to 90% of patients, with 25% to 30% of

Patricia Barry: *Psychosocial Nursing:*
Care of Physically Ill Patients and Their Families, 3rd ed.
© 1996 Lippincott–Raven Publishers

Table 21-1
Pain Management Resources

Resource	Address

AHCPR Clinical Practice Guidelines
  Acute Pain Management: Operative or Medical
  Procedures and Trauma (1992)
  (AHCPR 92-0032)
	U.S. Dept. of Health and Human Services
	Public Health Service, Agency for Health Care
	  Policy and Research
	2101 East Jefferson Street, Suite 501
	Rockville, MD 20852

AHCPR Clinical Practice Guideline
  Management of Cancer Pain (1994)
  (AHCPR 94-0592)
	address above

AHCPR Clinical Practice Guideline Management of Chronic Low Back Pain (1994)	address above
ONS Position Paper on Cancer Pain Assessment and Management (monograph)	Oncology Nursing Society 1016 Greentree Road Pittsburgh, PA 15220 (412) 921-7373
Principles of Analgesic Use in the Treatment of Acute Pain and Chronic Cancer Pain (1993)	American Pain Society P.O. Box 186 Skokie, IL 60076-0816
Pain: Clinical Manual for Nursing Practice (McCaffery & Beebe, 1989)	C.V. Mosby Co. 11830 Westline Industrial Drive St. Louis, MO 63146

---

patients describing pain as very severe (Bonica, 1990). The above statistics do not begin to capture the human suffering and social costs associated with pain.

Nurses have a contract with society to diagnose and treat human responses to health and illness (*Nursing: A Social Policy Statement,* 1980). Pain that is unrecognized and/or undertreated diminishes the quality of life, not only of the person experiencing pain, but of the family as well. Ferrell and colleagues (1991) have proposed pain management as a quality-of-care outcome. In this model, evidence of effective pain management skills is part of staff nurse performance criteria. Two important messages are conveyed in this model: 1) accountability and responsibility for effective pain management at the staff and managerial level, and 2) pain management as an institutional priority.

The North American Nursing Diagnosis Association (NANDA) lists both *pain* and *chronic pain* as accepted nursing diagnoses. Although many argue that pain is a collaborative diagno-

sis due to the interdisciplinary interventions necessary to treat it, nursing has played a pivotal role in pain assessment and diagnosis, and in the implementation of comprehensive treatment plans for people with pain. Pain may be more adequately defined as a nursing care syndrome. Inadequate pain management gives rise to a number of nursing diagnoses with pain as the etiologic factor (see Box 21-1). Effective treatment of pain leads to improved outcomes or complete resolution of the accompanying diagnoses.

BARRIERS TO EFFECTIVE PAIN MANAGEMENT

Numerous authors have described barriers to effective pain management. These barriers can be divided into three categories, as listed in Table 21-2 (Dahl et al., 1988).

While these barriers apply to acute and cancer pain, barriers to effective management

BOX 21-1	Nursing Diagnoses Associated With Pain as Etiologic Factor

Anxiety
Constipation
Fatigue
Impaired physical mobility
Fear
Powerlessness
Knowledge deficit
Self-care deficits: grooming, toileting, bathing
Sexual dysfunction
Spiritual distress
Social isolation
Altered thought process

(McCaffery & Beebe, 1989)

of chronic, nonmalignant pain include lack of rehabilitation focus and reliance on opioid analgesics, which can often perpetuate disuse and suffering (Fordyce, 1989). Other barriers include the invisibility of chronic pain, the social stigma and isolation associated with living with chronic pain, chronic disability, and a sense of learned helplessness or powerlessness (Schlesinger, 1993). In her study of women with chronic pain, Schlesinger found that successful coping often decreased the visibility of pain. This invisibility raised problems in terms of proving injury for insurance or disability, despite continued living with pain. This lack of validation reinforces negative pain behaviors.

McCaffery et al. (1990) reported data on nurses' knowledge of opioid analgesics and addiction, from a large sample of nurses at both basic and advanced workshops on pain management. In their sample of over 2000 nurses they found that only 25% could correctly identify the risk of addiction in patients being treated with opioids for pain. This study also found that nurses in this sample were unable to identify specific opioid drugs correctly. Implications for education emphasized the need for basic pain content in nursing education, as well as continuing education across specific care settings.

In a subsequent study, Ferrell, Eberts, McCaffery, and Grant (1991) extended their research by investigating clinical decision making and pain. They asked subjects to describe their process of assessment and documentation of pain intensity, what decisions were made with regard to pain medication and nonpharmacologic interventions, and what ethical conflicts and/or barriers were encountered. Results indicated that while 91% of

Table 21-2
Barriers to Effective Pain Management

HCP Barriers	Patient/Family Barriers	Systems Barriers

• Inadequate knowledge of pain management
• Poor pain assessment
• Concerns regarding regulation of controlled substances
• Fear of patient addiction
• Concern about side effects of analgesics
• Concern about development of tolerance to analgesics
	• Reluctance to report pain
	  fear of distracting physician from disease treatment
	  fear that pain means disease is worse
	  concern about not being a good patient
	• Reluctance to take pain medications
	  fear of addiction
	  fear of tolerance
	  worries about side-effects
		• Low priority assigned to pain management
		• Inadequate reimbursement
		• Restrictive regulation of controlled substances
		• Lack of access to or availability of appropriate treatment

AHCPR. (1994). *Management of cancer pain.* Clinical practice guideline, p. 17.

nurses asked the patient about pain intensity, only 45% considered this the most influential factor in pain assessment. Barriers to optimum pain relief cited in this study concur with those previously listed. Ethical conflicts arose when patients did not get adequate pain relief. Interestingly, 49% of nurses were concerned with overmedication, while 69% were concerned with undermedicating patients with pain.

Studies conducted over the past 20 years continue to demonstrate that, despite advances in knowledge, pain management is suboptimal. This problem is largely due to underprescription by physicians. In addition, nurses frequently undermedicate patients in the acute care setting (Cohen, 1982; Donovan, Dillon, & McGuire, 1987; Marks & Sachar, 1973; Paice, Mahon, & Faut-Callahan, 1991). The NIH consensus conference on pain (NIH, 1987) found that acute and cancer pain were undertreated with medication, while chronic, nonmalignant pain was overtreated with medication.

CONCEPTUAL FRAMEWORK

The International Association for the Study of Pain (IASP) has defined *pain* as an unpleasant sensory and emotional experience arising from actual or potential tissue damage or described in terms of such damage (IASP, 1979). McCaffery states that "pain is whatever the experiencing person says it is, existing whenever he says it does" (McCaffery, 1979). Both definitions

capture the subjective nature of pain. While there are multiple etiologies of pain, general principles apply across care settings.

It is important for nurses to understand the physiology of pain as well as theories that offer an understanding of the lived experience of both acute and chronic pain. This section of the chapter will briefly review pain physiology and then present an integrated view of the pain experience utilizing the Roy Adaptation Model of Nursing (1984). Discussion of the gate control theory will further facilitate an understanding of the experience of pain.

PAIN PHYSIOLOGY

Pain is a multidimensional phenomenon when viewed in the context of the whole person. The perception of pain and the individual's response to pain involve four processes (McGuire & Scheidler, 1990; Paice, 1991). Pain perception begins with stimulation of primary afferent fibers. Stimulation of these fibers can be the result of mechanical, thermal, or chemical stimuli. Table 21-3 provides information on myelinated and unmyelinated pain fibers, including pain descriptors.

Numerous biochemical mediators are released as a result of cellular injury, facilitating nociception (Payne, 1989a). Depolarization of the cell membrane after stimulation of the primary afferent fiber (nociceptor) is called *transduction*. The resultant change in the electrophysiology of the cell membrane produces an *action potential*. The generation of this action potential results in transmission of the pain

---

Table 21-3
Characteristics of Myelinated and Unmyelinated Pain Fibers

Type of Pain	Characteristics	Descriptors
Fast A-delta fiber (myelinated)	Results from mechanical injury	Sharp, pricking, acute, electric
Slow C-fiber (unmyelinated)	Results from tissue destruction caused by thermal or chemical injury	Burning, aching, throbbing, nauseating, chronic

Guyton, A.C. (1991.) *Textbook of Medical Physiology* (8th ed.). Philadelphia: W.B. Saunders.

message along the neuron. This pain message continues until it terminates in the dorsal horn of the spinal cord (Paice, 1991).

Within the dorsal horn, numerous neuropeptides and other substances are released, perpetuating transmission of the pain message within the central nervous system. *Substance P* has been identified as an important neuropeptide facilitating pain transmission in this area (Paice, 1991). It is important to note that the dorsal horn likewise is rich in opiate receptors. When these receptors are bound, by either endogenous or exogenous opiates, the release of substance P is inhibited, thereby halting pain transmission. Transmission continues along spinothalamic tract neurons within the anterolateral quadrant. A few fibers terminate in the reticular formation of the brain stem; most terminate in the thalamus, where they travel on to the somatosensory cortex and the association cortex (Guyton, 1991; Paice, 1991).

The descending analgesic system plays a major role in the individual's pain experience. It is comprised of three components: the periaquaductal gray area of the mesencephalon and upper pons; raphe magnus nucleus; and the pain inhibitory complex of the dorsal horn. These modulatory areas contain serotonin and norepinephrine, which inhibit pain transmission within the dorsal horn. The effect of tricyclic antidepressant drugs increases the availability of serotonin, thereby blocking pain transmission (Paice, 1991). Likewise, persons who have clinical depressions often have lower pain thresholds, presumably due to lower levels of serotonin.

Chronic pain sufferers often have significant depression, which compounds the pain experience. Depression is not the cause of pain. Modifying the pain experience by improving sleep and mobility have profound effects on the quality of life of persons suffering from chronic pain conditions. The role of noradrenergic agonists, such as clonidine, in the modulation of pain is still under investigation. The use of these agents intraspinally has been complicated by severe hypotension (Paice, 1991).

The modulation of pain by progressive muscle relaxation and guided imagery may be explained by the descending analgesic system. It

has been postulated that release of endogenous opioids activates the modulation of pain transmission described above. These and other nonpharmacologic interventions may indeed affect the transmission of pain as well as the perception of pain.

GATE CONTROL THEORY

Melzack and Wall proposed the *gate control theory of pain* in 1965. While some of its foundations have not been confirmed, it serves as the most comprehensive theory to date. It integrates both the sensory and emotional components of pain, allowing for unique individual expression. The basic tenets of the gate control theory are:

1. Afferent fibers transmit the pain impulse to the spinal cord, where a gating mechanism exists within the dorsal horn in the substantia gelatinosa.
2. The spinal gating mechanism is influenced by the activity in small-diameter and large-diameter fibers. Stimulation of large-diameter fibers tends to close the gate, whereas stimulation of small-diameter fibers opens the gating mechanism.
3. The gating mechanism is also influenced by nerve impulses from the brain.
4. A central control trigger activates higher cognitive processes that influence or modulate the gating mechanism by descending fibers.
5. When the output of the spinal cord transmission exceeds a critical level, it activates the action system responsible for the expression of pain (Jeans & Melzack, 1992).

Applying knowledge of ascending and descending analgesic systems will assist nurses in understanding the physiological basis of both acute and chronic pain. Table 21-4 highlights differences between acute and chronic pain experiences.

ROY ADAPTATION MODEL

A conceptual framework for nursing that provides a useful paradigm in assessing, treating,

Table 21-4 Differences Between Acute and Chronic Pain	
Acute Pain	**Chronic Pain**
• serves to warn of injury	• serves no useful purpose
• can be intense, short duration, but may also vary in intensity	• generally defined as pain of greater than 6 months duration
• has predictable end point, as healing occurs	• no predictable end point
• sympathetic nervous system responses, i.e., diaphoresis, increased heart rate, BP, RR	• adaptation of autonomic nervous system responses, therefore no change in vital signs as with acute pain
• anxiety	• depression, hopelessness, fatigue, and social isolation may occur
	• McCaffery and Beebe (1989) have further defined chronic or prolonged pain as follows:
	1. recurrent, acute pain (e.g., sickle cell crisis; migraine headaches; self-contained, recurrent pain)
	2. ongoing, time-limited pain (e.g., cancer pain, burn pain); may occur daily for months or years until condition is cured or controlled or may end with death of patient
	3. chronic, nonmalignant pain (i.e., rheumatoid arthritis, peripheral neuropathies, chronic low back pain); not life-threatening, but may cause considerable disability and may be lifelong

and evaluating patient outcomes for persons experiencing pain is the Roy Adaptation Model. The Roy model is a systems model based on the view of the person as a dynamic, biopsychosocial being, possessing the ability to adapt to changes in both external and internal environment (Roy, 1984, p. 30). The goal of nursing in this model is to promote adaptation. The response to various stimuli affecting a person is expressed through the adaptive modes—the physiological, self-concept, role function, and interdependence modes. Evaluation (assessment) of the adaptive modes are expressions of coping effectiveness. In the author's research, the adaptive modes were operationalized utilizing the quality-of-life tool developed by Padilla and Grant (1985) and revised by Ferrell, Wisdom, & Wenzl (1989).

Applying the concepts of adaptation and quality of life to the assessment and treatment of pain involves using successful adaptation as an outcome measure of effective pain management. Ferrell, Wisdom, Rhiner & Alletto (1991) and Wells (1994) have proposed that

quality of life be used as an outcome measure in evaluating pain treatment programs. Quality-of-life measurement tools have become an integral part of many treatment protocols, particularly in the area of cancer treatment. Figure 21-1 illustrates the conceptual relationships within the Roy Adaptation Model using chronic cancer pain as an example of environmental stimuli. The Roy model allows for integration of physiological concepts through the relationship of regulator and cognator processes, as illustrated in Figure 21-1.

It is important to remember to apply systems theory, as well, to the individual experiencing pain and his or her relationships to others. Particularly in the area of chronic pain, one must look at the role function and interdependence function in measuring the profound effects that chronic pain can have on role performance within the family, work environment, social network, and affiliations. Social isolation, powerlessness, and learned helplessness have a major impact on quality of life. Interventions must focus on restoration of function, pain re-

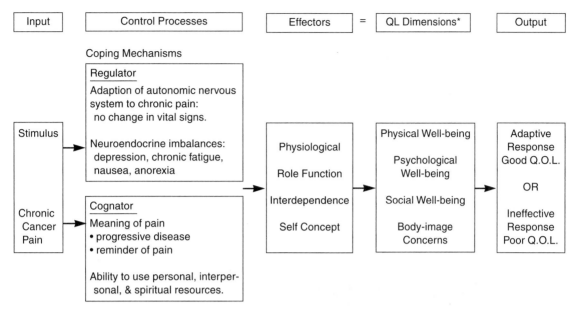

| Input | Control Processes | | Effectors | = | QL Dimensions* | Output |

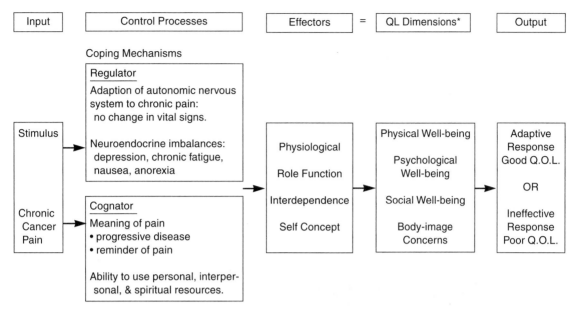

*As operationalized in the Quality of Life Index by Padilla & Grant (1985)

FIGURE 21–1. Conceptual relationships between chronic cancer pain and quality of life, using the Roy Adaptation Model.

lief, and empowerment in order to improve quality of life for persons with pain.

GENERAL PAIN MANAGEMENT PRINCIPLES

General principles of pain management focus on assessment, problem identification with etiologic factors, intervention, and evaluation of outcomes. It should be emphasized that assessment is not a one-time event; rather, it is ongoing. Lack of accurate assessment and reassessment is one of the most common causes of inadequate pain management. The single most reliable indicator of the existence and intensity of pain is the patient's self-report (AHCPR, 1992).

ASSESSMENT

Initial pain assessment should be included within the context of functional health pattern assessment as outlined in the Barry Holistic Systems Model in Chapter 8. Pain assessment

should include pain history: how the patient has responded to past experiences with pain; what he or she believes to be the cause of pain; what the patient believes will relieve pain; how he or she expresses pain.

McCaffery and Beebe (1989) have presented concise and easy-to-use assessment tools and flow sheets that can be used across care settings.

The components of pain assessment, as outlined by Donovan (1987), include location; intensity; factors influencing the occurrence of pain; observed behaviors, including vital signs; psychosocial modifiers; effects of pain; effects of therapy; and established patterns of coping. Diagrams of the front and back of the body are useful in allowing the patient to mark exact locations of pain. Assessment of intensity can be accomplished using numeric rating scales, visual analog scales, or word scales. Examples of these can be found in Figure 21-2. Next, have the patient describe the quality of pain. Many pain assessment tools provide word descriptors for patients to choose in describing their pain. The McGill

Pain Questionnaire has been widely tested in research settings and has been found to be a valid and reliable measurement tool in the assessment of pain (McGuire, 1987).

McCaffery and Beebe's (1989) assessment tool and flow sheet (see Fig. 21-3) can be readily used at the bedside. Use of a flow sheet allows for continuous monitoring and documentation of pain and its relief.

The pattern of pain—its onset, duration, and effect on activities of daily living—should be noted. Observation of the patient's behavior, social interactions, sleep patterns, and activity levels contribute valuable information on the patient's ability to function and cope with pain.

The patient may have noted a pattern of activity that causes pain or relieves pain. It is important to ascertain any of the treatments the patient has tried to reduce pain and note their effects. Likewise, note what has made the pain worse. Evaluating the effect of pain on other aspects of life—ability to work, relationships with others, sleep, mood, concentration—has major implications on quality of life. The use of pain diaries can assist patients in documenting some of these invisible effects of pain. Assessment of pain-relief strategies used by the

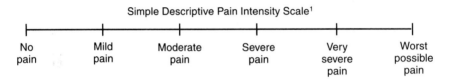

Simple Descriptive Pain Intensity Scale[1]

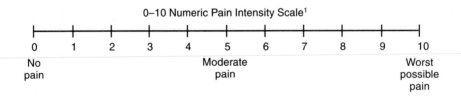

0–10 Numeric Pain Intensity Scale[1]

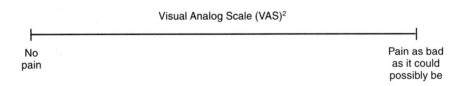

Visual Analog Scale (VAS)[2]

[1]If used as a graphic rating scale, a 10-cm baseline is recommended.
[2]A 10-cm baseline is recommended for VAS scales.

FIGURE 21–2. Pain intensity scales. (Agency for Health Care Policy and Research. [1992]. *Acute pain management: Operative or medical procedures and trauma.* Rockville, MD: Department of Health and Human Services, p. 116.)

patient should include consumption of alcohol and other recreational drugs. Judgmental inferences should be avoided. Often, unrelieved pain perpetuates a pattern of ineffective coping. Alcohol and other drug abuse may be more a symptom of unrelieved pain than of psychological dependence. Alcohol use has major implications for the use of nonopioid and opioid analgesics. Concomitant use of alcohol and acetaminophen can cause acute hepatic failure (Beaver, 1990). The CNS-depressant effects of alcohol can potentiate side effects due to opioids.

In practical terms, the acronym PAIN presented by Donovan (1985) provides an easy-to-use and readily accessible tool for ongoing pain assessment. It can be used across care settings and requires no special forms.

> *P:* Place. Identify any areas where pain exists on front and back view of the body.
> *A:* Amount. Using a numeric scale of 0–10 (0 = no pain, 10 = worst pain imaginable) rate present pain, at its worst and at its best. Note quality of pain and word descriptors.
> *I:* Interactions. What makes the pain worse?
> *N:* Neutralizers. What makes the pain better?

It is important to note the variety in cultural expression of pain. Nurses must recognize their own cultural biases in order to assess and treat patients of all cultures effectively. Cultural diversity requires that nurses assess patterns of pain expression, home remedies for pain relief, and beliefs about analgesic therapy and medical care in order to develop an acceptable plan of care for specific patients. Culture is comprised of socioeconomic status, ethnicity, and belief systems. Research exploring the influence of culture on pain perception and response to pain has been inconclusive due to small sample size and methodological flaws. More importantly, stereotyping of patients should be avoided. Gaston-Johansson, Albert, Fagan, and Zimmerman (1990) found that subjects of diverse educational and cultural backgrounds used similar terms to describe pain, *hurt* and *ache.*

Assessing what treatments have been effective in the past for patients assists in developing a plan that will build trust and compliance. A patient who states that only medication has helped in the past will be unlikely to respond positively to attempts to utilize focused breathing for a painful procedure, such as bone marrow biopsy. A plan that incorporates premedication with focused rhythmic breathing (provided by coach) will gain more acceptance from the patient.

It is equally critical to include assessment of the patient's significant other regarding the use of pain medications and causes of pain. The best-laid plans for adequate analgesia can be sabotaged at home by misunderstandings regarding normal side effects and management strategies, fear of addiction, or disbelief regarding pain severity.

Pain must be assessed and reassessed regularly, depending on the nature of the pain problem. A thorough physical exam, with specific attention to neurological exam and diagnostic testing as indicated, will assist in identification of the pain problem and appropriate treatment (AHCPR, 1994).

PHARMACOLOGIC APPROACHES TO PAIN MANAGEMENT

Pain should be treated aggressively and preemptively. For procedural or surgical pain, prevention of pain is an integral part of preoperative education and planning. Pain management associated with trauma or injury should be aimed at preventing further tissue injury or damage and minimizing patient discomfort and distress (AHCPR, 1992). Pharmacologic interventions are the cornerstone to pain management. Three major categories of drugs will be described: nonopioids, opioids, and adjuvant analgesics. The World Health Organization (WHO) recommends a three-step approach to the management of cancer pain, though this approach may be applicable to the management of other types of pain (Fig. 21-4).

Keep in mind the pharmokinetic principles of absorption, distribution, and elimination with respect to all drug therapies mentioned. Caveats for practice will be mentioned under each category of drug intervention.

Initial Pain Assessment Tool

Date _____

Patient's Name _____ Age _____ Room _____

Diagnosis _____ Physician_____

Nurse_____

I.   Location: Patient or nurse marks drawing

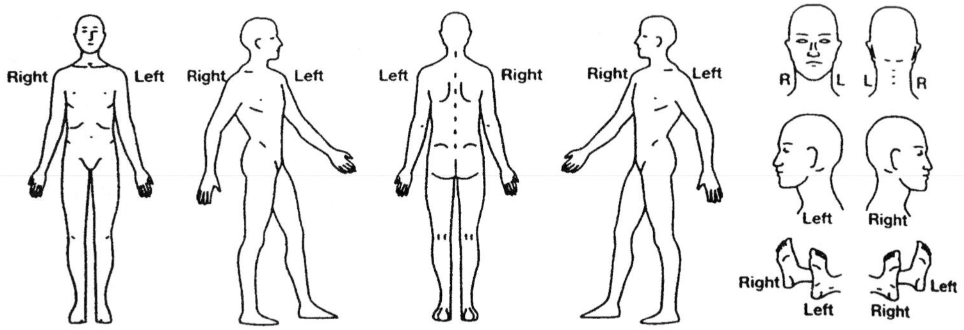

II. Intensity: Patient rates the pain. Scale used _____

Present: _____

Worst pain gets: _____

Best pain gets: _____

Acceptable level of pain: _____

III. Quality: (Use patient's own words, e.g., prick, ache, burn, throb, pull, sharp)

_____

IV. Onset, duration, variations, rhythms: _____

_____

V.   Manner of expressing pain: _____

VI. What relieves the pain? _____

VII. What causes or increases the pain?_____

VIII.Effects of pain: (Note decreased function, decreased quality of life.)

Accompanying symptoms (e.g., nausea) _____

Sleep _____

Appetite _____

Physical activity _____

Relationship with others (e.g., irritability) _____

Emotions (e.g., anger, suicidal, crying)_____

Concentration _____

Other_____

IX. Other comments: _____

_____

X. Plan: _____

_____

Note: May be duplicated and used in clinical practice.

FIGURE 21-3. Initial pain assessment tool and flowsheet for pain management documentation. (McCaffery, J., Beebe, A. [1989]. *Pain: Clinical manual for nursing practice.* St. Louis: CV Mosby, pp. 21, 27.)

Flowsheet for Pain Management Documentation

Patient's Name _____Date _____

Pain rating scale used _____

Purpose: To evaluate the safety and effectiveness of the analgesic(s)

Analgesics(s) prescribed: _____

Time	Pain rating	Analgesic	R	P	BP	Level of arovsal	Others[2]	Plan and comments

Note: May be duplicated and used in clinical practice.

[1]Pain rating: A number of different scales may be used. Indicate which scale is used and use the same scale each time.

[2]Possibilities for other columns: bowel function, activities, nausea and vomiting, and other pain relief measures. Identify the side effects of greatest concern to patient, family, physician, and nurse.

FIGURE 21-3. *(Continued)*

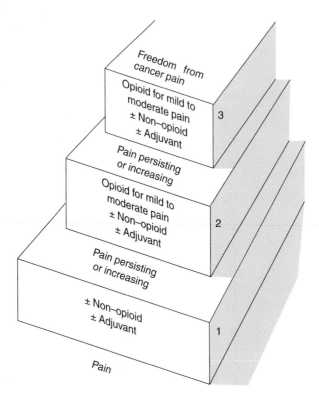

FIGURE 21-4. Three-step analgesic ladder. (Cancer pain relief and palliative care: Report of a WHO Expert Committee. [1990]. Geneva: World Health Organization, Technical Report Series, No. 804, Fig. 1.)

NON-OPIOIDS

Non-opioid drugs include nonsteroidal anti-inflammatory drugs (NSAIDs) and acetaminophen. They are widely used analgesics for several reasons: efficacy in controlling mild to moderate pain; wide availability (several are available over the counter); and few serious side effects. Generally, all NSAIDs provide three effects: antipyretic, anti-inflammatory, and analgesic. With the exception of acetaminophen, they accomplish these effects by blocking the biosynthesis of prostaglandins.

NSAIDs and acetaminophen work in the hypothalamus to regulate body temperature during febrile episodes, exerting an antipyretic effect (McCaffery & Beebe, 1989; Paice, 1992). Because NSAIDS work to block prostaglandin metabolism, they are ideally suited for the treatment of pain associated with tissue inflammation. Pain caused by dysmenorrhea, musculoskeletal injury, or bone metastases responds well to NSAIDs. Although acetaminophen does not appear to have anti-inflammatory effects, it does work peripherally to block pain transmission. It has been helpful for mild pain caused by osteoarthritis, headache, or musculoskeletal injury.

Side Effects of NSAIDS

The most common side effects of NSAIDs are gastrointestinal toxicity and bleeding problems. Prostaglandins provide protection of the lining of the stomach. In addition, many NSAIDs cause direct irritation of the gastric mucosa (Paice, 1992). Symptoms of toxicity can range from dyspepsia, nausea, and diarrhea, to ulceration and bleeding. Taking NSAIDs with meals or concomitant use of antacids can prevent some of these side effects. Use of misoprostol (cytotec) may also be indicated. Misoprostol is a prostaglandin analog specifically indicated in the prevention of

NSAID-induced gastric ulcers. It is absolutely contraindicated in pregnancy as it will induce abortion and potentially life-threatening bleeding (Katzung, 1989). Misoprostol is expensive and causes dose-limiting diarrhea, particularly in the elderly, for whom GI bleeding is a considerable risk. Continued assessment and follow-up is necessary to ensure safe analgesic administration and successful pain relief.

Central nervous system side effects include tinnitus, dizziness, visual disturbances, drowsiness, somnolence, and lethargy (Halpern & Davis, 1983). These are less common with newer NSAIDs.

Clinical decision making with respect to choosing NSAIDs should take into account risks for ulcers and bleeding, a patient's prior experience with NSAIDs, renal function, ease of dosing, and cost (McCaffery & Beebe, 1989). Nonacetylated salicylates, for example, do not interfere with platelet aggregation and cause less GI upset. Many of the newer NSAIDs are expensive and hold no advantage over cheaper, older NSAIDs. Ibuprofen, naproxen sodium, aspirin, and acetaminophen are available without prescription. Often, if one NSAID is ineffective in achieving adequate analgesia, switching to a different NSAID may offer increased relief (see Table 21-5). Numerous studies have demonstrated additive and opioid-sparing effects of NSAIDs in the management of postoperative pain and cancer pain (AHCPR, 1992; Ferrer-Brechner & Ganz, 1984; Stambaugh & Drew, 1988; Weingart, Sorkness, & Earhart, 1985).

OPIOIDS

Opioid analgesics have been around since the third century B.C. and are indicated in the management of acute pain, cancer pain and, in selected cases, chronic, nonmalignant pain.

Opioids are classified as full agonists, partial agonists, and mixed agonists-antagonists. Classification is dependent on receptor binding activity. Full agonists, such as morphine, exert maximum effect by complete binding with mu-opiate receptor. Partial agonists work by less effective binding. Mixed agonists-antagonists work by binding with one receptor while simultaneously blocking another (AHCPR, 1992). Mixed agonists-antagonists should *never* be given in close proximity to patients receiving an opioid agonist as they will precipitate withdrawal symptoms. It is important to note that the mixed agonists-antagonists have a ceiling effect and frequently cause psychomimetic effects. These limitations make them unsuitable for use in chronic pain and cancer pain management. Promising advances in basic science have led to discovery of opiate receptors in the periphery (Stein, 1991). New approaches to managing pain with opioids locally may be forthcoming.

Many barriers to effective pain management exist due to misunderstandings regarding addiction, tolerance, and physical dependence. Addiction is characterized by compulsion to obtain and use opioids for effects other than pain relief. Tolerance results when, after repeated administration, a drug dose begins to lose its effectiveness, requiring an increased dose. Tolerance is a physiological response and, in the case of cancer pain, may often indicate advancing disease.

Physical dependence occurs when abrupt withdrawal of the drug causes symptoms of abstinence syndrome characterized by yawning, rhinorrhea, sweating, and lacrimation, followed by restlessness, tremors, agitation, and anorexia. Late symptoms of withdrawal include nausea and vomiting, diarrhea, severe sneezing, chills, muscle spasm, and low back pain (McCaffery & Beebe, 1989). *Physical dependence* is not the same as *addiction*. Addiction is a voluntary behavior while physical dependence is involuntary.

Table 21-6 provides equianalgesic doses for commonly used opioids. Morphine is the standard for comparison and is generally considered the first-line, short-acting opioid for acute and cancer pain management. Lack of knowledge regarding equianalgesic dosing is a major cause for the undertreatment of pain (Foley, 1985). Equianalgesic tables provide a basis for comparison of doses when switching to an alternative opioid or route of administration. While equianalgesic dosing principles provide a guideline, they are no substitute for ongoing assessment and evaluation of analgesic effectiveness and side effects.

It is important to note that meperidine (Demerol) has an active metabolite, normeperi-

Table 21-5
Dosing Data for Acetaminophen and NSAIDs

Drug	Usual dose for adults ≥ 50 kg body weight	Usual dose for adults[1] < 50 kg body weight
Acetaminophen and over-the-counter NSAIDs		
Acetaminophen[2]	650 mg q 4 h	10–15 mg/kg q 4 h
	975 mg q 6 h	15–20 mg/kg q 4 h (rectal)
Aspirin[3]	650 mg q 4 h	10–15 mg/kg q 4 h
	975 mg q 6 h	15–20 mg/kg q 4 h (rectal)
Ibuprofen (Motrin, others)	400–600 mg q 6 h	10 mg/kg q 6–8 h
Prescription NSAIDs		
Carprofen (Rimadyl)	100 mg tid	
Choline magnesium trisalicylate[4] (Trilisate)	1,000–1,500 mg tid	25 mg/kg tid
Choline salicylate (Arthropan)[4]	870 mg q 3–4 h	
Diflunisal (Dolobid)[5]	500 mg q 12 h	
Etodolac (Lodine)	200–400 mg q 6–8 h	
Fenoprofen calcium (Nalfon)	300–600 mg q 6 h	
Ketoprofen (Orudis)	25–60 mg q 6–8 h	
Ketorolac tromethamine[6] (Toradol)	10 mg q 4–6 h to a maximum of 40 mg/day	
Magnesium salicylate (Doan's, Magan, Mobidin, others)	650 mg q 4 h	
Meclofenamate sodium (Meclomen)[7]	50–100 mg q 6 h	
Mefenamic acid (Ponstel)	250 mg q 6 h	
Naproxen (Naprosyn)	250–275 mg q 6–8 h	5 mg/kg q 8 h
Naproxen sodium (Anaprox)	275 mg q 6–8 h	
Sodium salicylate (Generic)	325–650 mg q 3–4 h	
Parenteral NSAIDs		
Ketorolac tromethamine[6,8] (Toradol)	60 mg initially, then 30 mg q 6 h Intramuscular dose not to exceed 5 days	

[1] Acetaminophen and NSAID dosages for adults weighing less than 50 kg should be adjusted for weight.
[2] Acetaminophen lacks the peripheral anti-inflammatory and antiplatelet activities of the other NSAIDs.
[3] The standard against which other NSAIDs are compared. May inhibit platelet aggregation for ≥ 1 week and may cause bleeding.
[4] May have minimal antiplatelet activity.
[5] Administration with antacids may decrease absorption.
[6] For short-term use only.
[7] Coombs-positive autoimmune hemolytic anemia has been associated with prolonged use.
[8] Has the same GI toxicities as oral NSAIDs.
Note: Only the above NSAIDs have FDA approval for use as simple analgesics, but clinical experience has been gained with other drugs as well.
Codes: q = every, tid = thrice daily.

Table 21-6
Dose equivalents for opioid analgesics in opioid-naive adults ≥ 50 kg[1]

Drug	Approximate equianalgesic dose		Usual starting dose for moderate to severe pain	
	ORAL	PARENTERAL	ORAL	PARENTERAL
Opioid agonist[2]				
Morphine[3]	30 mg q 3–4 h (repeat around-the-clock dosing); 60 mg q 3–4 h (single intermittent dosing)	10 mg q 3–4 h	30 mg q 3–4 h	10 mg q 3–4 h
Morphine, controlled-release[3,4] (MS Contin Oramorph)	90–120 mg q 12 h	N/A	90–120 mg q 12 h	N/A
Hydromorphone[3] (Dilaudid)	7.5 mg q 3–4 h	1.5 mg q 3–4 h	6 mg q 3–4 h	1.5 mg q 3–4 h
Levorphanol (Levo-Dromoran)	4 mg q 6–8 h	2 mg q 6–8 h	4 mg q 6–8 h	2 mg q 6–8 h
Meperidine[5] (Demerol)	300 mg q 2–3 h	100 mg q 3 h	N/R	100 mg q 3 h
Methadone (Dolophine, other)	20 mg q 6–8 h	10 mg q 6–8 h	20 mg q 6–8 h	10 mg q 6–8 h
Oxymorphone[3] (Numorphan)	N/A	1 mg q 3–4 h	N/A	1 mg q 3–4 h
Combination opioid/NSAID preparations[6]				
Codeine (with aspirin or acetaminophen)	180–200 mg q 3–4 h	130 mg q 3–4 h	60 mg q 3–4 h	60 mg q 2 h (IM/SC)
Hydrocodone (in Lorcet, Lortab, Vicodin, others)	30 mg q 3–4 h	N/A	10 mg q 3–4 h	N/A
Oxycodone (Roxicodone, also in Percocet, Percodan, Tylox, others)	30 mg q 3–4 h	N/A	10 mg q 3–4 h	N/A

[1]Caution: Recommended doses do not apply for adult patients with body weight less than 50 kg. For children and adults less than 50 kg, see Table 11, AHCPR Cancer Pain Guidelines.

[2]Caution: Recommended doses do not apply to patients with renal or hepatic insufficiency or other conditions affecting drug metabolism and kinetics.

[3]Caution: For morphine, hydromorphone, and oxymorphone, rectal administration is an alternate route for patients unable to take oral medications. Equianalgesic doses may differ from oral and parenteral doses because of pharmocokinetic differences.

[4]Transdermal fentanyl (duragesic) is an alternative. Transdermal fentanyl dosage is not calculated as equivalent to a single morphine dose. See package insert for dosing calculations. Doses above 25 μg/h should not be used in opioid-naive patients.

[5]Caution: Doses of aspirin and acetaminophen in combination opioid/NSAID preparations must also be adjusted to the patient's body weight. Aspirin is contraindicated in children in the presence of fever or other viral disease because of its association with Reye's syndrome.

[6]Caution: Codeine doses above 65 mg often are not appropriate because of diminishing incremental analgesia with increasing doses but continually increasing nausea, constipation, and other side effects.

Note: Published tables vary in suggested doses equivalent to morphine. Clinical response is the criterion that *must* be applied to each patient; titration to clinical response is necessary. Because of incomplete cross tolerance among these drugs, it is usually necessary to use lower than equianalgesic dose when changing drugs, and to re-titrate to response.

dine, that is a CNS stimulant with a half-life of 15 to 16 hours in persons with normal renal function. Accumulation of this active metabolite can precipitate seizures (Kaiko et al., 1983). Meperidine is contraindicated for the management of pain in persons with any of the following: impaired renal function, need for repeated (long-term) analgesic doses, and receipt of MAO inhibitors. Early signs of normeperidine toxicity include irritability, tremors, and restlessness.

Common Side Effects Of Opioids

Sedation. Sedation is a common and sometimes desirable effect in the treatment of pain. Sedation is a time-limited effect; tolerance to it appears to develop over a period of days. Do not mistake exhaustion from unrelieved pain as excessive sedation. Always assess the patient for pain relief and *know the patient's sleep history*. The patient may continue to have pain despite excessive sedation. A change to a lower dose of opioid or trial of an alternative opioid may be beneficial. In the case of persons with cancer, sedation may have other etiologies, such as hypercalcemia.

As a general rule of thumb, if sedation persists for more than a few days and other etiologies have been ruled out, switch to an alternate opioid. If sedation continues to be a problem despite titration down to the lowest tolerable dose (that dose which still relieves pain), a trial of psychostimulants may be beneficial. For cancer patients, the use of psychostimulants to combat excessive sedation can be useful. Methylphenidate (Ritalin) has been studied for use with opioid-induced sedation in cancer patients with pain (Bruera, Brennais, & Paterson, 1989). Evaluation of their use should take into consideration risks for agitation, palpitations, and psychosis. Use of caffeine (coffee, cola) can be helpful for both cancer patients and patients requiring short-term opioid therapy. Increasing caffeine intake for a few days after starting or increasing the dose of an opiod can mitigate symptoms of increased sedation.

It is important to note that sedation *always* precedes respiratory depression. Pasero (1994) has recommended grading sedation when documenting pain assessment and treatment on flow sheets. Use of a sedation rating scale,

such as the one presented in Box 21-2, can assist in adequate titration of opioids in both the acute and cancer pain settings and can easily be incorporated onto flow sheets or graphic sheets.

Constipation. Constipation is a predictable and universal side effect to opioids. Tolerance to this opioid side effect appears to develop slowly, if at all (Paice, 1992). Opioids induce constipation by binding to opiate receptors in the gut. The resultant decrease in motility also leads to increased water reabsorption from the stool. In pain management, a preventative approach to managing constipation is essential. Patient and family instruction about this side effect and effective treatment strategies includes both pharmacologic and nonpharmacologic approaches (Table 21-7).

Nausea and Vomiting. Nausea is a common side effect in patients on opioid analgesics. Opioids cause nausea and vomiting through several mechanisms: stimulation of the CTZ (chemoreceptor trigger zone); decreasing GI motility; and stimulation of vestibular complex. Persons who are ambulatory and just starting opioid therapy are at particular risk for nausea. It has been estimated that 40% to 70% of cancer patients starting opioids or increasing the dose of an opioid will experience nausea (Ferris et al., 1991). Fortunately, this is a time-limited side effect, with tolerance to the effect developing within a few days.

If nausea persists longer than a few days, consider looking for other causes or a trial of a different opioid. In the case of cancer patients

BOX 21-2	Sedation Rating Scale
S	sleeping, easy to arouse
1	awake and alert
2	occasionally drowsy, easy to arouse
3	frequently drowsy, arousable
4	somnolent, hard or difficult to arouse, if at all

Pasero, C. (1994). Pain control. *American Journal of Nursing, 94*(2), 22–23.

Table 21-7
Constipation Treatment Strategies

Nonpharmacologic Approaches	Pharmacologic Approaches
• Increase fluid intake to 8 large glasses of water per day	• Stool softeners (diocytl sodium sulfosuccinate)
• Increase ambulation and activity	• Bulk laxatives (psyllium, bran, methylcellulose)
• Increase dietary fiber (e.g., whole grains, fruits, dried fruits)	• Osmotic cathartics (magnesium salts, lactulose, sorbitol)
	• Contact cathartics (Senna, phenothalein, cascara, bisacodyl)

who have been on stable doses of opioids and who have persistent nausea, investigation should include evaluation for hypercalcemia and central nervous system metastases as potential etiologies of nausea. Antiemetic therapy may be helpful during the first few days of opioid therapy and should be aimed at preventing nausea and vomiting. This is particularly important in the postoperative setting.

Respiratory Depression. Respiratory depression is a rare side effect of opioid use and is more likely to occur in the following settings:

1. In the opioid-naive patient receiving the first few doses of an opioid.
2. In case of rapid titration of an opioid to relieve severe pain.
3. When pain is suddenly relieved (i.e., after neurolytic block, in a patient receiving opioids).

Pain appears to be a natural antidote to the respiratory depressant effects of opioids.

Fear of causing respiratory depression is a major reason for the undertreatment of pain across care settings. Careful assessment and use of flow sheets can assist nurses in providing safe and effective pain management. Again, remember that *sedation always precedes respiratory depression.* Use of naloxone should be judicious, especially in persons who have been on chronic opioid therapy. McCaffery and Beebe (1989) recommend diluting naloxone 0.4 mg in 10 cc of normal saline and administering by *slow* intravenous push until res-

piratory rate increases. The purpose is to reverse respiratory depression without reversing analgesia or precipitating withdrawal symptoms. Continued observation is essential and, depending on the half-life of the opioid drug involved, may require subsequent doses of naloxone (McCaffery & Beebe, 1989). Remember that naloxone has a short half-life, approximately 30 minutes.

In evaluating for respiratory depression, the importance of getting a baseline respiratory rate on the patient, particularly at sleep, cannot be overemphasized. An example from the author's practice best illustrates this point.

Mr. P was a 54-year-old Caucasian male with widely metastatic breast cancer, admitted with intractable pain due to bony mets and severe brachial plexopathy. He was being titrated on a morphine drip as well as adjuvant medications to manage his pain conservatively. At night, his respiratory rate dropped to 8 from a baseline RR of 12 when awake. Prior to initiating his morphine drip, his nighttime sleeping RR was 8 breaths per minute. For three nights, his night nurse had either stopped or significantly decreased his IV infusion rate due to respiratory depression to a rate of 8/minute. By afternoon, his pain was widely out of control and a vicious cycle of bolusing and increasing his drip to control his pain occurred. After speaking to his night nurse and holding a team conference to review the pain regime, we were able to achieve acceptable analgesia for this patient without perpetuating the cycle of increasing/decreasing IV drip without sustained pain control. ☙

Other Opioid Side Effects. Other opioid effects that can occur include myoclonus, seizures, and hallucinations, particularly at high doses (Bruera, Scholler, & Montejo, 1992). Urinary retention and pruritus also occasionally occur. Pruritus is a common side effect with intraspinal opioids.

Alternative Routes of Opioid Delivery

Many alternative routes of delivering opioids are now available. It is always preferable to use the oral route when the GI tract is functioning. For patients who need alternatives (postoperative, children, and some cancer patients) there are many options.

Intraspinal opioids are commonly used in the perioperative and postoperative settings with established safety and efficacy (Hurley & Johnson, 1990; Ready, 1990). *Transdermal fentanyl patches* (Duragesic) offer a noninvasive alternative to long-acting oral opioids in the management of cancer pain. Use of the fentanyl patch is not recommended for postoperative pain management.

The *intravenous route* for opioid delivery has been used with increased frequency. Both in the postoperative and cancer pain settings, its safety and efficacy have been well established (Barkas & Duafala, 1988; Citron et al., 1984; Portenoy, 1989a). Excellent guidelines for the use of opioid infusions are available in McCaffery & Beebe (1989) and Portenoy (1989b).

Use of *sublingual and buccal routes* in cancer patients unable to tolerate oral opioids have been reported (Paice, 1992). Because this route bypasses the first pass effect of the liver, dosing is similar to parenteral dosing.

The *rectal route* is an underutilized route to administering opioids (Cole and Hanning, 1990). Nurses practicing in hospice settings know the value of having rectal morphine or hydromorphone available for use in the home. Hospice nurses often develop alliances with pharmacists who are willing to compound various suppositories to manage symptoms in the home. Because this route bypasses the first pass effect of the liver, dosing, again, is equianalgesic to parenteral dosing (Paice, 1992).

The *subcutaneous route,* like the intravenous route, is indicated when the GI tract is non-functioning or when oral route at proper dose escalation is no longer able to control cancer pain. Common problems include plaque formation at needle site and skin irritation. Maximum concentration of morphine sulfate for subcutaneous use is 50 mg/ml. Hydromorphone is more soluble and more suitable for high dose infusions (Bruera, Brenneis, & MacDonald, 1987).

ADJUVANT ANALGESICS

Adjuvant analgesics may be indicated to improve pain relief in selected patients. They may be utilized at any step on the WHO analgesic ladder and may be indicated for specific pain syndromes. (AHCPR, 1994; American Pain Society, 1993).

Corticosteroids

Corticosteroids are helpful in the relief of pain associated with inflammation and nerve compression. In the case of cancer pain, cerebral metastases, spinal cord compression, and nerve root compression are indications for steroid use. The added benefits of improved mood, appetite stimulation, antiemesis, and improved sense of well-being make steroids very useful in terminal-phase pain management regimes (Ettinger & Portenoy, 1988). Untoward side effects include proximal myopathy, cushinghoid symptoms, and weight gain.

Tricyclic Antidepressants

Tricyclic antidepressants (TCAs) are useful adjuvants in the treatment of chronic pain and cancer-related pain. Most research has involved the use of amitriptyline (elavil), making it the logical choice when starting antidepressant therapy to treat pain. Neuropathic pain, particularly pain described as burning, constant, aching pain, responds well to the use of TCAs. Antidepressants enhance analgesia by blocking the reuptake of serotonin. Serotonin acts in the descending analgesic pathway to block pain transmission and enhance endorphins. TCAs also provide for normalization of sleep in patients with chronic pain (Foley, 1985; Marcus & Arbeiter, 1994).

Anticonvulsants

Anticonvulsants act as membrane-stabilizing agents to suppress neuronal firing. Pain that is neuropathic and described as electric, shooting, or lancinating pain may respond to drugs such as clonazepam, carbamazepine, and phenytoin. Examples of neuropathic pain syndromes include trigeminal neuralgia and postherpetic neuralgia.

Anxiolytics

Anxiolytics are occasionally useful as adjuvants to control other symptoms associated with pain. Diazepam is useful in relief of muscle spasm. It must be used cautiously when combined with opioids as it potentiates CNS depression. Hydroxyzine is a useful addition to opioids when anxiety or nausea is present. Both of these medications can cause tissue damage when administered parenterally. Midazolam has been used in terminal illness to manage agitation associated with pain. It is not a substitute for appropriate titration of opioids to relieve pain, but can help to relieve agitation. Bottomley and Hanks (1990) reported the use of midazolam, in combination with diamorphine, at doses of 10 to 20 mg/day by subcutaneous continuous infusion in advanced cancer patients with pain and agitation.

Neuroleptics

The use of phenothiazines is generally limited to the control of opioid-induced nausea. The CNS-depressant effects of phenothiazines and other neuroleptics potentiate those same effects from opioids. With the exception of methotrimeprazine, some phenothiazines actually possess antianalgesic properties. Methotrimeprazine has been used parenterally to control pain in selected patients. Foley and Inturrisi (1989) reported that methotrimeprazine, 15 mg intramuscularly, is equivalent to 10 mg of intramuscular morphine. This makes methotrimeprazine ideally suited for patients with bowel obstruction because it

is both a potent analgesic and an antiemetic. Foley and Inturrisi (1989) recommend that a test dose of 5 mg be administered to evaluate for hypotension. Excessive sedation and postural hypotension are dose-limiting side effects.

Butyrophenones, haloperidol, and droperidol have been helpful in managing nausea associated with the use of opioids in cancer pain management. Haloperidol is the drug of choice in managing acute psychoses or delirium in cancer patients (Foley & Inturrisi, 1989). Delirium has been estimated to occur in up to 85% of advanced cancer patients with a variety of potential etiologies; opioid analgesics are but one possible risk factor. Zimberg and Berenson (1990) provided an excellent guide on the assessment and treatment of delirium in cancer patients.

Psychostimulants

Psychostimulants, as mentioned previously, have a role to play in the management of sedation due to opioids. Their use is indicated only after attempts to titrate or switch to alternative opioids have been unsuccessful in managing this opioid side effect. Tolerance to the sedative effect of opioids usually takes a few days. It is critical to discontinue any other medication that may be contributing to sedation (Foley & Inturrisi, 1989).

Dextroamphetamine (2.5–7.5 mg po bid) and methylphenidate (5–10 mg po bid) have been used to counter the sedative effect of opioids when other strategies to manage this side effect have failed (AHCPR 1994).

Placebos

Placebos have no place in the management of pain. A placebo response is probably mediated by endogenous opioids and a positive response of pain relief does not offer any indication of real vs. psychogenic pain (AHCPR, 1994; McCaffery & Beebe, 1989). The use of placebos undermines patient-caregiver trust and places caregivers at risk for litigation for the undertreatment of pain. The American Pain Society and World Health Organization acknowledge that placebos are effective in a portion of people for a short period of time and *should not* be used in the management of cancer pain (AHCPR, 1994).

NONPHARMACOLOGIC APPROACHES TO PAIN MANAGEMENT

Nurses have used numerous nonpharmacologic approaches to pain management for years. These approaches have not always been well-documented and they have variable efficacy. The reader is referred to McCaffery & Beebe's (1989) excellent and in-depth practice guide for discussion of cutaneous stimulation, relaxation techniques, focused breathing, and guided imagery. They offer patient teaching tools ready for use in any practice setting.

For staff nurses in the acute care or home care settings unfamiliar with some of these techniques, consultation with an advanced practice nurse or consultant who can provide a short course of training in the use of these techniques will facilitate application to practice.

APPLICATION TO SPECIFIC PAIN PROBLEMS

ACUTE PAIN: POSTOPERATIVE PAIN

The treatment of postoperative pain has received greater priority in many acute care settings with the publication of the acute pain clinical practice guidelines in 1992 (AHCPR). Aggressive treatment of pain in the early postoperative period reduces morbidity, thereby speeding recovery, which translates into fewer hospital days (Wayslak, 1989). Unfortunately, undertreatment still persists.

Assessment and reassessment are critical, along with recognition by the health care team that pain treatment is a clinical and institutional priority. Ferrell (1994) advocated a top-down approach to making pain management an institutional priority. Continuous quality improvement projects can be targeted for postoperative pain management. Operationalizing a standard assessment form or adding pain intensity ratings to the bedside graphic sheet are

strategies for making pain and its relief visible.

There is not a more powerful tool for change than consumer demand. Education of the public regarding expectation of pain relief after surgery will force a consumer-driven wave of change. Nurses have a vital role to play in preoperative education, postoperative care, and patient and family education regarding expectations for pain relief. With shorter hospital stays and one-day surgical procedures, this is no small challenge. It requires a standard of care that incorporates the following:

1. Preoperative teaching regarding expected sensory experiences and standard assessment for comfort levels.
2. A plan for analgesia in the perioperative and postoperative period that takes into account the patient's past experiences with surgery or pain.
3. Discussion of the patient's responsibility in communicating with the team regarding pain and side effects.
4. A discharge pain regime that meets the patient's needs based on support at home, functional status, and availability of home services (insurance, access to care).

Early discharge of postoperative patients has placed a burden of care on family members who are expected to learn how to manage not only pain, but various dressing changes, drainage tubes, and other high-technology care. Accessibility to skilled home nursing care depends on third-party payers.

Nurses in acute care facilities can facilitate the transition to home for patients and their families by developing assessment and treatment plans that include family education throughout the hospital stay. Giving family members strategies to manage pain that are concrete and effective decreases their sense of helplessness.

CHRONIC PAIN

Chronic pain has been defined as pain that lasts at least 3 months past injury, with intensity ranging from mild to severe. The cause of pain may or may not be known. Pain in this circumstance serves no useful purpose (i.e., to warn against injury) and leads to untold suffering.

An estimated 80% of Americans will experience at least one episode of low back pain in their lifetime (Payne, 1989), with the majority of patients recovering within 1 to 3 months. The Agency for Health Care Policy and Research has recently released practice guidelines for the treatment of acute, low back pain. Their recommendations are that conservative treatment be employed to treat back pain, including the use of over-the-counter medications, 2 to 3 days bedrest, and early introduction of moderate exercise (Bigos, 1994). The majority of patients will make a full recovery using this approach. A relatively small percentage of patients do not recover and suffer chronic, disabling pain. Chronic back pain costs an estimated $60 billion annually (Mooney, 1991).

In addition to general assessment criteria previously outlined, there should be an in-depth assessment of the effect of pain on the patient's self-care abilities, roles and responsibilities, mood and overall coping abilities, sleep, and quality of life, as well as previous treatment and a workup of pain to date. The major focus should be on obtaining accurate assessment and defining a treatment strategy that is interdisciplinary. Accessibility to a pain treatment facility may be financially and geographically limited for some patients with pain. Movement away from specialty medicine will put the onus on primary care providers to be knowledgeable about appropriate assessment, treatment, and expected outcomes for patients with chronic pain. Outcome measures should focus on function and quality of life (Ferrell, Wisdom, Rhiner & Ailetto, 1991; Hazard, 1994; Wells, 1993).

The challenges of caring for persons with chronic pain are many. Several potential sources of conflict exist, arising from the person with pain, the health care providers, specifically nurses, and systems-oriented issues.

The person with chronic pain may continue to function in a biomedical model where diagnosis and cure are the focus (Weir & Crook, 1992). In this model, lack of definitive pathology leads to frustration in both the patient and provider, due to lack of successful pain relief. The patient embarks on a fruitless search for cause and cure when he or she would be better

served by a change of focus or model. The lack of pain relief, resulting in the demoralization of body and soul, leads to a sense of helplessness and loss of control.

A recent study by Toomey and colleagues found that patients with chronic pain were least likely to report predictable control of pain and demonstrated a higher chance dimension in pain locus of control. Their research suggests what many clinicians have observed in treating pain patients; cognitive appraisal of pain can effect treatment efficacy (Toomey et al., 1993). Patients with back pain were the most frequent consumers of unconventional medical therapy as defined by Eisenberg and colleagues in their evaluation of prevalence, cost, and patterns of use of unconventional medicine in the United States. The most commonly used unconventional therapies were relaxation techniques, chiropractic, and massage (Eisenberg et al., 1993).

When diagnostic evaluation has ruled out serious pathology, focus on regaining life by reducing the "life space occupied by pain" can increase a personal sense of control, reducing helplessness (Ryan, 1994). Ryan has her patients draw the amount of space occupied by pain in their life circle, at the beginning of a chronic pain support group. After training in techniques to enhance coping and reduce physiological distress associated with chronic pain, patients repeat this exercise, which serves as a wonderful technique for measuring the outcome of the group experience on patients. There is a growing body of patient-oriented literature to assist in empowering the patient with chronic pain. Box 21-3 lists a small sampling of consumer literature.

Several researchers have begun to explore the lived experience of chronic pain in women. Howell (1991) developed an evolving theory using a geode as a metaphor for coping with the transformation of a woman's life from the beginning of the pain experience through developing a new life of health with chronic pain. Critical to the progression from illness to health were patterns of validation of pain. Validation could come from the woman herself or from others. Schlesinger (1993) likewise found that validation of pain was necessary for effective coping. Interestingly, women who coped successfully, i.e., maintained a job or other role

BOX 21-3	PATIENT RESOURCES
	Marcus, N. & Arbeiter, J. (1994). *Freedom from Chronic Pain*. New York: Simon & Schuster Kabat-Zinn, J. (1990). *Full Catastrophe Living*. New York: Dell Moyers, B. (1993). *Healing and the Mind*. New York: Doubleday Cowles, J. (1992). *Pain Relief*. New York: Master Media, Ltd.

functions, were often penalized for the lack of visibility of their pain.

Families and the Person With Chronic Pain

Utilizing a systems approach to viewing the human experience of pain, one cannot ignore the impact of pain on the individual as well as his or her family. The pain experience interferes with all levels of human functioning, as outlined earlier in the Roy model.

Chronic pain interferes with physiological function, self-concept, role function, and interdependence. Chronic pain can destroy relationships. Unfortunately, in this era of cost containment, little if any insurance money is available for family treatment despite evidence that family and job status are critical external variables in determining treatment success for persons with chronic pain (Pawlicki, 1992). Pawlicki recommends that families accompany the patient to the initial visit/evaluation, which may be the only opportunity to establish a relationship and treatment goals that involve the whole family. The following steps should be undertaken by the clinician meeting with a chronic pain patient and family:

1. Support veracity of the patient's pain.
2. Give definition to the patient's pain, including what it is not.
3. Listen to the family, paying attention to what the family does when pain occurs and what it means to family members.
4. Differentiate between cure and rehabilitation (Pawlicki, 1992a).

Patient and family education should emphasize optimizing quality of life and learning new ways of coping in order to promote health within illness, in this case, chronic pain.

Controversial Use of Opioids in Chronic, Nonmalignant Pain

The use of opioid drugs can significantly improve functional status in persons with chronic, nonmalignant pain who have failed to respond to more conservative therapies. Zenz and colleagues (1992) described the use of opioids in 100 patients with chronic, nonmalignant pain who were experiencing neuropathic or back pain unresponsive to other therapies. Fifty-one patients had good pain relief as measured by visual analog and Karnofsky performance status. Twenty-eight had partial response and twenty-one had no beneficial response. Pain reduction was associated with increased performance status. There was no respiratory depression or addiction experienced by the patients.

Portenoy (1989c) offered the following guidelines for the use of opioids for chronic, nonmalignant pain:

1. Opioid maintenance should only be considered when all other attempts at analgesia have failed and when persistent pain causes serious functional impairments.
2. Substance abuse history is a relative contraindication.
3. One physician must take responsibility for management of opioid therapy.
4. Patients should give informed consent prior to embarking on opioid maintenance therapy, with specific delineation of goals of therapy.
5. After a period of titration, a maintenance dose should be selected with approximately four extra rescue doses per month (pain has periods of exacerbation; this approach allows for patient to make choices about rescue dosing).

Portenoy emphasized that any evidence of psychological dependence—i.e., drug-seeking behaviors, obtaining opioids from other physicians, or hoarding drugs—would result in stopping opioid therapy after an appropriate drug taper.

CANCER PAIN

Cancer pain is estimated to affect 3.5 million people daily across the world (WHO, 1986).

Bonica (1985) analyzed data from several studies and found that 30% to 40% of patients with early to intermediate-stage disease experienced significant pain. In advanced or terminal disease, 60% to 90% of patients experienced severe pain. Multiple sites of pain may exist in persons with advanced disease. Pain is one of the most feared and expected consequences of cancer (Cleeland, 1985), yet with the application of present knowledge regarding cancer pain management, the vast majority of cancer pain can be relieved (AHCPR, 1994; Portenoy, 1989b; WHO, 1986).

Causes of Pain in Cancer

Pain in patients with cancer may have numerous etiologies. Pain may be tumor-related, treatment-related, or caused by associated symptoms, such as constipation, or it may result from premorbid chronic pain syndromes (AHCPR, 1994; Foley, 1985). Specific pain syndromes associated with cancer have been identified (Portenoy, 1989b; Foley, 1985). The most common cause of pain in cancer patients is the result of direct tumor invasion of bone. Bone pain may result from primary or metastatic lesions. Because of its prevalence, bone pain will be the focus for the discussion of pain management in cancer.

Populations at risk for developing bone pain secondary to cancer include patients with the following malignancies (Spross & Singer, 1992):

1. Primary bone tumors (i.e., osteogenic sarcomas)
2. Breast carcinomas
3. Lung carcinomas
4. Prostate carcinomas
5. Multiple myelomas

The prevalence of breast, lung, and prostate cancer in the United States contributes to the clinical significance of cancer-related bone pain in oncology nursing practice. Assessment and treatment strategies outlined in the section on general pain management principles can be applied in the management of bone pain due to metastatic cancer. Table 21-8 presents a nursing care standard for the treatment of cancer-related bone pain, with specific outcome criteria. The overall goal of treatment is for the patient to achieve optimal pain control with minimum analgesic side effects and maximal quality of life.

Pharmacologic strategies should include the use of measures outlined in the WHO analgesic ladder, specifically NSAIDs with or without opioids and adjuvant analgesics as indicated. Nonacetylated salicylates have been advocated as first-line NSAIDs in patients with pain due to bone metastases (Beaver, 1990; Wilkie, 1990).

Radiation therapy, chemotherapy, and hormonal therapy can be effective in the palliation of bone pain.

Encourage physical activity as tolerated. Collaborative interventions with orthopedics (to ensure the stability of weight-bearing bones) and physical and occupational therapy can facilitate maximum functional mobility. Mobility and weight bearing can reduce calcium demineralization, improve functional status, and reduce associated symptoms, providing that pain is well-managed.

Nonpharmacologic interventions include relaxation techniques, application of heat/cold, gentle massage (avoid areas of bony involvement), facilitation of adequate sleep, and spiritual support.

Important areas for patient and family education include the following:

1. Pain regime and preventative approach to pain management
2. Review of safety issues to prevent complications
3. Individualized, anticipatory guidance regarding pain management at home ("what ifs"), including pain emergencies and side effect management
4. Instruction on what to report to providers and the use of a diary, if desired

Table 21-8
Cancer-Related Bone Pain

Etiologies or Risk Factors	Process Criteria	Outcome Criteria
Amenable to independent action: a. impaired mobility b. sleeplessness c. learning needs related to pain medication regime, side-effect management d. spiritual distress e. anxiety	Perform baseline and ongoing assessment of pain: a. location of pain(s) b. quality and intensity c. duration, frequency d. associated symptoms (i.e., nausea, anorexia, fatigue) e. relief measures taken (pharmacologic, including over-the-counter remedies, alcohol and recreational drugs, and nonpharmacologic) f. changes in roles and relationships g. mood h. functional status i. past and present experiences with pain and coping style j. meaning of pain k. sleep patterns	The patient will: a. communicate comfort level daily until effective pain control is achieved. b. identify measures to modify factors that influence comfort. c. describe treatment plan and expected outcomes.* Patient/caregiver will state knowledge of pain regime, including pharmacologic and nonpharmacologic interventions. Patient/caregiver will identify side effects of analgesics and plan for managing same at home.

Amenable to collaborative action:
a. bone metastases
b. pathological fracture
c. spinal cord compression
d. hypercalcemia
	Monitor patient for signs and symptoms of complications related to bone metastases.
	a. acute change in quality or intensity of pain (new onset of severe, sharp pain may be indicative of fracture)
	b. hypercalcemia
	Symptoms include:
	  1. lethargy
	  2. nausea
	  3. constipation
	  4. dehydration
	  5. flaccidity
	c. spinal cord compression (SCC)
	  1. back pain is heralding symptom in 90% of patients with SCC.
	  2. radiation and steroids
		Patients receiving opioid analgesics will state preventative plan for managing constipation.
		Patient/caregiver will identify symptoms to report to health care provider:
		1. increased or unrelieved pain
		2. change in mental status
		3. constipation > 2 days
		4. inability to tolerate current analgesic regime (i.e., excessive nausea and vomiting, inability to swallow due to stomatitis, esophagitis)

*American Nurses Association & Oncology Nursing Society (1987).

5. How to use nonpharmacologic approaches, tailored to the individual patient

It is also important to implement measures to reduce side effects of analgesic therapies including constipation, nausea and vomiting, disturbance of sleep patterns, and impaired cognition.

Caring for Persons With Terminal-Phase Cancer and Pain

Unrelieved cancer pain is an oncologic emergency (Spross, 1985). During advanced stages of cancer, pain is quite prevalent, often with more than one site of pain (Twycross & Fairfield, 1982). The relief of cancer pain is a clinical priority for nurses caring for patients in acute care settings and in the home. The severity of pain and other symptoms can vary in patients with terminal-phase disease.

The majority of patients can achieve adequate pain relief by applying the pain relief measures already described. It must be emphasized that accurate assessment and reassessment is critical to maintaining pain relief and insuring maximal quality of life. For patients who do not respond to conservative pain management strategies, use of high-technology may be warranted. Please refer to the Oncology Nursing Society's position paper on the use of high-technology interventions in the management of cancer pain (Whedon & Ferrell, 1991). Utilization of resources, such as specialized pain teams and advanced practice nurses skilled in oncology care, can assist in developing plans of care for difficult-to-manage pain problems. Developing a strong knowledge base regarding the use of analgesic therapies, including equianalgesic dosing principles, will also assist nurses in caring for patients with advanced cancer pain.

A study by Coyle, Adelhardt, Foley, & Portenoy (1990) investigated the character of advanced cancer in the last 4 weeks of life. In their sample of 90 patients, 100% of the patients experienced pain. In the last 4 weeks of life, 53% of this sample used more than one route of opioid administration, with only 21% of the sample being able to maintain oral dosing on the last day of life. Patterns of opioid dosing varied. High-dose opioids were required for some patients, with one patient requiring 35,164 morphine equivalent mg per day. In a similar report of pain and opioid use in advanced cancer, Brescia et al. (1992) found wide variability in opioid dosing in 1103 patients admitted to the hospital with advanced cancer. The majority of patients did have stable dosing patterns, but the variability underscored the need for frequent and ongoing clinical assessments.

A multitude of other symptoms can occur in patients with advanced cancer including fatigue, sleeplessness, restlessness, confusion, shortness of breath, anxiety, nausea, and constipation. Supportive care should focus on symptom control utilizing pharmacologic and nonpharmacologic approaches and should address the symptoms patients find the most distressing. Teaching a family member how to coach a patient through a breathing exercise or how to apply heat and cold accomplishes two goals. It assists the patient in obtaining relief of pain while also giving the family member an active role in relieving pain. Being able to do something serves to decrease helplessness. Patient teaching should always include family members or other primary caregivers in order to provide them with information to make pain management decisions in the home. Teaching nonpharmacologic approaches in a structured fashion increases their perceived worth as a pain relief strategy. A combined approach that includes analgesics as well as relaxation, cutaneous measures, and imagery gives the patient more freedom in individualizing a pain relief plan. Rhiner, Ferrell, Ferrell, and Grant (1993) reported the use of a structured, nondrug intervention plan for managing cancer pain in elderly cancer patients in the home.

Hospice services provide a much-needed answer to the problems of patients with advanced cancer. While assisting patients and their families in dealing with terminal illness, they also provide expert symptom management and support. Warner (1992) found that teaching family members specific pain management strategies in a hospice setting facilitated not only patient's pain relief, but reduced family stress and distress. Family caregivers felt a sense of control and increased self-efficacy.

Effects of Cancer Pain on Family Caregivers

Cancer is an illness that affects families, not just individual patients. Families, depending on the developmental stage of family members, face many difficult crises in dealing with cancer as a chronic and sometimes terminal illness. The potential loss of a loved one, the shifts in roles and relationships, and the burdens of physical care pose formidable challenges for the strongest of families. Ferrell et al. (1993) noted that cancer is an all-consuming experience, altering the meaning of life for both the patient and family. As the patient suffers, so, too, does the family.

Nurses caring for patients must attend to the needs of both patient and family in order to guide them through the process of living with cancer. For those patients who are dying, the nurse has the privilege of sharing an intimate transition, providing physical and emotional comfort to the patient and family—a midwife at the other spectrum of life. Pain management plays an integral part in terminal care, for the memories of pain or comfort will blaze forever in the family members reliving of the experience.

CONCLUSION

Pain management is perhaps the greatest challenge in caring for patients across care settings. Whether caring for the neonate or the older adult, nurses have a responsibility and accountability for ensuring comfort, regardless of the cause of pain. Critical skills include knowledge of pain physiology, assessment, analgesic pharmacology, nonpharmacologic approaches, and most importantly, evaluation of the effectiveness of interventions. We must develop centers of nursing excellence in pain management, so that we not only make pain visible, but also make the expertise of the nurse in managing pain visible.

BIBLIOGRAPHY

Agency for Health Care Policy and Research. (1992). *Clinical practice guideline for acute pain management: Operative or medical procedures and trauma.* Rockville, MD: Department of Health and Human Services.

Agency for Health Care Policy and Research. (1994). *Clinical practice guidelines for management of cancer pain.* Rockville, MD: Department of Health and Human Services.

American Nurses Association & Oncology Nursing Society (1987). *Standards of Oncology Nursing Practice.* Kansas City: American Nurses Association.

American Pain Society (1993). *Principles of analgesic use in the treatment of acute pain and chronic cancer pain: A concise guide to medical practice* (3rd ed.). Skokie, IL.

Barkas, G., & Duafala, M. E. (1988). Advances in cancer pain management: A review of patient controlled analgesia. *Journal of Pain and Symptom Management, 3,* 150–160.

Beaver, W. T. (1990). Nonsteroidal anti-inflammatory analgesics in cancer pain. In K. M. Foley, J. J. Bonica, & V. Ventafridds (Eds), *Advances in pain research and therapy. Vol. 16–Proceedings from the Second International Congress on Cancer Pain.* New York: Raven Press.

Bigos, W. (1994). *Agency for Health Care Policy and Research: Clinical practice guidelines for the management of acute low back pain.* Rockville, MD: Department of Health and Human Services.

Bonica, J. J. (1985). Treatment of cancer pain: Current status and future needs. In H. L. Fields, R. Dubner, & F. Cervero (Eds.), *Advances in pain research and therapy. Vol. 9. Proceedings of the Fourth World Congress on Pain.* New York: Raven Press.

Bonica, J. (1990). Cancer pain, In Bonica, J. (Ed.) *The management of pain* (2nd ed.). Philadelphia: Lea and Febiger, 400–460.

Bottomley, D. & Hanks, G. (1990). Subcutaneous midazolam infusions in palliative care. *Journal of Pain and Symptom Management 5*(4), 259–261.

Brescia, F. J., Adler, D., Gray, G., Ryan, M. A., Cimino, J., & Mamtani, R. (1992). Hospitalized advanced cancer patients: A profile. *Journal of Pain and Symptom Management, 5*(4), 221–227.

Bruera, E., Brenneis, C., & MacDonald, R. N. (1987). Continuous subcutaneous infusion of narcotics for the treatment of cancer pain: An update. *Cancer Treatment Reports, 71*(10), 953–958.

Bruera, E., Brenneis, C., & Paterson, A. H. (1989). Use of methylphenidate as an adjuvant to narcotic analgesics in patients with advanced cancer. *Journal of Pain and Symptom Management, 4*(1), 3–6.

Bruera, E., Schoeller, T., & Montejo, G. (1992). Organic hallucinosis in patients receiving high doses of opiates for cancer pain. *Pain, 48*(3), 397–399.

Cancer facts and figures–1994. (1994). Atlanta, GA: American Cancer Society.

Christenson, J. L. (1993). Chronic pain: Dynamics and treatment strategies. *Perspectives in Psychiatric Care, 29*(1), 13–17.

Citron, M., et al. (1984). Safety and efficacy of continuous intravenous morphine for severe cancer pain. *American Journal of Medicine, 77,* 199–204.

Cleeland, C. (1984). The impact of pain on patients with cancer. *Cancer, 54,*2635-41.

Cohen, F. L. (1982). Postsurgical pain relief: Patients' status and nurses' medication choices. *Pain, 9,* 265–274.

Cole, L., & Hanning, C. D. (1990). Review of the rectal use of opioids. *Journal of Pain and Symptom Management, 5*(2), 118–126.

Coyle, N. (1989). Continuity of care for the cancer patient with chronic pain. *Cancer, 63,* 2289–2293.

Coyle, N., Adelhardt, J., Foley, K., & Portenoy, R. (1990). Character of terminal illness in the advanced cancer patient: Pain and other symptoms during the last four weeks of life. *Journal of Pain and Symptom Management, 5* (2), 83–93.

Dahl, J. L., Joranson, D. E., Engber, D., & Dorsch, D. (1988). The cancer pain problem: Wisconsin's response. *Journal of Pain and Symptom Management, 3*(1), S2–S8.

Daut, R. L., & Cleeland, C. S. (1982). The prevalence and severity of pain in cancer. *Cancer, 50* (9), 1913–1918.

Donovan, M. I. (1985). Nursing assessment of cancer pain. *Seminars in Oncology Nursing, 1*(2), 109–115.

Donovan, M. I. (1987). Clinical assessment of cancer pain. In D. B. McGuire & C. H. Yarbro (Eds), *Cancer pain management.* Orlando, FL: Grune & Stratton, Inc.

Donovan, M. I., Dillon, P., & McGuire, L. (1987). Incidence and characteristics of pain in a sample of medical-surgical in-patients. *Pain, 30,* 69–78.

Eisenberg, D. M., et al. (1993). Unconventional medicine in the United States: Prevalence, costs and patterns of use. *New England Journal of Medicine, 328*(4), 246–252.

Ettinger, A. B., & Portenoy, R. K. (1988). The use of corticosteroids in the treatment of symptoms associated with cancer. *Journal of Pain and Symptom Management, 3,* 99–103.

Ferrell, B. R. (1994). An institutional commitment to pain management. *APS Bulletin, 4*(2), 16, 17, 20.

Ferrell, B., Taylor, E., Grant, M., Fowler, M. & Corbisero, R. (1993). Pain management at home: Struggle, comfort & mission. *Cancer Nursing,* 16, 169–78.

Ferrell, B. R., Eberts, M. T., McCaffery, M., & Grant, M. (1991). Clinical decision making and pain. *Cancer Nursing, 14*(6), 289–297.

Ferrell, B. R., Rhiner, M., & Grant, M. (1991). Pain management: Nursing contributions through pain research. *Pain Management Issues in Research and Practice,* Proceedings of the Sixth National Conference on Cancer Nursing.

Ferrell, B. R., Wisdom, C., Rhiner, M., & Alletto, J. (1991). Pain management as a quality of care outcome. *Journal of Nursing Quality Assurance, 5*(2), 50–58.

Ferrell, B., Wisdom, C., & Wenzl, C. (1989). Quality of life as an outcome variable in the management of cancer pain. *Cancer, 63,* 2321–2327.

Ferrer-Brechner, T., & Ganz, P. (1984). Combination therapy with ibuprofen and methadone for chronic cancer pain. *American Journal of Medicine, 77*(Suppl. 1A), 78–83.

Ferris, F. D., Kerr, I., Sone, M., & Marcuzzi, M. (1991). Transdermal scopalamine use in the control of narcotic induced nausea. *Journal of Pain and Symptom Management, 6*(6), 389–393.

Foley, K. M. (1985). The treatment of cancer pain. *New England Journal of Medicine, 313,* 85–95.

Foley, K. M. & Inturrisi, C. E. (1989). Pharmacologic approaches to cancer pain. In K. M. Foley & R. Payne (Eds), *Current therapy of pain.* Toronto: B. C. Decker.

Foley, K. M., & Payne, R. (Eds). (1989). *Current therapy of pain.* Toronto: B. C. Decker.

Fordyce, W. E. (1989). Cognitive and behavioral treatment of chronic pain and disability. In K. M. Foley &

R. Payne (Eds.), *Current therapy of pain.* Toronto: B. C. Decker.

Gaston-Johansson, F., Albert, M., Fagan, E., & Zimmerman, L. (1990). Similarities in pain descriptors of four different ethnic-culture groups. *Journal of Pain and Symptom Management, 5*(2), 94–100.

Gordon, M. (1991). *Manual of nursing diagnosis.* St. Louis: Mosby Year Book.

Guyton, A. C. (1991). *Textbook of medical physiology* (8th ed.). Philadelphia: W. B. Saunders.

Halpern, J. S., & Davis, J. W. (1983). Nonsteroidal anti-inflammatory drugs. *Journal of Emergency Nursing, 9*(2), 104–108.

Hazard, R. (1994). Occupational low back pain: The critical role of functional goal setting. *APS Journal, 3*(2), 101–106.

Howell, S. L. (1991). Validating women's experiences of living with chronic non-malignant pain. Doctoral Dissertation. University of Colorado Health Science Center, Denver, CO.

Hurley, R. J., & Johnson, M. D. (1990). Spinal opioids in the management of obstetric pain. *Journal of Pain and Symptom Management, 5*(3), 146–153.

International Association for the Study of Pain (IASP). (1986). Pain terms: A current list with definitions and notes on usage. *Pain, 3,* S216.

International Association for the Study of Pain, subcommittee on taxonomy, part II (1979). Pain terms: A current list with definitions and notes on usage. *Pain, 6,* 249–52. (Updated 1982, 1986.)

Jeans, M. E., & Melzack, R. (1992). Conceptual basis of nursing practice: Theoretical foundations of pain. In J. Watt-Watson & M. Donovan (Eds.), *Pain management: Nursing perspectives.* St. Louis: Mosby-Year Book.

Kabat-Zinn, J. (1990). *Full catastrophe living.* New York: Dell Publishing.

Kaiko, R. F., Foley, K. M., Grabinski, P. Y., Heidrich, G., Rogers, A. G., Inturrisi, C. E., & Reidenberg, M. M. (1983). Central nervous system excitatory effects of meperidine in cancer patients. *Annual of Neurology, 13*(2), 180–185.

Katzung, B. (1989). *Basic and clinical pharmacology.* Norwalk, CT: Appleton & Lange.

Levick, S., Jacobs, C., & Loukas, D. (1988). Naproxen sodium in the treatment of bone pain due to metastatic cancer. *Pain, 35:* 253–258.

Marcus, N. & Arbeiter, J. (1994). *Freedom from chronic pain.* New York: Simon & Schuster, 129–130.

Marks, R., & Sachar, E. (1973). Under treatment of medical inpatients with narcotic analgesics. *Annals of Internal Medicine, 78*(2), 173–181.

McCaffery, M. (1979). *Nursing management of the patient with pain.* Philadelphia: J. B. Lippincott.

McCaffery, M., & Beebe, A. (1989). *Pain: Clinical manual for nursing practice.* St. Louis: C.V. Mosby Co.

McCaffery, M., Ferrell, B. R., O'Neil-Page, E., Lester, M., & Ferrell, B. (1990). Nurses' knowledge of opioid analgesics and addiction. *Cancer Nursing, 13,* 21–27.

McGuire, D. B. (1987). The multidimensional phenomenon of cancer pain. In D. B. McGuire & C. H. Yarbro (Eds.), *Cancer pain management.* Orlando, FL: Grune & Stratton, Inc.

McGuire, D. B., & Scheidler, V. R. (1990). Pain. In S. L. Groenwald, M. Frogge, M. Goodman, & C. Yarbro

(Eds.), *Cancer nursing: Principles and practice* (2nd ed.). Boston, MA: Jones and Bartlett Publishers.

Melzack, R. & Wall, P. (1965). Pain mechanisms: A new theory. *Science, 150,* 971–979.

Mooney, N. E. (1991). Pain management in the orthopedic patient. *Nursing Clinics of North America, 26*(1), 73–84.

National Institutes of Health. (1987). NIH Consensus Conference on Pain. *Journal of Pain and Symptom Management, 2*(1), 35–44.

Nursing: A social policy statement. (1980). St. Louis: American Nurses Association.

Padilla, G., & Grant, M. (1985). Quality of life as a cancer nursing outcome variable. *Advances in Nursing Science, 8*(1), 45–60.

Paice, J. (1992). Pharmacological management. In J. Watt-Watson & M. I. Donovan, *Pain management: Nursing perspectives.* St. Louis: Mosby-Year Book.

Paice, J. A. (1991). Unraveling the mystery of pain. *Oncology Nursing Forum, 18*(5), 843–849.

Paice, J., Mahan, S., & Faut-Callahan, M. (1991). Factors associated with adequate pain control in hospitalized post surgical patients diagnosed with cancer. *Cancer Nursing, 14*(6), 298–305.

Pasero, C. (1994). Pain control. *American Journal of Nursing, 94*(2), 22–23.

Pawlicki, R. (1992). A neglected issue: The family of the chronic pain patient. *APS Bulletin, 2*(4), 5–6.

Payne, R. M. (1989a). Cancer pain: Anatomy, physiology and pharmacology. *Cancer, 63,* 2266–2274.

Payne, R. M. (1989b). Low back pain. In K. M. Foley & R. M. Payne, *Current therapy of pain.* Toronto: B. C. Decker.

Portenoy, R. K. (1989b). Cancer pain: Epidemiology and syndromes. *Cancer, 63,* 2298–2307.

Portenoy, R. K. (1989a). Intravenous infusion of opioids for cancer pain. In K. M. Foley & R. Payne (Eds.). *Current therapy of pain.* Toronto: B. C. Decker.

Portenoy, R. K. (1989). Opioids in non-malignant pain. In K. M. Foley & R. Payne (Eds.), *Current therapy of pain.* Toronto: B. C. Decker.

Porter, J., & Jick, H. (1980). Addiction rare in patients treated with narcotics. *New England Journal of Medicine, 302*(2), 123.

Ready, L. B. (1990). Spinal opioids in the management of acute and post-operative pain. *Journal of Pain and Symptom Management, 5,* 138–145.

Rhiner, M., Ferrell, B. R., Ferrell, B. A., & Grant, M. (1993). A structured non-drug intervention program for cancer pain. *Cancer Practice, 1*(2), 137–143.

Roy, C. (1984). The Roy Adaptation Model of Nursing. In C. Roy (Ed.), *Introduction to nursing: An adaptation model* (2nd ed.). Englewood Cliffs, NJ: Prentice Hall.

Ryan, L. (1994). Cognitive-behavioral interventions for managing pain. Presented at MNA sponsored workshop on cancer pain management, Nov. 5, Chatham Bars Inn, MA.

Schlesinger, L. (1993). Pain, pain management, and invisibility. *Research in the Sociology of Health Care, 10,* 233–268.

Spross, J. A. (1985). Cancer pain and suffering: Clinical lessons from life, literature and legend. *Oncology Nursing Forum, 12*(4), 23–32.

Spross, J. A., McGuire, D. B., & Schmitt, R. M. (1990). *Oncology Nursing Society position paper on cancer pain.* Pittsburgh: Oncology Nursing Press.

Spross, J., & Singer, M. (1992). Patients with cancer pain. In J. H. Watt-Watson & M. I. Donovan (Eds.), *Pain management: Nursing perspectives.* St. Louis: Mosby-Year Book.

Stambaugh, J. E., & Drew, J. (1988). The combination of ibuprofen and oxycodone/acetaminophen in the management of chronic cancer pain. *Therapeutics in Clinical Pharmacology, 44,* 665–669.

Stein, C. (1991). Peripheral analgesic actions of opioids. *Journal of Pain and Symptom Management, 6*(3), 119–124.

Toomey, T. C., Mann, J. D., Abashian, S. W., Carnicke, C. L., & Hernandez, J. T. (1993). Pain locus of control scores in chronic pain patients and medical clinic patients with and without pain. *Clinical Journal of Pain, 9*(4), 242–247.

Twycross, R. G. & Fairfield, S. (1982). Pain in far advanced cancer. *Pain, 14,* 303–310.

Warner, J. E. (1992). Involvement of families in pain control of terminally ill patients. *Hospice Journal.*

Wayslak, T. J. (1992). Surgical pain management. In J. Watt-Watson & M. I. Donovan (Eds.), *Pain management: Nursing perspective.* St. Louis: Mosby-Year Book.

Weingart, W. A., Sorkness, C. A., & Earhart, R. H. (1985). Analgesia with oral narcotics and added ibuprofen in cancer patients. *Clinical Pharmacology, 4*(1), 53–58.

Weir, R. E. & Crook, J. M. (1992). Chronic pain and the management of conflict. In J. H. Watt-Watson & M. I. Donovan (Eds.), *Pain management: Nursing perspectives.* St. Louis: Mosby-Year Book.

Wells, N. (1994). Quality of life issues in pain management research. *APS Bulletin, 4*(3), 6–9.

Western Consortium for Cancer Nursing Research. (1987). Priorities for cancer nursing research: A Canadian replication. *Cancer Nursing, 10,* 319–327.

Whedon, M., & Ferrell, B. (1991). Professional and ethical considerations in the use of high-tech pain management. *Oncology Nursing Forum, 18*(7), 1135–1142.

Wilkie, D. J. (1990). Cancer pain management: State of the art nursing care. *Nursing Clinics of North America, 25*(2), 331–343.

World Health Organization. (1986). *Cancer pain relief.* Geneva.

Zenz, M., Strumpf, M., & Tryba, P. (1992). Long term opioid therapy in patients with chronic non-malignant pain. *Journal of Pain and Symptom Management, 7*(2), 69–77.

Zimberg, M., and Berenson, S. (1990). Delirium in patients with cancer: Nursing assessment and intervention. *Oncology Nursing Forum, 17*(4), 529–538.

CHAPTER 22

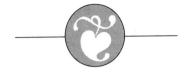

The Use of Therapeutic Touch to Reduce Mind-Body-Spirit Distress

Ann Minor

Therapeutic Touch is a holistic healing modality that facilitates the natural healing process. While the phrase suggests the use of a person's hands to help or to heal, the practitioner need not actually "touch" the person to facilitate healing.

Florence Nightingale (1859) said that nature alone cures:

> It is often thought that medicine is the curative process. It is no such thing; medicine is the surgery of functions, as surgery proper is that of limbs and organs. Neither can do anything but remove obstructions; neither can cure; nature alone cures. Surgery removes the bullet out of the limb, which is an obstruction to cure, but nature heals the wound. So it is with medicine; the function of an organ becomes obstructed; medicine, so far as we know, assists nature to remove the obstruction, but does nothing more. And what nursing has to do in either case, is to put the patient in the best condition for nature to act upon him. [pp. 74–75]

HISTORY OF THERAPEUTIC TOUCH

Therapeutic Touch (TT) is a contemporary interpretation of several ancient healing practices. Healing, as defined by Macrae (1987), is the tendency to integrate the individual as a whole, by addressing the body, mind, and spirit. During Therapeutic Touch, the focus of healing is on the process of balancing the energies of the whole person rather than on treating only the specific physical disease.

Dolores Krieger, R.N., Ph.D., co-founder of TT, was a nursing professor at New York University. Krieger, a nurse scientist, held a special interest in neurophysiology and in healing. After several years of observation and study of the healing act, Krieger discovered that, contrary to the religious laying-on-of-hands, the

Patricia Barry: *Psychosocial Nursing: Care of Physically Ill Patients and Their Families,* 3rd ed. © 1996 Lippincott–Raven Publishers

healer did not need to have a religious belief in order for healing to occur. In 1969 Krieger joined together with Dora Kunz and the two began to develop the technique that was subsequently named Therapeutic Touch.

Later that year, Krieger used her nursing research skills to measure the biochemical changes in patients receiving Therapeutic Touch. She conducted her first pilot research study to examine the effects of Therapeutic Touch on the hemoglobin levels of hospitalized patients. In 1972 she did a full-scale study and in 1973 she replicated her research. All three studies consistently demonstrated that subjects' hemoglobin levels could be raised through Therapeutic Touch intervention (Krieger, 1975). This was the first scientific research study that gave Therapeutic Touch the validation necessary for acceptance into the medical and nursing community.

Krieger (1991) continued to develop and support TT as an effective nursing intervention and encouraged its use as a healing technique within hospitals and health care institutions. She states that, over the years of research and practice, four highly reliable clinical changes have been demonstrated to occur in the healee during the practice of Therapeutic Touch. These consistent changes are:

1. A rapid relaxation response
2. A significant reduction in pain
3. An acceleration of the healing process
4. Alleviation of psychosomatic illness

BASIC ASSUMPTIONS OF THERAPEUTIC TOUCH

Many healing practices are based on the use of one, or all, of the five senses of sight, smell, taste, hearing, and physical touch. Janet Macrae (1987), a practitioner and instructor of Therapeutic Touch, describes how the practice of Therapeutic Touch involves opening oneself to a new dimension or mode of perceiving:

> The practice of Therapeutic Touch, however, is based on the concept of a subtle, non-physical energy, which sustains all living organisms. This energy is not an abstraction but a vitalizing, universal force, which is always present and available. The practice of Therapeu-

tic Touch represents a conscious effort to draw upon this universal life energy and direct its flow for healing. (p. xii)

The science-based practice of nursing utilizes conceptual systems to provide rationales for practice. Originally Therapeutic Touch was developed by Krieger and Kunz using the assumption that an energy field interaction occurs between the nurse and the patient during the Therapeutic Touch process (Krieger, 1975). According to Jurgens, Meehan, and Wilson (1987), Krieger originally cited an Eastern philosophical system common to Buddhist, Hindu, and Taoist thought. The fundamental assumption of Krieger's system is that there is a universal life energy, and that the universe is composed of mutually penetrating forms of energy through which all matter and consciousness are interconnected.

Martha Rogers' science of unitary human beings provides a conceptual system in which Therapeutic Touch is an example of her system at work. Meehan (1993) examined the nursing practice of Therapeutic Touch from a Rogerian perspective: "A nursing intervention is viewed as knowledgeable and purposive patterning of nurse-environmental/patient-environmental energy field mutual process which seeks to strengthen the coherence and integrity of the patient-environmental field process for realization of maximum patient healing and well-being." (p. 70)

In their development of Therapeutic Touch, Krieger and Kunz based their rationale of its healing efficacy on four scientific premises (Krieger, 1993):

1. All the life sciences agree that, physically, a human being is an open energy system.
2. Anatomically, a human being is bilaterally symmetrical.
3. Illness is an imbalance in an individual's energy field.
4. Human beings have natural abilities to transform and transcend their conditions of living.

SUN, LIGHT, ENERGY, AND HEALING

Krieger studied the Eastern health practices of yoga, Ayurvedic medicine, Tibetan medicine, and Chinese medicine, and concluded that *prana*, an Indian Sanskrit word meaning vitality, is the subsystem of energy and the base of the human energy transfer in the healing act. Krieger's research into Eastern literature found that *prana*, which is derived from the sun, is thought to be responsible for the phenomena of regeneration and wound healing. In addition, she found that it is believed that normally healthy persons have an excess of *prana*, that ill persons have a deficit of *prana*, and that *prana* can be transferred from one individual to another (Krieger, 1979). Krieger's findings bridged the teachings of East and West:

> As one goes deeper into the study of *prana*, one finds that the literature of these ancient people makes statements that can be in consonance with some of the most contemporary theory of the West. The literature of the East, for instance, says that *prana* derives from the sun. This statement is not at all at variance with our current recognition that the crucial chemical base of the life process in man is dependent upon sunlight, for the photons coming from the sun set off the process of photosynthesis, which is the driving force for the primary synthesis of organic matter. [Krieger, 1979, p. 12]

The Need for Light

Florence Nightingale (1859) believed that light was healing:

> It is the unqualified result of all my experience with the sick, that second only to their need of fresh air is their need of light; that, after a close room, what hurts them most is a dark room. [p. 47–48]
>
> One of the greatest observers of human things (not physiological), says, in another language, "Where there is sun there is thought." All physiology goes to confirm this. Where is the shady side of deep valleys, there is cretinism. Where are cellars and the unsunned sides of narrow streets, there is the degeneracy and weakliness of the human race—mind and body equally degenerating. Put the pale withering plant and human being into the sun, and, if not too far gone, each will recover health and spirit. [p. 49]

Krieger and Nightingale refer to the healing effects of light from the sun. There is another source of light which comes from deep within every person. This beautiful light is the source that connects to the inner self. The nurse who sees light as the basis of all life and of all healing can see this light. In some individuals, this light has been covered over by layer after layer of physical, mental, and emotional hurt. Many physically and emotionally ill people have a sense of darkness around themselves. They have closed themselves off, feeling disconnected from the light. Their light is there, but they may not have been able to connect with it for a very long time. And for some, they may have forgotten altogether that it exists. Therapeutic Touch is a way to help a person spiritually connect with the light within. Reconnecting spiritually helps to restore hope when hope seems impossible and bring peace when turmoil is ever-present. Therapeutic Touch nurtures the physically ill body in its struggle to become whole and to heal.

CASE EXAMPLE*

I was asked to see Sara T for a Therapeutic Touch consult for the purpose of pain management. Sara, a 38-year-old mother of three young children, has suffered from lupus and fibromyalgia for several years. Over the past several years she has undergone a variety of treatments, including large doses of steroids and chemotherapy. Due to the abnormally high doses of medication that she has received, several organs of her body have been damaged. Sara now suffers from pathogenic spinal fractures and chronic, excruciating joint and abdominal pain. She is unable to eat due to persistent nausea and open sores in her mouth. She has a central line for hyperalimentation, a gastrostomy tube for tube feedings, and a Foley catheter. Sara's psychosocial history includes being married and divorced twice, physical abuse from one of her husbands, and recent memories of childhood molestation. Sara has custody of her three young children, two of whom are also survivors of sexual abuse from their father.

Sara's medical physician, afraid that she had become addicted to her pain medication,

---

*The name and age of the patient has been changed to protect her privacy.

tried to wean her from the morphine that she had been taking regularly for the past 2 years. The Toradol which was ordered for pain was not effective. When I first met Sara, she was lying in bed, angry, frustrated, and in pain. I introduced myself and explained the purpose and procedure of Therapeutic Touch. Sara was receptive to trying it, anxious to do anything that might help to decrease her pain and distress. The first treatment helped Sara to relax, but her pain lessened only slightly. The next day I repeated the Therapeutic Touch procedure and Sara experienced similar results with the pain; however, this time she was able to sleep for 30 minutes after the treatment. I continued to see Sara daily for Therapeutic Touch treatments and each time Sara would experience a deep relaxation response but her pain remained mostly the same. She was becoming withdrawn, depressed, and without hope.

One week after the beginning of the Therapeutic Touch treatments, a shift in Sara began to occur. I entered her room expecting to see her in pain, but instead, she was sitting up and waiting to talk. She told me that the pain was still the same but it didn't matter as much anymore. She said that after the last Therapeutic Touch treatment she was resting in bed with her eyes closed, and suddenly she began to see light inside of her. She said that the light felt familiar, but because she hadn't seen it for such a long time, she had forgotten that it was there. She then began to talk about her religious and spiritual beliefs and about several significant spiritual experiences that had occurred to her over the past several years.

Sara was discharged from the hospital (G tube and Foley catheter in place) 3 days later. Her pain was less, she wanted to be home with her children, and she had hope. Sara had reconnected with the light within, the source of all healing. ❧

THE THERAPEUTIC TOUCH PROCESS

There are four phases to the Therapeutic Touch process:

1. Centering
2. Assessment
3. Rebalancing
4. Reassessment

PHASE 1: CENTERING

The *centering* process is the act of becoming quiet and focused within. It is a state of quiet and calm in which the practitioner is present in the moment. Centering is attained prior to the beginning of the Therapeutic Touch treatment and is maintained throughout the treatment. Dora Kunz, the cofounder of Therapeutic Touch, states:

> If we are upset and in a state of inner turmoil, we may try to reach out and send feelings of compassion to the patient, but the effort may be distorted by an undercurrent of turbulent emotion. Through centering, we become aware of our own disturbed emotions and consciously disassociate ourselves from them by focusing all our energies in the heart center, which is the seat of compassion and of wholeness. This fosters two qualities which are important in the healing process: rootedness and detachment. [Kunz, 1991, pp. 161–2]

Centering is learned, and practiced, in a variety of ways. A centered state can be achieved through meditation, breath, and/or visualization. As with any art form, the more centering is practiced, the easier it is to attain. Experienced Therapeutic Touch practitioners are able to center spontaneously and quickly, thus enabling them to use Therapeutic Touch at any time and in any place. This is especially important when in the midst of a crisis or an emergency.

Krieger, in her workshops, teaches students the importance of maintaining a centered state throughout the Therapeutic Touch process. "Under any circumstances, and particularly while you are learning Therapeutic Touch, the key to eventual success is always to return to that centering place within yourself. It is this place that is the learning and testing ground for your growing understanding of the many facets of your consciousness" (Krieger, 1993).

The following is a story that involves my own experience as a Therapeutic Touch practitioner.

CASE EXAMPLE

It was 11 PM at night and my husband and I heard the screeching of tires, a loud sound of automobile metal crumpling, glass breaking, and a piercing scream. I sent my husband out to the scene, called the EMS (emergency medical service), and gathered up my medical supplies.

On my way down the driveway I knew that I must become calm, and maintain my calm. I took a deep breath and centered myself, not knowing what tragedy I might see. When I arrived at the scene, there were three injured teenagers. The driver of the car had been speeding, lost control, and crashed into a cement bridge abutment. Two of the injured were out of the car and my husband was attending to them, so I went to the third. A young girl was lying in the middle of the road, crying that her leg was broken—it was her scream that we had heard earlier. I did a nursing assessment and concluded that she did not have any obvious life-threatening injuries, her legs did not appear fractured, but she was hysterical. There was nothing else that I could do for her at this time, so I sat down on the road beside her, explained what I was going to do, and began to do Therapeutic Touch. I concentrated my efforts on smoothing out and rebalancing (unruffling) the energy field around her chest and over both legs, while continuously thinking thoughts of peace and calm. I knew that the best thing that I could do for her at that time was to help her release the panic and become calm. After a few minutes of Therapeutic Touch, she stopped crying. I continued to do Therapeutic Touch, maintaining my centered state by periodically taking deep, focused breaths. Approximately 10 minutes later, when the ambulance arrived, she had stopped crying, was no longer complaining about her leg, and walked to the ambulance. ❧

PHASE 2: ASSESSMENT

The *assessment* phase of Therapeutic Touch involves the practitioner gently moving his or her hands in a symmetrical pattern, from head to feet, approximately 3 to 5 inches above the surface of the body. Using the palms (*chakras*)

of the hands as sensors, the practitioner is able to feel, or sense, differences (cues) in the human energy field. This process is quick and usually only takes 1 to 2 minutes. Krieger, in describing how to feel energy with the hands, explains it in this way:

> Although we do not recognize it in our culture, other cultures recognize several energy centers in the body. In the East, two of these energy centers are recognized to be in the palms of the hands. If you turn your hand palm up, you will notice that the center of the palm is depressed. This well or depression in the center of the palm is considered to be the physical locus for these hand energy centers (called *chakras* in Sanskrit). From my reading of the literature of the Ayurvedic medicine of India, it seems to me that it is these *chakras,* one in each hand, that are the functional agents in all therapeutic uses of the hands. [Krieger, 1979, p. 46]

The assessment phase is used to identify areas of the human energy field in which the field pattern is imbalanced or the flow is blocked. Using assessment as a guide, the informed practitioner then moves on to the next step, which is rebalancing.

PHASE 3: REBALANCING

The third phase of the Therapeutic Touch process is called *rebalancing*. The purpose of rebalancing is to remove blockages in the energy flow, to direct energy, and to reestablish balance. Again, using the *chakras* of the hands, the practitioner gently moves his or her hands in a symmetrical pattern, from head to feet, approximately 3 to 5 inches above the surface of the body. This process, described above, is called unruffling and usually takes between 5 to 10 minutes to complete. It is often during the unruffling phase that a rapid relaxation response occurs in the patient. Following unruffling, energy may then be directed to the area of the patient's body that is ill or injured by holding the hands close to the body and visualizing energy moving through the hand *chakra*.

Janet Macrae, an experienced Therapeutic Touch practitioner, talks about energy blockages:

If life is characterized by an interchange of various qualities of energy, it can be assumed that any form of obstruction—either within the organism or between the organism and the environment—is contrary to Nature's tendencies and therefore unhealthy. We can find many physical examples of this fact: blockages in the respiratory system, the digestive system, the urinary system, and the circulatory system are all associated with ill health. When you learn Therapeutic Touch, you will discover that obstructions in the flow of the life energy also result in a diminution of well-being. We know that mental and emotional blockages not only hinder mature development but also lead to physical disease. On any level, obstructions fragment the wholeness of the individual. [Macrae, 1987, p.16]

PHASE 4: REASSESSMENT

The final step of the Therapeutic Touch process is *reassessment and closure*. The assessment phase is repeated as the practitioner scans the patient's entire body again, feeling for differences in the energy field. Quite often, the patient's energy flow has been reestablished and changes are felt. At this time, the practitioner ends the treatment. The entire Therapeutic Touch treatment usually lasts approximately 25 minutes.

SPECIAL CONSIDERATIONS

LESS IS BETTER.
IF YOU DON'T KNOW, DON'T DO IT.

When practicing Therapeutic Touch, there are special considerations to know about. "Therapeutic Touch is a process that is always individualized and usually does not exceed 30 minutes. In general neonates, children, pregnant women, people with psychiatric disorders, the elderly and/or debilitated are more sensitive to the interaction" (NHPA, 1991). It is recommended that health care professionals learn Therapeutic Touch from experienced Therapeutic Touch instructors and practice this technique under the guidelines of a policy and procedure. Guidelines for Therapeutic Touch policy and procedure for health professionals

are available from Nurse-Healers Professional Associates, Inc. (NHPA, 1991).

Dolores Krieger gives the following advice regarding Therapeutic Touch:

Hippocrates's admonition "Do no harm" has been passed down for twenty-five hundred years as excellent advice for anyone who would help or heal others. Harm most frequently occurs because of ignorance. Therefore, if you don't know what to do, refer the healee to someone who does. Or, if upon reassessment you pick up no further cues in the healee's energy field, do not persevereate; assure yourself of the healee's comfort and safety, and stop the Therapeutic Touch interaction. [Krieger, 1993, p. 169]

NURTURING THE NURSE

Therapeutic Touch is a powerful way to help nurture the nurse. During this time of numerous changes in the health care field, many nurses are feeling misplaced, uncertain, and overworked. The practice of Therapeutic Touch, in which one reaches out to another in compassion and concern, nurtures the nurse as well as the patient. As one learns and practices Therapeutic Touch, and quiet inward focusing occurs, transpersonal changes often follow. For many nurses, this experience produces an inner calm which extends beyond the clinical setting.

CLINICAL APPLICATIONS

TT: THEORY AND ASSUMPTION OF AN ENERGY EXCHANGE

In our Western culture, most traditional medical practices are based on the results of scientific research. The concept of using *prana* to restore energy and promote healing is not readily accepted by some. A barrier to the acceptance of Therapeutic Touch in hospital or healthcare systems is the objection by some to the claim that Therapeutic Touch promotes healing by way of an energy exchange. This objection stems from the lack of current scientific evidence necessary to support an energy exchange theory.

Quinn (1989) replicated and extended a previously published research study that she had done (Quinn, 1984). The original results indicated that TT involves an energy exchange. The findings in the second study did not show significance, however. Quinn acknowledges the need for further scientific research in this area of TT but advises caution: "There is a need to be cautious and creative in conducting this scientific study lest, like the butterfly that is pinned down for closer inspection, the phenomenon is destroyed in the attempts to understand it" (p. 87).

When talking about Therapeutic Touch, it is important not to predict results that have not been proven. At present, Therapeutic Touch is based on a theory and an assumption of an energy exchange. It is best to report about the many positive research findings on the efficacy of Therapeutic Touch and to be clear about the limitations of the scientific knowledge that demonstrates the actual energy exchange.

IMPLEMENTING THERAPEUTIC TOUCH IN THE HOSPITAL

Nurses who want to implement Therapeutic Touch in their hospital or health care facility should be knowledgeable about Therapeutic Touch and the research that has been done. Nursing scholars have produced a large body of scientific research related to Therapeutic Touch. In 1985, Therapeutic Touch was assigned a category of its own in MEDLINE, a major computer retrieval system for literature significant to the health profession.

Some of the nursing research projects include psychoimmunologic effects (Quinn & Strelkauskas, 1993); theory-based mental health nursing (Hill & Oliver, 1993); Therapeutic Touch and the elderly (Quinn, 1992; Simington, 1993); the experience of receiving Therapeutic Touch (Samarel, 1992); pain management (Bzdek & Keller, 1986; Meehan, 1993; Owens & Ehrenreich, 1991; Wright, 1987); energy field assessment (Wright, 1991); relaxation response (Heidt, 1991); and Therapeutic Touch applied to the treatment of addiction (Macrae, 1989).

When nurses want to propose a Therapeutic Touch program at their hospital, the following questions should be reviewed before approaching the institution's administration:

What is Therapeutic Touch?
What are its benefits?
How is it explained to a patient?
How is Therapeutic Touch documented in the patient's chart?
How do caregivers become qualified to practice Therapeutic Touch?

THERAPEUTIC TOUCH: A COMPLEMENTARY HEALING MODALITY

Nurses can use Therapeutic Touch as a complementary healing modality in the home, hospital, community health organization, mental health institution, and extended-care facility. There are many clinical applications. The most common uses for Therapeutic Touch are relaxation, pain reduction, and acceleration of the healing process. Some areas in the hospital where Therapeutic Touch has been used are the preadmission testing unit, ambulatory surgery unit, operating room, postanesthesia care unit, emergency room, intensive care unit, inpatient units, labor and delivery, newborn nursery, neonatal intensive care unit, and mental health units.

BODY, MIND, SPIRIT

The patient receiving Therapeutic Touch does not need to believe in its efficacy or to understand its actual mechanisms. He or she must, however, be willing to receive it. The following case example tells the story of a patient who requested Therapeutic Touch initially for the purpose of helping her to prevent nausea and vomiting while receiving chemotherapy treatments. She admitted that she didn't believe in Therapeutic Touch; however, she was feeling desperate and willing to give it a try based on the positive experiences that she had heard from others. Her husband, also frightened and frustrated, was uncertain of the effectiveness of Therapeutic Touch. Later, he shared his experience.

CASE EXAMPLE*

Joan, age 62, was diagnosed with cancer at the age of 58. Joan was a daughter, sister, wife, mother, grandmother, and registered nurse. She was determined to live and to "beat this thing." In her own words, she expressed her determination to overcome this disease and her desire to live: "I don't have time to die right now." Joan's journey was remarkable. Her initial response to chemotherapy was positive, her attitude constantly optimistic, and her physical stamina exceptional. She did beat the projected odds; her expected prognosis of death within 6 months was surpassed by more than 4 years. Joan was determined not to die until she was ready, and she wasn't planning on being ready for a long time.

Joan came to see me for Therapeutic Touch 4 years after she had been diagnosed with liver cancer and 2 weeks after she had been diagnosed with metastatic bone cancer. She was going on vacation and when she returned she would start chemotherapy again. She said to me, "I need the big guns this time and I don't want to be sick. I don't know if I believe in Therapeutic Touch but I want to try it. Can you help me?"

Four years and three months after the initial diagnosis of liver cancer, Joan died. The last 2 months of her life were filled with pain, anger, desperation, anxiety, sorrow, longing, peace, hope, and joy. How could Joan experience such a diversity of feelings, such a range of emotions? How could she feel peace, hope, and joy, in the midst of pain and dying? It was through Therapeutic Touch that Joan was able to feel and to be. The complementary use of Therapeutic Touch became part of the process that assisted Joan to be able to make right relationships with her family, her environment, herself, and her God. Before she died, Joan spoke about her feelings of peace. Her physical body was not cured, but her mind and her spirit were freed. Joan died when she was

ready and she claimed that Therapeutic Touch helped prepare for her readiness. ❦

Two weeks after Joan's death, I received this letter from her husband:

Dear Ann,
Yours is the last and the hardest letter I have to write regarding Joan's death. Joan was a very strong-willed individual, as you probably already know. At no time during her illness did the word *dying* pass her lips. In October, when Joan was hospitalized with the fractured ribs, I was surprised to see her seek out alternate means of support and relief from pain. Since last May when Joan was operated on for the last time, she had slowly lost her strength, but not her will to live. It wasn't until we were in Florida, vacationing, that I saw how much she was failing. She had kept her weakness well hidden from all of her family.

One evening during her October stay in the hospital, Joan turned the conversation to Therapeutic Touch, and the relief that it gave her from the continuous pain she was in at that time. Also for the first time in four years, she talked of death. Not a statement, "I'm dying," but of the peace of mind that your conversations with her were helping Joan prepare for another life. Then Ann, I met you and saw for myself the relief that your hands were capable of giving Joan. I continued to see the relief in her face and body through her final hours. Not only were your thoughts for Joan, but in her final hours, your presence felt the pain within me. Your touch helped me through a very difficult time, and is still helping. I cannot repay you for your kindness on this earth. Our many thanks, Michael.

CONCLUSION

The above testimony is unique in its story, but universal in its truths. Nurse healers around the world help their patients to heal through the use of Therapeutic Touch. Today's nurses can bring light to the world as they use their hands to help and to heal.

Practitioners of this healing art believe that the ability to do Therapeutic Touch is a natural human potential. Those who are willing to learn, and have the intent to help and to heal, can learn Therapeutic Touch.

---

*The names of the patient and her husband have been changed to protect their privacy. In addition, the patient's age and type of illness have been changed. Permission was obtained from Joan's husband (Michael) to reprint this letter.

BIBLIOGRAPHY

Boguslawski, M. (1980). Therapeutic Touch: A facilitator of pain relief. *Topics in Clinical Nursing, 2,* 27–37.

Bzdek, V., & Keller, E. (1986). Effects of therapeutic touch on tension headache pain. *Nursing Research, 35*(2), 101–106.

Heidt, P. (1990). Openness: A qualitative analysis of nurses' and patients' experiences of therapeutic touch. *Image: Journal of Nursing Scholarship, 22*(3), 180–186.

Heidt, P. (1991). Helping patients to rest: Clinical studies in therapeutic touch. *Holistic Nursing Practice, 5*(4), 57–66.

Hill, L., & Oliver, N. (1993). Therapeutic touch and theory-based mental health nursing. *Journal of Psychosocial Nursing, 31*(2), 19–27.

Jurgens, A., Meehan, T., & Wilson, H. (1987). Therapeutic touch as a nursing intervention. *Holistic Nursing Practice, 2*(1), 1–13.

Krieger, D. (1975). Therapeutic touch: The imprimatur of nursing. *American Journal of Nursing, 75*(5), 784–787.

Krieger, D. (1979). *The therapeutic touch.* Englewood Cliffs, NJ: Prentice-Hall.

Krieger, D. (1991). Therapeutic touch: Toward an understanding of unitary human be-ness. *Cooperative Connection,* Winter. XII (1), 1–11.

Krieger, D. (1993). *Accepting your power to heal.* Sante Fe, NM: Bear & Company.

Kunz, D. (1991). *The personal aura.* Wheaton, IL: The Theosophical Publishing House.

Macrae, J. (1987). *Therapeutic touch: A practical guide.* New York: Knopf.

Macrae, J. (1989). Principles of therapeutic touch applied to the treatment of addiction. *Addictions Nursing Network, 1*(2), 11–15.

Meehan, T. (1993). Therapeutic touch and postoperative pain: A Rogerian research study. *Nursing Science Quarterly,* Summer, 6(2), 69–78.

NHPA: Nurse Healers Professional Associates, Inc. (1991). Allison Park, PA.

Nightingale, F. (1859). *Notes on nursing.* Philadelphia: J. B. Lippincott.

Owens, K., & Ehrenreich, D. (1991). Literature review of nonpharmacologic methods for the treatment of chronic pain. *Holistic Nursing Practice, 6*(1), 24–31.

Quinn, J. (1984). Therapeutic touch as energy exchange: Testing the theory. *Advances in Nursing Science, 6*(2).

Quinn, J. (1989). Therapeutic touch as energy exchange: Replication and extension. *Nursing Science Quarterly, 2*(2), 79–87.

Quinn, J. (1992). The senior's therapeutic touch education program. *Holistic Nursing Practice, 7*(1), 32–37.

Quinn, J., & Strelkauskas, A. (1993). Psychoimmunologic effects of therapeutic touch on practitioners and recently bereaved recipients: A pilot study. *Advances in Nursing Science, 15*(4), 13–26.

Samarel, N. (1992). The experience of receiving therapeutic touch. *Journal of Advanced Nursing, 17*(6), 651–657.

Simington, J. (1993). Therapeutic touch for the elderly. *Nurse Practitioner, 18*(11), 23–24.

Thayer, B. (1990). Touching with intent: Using therapeutic touch. *Pediatric Nursing, 16*(1), 70–72.

Wright, S. (1987). The use of therapeutic touch in the management of pain. *Nursing Clinics of North America, 22*(3), 705–714.

Wright, S. (1991). Validity of the human energy field assessment form. *Western Journal of Nursing Research, 13*(5), 635–647.

CHAPTER 23

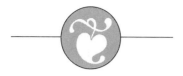

Psychosocial Aspects of Complex Responses to Cancer

Anne Cloutier
Sheila Ferrall

At any one moment countless individuals are surviving cancer, facing the challenges of diagnosis and treatment, or in the throes of the terminal trajectory. The American Cancer Society (1994) estimates that 1,208,000 new cases of cancer will be diagnosed in 1994, and 538,000 people will die from the disease. In addition, there are currently over 8 million persons living with a history of cancer. Regardless of their place on the cancer continuum, patients and families must deal with a multitude of stressors including loss of independence and control; feelings of helplessness and worthlessness; alterations in body image and functions; and fear of death, dying, and an uncertain future.

Cancer care, traditionally offered on inpatient units, has responded to the mandate for cost containment by shifting care to outpatient settings. Technological advances have allowed treatments that were exclusively administered to inpatients to be delivered in ambulatory and home care arenas. This transition has expanded the role of nurses in these settings and placed greater responsibilities for care on patients and families. Discussing fears and making treatment decisions must now take place during a few brief, often hurried, outpatient visits. The need for nurses to develop trusting relationships and effective communication patterns with patients and families experiencing cancer has become paramount.

INDIVIDUAL RESPONSES ALONG THE CONTINUUM OF CARE

The subjective experience of cancer patients can be positively affected by integrating good

Patricia Barry: *Psychosocial Nursing:*
Care of Physically Ill Patients and Their Families, 3rd ed.
© 1996 Lippincott–Raven Publishers

psychosocial care into the medical plan of care. This requires early identification of those who are at risk for more distress, recognition of signs of psychosocial suffering, and strategies to manage these problems. Those who face cancer with a prior history of emotional problems, a lack of personal or social resources, and more advanced illness may encounter more difficulty with coping. When evaluating patients with psychosocial distress, it is important to consider physical causes that may affect mood, thought and behavior, such as central nervous system involvement, metabolic abnormalities, and neuropsychiatric effects of therapy.

RECURRING RESPONSES ALONG THE CONTINUUM

Although particular responses can be expected at disease transition points, several are known to recur during the course of cancer, with anxiety and depression being the most common.

Anxiety

Anxiety occurs at varying levels throughout the course of illness. People describe tension, nervousness, feeling upset, and insomnia. Anxiety is most prevalent while awaiting diagnosis or reports of diagnostic testing, hearing the diagnosis of cancer, anticipating and completing treatment, learning of recurrence, and during advanced illness. Specific aspects of the cancer experience associated with anxiety include uncontrolled pain or other symptoms, phobias related to needle use, and conditioned nausea and vomiting associated with chemotherapy. For survivors, anxiety recurs at follow-up appointments and the presence of any symptom that may mean a return of the cancer. Although anxiety may be unpleasant, minimal to moderate levels may be motivating for some patients (Clark, 1993). For those who have persistent, severe anxiety, nursing interventions can be helpful, although psychiatric consultation may be necessary.

Prior to initiating nursing care, an accurate assessment of the presence of anxiety begins with validating observed perceptions to estab-

lish a plan that addresses the patient's actual response. Further questioning about how a patient usually experiences, expresses, and copes with anxiety can be useful for subsequent encounters when anxiety may recur.

The focus of anxiety for cancer patients may be critical to planning appropriate management strategies. Stress related to the cancer experience makes it difficult for patients to embrace all that they must be told, necessitating reinforcement of patient instructions and clarification of misconceptions regarding treatment, prognosis, and disease status. Nursing interventions are directed at helping patients to identify and recognize their feelings, as well as what is prompting them. Demonstrating interest in the patient's feelings by using open-ended questions and an unhurried approach is helpful. Validating that anxiety related to cancer is quite normal is also helpful. For others, perceiving the potential threat differently can reduce anxiety. Finally, for those who are unable to identify the source of their apprehension, but rather sense a generalized, nonspecific feeling, nurses can help activate previously used coping strategies or learn new ones. Such strategies include music therapy, relaxation therapy, problem-solving skills, and participation in self-help or support groups. Nurses in all settings need to be attuned to the possibility of recurring anxiety, especially at critical junctions in the cancer continuum.

Denial

While anxiety usually causes distress for patients, it is the use of *denial* that provokes distress in health care providers. Nurses frequently view denial as maladaptive. However, denial may be the only effective defense mechanism a patient has to deal with an overwhelming situation. Denial and acceptance fluctuate during the course of cancer, especially at the initial diagnosis, relapse, and terminal stages. Many patients with cancer use some degree of denial. Patients may show acceptance of some aspects of their situation while rejecting others. Lederberg and Massie (1993) differentiate between *instrumental* and *affective* denial. The former prevents a patient from seeking or complying with treatment while the latter allows an individual to be more hopeful, yet make appropriate decisions regarding his or her medical needs. Affective denial is often seen at the time when a diagnosis is confirmed, as a patient prepares to deal with all the ramifications of the illness. When a patient's condition worsens, this form of denial can facilitate an improved quality of life in spite of a shortened survival (Jalowiec & Dudas, 1991; Lederberg & Massie, 1993).

Excessive denial is associated with delays in seeking treatment, noncompliance with prescribed regimens, poorer adjustment to the cancer diagnosis, and lack of utilization of available resources. Denial is most effective when used as a short-term coping strategy.

In assessing denial in patients, it is important to determine what benefit the patient is receiving and the characteristics of the denial. *What* the patient is specifically denying and to what extent can make a difference in the impact of the denial. The myth that all patients experiencing cancer must be forced to face the grim reality of their situation must be dispelled. Rather, the patient who uses denial is asking health care professionals to adjust their pace to his or her own. The use of denial to facilitate a hopeful attitude should be encouraged. Intervening for denial occurs only when it poses a problem related to the patient's treatment or other necessary planning.

Anger

Anger, a common response to loss, masks feelings of powerlessness for persons with cancer. Initially, anger may be accompanied by a sense of unfairness: "Why me? Why now?" Frustration and anger are common in those who feel they have led a healthy life, yet got cancer. Thoughts of forced dependency create anger for others who value being active and independent. Some people direct their anger inwardly for not having changed behaviors, while others focus anger at health care professionals or the system. At the time of recurrence, questions arise about the appropriateness and effectiveness of treatments as well as health surveillance activities. Anger is associated with a patient's search for meaning and occurs commonly with increased dependency and physical distress (Taylor et al., 1993). On-

going anger depletes patients of energy to handle the situation constructively and isolates them from family and friends.

Nursing care focuses on helping patients to identify feelings, perceptions, and interpretations so that they can be appraised in a new context. Maintaining a diary of feelings and precipitating factors to be shared with a nurse or psychosocial professional should be encouraged. Patients need help recognizing their acceptable and unacceptable behavioral responses to anger. Teaching patients new ways to manage their anger is effective when coupled with understanding and reinforcement. Many individuals are afraid to express their anger for fear of abandonment by health care providers or family members. Nurses need to be alert for subtle clues that a patient may be holding back hostile feelings. These feelings should be expressed and, if necessary, directed into more constructive channels. Validating the normalcy of these feelings can be accomplished with a self-help group, veteran patient visitor program, or by the nurse. Anger is seen less commonly than other psychosocial responses to cancer but requires effective nursing strategies to improve a patient's ability to cope with these feelings.

Depression

Another challenge of the cancer experience is maintaining hope in the face of uncertainty. Hopelessness and depression are quite common in persons with cancer and can pose formidable obstacles to coping and completing therapy. Hopelessness recurs as changes in health, relationships, and spirituality are realized. A sense of hopelessness in cancer patients contributes to the development of depression.

Those who are hopeless and depressed have a lower self-esteem and unrealistic, negative expectations of the future. It is common to see an acute stress response to cancer during the first 7 to 14 days after diagnosis, manifested by complaints of feelings of depression, anxiety, and irritability; difficulty concentrating; insomnia; and anorexia. Although depression is the most common psychosocial response to cancer, most individuals resolve this acute stress response within a couple of weeks (Holland, 1989). For others, certain risk factors predispose them to a more problematic response: prior emotional difficulties, prior history of depression, lack of a social support network, advanced illness, uncontrolled pain, and certain disease sites (pancreas, endocrine and ectopic, hormone-producing tumors) (Lederberg & Massie, 1993). Even though depression is prevalent in cancer, it is underrecognized and untreated. Many wrongly consider depression to be appropriate in cancer patients and do not intervene to manage it.

Due to the nature of cancer care, nurses establish and maintain significant relationships with patients. This places them in a pivotal role to identify subtle changes that might indicate depression. Tearfulness, decreased interest in family members or usual activities, decreased appetite, and insomnia are common. Failure to engage in restorative activities can be seen in cancer patients experiencing depression. The vegetative signs of depression—sleep and appetite disturbances and loss of energy and weight—are common symptoms of cancer or side effects of its treatment. To assess depression accurately in those with cancer, psychological symptoms are more reliable indicators. These include sadness, anxiety, and feelings of hopelessness, helplessness, and worthlessness.

A review of nursing interventions to deal with hopelessness will be discussed later in this chapter. For cancer patients experiencing depression, offering premature reassurance is of no value and stifles the person from expressing his or her feelings.

Acknowledgment of feelings is a first important step. Verbalization should be encouraged using effective communication techniques including good eye contact, attentive listening, and a caring touch. Once ventilation has occurred, reassurance and realistic appraisal of the situation can take place.

Reflecting back feelings helps the patient to identify, admit, and accept them. Depressed patients need encouragement and permission to reveal these painful feelings. Open-ended, feeling questions can also help to elicit this information. Depressed individuals can often sense others' reluctance or discomfort when they try to initiate conversation about their depressed mood.

Suicide Risk

Cancer patients experience many ups and downs related to their illness, and need nursing support at each hurdle. Patients may experience depression while in the hospital or at home. Nurses play a key role in assessment and management of depression for those experiencing cancer and need to consider suicide risk in cases of severe depression.

The risk of suicide in cancer increases with uncontrolled pain, depression, delirium, advanced disease, and poor prognosis. Mild impairments in mental ability and judgment are associated with a higher rate of suicide, while the risk decreases with more severe cases of delirium as the individual is unable to execute a plan. Those with inadequate pain control who have committed suicide had previously asked for better symptom management. Suicidal ideas or actual preparations often precede suicides (Valente, Saunders, & Grant, 1994).

The actual rate of suicide in cancer is difficult to define since an unknown number of suicides may be concealed by family members and health care providers. Even among high-risk groups, consummated suicides are thought to be infrequent.

Certain characteristics are common in those with cancer who commit suicide: unmarried, living alone, age younger than or older than 60, increased emotional distress, family difficulties, insomnia, alcohol abuse, exhausted resources, and paranoid thinking (Saunders & Valente, 1988; Valente, Saunders, & Grant, 1994).

Assessment of those at risk for suicide is a neglected area of nursing practice. Some key questions will help identify those at risk. For instance, one might progress with questions in the following manner:

Does your situation discourage you?
Do you feel like crying?
Are there times when life doesn't feel worth living?
Have you gone so far as to think of how you would actually end your life?
Have you begun making arrangements for this?

Nurses should also listen for comments such as "I'd rather be dead." These may be merely expressions of frustration, but should be evaluated for suicidal ideation. Those who are depressed, chronically ill, and have a suicide plan and the means are at significant risk for suicide and need psychiatric evaluation. Although suicide in the oncology population may seem rational to some, nurses are legally obligated to do all that they can to prevent it.

THE CANCER CONTINUUM

DIAGNOSTIC EVALUATION AND PLANNING FOR TREATMENT

The initial phase of the cancer continuum begins with a suspicion that cancer is a possibility and continues through the diagnostic evaluation and treatment planning stages. Patients vacillate from believing that nothing is wrong to worrying that it is the worst of all possible nightmares: *cancer.* Patients recall the period of not knowing the diagnosis as the worst time in their experience with cancer, a time when many personal decisions are suspended and all of life is in limbo (Northouse & Lancaster, 1994). Although reactions vary from person to person and in the same individual over time, some common themes are known. All persons facing a cancer diagnosis experience significant emotional turmoil that includes difficulty concentrating, insomnia, loss of appetite, and/or feelings of panic, anxiety, depression, and despair (Holland, 1989; Jalowiec & Dudas, 1991; Lederberg & Massie, 1993; Mood, 1991). Past experiences of others who have had cancer or, worse, died from it, pervade an individual's thinking.

Once the diagnosis of cancer is confirmed, shock, numbness, and denial are common. During this time, thoughts of life and death predominate. Weisman and Worden (1976), in their classic work on the first 100 days after diagnosis, describe this as the existential plight in cancer. Cancer brings an awareness of personal mortality and vulnerability, accentuated by advanced illness and more symptoms. Strong interpersonal support, an optimistic outlook, and openness reduce psychosocial distress. Those individuals who have regrets about the past, marital problems, minimal social support, and a pessimistic attitude have more existential distress. These existential concerns diminish over the second 100 days as patients come to terms with their situation.

Many individuals search for meaning in their cancer experience. O'Connor, Wicker, and Germino (1990) conducted interviews with 30 patients recently diagnosed with cancer. Six themes were prevalent:

Seeking an understanding of the personal significance of the disease
Looking at the consequences of the diagnosis
Reviewing life
Changes in outlook toward self, life, and others
Living with cancer
Hope

In addition, two factors were influential: faith and social support.

Attributing a cause to illness is a highly adaptive process, enabling people to have a sense of mastery over their predicament (Holland, 1989; Mood, 1991). Nurses can help patients to examine what their illness means to them, and how cancer has impacted their lives. Identifying what offers a sense of hope for individuals and what helps them to live with the diagnosis are also important. Some persons focus on past aspects of their life, while others concentrate on current relationships. Searching for meaning is an important facet of adjustment to cancer and nurses can be instrumental by acknowledging and legitimizing its significance.

During the diagnostic and treatment planning phase, patients have frequent interactions with the health care system, although they are usually outpatients. Many of their fears and decisions occur at home, making each ambulatory encounter critically important. Weighing the potential risks, benefits, and losses of a complex treatment plan at a time of great stress creates conflict for many people. Patients and families need an advocate in the health care system who is readily available as concerns and questions arise, and provides information in a timely manner.

TREATMENT FOLLOWED BY CURE

After treatment ensues, living with cancer and the repercussions of treatment become the focus. Attempts are made to restore normalcy and adapt to changes in roles and lifestyles by reallocating responsibilities and balancing the needs of patient and family. When treatment is complete, individuals are often surprised at how ambivalent they feel. Dependence on the health care system for the past months comes to an end, creating feelings of anxiety and concern about the future. Feelings of uncertainty again arise. Many individuals experience intermittent anxiety and depression which disappoints them. Reassurance and rehabilitation may be necessary for sequelae of the disease or its treatment. Many individuals may be returning to work for the first time, encountering friends' and colleagues' reactions. Acknowledgment of the difficulties confronted by cancer survivors can help patients prepare for them and accept their own changing emotional reactions to what they may think should be a time of celebration.

REMISSION FOLLOWED BY RECURRENCE

Despite the fact that recurrence is no longer synonymous with being terminal, patients react with profound disappointment and interpret recurrence to be the end of any hope for cure. Those who are most surprised about recurrence experience the most distress. Age, social role, and developmental stage are also known to influence an individual's perception of recurrence (Mahon, 1991). At this painful time, threat to life cannot be denied and patients are often left with less than optimal treatment choices. They again experience acute emotional turmoil similar to the initial diagnostic period, but many report that it is worse. In addition to the aspects described earlier, patients often blame themselves or their physician for failure of the treatment (Holland, 1989). Planning for suicide counteracts fears of a painful death, a concern that should be addressed at this time.

Patients who have a recurrence may seek alternative therapies, especially if they are told that nothing can be done for their cancer. They worry that the physician and health care system will not continue to treat their cancer aggressively and need an opportunity to ask questions and explore possible scenarios that they might have imagined.

Interactions with the health care system again increase as do recollections of prior events. Although the patient may be experienced at cancer treatment, recall of all necessary information should not be assumed. Providing referrals to community resources, clarifying misconceptions, and explaining normal emotional reactions are important interventions. A major challenge for patients and caregivers is the maintenance of hope. Patients have been found to be much less hopeful at the time of recurrence than at initial cancer diagnosis (Mahon, 1991). Coping with recurrence is easier if one has less extensive disease and more optimism and support from others.

PROGRESSIVE DISEASE AND TERMINAL TRAJECTORY

Although survival rates have improved, many will eventually succumb to cancer. When treatment fails or no primary treatment is available, patients may be offered therapies aimed at controlling, not curing their disease. This is discouraging and a new period of adjustment must take place. Relationships with health care providers take on special meaning as patients and families hang on every word and conversation, looking for clues that something has changed in their situation. As disease progresses, issues surface regarding dependency and intimacy. Patients feel helpless as disability and weakness increase and feel like they are an enormous burden on their loved ones.

Those facing death generally share the same concerns as those who are living, with the additional burdens imposed by physical and mental deterioration. Self-expression, self-worth, affection, and social interaction continue to be important. Although fears of telling the dying person too much continue to be prevalent, people are generally more frightened by the unknown. Common sense, compassion, sensitivity, and knowledge of a patient's wishes should guide interactions. It is critical to remember that the dying patient is the same person as before and that inquiring about his or her past can help patients reminisce and enjoy past memories. Showing respect and concern for the situation as well as an openness to discuss other aspects of a person's life will afford the dying person more opportunities for meaningful interaction.

Many terminally ill persons withdraw into a period of isolation, depression, and fear. Existential concerns and finding meaning in their suffering are especially important. The quality of a person's remaining time influences his or her adjustment. It is also common for patients to use partial denial, knowing on the one hand that they are terminally ill, yet maintaining a positive outlook regarding the future. Those who are religious and have relied on spiritual beliefs in the past will continue to do so. Just as there is no one way to respond to death, there is no one way to approach dying persons.

As patients come closer to death, problems with symptom management may become paramount. Without adequate control of pain, nausea, or dyspnea, patients are unable to enjoy any quality of life or deal with closure issues. Nurses must anticipate symptoms that may occur and be skilled and comfortable in assessing and managing them. For a detailed account of pain management interventions for those with progressive cancer, see Chapter 20. Family members who act as primary caregivers require education and preparation to address potential attitudinal barriers related to using narcotics and fears of addiction. It is important to clarify these misconceptions early so that needless suffering does not occur for both patient and family.

Patients and/or their families must also be instructed about changes that occur when death is imminent and ways that they will be supported. It is helpful to discuss situations that may prompt family members to call for emergency help and the possibility of resuscitative efforts. As a person's condition deteriorates, increased contact with family caregivers provides opportunities to address issues and reinforce instructions. With most home care hospice programs a vigil is maintained for a period of time prior to death, to provide additional support to family caregivers. For those who die in a hospital, involvement of family members is no less important. They still play a primary role in caregiving and require the same preparation and instructions of what to expect.

Issues concerning the use of life support still predominate for terminally ill patients. The Patient Self Determination Act, passed in 1991, requires hospitals to ask patients on admission about their wishes regarding resuscitation and life support. Unfortunately, many patients are acutely ill, anxious, and under stress at the time of admission and are not prepared to make this decision even when given the opportunity. Others refrain from such a decision due to religious, racial, or cultural beliefs. Ideally, the issue of advance directives should be discussed prior to a health crisis and with someone who knows the person well. Nurses can act as advocates for patients and assist them with this difficult process. Assessment and education regarding advance directives should be part of an initial visit for cancer patients, so that ongoing dialogue can occur as a relationship is established. Helping patients to sort out the differences and implications of available health care technologies and advance directives is critical. For those who have prepared advance directives, it is essential to review their content and intentions with patients and families in case any changes need to be made.

PSYCHOSOCIAL RESPONSES TO SPECIFIC TREATMENTS

SURGERY

Individuals have emotional reactions to their diagnosis, prognosis, and the method of cancer treatment chosen. Surgery, the oldest form of cancer treatment, can accomplish a variety of goals: definitive treatment, debulking, removal of metastatic disease, treatment of oncologic emergencies, palliation of symptoms, reconstruction, and prevention of malignant transformation (Jacobsen & Holland, 1989). The functional and cosmetic deficits from surgery as well as the site of disease can affect a person's adjustment. All patients facing surgery experience anxiety and fear, but those anticipating cancer surgery are more distressed.

Breast surgery has been associated with loss of self-esteem, sexual dysfunction, altered body image, anxiety, and depression. Breast-conserving procedures have improved the psychological outcome of surgery. Colostomy surgery can cause people to feel disgust, anger, embarrassment, and shame and precipitate sexual dysfunction, as well as social isolation. Equipment improvements and better preparation for the procedure via consultation with an enterostomal therapist have resulted in less psychosocial morbidity. For those who have head and neck cancer surgery, attractiveness, communication, and social interaction are assaulted with these procedures. Concerns about rejection and reactions of others are prevalent in the postoperative period. Those who are predisposed to head and neck cancer usually have a history of alcohol and tobacco abuse which may complicate their psychosocial picture.

Limb amputation often occurs in a younger population afflicted by osteogenic sarcoma resulting in loss of function and future goals and phantom limb pain. Limb-sparing procedures have become part of the repertoire of standard approaches for this disease to attempt to minimize disability. Genitourinary cancers can raise misconceptions regarding cancer causation related to sexual history and distress regarding altered sexual function, body image, self-esteem, and infertility. Some patients and their partners worry that continuing sexual relations will spread the cancer. Response to surgical treatment is quite variable. Those who have a history of psychiatric problems, a high degree of preoperative anxiety, or depression and suicidal risk should be referred to a psychosocial clinician.

RADIATION THERAPY

Radiation therapy is useful in a variety of cancers for cure, palliation, prophylaxis, and management of structural emergencies. The public associates radiation therapy with palliation and horrific side effects, such as radiation burns and poisoning. They also must differentiate the effects of radiation disasters such as Chernobyl from therapeutic radiation. In addition, the nature of this treatment prompts fear in many who misinterpret their radioactive state and ability to harm others.

The need to receive radiation therapy on a daily basis is problematic for patients who have an insufficient support network. As treatment continues, fatigue increases and patients may be unable to drive themselves for treatment. Preparing patients for this treatment requires detailed information regarding the equipment and procedures used, including tattooing. Tattoos which mark the area to be treated can make patients feel stigmatized and serve as a reminder of their cancer. Although each treatment takes a very short time, the initial treatment-planning visit can be quite long. During the treatment, patients are alone in a room with a large, overwhelming machine wrapped around them in some fashion. It is imperative that they feel confidence in the ability of the therapist to observe and communicate with them at all times. A tour through the radiation therapy department with special attention to some of these details can allay anxieties.

CHEMOTHERAPY

Chemotherapy, like radiation therapy, prompts fear in many who have heard frightening stories of its side effects. Indeed, the side effects of chemotherapy are problematic and variable. It too is thought of as a last resort by the public, even though it plays a significant role in the cure and control of many cancers.

Since chemotherapy may be harmful to health care workers and others if ingested, absorbed, or inhaled, precautions are taken, including gloves, gowns, and/or goggles or glasses when administering drugs or handling body fluids. Family caregivers may also need to be instructed in safety precautions. A careful explanation to patients will prevent them from thinking they are "radioactive-like" and harmful to others.

Alopecia is a side effect that causes most patients to dread treatment. This side effect is not universal and patients must be prepared regarding the degree and timing of alopecia, if it is likely to occur. Hair loss is ranked high as one of the most distressing side effects of chemotherapy. There are few interventions for this problem and none that prevent it from occurring. Patients are instructed to purchase wigs and consider attending the *Look Good Feel Better Program* of the American Cancer Society, in which trained cosmetologists provide beauty tips to counteract the effects of chemotherapy on hair and skin.

Nausea and vomiting, an unpleasant side effect, varies with drug, combination, and dosages of chemotherapy. Patterns of nausea and vomiting include acute (within a few hours), subacute (6–12 hours later) and delayed (24–72 hours later). Some patients experience anticipatory nausea and vomiting as a conditioned response when management is less than adequate. This is especially prevalent in patients under 40 and responds well to lorazapam (Ativan) and/or relaxation training prior to treatment. Refractory nausea and vomiting have in the past prompted patients to withdraw from treatment. Today, a vast array of effective antiemetics, that work in differing ways, are available. Antiemetics, however, are underused by patients. In fact, patients rarely take them to prevent nausea and vomiting, but rather wait until it occurs to treat it. Although data exists to help predict emetogenic risk, individualized assessment must also occur. Antiemetics used in an around-the-clock manner are more effective. Patients need encouragement to take these medications and avoid needless suffering.

Fatigue and weakness associated with chemotherapy range from mild to debilitating. Some patients are unable to continue fulfilling roles and responsibilities and must cope with this temporary or permanent loss. Daily routines and goals are interrupted. Patients are also troubled by changes in weight, skin discolorations, peripheral neuropathies, and bowel dysfunction. The degree of psychosocial distress varies greatly and is influenced by patients' premorbid characteristics as well as the array and severity of side effects experienced.

BIOTHERAPY

Biotherapy is a fourth type of cancer treatment. The most common biologics used are interferons and interleukins. As they are approved only for limited uses, many patients receive these treatments in clinical trials. Because biologics are considered investigational in many situations, reimbursement is limited. Clinical trials may force patients to travel a great distance and some trials have a waiting list for entry (Tsevat & LaCasse, 1992). Patient preparation for biotherapy includes side effect management, schedule, and reimbursement information. Sometimes, self-injection instructions are also required.

Biotherapy carries a significant risk of neuropsychiatric side effects. These effects progress from mild to severe and include changes in cognition, orientation, attention span, wakefulness, psychomotor behavior, and mood (Sparber & Biller-Sparber, 1993). Intermittent bouts of crying reflect alterations in mood. For mild cases, interventions include rest, emotional support, and orientation. More severe toxicity may require critical care. It is important to reassure patients and families that changes in cognition are temporary. Due to the nature and degree of these toxicities, patients may reconsider their desire to complete therapy and need assistance with this difficult decision.

BONE MARROW TRANSPLANT

Although they have endured prolonged hospitalization, isolation, and life-threatening toxicities, bone marrow transplant (BMT) survivors report only mild to moderate psychological distress. A phenomenon of feeling lucky to be alive is prevalent since many of these patients have previously experienced chemotherapy, radiation therapy, failure of treatment, and disease recurrence (Ahles & Shedd, 1991; Whedon & Ferrell, 1994).

BMT is performed for hematologic malignancies as well as solid tumors and can involve marrow harvested from others (i.e., a sibling or family members), as well as from the patient. All patients receive very high-dose chemotherapy, with or without total body irradiation. Toxicities associated with BMT are severe, especially immunosuppression. For this reason, patients are placed in protective isolation rooms for their hospital stay, which ranges from 3 to 6 weeks.

As patients face BMT, they hope for cure in spite of knowing the high mortality and morbidity associated with this procedure. Making a decision regarding this approach is quite difficult and patients benefit from psychosocial assistance. During hospitalization, patients must deal with side effects that are often worse than those experienced with standard dose therapy, prolonged isolation and hospitalization, neuropsychiatric effects of the treatment, and profound family stress. Depression and chronic anxiety are the most common psychosocial problems associated with BMT. Body image concerns are paramount as the effects of this treatment can be devastating. For these reasons, psychological assessment and support are considered integral to any BMT program.

CANCER REHABILITATION AND SURVIVAL

As survival rates continue to increase, long-term issues related to the experience of cancer are further described. Posttreatment concerns include development of secondary malignancies, organ dysfunction, and infection secondary to immunosuppression, as well as residual fatigue, disabilities, and disfigurements. Those experiencing more significant physical disabilities or disfigurements express the most psychosocial distress.

Concern that physical symptoms may herald a recurrence leads some survivors to a state of chronic anxiety, fear, and hypochondriasis. Others choose to avoid thinking about illness and may discontinue appropriate follow-up care. This residual response to diagnosis and treatment, coupled with a close encounter with mortality, serves to make the cancer survivor feel a pervasive sense of uncertainty and vulnerability. Reliving the diagnosis and treatment at anniversaries of key events heightens anxiety even years later. In contrast, some survivors develop a renewed zest for life and refocus their priorities consistent with this enhanced appreciation.

Reentry issues emerge for many cancer survivors, related to resuming roles and responsibilities, employment, and/or insurance concerns. Many find planning for the future creates interpersonal distress and postponing of goals.

Although most people with cancer return to work, job problems do occur. Overt discrimination in the form of dismissal or demotion is prohibited by laws at the federal and state levels. Co-workers, however, may be antagonistic because of increased work burdens that might have occurred during treatment. The most common employment problem is "job lock" (Tross & Holland, 1989). Survivors fear losing benefits, especially health insurance coverage, and do not make career changes, destroying their options for advancement and job security.

The financial burden of cancer extends beyond the costs of therapy to transportation expenses, home care expenses, lost wages, copayments, and deductibles. Many persons experience significant deterioration in their financial health (Glajchen, 1994).

It is critical that a rehabilitation framework be adopted for acute care of persons with cancer. By preparing patients to function optimally in the future, many of these issues can be addressed. Nurses in all settings can be pivotal in this plan by educating patients and families about the potential psychosocial distress they may encounter, signs and symptoms of recurrence, potential secondary effects of treatment, employment and insurance concerns, and ways to obtain support and assistance. Although many potential psychosocial concerns have been described, the majority of cancer patients do adjust to their illness, either independently or with the aid of health care professionals. Early recognition of these potential sequelae by nurses and others can facilitate appropriate management.

CHALLENGES FOR INDIVIDUALS COPING WITH CANCER

An individual's psychosocial response to cancer and its treatment revolves around three main areas:

1. Altered relationships

2. Independence-dependence issues
3. Body image and integrity alterations

Within each of these major categories the patient faces issues and challenges to recognize and address.

ALTERED RELATIONSHIPS

Facing cancer requires an enormous amount of personal reserve, both on the part of the patient and significant others. Interpersonal relationships undergo tremendous stress during this critical period, when their stability is challenged. Both patients and family members harbor feelings of frustration, anger, fear, and uncertainty of what the future will hold.

Isolation

Patients with cancer frequently describe a lack of social interaction because of their diagnosis. Friedman, Florian, and Zernitsky-Shurka (1989) suggest four explanations for the cancer patient's lack of social interaction:

1. Social stigma associated with cancer: cancer may cause aversive physical changes and inspire fear of contagion.
2. Lack of open communication about the disease.
3. Conflicting feelings of significant others: significant others may be angry with the patient for developing the disease or hold them responsible for becoming ill, while trying to be cheerful and supportive.
4. Disability arising from the cancer may prevent patients from participating in social activities.

These factors work together to make the cancer patient feel isolated and alone at a time when they need psychosocial interaction the most.

Feelings of isolation or loneliness may contribute to the painful dilemma of dealing with cancer. It is difficult to maintain hope and optimism in the face of loneliness and despair. The nurse is in a position to assess the cancer patient's psychosocial response to cancer and its effects on interpersonal relationships. Through identifying patients at risk for feelings of loneli-

ness and appropriate referrals to support groups, the nurse may help relieve some of the trauma associated with the experience.

Sexuality

Another area that can be affected in the individual with cancer is sexuality or sexual health. The World Health Organization (1975) describes sexual health as the "integration of the somatic, emotional, intellectual, and social aspects of sexual beings in ways that are positively enriching and that enhance personality, communication and love." Similarly, Lamb and Woods (1981) suggest sexuality is a "complex phenomenon which pervades our biological being, our sense of self, and the ways in which we relate to others."

The disease process of cancer can alter sexuality through a variety of means. Fatigue or general malaise is an accompanying symptom of many cancers and can result in decreased sexual desire. Pain or neurologic dysfunction may prevent usual expressions of sexuality. In a study of women with endometrial cancer, Lamb and Sheldon (1994) identified bleeding, fatigue, and pain as the symptoms most likely to disrupt sexual health. Issues such as fear of contagion and resentment toward the person with cancer may inhibit the patient's spouse from his or her usual manner of sexual expression.

Treatment for cancer can result in a range of difficulties related to sexual functioning. Surgery may be especially disfiguring or may structurally modify the genitalia, resulting in altered functioning. Fertility is frequently impaired as a result of cancer treatment. Many types of cancer require multimodal treatment, each one having a different effect on sexuality. Gynecologic cancers, for example, often require surgery which might involve structural changes and infertility. Radiation therapy to the female pelvis results in thinning of the vaginal wall, loss of elasticity, and decreased lubrication, which can contribute to dyspareunia. Chemotherapy may cause temporary or permanent sterility and resulting fatigue can contribute to overall loss of desire.

The Oncology Nursing Society, a professional organization of specialized nurses, issued an outcome standard on sexuality (ANA

& Oncology Nursing Society, 1987) recognizing this aspect as an integral component of individual well-being. Nurses can play a key role in helping cancer patients deal with altered sexuality; however, many are afraid to address this subject. Failure to assess sexuality in patients may allow issues or problems that impact quality of life to be ignored. Nurses should examine their own knowledge, attitudes, and values in the area of sexuality and strive to develop an assessment approach that allows patients to feel comfortable discussing sexuality. Open-ended questions are recommended, such as "How has treatment affected your role as mother, wife?" "Has cancer affected your relationship with your spouse?" and, more directly, "Has your illness changed your sexual function?" Asking specific questions about patients' sexuality gives them permission to discuss this sensitive subject.

Nurses need not be sex therapists or counselors to assist patients in maintaining sexual health. Many problems can be resolved by listening, giving information, clarifying myths and misconceptions, and fostering communication. Nurses should discuss the impact of cancer on sexuality and help the patient and spouse to identify methods to prevent or cope with changes. Recognizing the importance of sexuality and allowing the patient to ask questions, seek support, and gain insight can contribute significantly to maintaining sexual identity.

INDEPENDENCE-DEPENDENCE ISSUES

Spouse, parent, employee, student are but a few of the roles an individual may enact at any given period of time. Cancer affects these roles in many ways. When one first learns of the cancer diagnosis, responsibilities may be essentially the same, but as disease progresses and treatment ensues, shifting of roles and responsibilities occurs.

Both the debilitating effects from disease and the side effects from cancer treatment necessitate modifications in daily activities. Consider some of the problems John faced as a result of his disease and treatment.

John was a 35-year-old diagnosed with non–Hodgkin's lymphoma and treated as an outpatient. Fatigue was his most debilitating side effect from chemotherapy. As a result of his fatigue he was forced to relinquish the running of his business to his wife and assume the role of primary caregiver for their three children. Suddenly, this man who owned and operated a business was unable to fulfill that role and his wife, who had devoted her time to caring for their children, stepped into his place. They both spoke of how difficult it was to exchange roles. Each morning, John would get the children ready and off to school, then collapse in exhaustion, while his wife went off to work.

While some patients who receive outpatient treatment are able to maintain their previous roles to some degree, many patients are unable to sustain all of their previous roles throughout their illness and treatment. John's situation is a frequently occurring example of how roles and responsibilities can become rearranged as a result of cancer and its therapy.

BODY IMAGE AND INTEGRITY ALTERATIONS

When one thinks of body image as associated with the cancer patient, one immediately considers the range of obviously disfiguring surgeries that a patient may undergo as treatment for the disease. Changes in body image, however, are not only linked to mutilating surgeries, but to the entire scope of cancer treatment. Radiation therapy and chemotherapy offer a host of side effects that may result in body image disturbances. Hair loss, skin changes, stomatitis, changes in bowel and bladder function, pain, fatigue, nausea, and vomiting are but a few of the consequences that may produce profound effects on body image.

Closely linked to the concept of body image is that of self-esteem. Self-esteem is defined by Rosenberg (1965) as a positive or negative attitude toward oneself based on evaluation of self characteristics, and includes feelings of self-satisfaction and self-acceptance. Indeed, self-esteem can be affected by body image. That is, a disruption in body image may contribute to lowered self-esteem. Research has linked self-esteem with quality of life.

A recent study examined the concept of self-esteem as it related to female cancer patients prediagnosis and during treatment-induced alopecia (Carpenter & Brockopp, 1994). Participants in the study were asked to complete two self-esteem scales on the day of their interview and retrospectively prediagnosis. The findings showed a significant decrease in self-esteem levels from the prediagnosis period to the time of experiencing treatment-induced alopecia. The researchers suggest that a cancer diagnosis and treatment may lower self-esteem in women and should be considered an area for assessment and intervention.

Nurses are in the best position to assess changes in body image and self-esteem. Extended patient contact on inpatient units and repeated exposure during outpatient visits allows ample time to approach these issues with cancer patients. Providing an opportunity to discuss perceived losses and giving permission to grieve are appropriate interventions. Nurses must explore their reactions to changes in body image and avoid conveying negative reactions to patients. Preparing patients for changes in structure and function and referring to appropriate support groups can enhance adaptation to changes. Nurses also have responsibility to observe and intervene for self-destructive and/or suicidal behavior.

CHALLENGES FOR FAMILIES COPING WITH CANCER

Cancer is a disease that strikes families as well as individuals. The term *family* has been defined by Gillis, Highley, and Roberts (1989) as "a group of two or more individuals usually living in close geographic proximity; having close emotional bonds; and meeting affectional, socioeconomical, sexual, and socialization needs of the family group or the wider social systems" (p. 72). Families' responses to cancer and its treatment revolve around four major areas:

1. Family coping and adjustment
2. Issues affecting specific family members
3. Needs of family caregivers
4. Grief and bereavement

Within each of these major areas, the family is faced with issues and challenges that must be recognized and addressed.

FAMILY COPING AND ADJUSTMENT

Jassak, in a lecture entitled "Families: An Essential Element in the Care of the Patient with Cancer,"(1992) discusses three consistent research findings with respect to families coping with cancer:

1. The family affects the patient's adjustment to cancer.
2. Family members do not necessarily share the same concerns about cancer; concerns may vary according to the age and role of family members and specific characteristics of the disease.
3. Family members cope with cancer in different ways.

Whatever the diagnosis, the family is challenged with managing the inevitable changes that occur.

Multiple issues must be considered when evaluating the effect of cancer in terms of family adjustment (Jassak, 1992). Changes in roles and responsibilities affect not only individuals with cancer, but families as well. Members must deal with assuming responsibility for the patient's previous roles, yet remain flexible enough to let the patient perform them as able. Physical requirements of care become important as disease progresses and treatment side effects begin. Family members report emotional strain, fear of death or letting go, and uncertainty. For most families, financial concerns are inevitable. Sometimes family members are unsure how to approach or support the patient. Frequently families are not aware of support services that are available or how to access those resources. Family members' needs and concerns may be different from the patient's and an individual's diagnosis of cancer may prompt other family members to examine their spiritual beliefs.

Assessment of four main factors will yield information with respect to family coping (Hill & Hansen, 1964):

1. What is the family's perception of the illness?

2. What is the perceived threat to the family unit?

3. What resources are available for financial and psychosocial support?

4. What is the family's previous experience with similar crisis situations?

Evaluation of these four areas will enable the nurse to assess the impact of cancer on the family and determine appropriate interventions.

Jassak (1992) identifies six critical interventions that facilitate family adaptation to living with cancer:

1. *Seek family input:* Ask patient and family what they perceive their needs are.

2. *Decrease ambiguity:* Allow families to raise questions about what can be expected.

3. *Provide information to the family as a unit:* Consider including the patient and family as part of patient care conferences; consistently verify information discussed.

4. *Identify resources:* Whenever possible, involve all family members in care; identify appropriate resources at each phase of illness.

5. *Provide feedback:* Help the family to recognize the integral role that they play in individual and family coping with cancer.

6. *Periodically evaluate family response:* Cancer is often viewed as a pervasive element in family lives, yet needs change over the course of illness and family adaptation must accommodate the changes.

These six critical interventions provide the framework for family intervention. Adaptation of the family and individual and collective coping can be enhanced through the careful assessment and intervention of the nurse.

ISSUES AFFECTING SPECIFIC FAMILY MEMBERS

A myriad of research has been conducted evaluating the specific concerns of spouses of patients with cancer (Northouse & Peters-Golden, 1993). Three issues surface repeatedly in the literature and are of utmost concern to the spouses of cancer patients. First is the fear associated with a cancer diagnosis. This fear contributes to patients' and spouses' anxiety, helplessness, and loss of control. Second, spouses feel unprepared for dealing with the emotional trauma associated with the cancer diagnosis.

A third issue is the ability to deal with the daily disruptions caused by the disease. As a result of the cancer and treatment, spouses frequently report disruption in employment, household schedules, child-care arrangements, and social involvement.

Support of the spouse is crucial when dealing with the cancer patient. Research has demonstrated that social support by family members plays an important role in the cancer patient's perceived quality of life. Fuller and Swenson (1992) examined marital quality and quality of life among cancer patients and their spouses. The results revealed that patients identified being close with their spouse as the best predictor of their quality of life, while partners reported coping with marital situations or problem solving was the most important indicator of quality of life. The researchers point out the importance of this information in terms of supporting the patient and family with cancer. Clearly, nurses need to attend to the different needs of patients and spouses while helping them to recognize those differences.

Hymovich (1993) recently described another aspect of the cancer experience, that is, the childrearing concerns of the patient with cancer. This qualitative research identified parents' perceptions of stressors and coping strategies related to childrearing; specifically, family relationships, communication, and the child's response to illness were areas identified. Hymovich suggested the following nursing interventions to help the cancer patient and spouse cope with childrearing (p. 1359):

1. Recognize the importance of potential childrearing stressors in the early postdiagnosis period.

2. Provide support regarding parenting roles.

3. Provide developmentally appropriate information to children.

4. Help parents prepare children for changes in the family.

5. Encourage discussion of childrearing concerns.

6. Identify issues that parents may not be aware of (e.g., separation anxiety).
7. Utilize written patient education materials.
8. Suggest participation in support groups.
9. Prepare children for change in their parents.
10. Help parents understand how children respond to stress.

Hymovich recommended that further research be conducted to determine the most effective strategies to assist parents affected by cancer with childrearing practices.

NEEDS OF FAMILY CAREGIVERS

The trend for cancer care to be delivered more frequently in an outpatient environment has resulted in a dramatic increase in family members' responsibility for caring for the patient. Patients who receive treatment on an outpatient basis spend relatively little time with health care providers. Likewise, with shortened hospital stays and early discharge, more responsibility to meet patients' needs has shifted to the caregiver at home. A caregiver is defined as "the individual responsible for the majority of caregiving tasks, including emotional support and supervision of the family member with cancer" (Laizner et al., 1993, p. 114). Caregivers are more frequently women and often are employed outside the home. Caregivers are typically responsible for assisting the patient with self-care, providing transportation, helping with procedures, and assisting with medications and symptom management (Laizner et al., 1993).

As the link between family support and quality of life for patients has been identified, it has become apparent that the needs of caregivers must be recognized. Hileman, Lackey, and Hassanein (1992) attempted to identify, categorize, and assess the importance of needs expressed by caregivers and to determine how well these needs were satisfied. The greatest unsatisfied needs identified by caregivers were, first, informational and, second, psychological. Caregivers wanted information about symptoms, side effects from treatment, community resources, and the future. Patient care issues were identi-

fied as the third greatest need. The researchers suggest that nurses should continue to place increased focus on meeting the informational and psychological needs of patient caregivers.

Another concept related to families is that of *caregiver burden.* Caregiver burden is defined as a "two dimensional phenomenon embracing on the one hand the extent of disruption or change in various aspects of the caregiver's life (objective burden) and on the other hand the caregiver's attitudes toward, or emotional reactions to, the caregiving experience (subjective burden)" (Schott-Baer, 1993, p. 231). One recent study (Schott-Baer, 1993) indicated that increased length of time in the caregiver role resulted in increased subjective burden. Older persons in the caregiver role reported less subjective burden. In a study by Carey, Oberst, McCubbin, and Hughes (1991), caregivers identified giving emotional support as their most difficult and time-consuming role. Participants also reported spending time assisting with household tasks, errands, and transportation. Patient dependency was the main contributor to caregiving burden. The authors point out that evidence of patient dependency should alert the nurse to caregivers who are at high risk for caregiving burden.

GRIEF AND BEREAVEMENT

Families need time to experience the death event on their own terms. When family members have the opportunity to prepare for the death of a loved one at home, they are also preparing themselves. This type of preparation is referred to as *anticipatory grieving.* Gordon (1993) defines anticipatory grief as "expectation of disruption in familiar patterns or significant relationships" (p. 287). Nurses have the opportunity to facilitate this process by encouraging family members to approach unresolved issues with the dying person. Family members should be encouraged to say those things to the patient they haven't said or believe they haven't said often enough.

Finally, the nurse should discuss with families what feelings may be expected as a result of the loss.

Grief is an expected, normal reaction to a real or perceived loss. Worden (1982) identifies four tasks that must be resolved for the normal grief process to progress:

1. To accept the reality of the loss.
2. To experience the pain of grief.
3. To adjust to the environment in which the deceased is missing.
4. To withdraw emotional energy, and replace it with another relationship.

The grief process is highly individualized and resolution takes place gradually over a period of time. The nurse can play an important role in supporting the grief process by listening to subjective responses to the loss, allowing expression of negative emotions, validating perceptions of responses, and giving permission to grieve and resolve the loss.

SPECIAL ISSUES RELATED TO CANCER DIAGNOSIS AND TREATMENT

INFORMED CONSENT AND TRUTH TELLING

Oncology nurses have long had to deal with the challenges of truth telling and informed consent. In the past, revealing the diagnosis of cancer was limited by professional attitudes and protective families. This failure to communicate openly and honestly with patients created ethical dilemmas for nurses.

The 1970s brought a dramatic shift in the approach to disclosure of a cancer diagnosis. In 1961, 88% of physicians surveyed said that they never revealed a cancer diagnosis to patients, while in 1979, only 2% of those surveyed indicated this practice (Holland, 1989). As we learned more about coping, it became clear that open communication contributed to the development of trusting, healthy relationships with caregivers. Paternalistic attitudes diminished while confidence in patients' abilities to adjust to this diagnosis increased.

Current values focus on respect for patients' right to know and right to self determination. Competent patients, indeed, have the right to decide how much they know, who tells them, and who else should be involved. Family wishes should not limit truth telling; rather, a patient's choice is the most important consideration. Open communication facilitates sharing of fears, concerns, and wishes between patients and family members and, in fact, can be very therapeutic. Health care providers face the challenge of giving hope within the context of the reality of the illness and limitations of treatment.

As emphasis has been placed on patients' autonomy, patients have become active participants in treatment decisions. Unfortunately, treatment decisions are usually made soon after the cancer diagnosis is confirmed, a time when patients are most anxious and least able to comprehend this complex information. Informed consent refers to the process of competent patients receiving and comprehending adequate information to make a voluntary decision regarding treatment. The proposed treatment, risks, benefits, alternative treatment options, right to confidentiality and optimal care, and freedom to withdraw at any time are usually disclosed in an informed consent document. These documents should complement, not replace, the verbal discussion among patient, family, and physician.

Often the nurse is at the patient's side when the full impact of the cancer diagnosis is realized. This places the nurse in a key position to provide ongoing emotional support, reassurance, and clarification of questions and concerns. The nurse acts as a liaison between patient, family, and physician, ensuring that unanswered questions are addressed.

INVESTIGATIONAL THERAPY

The decision to participate in investigational treatments can complicate the informed consent process and increase psychosocial stress. Patients are sometimes offered investigational therapies when standard treatments are no longer effective. In their desire to survive, patients consent to participate in clinical trials.

Cancer treatments are evaluated through three phases of clinical trials which systematically evaluate effectiveness, safety parameters, and toxicities, as well as compare new treatments with standard approaches. Preparation of patients focuses on helping them to understand the study's purpose, which sometimes does not involve cure, and, when needed, randomization procedures, in which neither physician nor patient control the choice of therapy. Reviewing goals for participation in investigational trials occurs initially and throughout the trial as patients deal with the anxiety and stress of chronic or progressive cancer. Nurses act as educators, direct caregivers, and patient advocates, assisting patients to define their own goals for participating.

ALTERNATIVE THERAPIES

According to Herbert (1980), "unorthodox (unproven, alternative or questionable) treatments or methods are ones that have not been objectively, reliably, responsibly, and reproducibly demonstrated in the peer reviewed literature to be more effective than no treatment." Biological products, devices, herbal concoctions, dietary and vitamin approaches, faith healing, and psychological approaches are considered by the American Cancer Society (1993) to be questionable methods which typically claim to cure or control cancer using patient testimonies versus scientific data. Marketing strategies often describe them as natural and nontoxic, making them more appealing than traditional cancer treatments with their myriad side effects and toxicities.

When patients are confronted with recurrence or progression of their cancer, they may seek any treatment that offers hope. Patients' fears, however, may be exploited in light of this period of intense vulnerability and feelings of desperation. Choosing these therapies can enhance patients' sense of personal control over an otherwise grim situation. Concern that health care providers will negatively judge their exploration of questionable methods often prevents patients from broaching the subject.

Yarbro (1993) recommends the following steps to assist nurses in providing appropriate care and support to patients seeking alternative therapy: identification of quackery, assessment of communication channels and patient motivations, maintenance of positive communication channels, and maintenance of patient participation in health care decisions. As patient advocates and educators, nurses can act

as a powerful deterrent toward controlling the use of unproven methods.

STRATEGIES TO FACILITATE COPING

Many psychosocial interventions are applicable and effective for persons with cancer. Three areas of particular concern have been selected for discussion: providing informational support, promoting hope, and mobilizing support systems.

PROVIDING INFORMATIONAL SUPPORT

Information seeking is a coping strategy commonly used to deal with the diagnosis of cancer. Patients who take an active role in their treatment generally have more hope, a sense of control, and less psychosocial distress. Patient education helps patients to adjust to their illnesses, carry out prescribed regimens, and recognize and manage side effects. Cultural background, educational level, learning style, age, sensory abilities, and personality all play a role in how a patient learns (Villejo & Meyers, 1991). There are many potential learning barriers to cancer patient education including stress and anxiety related to diagnosis, physical condition, lack of interest and motivation, and amount of information necessary. For these reasons, it is important to plan educational strategies with these barriers and the phase of illness in mind.

Early in the diagnosis, patients will be overwhelmed by new information as well as their emotional responses and will only be able to accomplish short-term acquisition of facts. Later, as patients adjust to the situation, retention and transfer of information, including concepts, principles, attitudes, and behaviors can be expected (Watson, 1982). When developing a teaching plan, priorities must be set regarding what information is essential for the patient's health and safety and what methods will be used to assist them in understanding the content. At the time of diagnosis and treatment planning, patients must learn about laboratory and diagnostic testing that will be done, including preparation and precautions, and the treatment regimen, including type of therapy, schedule, side effects, self-care measures, and goals. Information on sensations the patient will experience decreases discomfort associated with procedures.

A simple assessment of patients' readiness, willingness, and ability to learn can establish a successful plan for accomplishing this (Reiger & Rumsey, 1992). It is also helpful to ask patients how they like to learn and if they would like family members to be involved. Teaching must be done in an appropriate atmosphere where patients' goals and expectations are considered and information sharing is a two-way communication. A working knowledge of adult learning principles and methods to evaluate readability levels of written materials can assist nurses with their patient education endeavors. Due to the complexity of the content and emotional state of the patient, information usually needs to be repeated at subsequent visits and offered in a variety of approaches.

A myriad of printed materials, audiovisual programs, and computer-assisted instruction programs are available from the American Cancer Society, National Cancer Institute Office of Cancer Communications, professional organizations, and pharmaceutical companies. Most of these materials are free of charge and can be ordered in quantities for patient use. Printed matter should be aimed at the fifth- to seventh-grade reading level, a difficult accomplishment when dealing with medical jargon. In addition, information services are available nationally through the National Cancer Institute and American Cancer society, as well as locally via Cancer Answers® and Cancer HELPLINK® provided by various hospitals. These information services are staffed by trained volunteers or registered nurses who can assist patients and families with any questions relating to cancer as well as offer them suggestions for resources in their community. Many people appreciate the anonymity these programs offer, with an opportunity to ask questions they might not ask their health care providers. Information on clinical trials and research developments are usually available through these programs as well.

Nurses are responsible for the bulk of cancer patient education, supported by informa-

tion from physicians, social workers, therapists, pharmacists, and others. Skill in this area is required to practice effectively and meet critical patient needs. Nurses often neglect using the nursing process when considering learning needs. Just as with any other patient care problem, a thorough assessment, plan, and evaluation of achievements can help meet expected outcomes and identify unmet needs. Lack of time and resources can be deleterious to this vital area of nursing practice.

PROMOTING HOPE

While hopefulness in cancer patients is correlated with better adjustment and coping, it is difficult to maintain in the face of an uncertain future. Those who are hopeful enjoy a better quality of life and often work harder to achieve their goals. Too often, health care professionals are focused on eradicating negative responses to cancer and neglect this useful resource (Callan, 1989).

Callan (1989) delineates three types of hope that should be encouraged in working with cancer patients: hope for cure, hope for more attainable future goals, and transcendent hope based on meaning. He suggests using open-ended questions to begin discussions on hope, such as "Tell me about your hope," and "In addition to cure, what other things do you hope for?" These questions can assist individuals in identifying hope as well as expanding their concept of it.

Hope has a unique and personal meaning for each person and is affected by developmental stage. For young adults, hope is related to potential for the future and the development of important relationships. Those a bit older are concerned with settling down and establishing their niche. Midlife brings productivity and increasing success in one's personal and work roles. Late adulthood is a time of looking forward to retirement and its rewards. Cancer and its treatment are a threat to hope at any stage in life. Most individuals are able to adjust their hope as changes from illness become a reality.

Clark (1993) suggests four areas of concentration regarding interventions to promote hope: assisting with reality surveillance, reinforcing personal power and ability, encouraging supportive relationships, and creating a future perspective. Nurses can help patients to review their health status, including their perceptions and any misconceptions needing correction. Communicating confidence in the treatment regimen and including the patient in planning goals, schedules, and care are vital. Once a relationship is established, nurses can help patients to analyze their strengths and review past successful coping strategies used during stress. Encouraging the use of needed resources and reaffirming their value help to reinforce control over the situation. As part of a nursing assessment, supportive relationships should be evaluated. Patients may need motivation to continue these relationships as well as assistance in asking for help. Nurses can guide patients in setting realistic, measurable, short-term goals and can provide valuable ongoing feedback regarding achievement. At times, hope may need to be redirected to short-term possibilities. Enthusiastic interactions with patients and interest in their future hopes and dreams will help motivate them to be more expressive. Lastly, nurses can help patients recognize the many small things in life there are to enjoy (Clark, 1993; Jalowiec & Dudas, 1991).

MOBILIZING SUPPORT SYSTEMS

The value of social support in buffering the effects of stress associated with cancer has been well-documented. How social support works is unclear, but it reduces distress and enhances self-esteem, adjustment, and well-being. Social support takes on a variety of forms; family and friends are the most common source.

Including family members in treatment planning from the start points out their important involvement. Simple measures such as planning conferences to discuss changes in condition or treatment when family members can participate help sustain their involvement. The patient's desire for assistance and support from family members is first established, pointing out the benefits of their inclusion. Again, patients feel like a burden and may need some encouragement in understanding the effect of their illness on the entire family. Families often feel helpless and need to be involved. Encouraging patients and families to attend support programs together, such as "We Can Weekend" and "I Can Cope," sponsored by the American Cancer Society, helps establish their partnership in fighting this illness. As family members are included, it is important to assess their needs, as an individual's issues may differ from the patient's.

The benefit of family interaction was studied by Gotcher (1992) using self-report data from 102 patients with cancer. The relationship between patient/family communication and psychosocial adjustment to cancer was specifically investigated. Results demonstrated that interactions with family were important, especially the frequency of interaction and emotional support received during interactions. Honesty and discussion of unpleasant topics were not found to be significant variables and the author postulated that patients often sense the reluctance of others to discuss openly cancer and dying, which could have affected these results.

Patients also may receive support from friends, co-workers, neighbors, and members of their church or other spiritual center. When these informal systems of support aren't sufficient, people turn to more formal systems, such as hospitals, health care professionals, and community and home care agencies. Specific technical assistance in caring for a cancer patient at home may require the aid of home care nurses. Today, many cancer patients are discharged still requiring high-tech care, such as infusions, chemotherapy, and wound and tracheostomy care. Families often assume these responsibilities, but need support initially after discharge. Home care instructions should begin while the patient is in the hospital and be coordinated with the agency that will be providing care at home to ensure consistency. Additional stress is placed on families who may already be assuming other responsibilities the patient cannot perform. Home care agencies offer nursing, homemaker, and other support services, such as social work, counseling, and physical therapy. Patients and families should be encouraged to avail themselves of whatever support is needed. Support groups specifically for family members of cancer patients can aid in reducing psychosocial distress.

In addition, patients and families may receive support from individual counselors, therapists, or clergy referred by their physician, nurse, or other contact. Oncology caregivers should maintain a referral list of psychosocial professionals in their community who specialize in working with cancer patients and families. Larger cancer programs typically have psychosocial clinicians on staff who see patients individually or conduct group interventions. Veteran patient visitor programs, such as "Reach to Recovery" offered by the American Cancer Society for breast cancer patients, can be extremely helpful for the patient who needs to see someone who has survived the experience but does not feel inclined to attend a group or is unable to do so.

Self-help, support, and psychotherapy groups are also available. The first is under the control and direction of individual members, who all share the same situation or condition. Usually, health care professionals are not involved, although consultation or guest speaking is sometimes requested. Self-reliance, hope, and improved morale are goals of these groups.

Support groups, in contrast, are initiated, organized, and led by health care professionals who use selected psychotherapy knowledge and skills to conduct sessions. Certain behavioral expectations exist for members and leaders, who play very different roles. Support groups also encourage self-reliance, hope, and improved morale. In addition, participants may acquire new knowledge and skills, advice, a confidante, assistance with financial aid, help with duties or responsibilities, encouragement, and feedback on behavior. Normalization of the experience is important and groups are very effective in acknowledging and validating individual's interpretations of events. Members are encouraged to focus on attainable goals and observe modeling of effective coping by others with the same experience. Group members play an advocacy role and encourage expression of feelings (Jalowiec & Dudas, 1991; Lederberg & Massie, 1993). The shared experience and sense of knowing contribute to the development of important relationships in groups. Sanction and recommen-

dation by health care providers are critically important and motivate many individuals to participate.

Although social support is known to be beneficial, it does carry the risk of negative consequences as well. Invasion of privacy, unkept promises, unwelcome advice, forced dependency, and encouraged noncompliance with treatment are examples (Jalowiec & Dudas, 1991). Nurses must continue to assess the benefit of social support systems, monitoring for negative outcomes. Clearly, the value of social support outweighs the potential negative effects and nurses are in an excellent position to help mobilize resources for patients and their families.

CHALLENGES FOR THE FUTURE

Much of the information on psychosocial distress associated with cancer is based on research studies using instruments designed for the psychiatric population. To better evaluate the incidence of psychosocial sequelae in cancer patients and families, instruments should be developed and tested with this group. Once the problem is better defined, routine approaches for ongoing assessment can be integrated into practice.

In addition to having cancer-specific tools for research and assessment, health care providers must develop the appropriate mindset for dealing with this issue. Psychosocial distress is not an acceptable corollary to the cancer experience; rather, it deserves the same commitment to evaluate and design effective interventions as do physical aspects of the disease. Next steps include developing interventions to facilitate coping and adjustment; minimize fear, anxiety, and depression; and counteract the multiple losses associated with the diagnosis and treatment of cancer.

CONCLUSION

A myriad of complex psychosocial responses are known to occur as patients and families learn to deal with cancer. Anxiety, anger, depression, hopelessness, and denial can be problematic, requiring psychosocial consultation and intervention. Many individuals, however, cope with the issues, problems, and challenges of cancer with the steady support of their health care team. Nurses assist patients and families to adjust to changes in roles and relationships as well as physical deficits and disabilities.

Providing information, promoting hope, and mobilizing support are strategies commonly used to counteract the potentially devastating effects of cancer and its treatment. Although great strides have been made in the management of cancer and increasing emphasis has been placed on psychosocial issues and quality of life, there is much work yet to be done.

BIBLIOGRAPHY

Ahles, T. A., & Shedd, P. (1991). Psychosocial impact of bone marrow transplantation in adult patients: Prehospitalization and hospitalization phases. In M. B. Whedon (Ed.), *Bone marrow transplantation: Principles, practice and nursing insight.* Boston: Jones & Bartlett.

American Cancer Society. (1993). *Questionable methods of cancer treatment.* (93-25M-No. 3023). Atlanta, GA: American Cancer Society.

American Cancer Society. (1994). *Facts and figures–1994.* Atlanta, GA: American Cancer Society.

American Nurses Association & Oncology Nursing Society. (1987). *Standards of oncology nursing practice.* Kansas City, MO: American Nurses Association.

Callan, D. B. (1989). Hope as a clinical issue in oncology social work. *Journal of Psychosocial Oncology,* 7(3), 31–46.

Carey, P. J., Oberst, M. T., McCubbin, M. A., & Hughes, S.H. (1991). Appraisal and caregiving burden in family members caring for patients receiving chemotherapy. *Oncology Nursing Forum,* 18(8), 1341–1348.

Carpenter, J. S., & Brockopp, D. (1994). Evaluation of self esteem of women with cancer receiving chemotherapy. *Oncology Nursing Forum,* 21(4), 751–757.

Clark, J. (1993). Psychosocial responses of the patient. In Groenwald, S. L., Frogge, M. H., Goodman, M., & Yarbro, C. H. (Eds.). *Cancer nursing: Principles and practice.* Boston: Jones & Bartlett.

Friedman, G., Florian, V., & Zernitsky-Shurka, E. (1989). The experience of loneliness among young adult cancer patients. *Journal of Psychosocial Oncology,* 7(3), 1–15.

Fuller, S. T., & Swensen, C. H. (1992). Marital quality and quality of life among cancer patients and their spouses. *Journal of Psychosocial Oncology,* 10(3), 41–56.

Gillis, C. L., Highley, B. L., & Roberts, B. M. (1989). *Toward a science of family nursing.* Menlo Park, CA: Addison-Wesley Publishing.

Glajchen, M. (1994). Psychosocial consequences of inadequate health insurance for patients with cancer. *Cancer Practice,* 2(2), 115–120.

Gordon, M. (1993). *Manual of nursing diagnosis.* St. Louis: C. V. Mosby.

Gotcher, J. M. (1992). Interpersonal communication and psychosocial adjustment. *Journal of Psychosocial Oncology,* 10(3), 21–39.

Herbert, V. (1980). Unproven (questionable) dietary and nutritional methods in cancer prevention and treatment. *Cancer,* 58: 1930–1941.

Hileman, J. W., Lackey, N. R., & Hassanein, R. S. (1992). Identifying the needs of home caregivers of patients with cancer. *Oncology Nursing Forum,* 19(5), 771–777.

Hill, R., & Hansen, D. A. (1964). Families under stress. In Christensen, H. T. (Ed.), *Handbook of marriage and the family.* Chicago: Rand McNally.

Holland, J. C. (1989). Clinical course of cancer. In J. C. Holland & J. H. Rowland (Eds.), *Handbook of Psychooncology.* New York: Oxford University Press.

Hymovich, D. P. (1993). Child-rearing concerns of parents with cancer. *Oncology Nursing Forum,* 20(9), 1355–1360.

Jacobsen, P., & Holland, J.C. (1989). Psychological reactions to cancer surgery. In J. C. Holland & J. H. Rowland (Eds.), *Handbook of psychooncology.* New York: Oxford University Press.

Jalowiec, A., & Dudas, S. (1991). Alterations in patient coping. In S. Baird, R. McCorkle, & M. Grant, *Cancer nursing: A comprehensive textbook.* Philadelphia: W. B. Saunders.

Jassak, P. F. (1992). Families: An essential element in the care of the patient with cancer. *Oncology Nursing Forum,* 19(6), 871–876.

Laizner, A. M., Yost, L. M. S., Barg, F. K., & McCorkle, R. (1993). Needs of family caregivers of persons with cancer: A review. *Seminars in Oncology Nursing,* 9(2), 114–120.

Lamb, M. A., & Sheldon, T. A. (1994). The sexual adaptation of women treated for endometrial cancer. *Cancer Practice,* 2(2), 103–113.

Lamb, M. A., & Woods, N. F. (1981). Sexuality and the cancer patient. *Cancer Nursing,* 4(2), 137–144.

Lederberg, M., & Massie, M. J. (1993). Psychosocial and ethical issues in the care of cancer patients. In V. DeVita, S. Hellman, & S. Rosenberg (Eds.), *Cancer: Principles and practice of oncology.* Philadelphia: J. B. Lippincott.

Mahon, S. (1991). Managing the psychosocial consequences of cancer recurrence: Implications for nurses. *Oncology Nursing Forum,* 18(3), 577–583.

Mood, D. (1991). The diagnosis of cancer: A life transition. In S. Baird, R. McCorkle, & M. Grant, *Cancer nursing: A comprehensive textbook.* Philadelphia: W. B. Saunders.

Northouse, L. L., & Lancaster, D. (1994). Coping. In J. Gross & B. L. Johnson (Eds.), *Handbook of oncology nursing.* Boston: Jones & Bartlett.

Northouse, L.L., & Peters-Golden, H. (1993). Cancer and the family: Strategies to assist spouses. *Seminars in Oncology Nursing,* 9(2), 74-82.

O'Connor, A. P., Wicker, C. A., & Germino, B. B. (1990). Understanding the cancer patient's search for meaning. *Cancer Nursing,* 13(3), 167–175.

Reiger, P. T., & Rumsey, K. (1992). Responding to the educational needs of patients receiving biotherapy. In R. M. Carroll-Johnson (Ed.), *The biotherapy of cancer:*

Proceedings of a symposium. May 10, 1991, San Antonio, TX.

Rosenberg, M. (1965). *Society and the adolescent self image.* Princeton, NJ: Princeton University Press.

Saunders, J. M., & Valente, S. M. (1988). Cancer and suicide. *Oncology Nursing Forum, 15*(5), 575–581.

Schott-Baer, D. (1993). Dependent care, caregiver burden, and self care agency of spouse caregivers. *Cancer Nursing, 16*(3), 230–236.

Sparber, A. G., & Biller-Sparber, K. (1993). Immunotherapy and neuropsychiatric toxicity. *Cancer Nursing, 16*(3), 188–192.

Taylor, E. J., Baird, S. B., Malone, D., & McCorkle, R. (1993). Factors associated with anger in cancer patients and their caregivers. *Cancer Practice, 1*(2), 101–109.

Tross, S., & Holland, J.C. (1989). Psychological sequelae in cancer survivors. In J. C. Holland & J. Rowland (Eds.), *Handbook of psychooncology.* New York: Oxford University Press.

Tsevat, J. G., & LaCasse, C. L. (1992). Understanding the special needs of patients receiving biotherapy: A conceptual model. In R. M. Carroll-Johnson (Ed.), *The biotherapy of cancer: Proceedings of a symposium.* May 10, 1991, San Antonio, TX.

Valente, S. M., Saunders, J. M., & Grant, M. (1994). Oncology nurses knowledge and misconceptions about suicide. *Cancer Practice, 2*(3), 209–216.

Villejo, L., & Meyers, C. (1991). Brain function, learning styles, and cancer patient education. *Seminars in Oncology Nursing, 7*(2), 97–104.

Watson, P. (1982). Patient education: The adult with cancer. *Nursing Clinics of North America, 17*(4), 739–752.

Weisman, J., & Worden, W. (1976). The existential plight in cancer: Significance of the first 100 days. *International Journal of Psychiatry in Medicine, 7*(1), 1–15.

Whedon, M. B., & Ferrell, B. R. (1994). Quality of life in adult bone marrow transplant patients: Beyond the first year. *Seminars in Oncology Nursing, 10*(1), 42–57.

Worden, J. W. (1982). *Grief counseling and grief therapy.* New York: Springer.

World Health Organization. (1975). *Education and treatment in human sexuality: The training of health professionals.* Geneva, Switzerland: World Health Organization Technical Report.

Yarbro, C. H. (1993). Questionable methods of cancer therapy. In S. Groenwald, M. H. Frogge, M. Goodman, & C. H. Yarbro (Eds.), *Cancer nursing: Principles and practice.* Boston: Jones & Bartlett.

CHAPTER 24

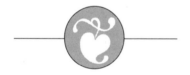

Interventions with the Dying Patient and the Family

Patricia Barry

Dying is a complex process. It usually happens over time and involves the dying person, family, friends, co-workers, the caregiving team of physicians, nurses, and social workers, and all others who come in contact with the terminally ill person.

There are many subsystems involved in the process. One subsystem is the dying person's psyche. Each person is a complex being with intrapsychic reactions occurring as a response to dying, involving a range of beliefs about death. A second subsystem is the dying person's body, which is changing both internally and externally. Awareness of these changes feeds back into the psyche and is constantly adding stress to one's ability to maintain self-esteem and body image.

A third subsystem is the family unit. It is made up of two or more people, all of whom are accustomed to filling certain roles and relating with other members in specific ways; these constitute the normal dynamics of the family. The threat of death to one of the family members can cause major shifts in family functioning. It is one of the most critical events that can happen to a family (Aguilera, 1994).

The fourth major subsystem is the caregiving subsystem, which is made up of many parts: the people who constitute it and the technical capacity of the institution to give quality care. A critical factor in quality of care is the philosophy of the institution (Clemence Vaillot, 1966). In addition, the availability of caring and competent home care personnel can make it possible for the individual and family to give quality care in the home environment. The philosophy of an institution about the dying process can be one of the most important factors in the quality of a patient's death. "Philosophy" is an abstraction, but it is made up of the beliefs of the administrative personnel in management, medicine, and nursing, which can promote or undermine a policy of support to the dying person and his or her family (Carroll, 1993; Hover, 1993; May,

Patricia Barry: *Psychosocial Nursing:*
Care of Physically Ill Patients and Their Families, 3rd ed.
© 1996 Lippincott–Raven Publishers

1993; Pickett, 1993; Pilkington, 1993; Waltman & Zimmerman, 1991).

Because of the multiple factors affecting the dying person, the dying process can be called dynamic. Elisabeth Kubler-Ross (1981, p. 1) has said that "the key to the question of death unlocks the door of life.... For those who seek to understand it, death is a highly creative force."

This chapter deals with theory about the effects of dying on the patient and family, presents intervention recommendations for the nurse to use in caring for dying patients, and discusses the effects that caring for dying patients has on the nurse. The nurse's needs during this time must be recognized as well. Many authors have identified the nurse as the person in the hospital environment who is best able to give emotional support to the dying patient (Carroll, 1993; Funk, 1992; Nyatanga, 1993; Parkinson, 1992; Tradimus, 1991; Widdrington, 1992).

UNDERSTANDING THE EMOTIONAL EFFECTS OF THE DYING PROCESS

WHAT DOES DEATH MEAN TO A DYING PERSON?

In order to understand how a dying person feels about dying, it is important to be aware that death has different meanings depending on the person's age. This difference in the way death is conceptualized extends also to family members.

Children and Adolescents

The memory of death to children and adolescents is described in Chapter 26.

Adulthood

The person in young and middle adulthood thinks of, and has concerns about, the dying process. The actual death is not as great a concern as how one dies. The fears associated with dying are related to pain, loss of control, abandonment, and the unknown. Adults are not as certain as they were in adolescence about whether there is life after death (Castles &

Murray, 1979; de Vries, Bluck, & Birren, 1993; Steinmetz et al., 1993).

Old Age

Many elderly people approach their inevitable deaths with a tranquility that is unusual in younger people. This can be due to their desire to avoid a long, painful, and gradually helpless physical condition. They may welcome death as an alternative to being useless and unwanted members of society (Claxton, 1993; Creagan, 1993; McCarthy, 1980; Zisook et al., 1993).

FEARS OF THE DYING

Pattison (1978) has described the period between the patient's becoming aware that death is inevitable and his or her actual death as the *living–dying interval*. During this time, the patient may experience many or all of the Kubler-Ross (1981) stages, which include:

1. Denial or shock
2. Anger
3. Bargaining
4. Depression
5. Acceptance

While working through these stages, a patient can experience the following specific fears (Pattison, 1978):

1. Fear of the unknown
2. Fear of loneliness
3. Fear of sorrow
4. Fear of loss of body
5. Fear of loss of self-control
6. Fear of suffering and pain
7. Fear of loss of identity
8. Fear of regression

THE FAMILY'S REACTION TO ANTICIPATED LOSS OF A LOVED ONE

Family members as well as the dying person experience the stages of grief outlined by Kubler-Ross and Bowlby (see Chapter 9). The patient and family may not experience these stages simultaneously, however.

For example, a spouse or family member may be at the anger stage and be hostile, while the patient is in the bargaining or depressed stage. Similarly, the patient may have slowly and painfully traversed the preliminary stages of coping and have reached the final acceptance stage after long months of introspection, while the spouse may still be fixated at the stage of denial. Because of the spouse's rigid denial, there may be little or no communication between them about the patient's impending death. This is frequently so when the subject of death raises the anxiety level of the patient or family, or both, to a point where avoiding discussion of death reduces anxiety. Avoidance of discussion also occurs when each spouse tries to protect the other and avoids bringing up the subject (Levine, Rudy, & Kerns, 1994; Robinson, 1993).

Aldrich (1974) suggests that one of the reasons why denial may be more prolonged in family members than in patients is because of the family's feelings of ambivalence toward the dying family member. *Ambivalence* is the presence of conflicting feelings about the same object. This is caused in part by the element of hope that is present in anticipatory grief. In conventional grief, the family member has already died; there is no hope. There is ambivalence in anticipatory grief because the patient is still alive. Because the patient is alive, the family member believes that he or she must take action to help the dying family member: spend more time with the patient, change physicians, seek a miracle cure, and protect the patient (Carroll, 1993; May, 1993; Miles, 1993; Thompson, 1992).

Guilt may be the cause of ambivalence in both anticipatory and conventional grief. A person may feel guilt if he or she does not take all action possible to "save" the dying family member. The family member may feel guilt because it seems wrong to accept the death of someone dear. Or, the family member may feel anger toward the dying person, which is intolerable. The family member may also feel guilt about being a survivor, and ask the question, "Why is he dying and not me?"

Ambivalence may be one of the most important reasons why family members become fixated at the denial stage. The result is a failure to work through and accept the coming death of their loved one. The tragedy is especially poignant if the patient has been able to accept death, but there is no one in the social system, neither family member nor health professional, with whom the patient can share this acceptance (Miles, 1993; Zisook et al., 1993).

The ideal situation is for the patient and spouse or family member to arrive at the stage of acceptance at the same time. When this occurs, Parkes (1972, p. 131) found the following in his work with terminal patients:

> It is sometimes possible for a husband and wife to work together towards an acceptance of the approaching death of one of them. If the circumstances are right they can share some of the anticipatory grief which each needs to feel. The striking thing about such cases is that, despite the sadness which is an inevitable component of anticipatory grieving, couples who choose to face the future in this way often seem to win through to a period of calm and contentment which persists to the end. After bereavement has occurred, the surviving spouse is likely to look back on this period with a satisfaction that contrasts with the dissatisfaction expressed by many who have chosen to hide the truth.

Families and their dying members do not always choose to hide the truth, but conscious or unconscious denial of the intolerable truth engendered by the anxiety of the patient, family, and professional caregivers may prevent this sharing of the process of final acceptance. The medical and nursing staffs can unintentionally join with the patient and family in the denial process and compound it (Steinmetz et al., 1993; Waltman & Zimmerman, 1991).

THE EFFECT OF THE SOCIAL ENVIRONMENT ON THE GRIEVING PERSON

Western culture rarely tolerates a grieving person's expressions of feelings for more than a few weeks after the death of a loved one. A bereaved person is expected to adjust and cease talking about feelings about the loss very soon. Friends and family members usually do not object to a bereaved person's mentioning the loss, but repeated descriptions of sadness, hopelessness, inability to sleep, and so on eventually meet with cues that the listener does not want to hear any more. In general, Western society usually commends the bereaved person who "holds up well" and shows little or no emotion or distress during the dying process, funeral, and the weeks after the loss. Actually, this person may experience much more painful distress later due to a maladaptive grief response. Wide variations in grief responses are possible when considering ethnic differences in coping with death and dying (Brotzman & Butler, 1991; Martinson, Chang, & Liang, 1993; Pickett, 1993). Chapter 5 describes the assessment of cultural variations in grief responses.

In order for the hospital care system to facilitate the patient's and family's acceptance of death, caregivers need to understand the normal reactions experienced during the stages of bereavement. It is frequently the caregiver's discomfort in listening to patients' and family members' anticipatory grief that causes distancing and avoidance to occur. By understanding the normal feelings of a grieving person, nurses may be able to encourage and validate these emotions (Crawley, 1991; Ufema, 1993; Widdrington, 1992).

NORMAL EMOTIONAL RESPONSE TO LOSS

Responses to loss will vary with each person. The following descriptions of the feelings associated with a major loss are the same for a patient anticipating his or her own death and for family members preparing for the loss of their loved one or who have already experienced the loss.

The usual response to a major loss is disbelief. The ego will not accept this sudden, terrible information. In an emergency room, for example, if parents are told that their child did not survive a school bus accident, they will react with cries of, "No, no, no," "I can't believe it," or "Are you sure?" The other reaction may be one of shock; the news does not seem to penetrate (Davidhizar & Kirk, 1993).

When a patient or bereaved person "holds up well," it may be because the person is in denial or has repressed the news. Family members and friends usually are relieved. They compliment the person's stoicism, courage, and so on, thus positively reinforcing the behavior. In a few weeks, when the repression disappears and the person has full awareness, true feelings may emerge. The person may be afraid to express them, despite feeling that he or she is "bursting" with grief. The social system, in effect, tells the patient or bereaved person, "We cannot tolerate these feelings in you." After all, the person has been complimented for being courageous (Carroll, 1993; Parkinson, 1992).

A normal feeling that emerges after a loss is an overwhelming sadness accompanied by crying and sobbing. The grieving person feels unable to control when the waves of sadness will occur. Seeing an item that belonged to the loved person, or thinking of the loved person, will bring on greater depths of sadness. Because being stoic is the socially reinforced behavior, most people fear losing control entirely. The feelings are frightening because of their intensity (Carroll, 1993; McCallum, Piper, & Morin, 1993; Pilkington, 1993).

For family members in anticipatory or conventional grief, the period of *awareness*, when the full realization of the loss occurs, represents the beginning of grief work. This marks the beginning of the middle stage of bereavement (Bowlby, 1980). During this phase, the lost person is idealized. The bereaved has a great need to talk about the lost person and is preoccupied with thoughts of this person. Illusory phenomena are very common. For example, the bereaved may think he or she sees the lost person driving a car, in a crowd, or at any specific place where the two of them often interacted. These illusory phenomena, accompanied by frequent nightmares, cause the bereaved to think he or she is losing sanity (Bowlby, 1980). The feeling of losing one's sanity is not unusual. This fear is so frightening that it is rarely shared with others (Thompson, 1992; Zisook et al., 1993).

A similar process can occur for the dying person, except that these thoughts and feelings are experienced about the self. The dying person usually reviews his or her life, relationships, work, and so on. The dying person may experience episodes of *derealization*. These are profound emotional periods when the person feels detached from the world around him or her (Nuland, 1994; Parkinson, 1992; Pickett, 1993).

During this time, neurovegetative signs of reactive depression may occur, including insomnia, loss of appetite, and loss of energy. The grieving person sighs frequently (Bowlby, 1980). He or she may feel overwhelming anxiety, which further adds to the feeling of loss of control and feelings of "going crazy." Dying people experience anger about their illness. The accompanying feelings of helplessness and hopelessness may be projected onto family and caregivers (Carroll, 1993; Creagan, 1993).

Another normal emotional response in family members is one of anger toward the lost person. The anger is caused by the feeling that the dead person has abandoned them. These feelings of anger are abhorrent to grieving people and strong guilt is the result (McCallum et al., 1993; Wolfelt, 1991).

It is not unusual for feelings of acute grief to continue for over a year. The feelings described above may be quite intense for many months, accompanied by marked mood swings and ambivalence. The pain and yearning for the lost person may intensify prior to the one year anniversary (Engel, 1975) and gradually diminish. Following the anniversary, the experience of acute grief and moderate-to-severe mood swings slowly come under control. A family member may begin to feel more at peace as the intrapsychic conflicts created by the grief process begins to diminish (Carroll, 1993; McCallum, Piper, & Morin, 1993).

FAMILY SYSTEM RESPONSES TO A DYING MEMBER

When a family learns that one of its members is dying, it is immediately subject to a variety of new stresses. These stresses affect all the dynamics in the family system. Whether a family is "healthy" or has many pathological coping patterns, the stress can be severe. One factor that immediately determines the severity of this stressor is the role the dying member fills in the family (Aguilera, 1994; Carroll, 1993; Creagan, 1993; Hansen, 1984; Schneider, 1984).

There are obvious roles that are highly valued in a family: the role of mother or father in an active family, the role of a child of any age, the role of a loved grandparent. Another role less-recognized by many caregivers is that of the person who maintains equilibrium in the family. For example, the role could be filled by a single uncle who has been involved in a family that is fatherless or in which the father is weak and nonsupportive. Another example is that of an elderly woman who always encouraged her children's dependency. Accordingly, even though her children may be in their 50s or 60s, her loss may be highly threatening to one or more of them.

FAMILY AS SUPPORT SYSTEM

One of the most important factors in a person's ability to cope with grief is the effectiveness of his or her psychological defenses. These defense mechanisms will determine if the person's coping is adaptive or maladaptive. Another important factor is the way the family system normally manages stress. The anticipated or actual loss of a family member is one of the most stressful events a family experiences (Aguilera, 1994). If the family's coping ability fails, it will have a definite impact on the patient's coping strength (Davies, 1993; Miles, 1993; Wolfelt, 1991).

The coping pattern of each of its members strongly affects the way a family responds to stress. If the members are accustomed to dealing with threatening events by using immature defenses, the family is at greater risk for maladaptation. If only a few members respond maladaptively, the more mature coping responses of the other members can help to promote the adaptation of the entire family (Creagan, 1993; Smith & Regnard, 1993). More likely, however, family members respond similarly.

Research on families in crisis has indicated that the family coping response to a threatening event becomes formed by 1 to 4 weeks after the initial threat occurs (Aguilera, 1994). During this time, it is possible to see both adaptive and maladaptive defenses working. A list of defense mechanisms appears in Chapter 3.

ANNIVERSARY REACTION

An *anniversary reaction* to the date of death or the date when the illness was originally diagnosed is an important phenomenon that occurs in most people. It occurs whether the grief resolution was normal or pathological. In an anniversary reaction, someone who has lost a significant person will experience an emotional or physical reaction around the time of the anniversary of the loss. A person usually is at a loss to explain what is going on (Engel, 1975; Kaplan & Sadock, 1994, 1995). The following case example will help to clarify this concept.

CASE EXAMPLE

A general hospital patient was admitted for a respiratory ailment in March. Her medical history revealed that she had been admitted to the hospital during February or March each year during the previous 6 years because of various ailments: hernia repair, cholecystectomy, abdominal pain, and so on. Questioning by the nurse revealed that one of her children had died on March 20 years earlier. Her husband's birthday was in March. She had been divorced from him in March, and he later died in March. ❦

The month of March was highly significant to this woman. She had been unaware of the relationship between the month of March and the repressed painful memories it recalled at an unconscious level, and her numerous health problems.

George Engel, one of the leading liaison psychiatrists in the United States, wrote a sensitive article about his own anniversary reactions to the deaths of his twin brother and father, with whom he had close relationships. Engel's brother died of a heart attack in the summer of 1963. Following the death, Engel experienced most of the disquieting symptoms of grief reaction described above. He also became obsessed with the idea that he, too, would experience a heart attack. Three weeks short of the first anniversary of his brother's death his prediction was fulfilled.

Immediately after the death of his brother and on significant anniversaries, Engel had dreams that gave him remarkable insights into his relationship with his brother and his reaction to the deaths of his brother and father. His father died at age 58. In Engel's own 58th year he had unusual psychological and physical experiences that were strongly associated with his brother and father (Engel, 1975).

It is easy to understand that people can be aware of upcoming anniversaries of losses of significant people. It is more difficult to understand that the anniversary reactions described in the examples above were unconscious. People repress their awareness of these anniversaries, yet the unconscious mourning process is an active one. To the unaware person, the outward manifestations may take many forms that are never connected to the original loss.

MALADAPTIVE GRIEVING PROCESS

If a person does not proceed through the stages of grief outlined above, it is possible for a maladaptive grieving process to occur. A maladaptive grieving process, also known as *pathological bereavement*, is characterized by maladaptive coping in response to a significant loss. There is either excessive repression of grief or an excessive and prolonged emotional response that extends beyond 1 year (Carroll, 1993; McCallum, Piper, & Morin, 1993; Wolfelt, 1991; Zisook et al., 1993).

Maladaptive grieving can be manifested in many ways. Some people become fixated in denial. Although they are intellectually aware of the death of the person, there is little or no affective or feeling response. This is caused by the defense mechanism called *isolation* (see Chapter 3). The feelings of grief are repressed or are delayed indefinitely. Sometimes, years later, another loss will trigger the emotional response that was denied during the first loss (Parkes, 1972). In other cases, the feelings of grief may never surface, but the person may become socially guarded and isolated.

Such persons may not feel sadness or display the range of emotions usually associated with a major loss. Their feelings are deeply repressed. Some of the ways maladaptive grief may be demonstrated are by prolonged immobility and withdrawn states; hyperactivity, a flurry of activity that helps the bereaved to avoid the pain; excessive spending of money and pleasure seeking; and alcohol or tranquilizer abuse (Carroll, 1993; Pilkington, 1993).

Depression may also occur many months or years after the original loss. When it occurs years later, it may be misdiagnosed as endogenous depression (Bowlby, 1980). Another outcome of maladaptive grieving is that the bereaved may display excessive and inappropriate anger toward some person in his or her social system. This person becomes the focus of the bereaved's rage. This anger can also be turned inward and be expressed by a physical symptom (Cassem & Barsky, 1991).

CONSEQUENCES OF UNRESOLVED GRIEF FOR FAMILY MEMBERS

Most families have periods of several weeks to several years to begin to accept the impending loss of a family member. If the opportunity to work through the death of a person is not developed before the loss occurs, it is possible that the coping strategies developed by family members during the conventional grief stage may become more maladaptive and prolong the bereavement process (Pilkington, 1993; Wolfelt, 1993; Zisook et al., 1993). Unresolved grief may lead to abnormal psychopathology. Studies have found that unresolved grief led to a greater than normal incidence of physical and mental illness in bereaved family members (Aguilera, 1994; Davies, 1993).

Engel (1961) theorized that the experience of grief imposes psychological stress that disturbs the total adjustment of the person left behind; the biochemical, physiological, and psychological spheres all can be involved in the normal as well as the abnormal bereavement response. Engel's theories are compatible with Selye's stress theory, presented in Chapter 6.

In a major study of widowed people, Rees and Lutkins (1967) found that their mortality was 15 times higher than normal during the 2-year period following the loss of their spouses. Jagger and Sutton (1991) found a higher-than-average risk of mortality for bereaved widows during the first 6 months following the deaths of their spouses. It has also been suggested

that a history that includes unresolved loss is a significant finding in a majority of cancer patients (Bahnson, 1981).

Another type of unresolved grief reaction is one in which the lost person preoccupies the grieving person's mind more than a year after the loss occurred. Some of the causes of a delayed grief resolution are an inability to express rage or cry about the loss, lack of supportive persons in the environment, overidentification with the dead person, anger and ambivalence toward him or her, an earlier unresolved grief reaction, and prolonged encouragement by a social system of the bereaved's grief reaction (secondary gain) (Parkes, 1972). As mentioned above, it is not unusual for a delayed grief reaction to occur at or near the time of the first or a subsequent anniversary of the death (Engel, 1975; Kaplan & Sadock, 1994).

The following research findings emphasize the effects of unresolved grief. Rosenbaum (1981), in a study of medication use of widows and widowers, discovered many significant facts about the ways they maladaptively coped with their spouses' deaths. A partial list of findings is as follows:

1. There was an increase in the use of psychotropic medication (tranquilizers, antidepressants, hypnotics) following the loss of their spouse. Although a slight leveling-off occurred, the amount of medication used remained higher than it was before the loss.
2. The most common reasons given for taking such medications was "to help relax" and "to help with sleep."
3. These people continued using psychotropic drugs, some of them for many years.
4. Most subjects reported that refills for these medications were obtained by calling the physician's office and talking to the nurse or receptionist. They were given either "no instructions" or "unsatisfactory instructions" regarding their use.
5. Of those subjects who knew their spouse was dying, only 4 of 26 had free and open discussion with their spouse about the impending death. Of those who had free

discussions, none of the spouses was taking medication after the death.*

These and other studies reported in this chapter poignantly illustrate the great need for caregivers to be able to identify the maladaptive coping responses of dying people and their families. Too often, caregivers assume that these responses are temporary and that after the patient's death the problems will decrease. This is not usually so. The long-term consequences of unresolved grief are of major significance.

Unless some perceptive person recognizes the problem, these people will experience a changed existence because of maladaptive coping. Their quality of life can be diminished for years, both during the terminal illness and after the death of their loved one. This maladaptation can persist through the rest of their lives (Carroll, 1993; Creagan, 1993; Pickett, 1993; Wolfelt, 1991; Zisook et al., 1993).

Home care nurses and nurses in primary and outpatient care settings are more likely to see people with unresolved and maladaptive grief than are nurses in inpatient settings. These patients should be referred for individual or family consultation (Baile et al., 1993; Waltman & Zimmerman, 1991).

NURSING DIAGNOSIS OF INEFFECTIVE COPING IN FAMILY MEMBERS

In general, hospital nurses usually are the first to observe distress in the families of dying people. The following diagnoses, approved by the National Group for the Classification of Nursing Diagnosis, could be used when identifying an ineffective response in one or more grieving family members:

Adjustment, Impaired
Anticipatory Grieving
Anxiety
Body Image Disturbance
Caregiver Role Strain
Caregiver Role Strain, Risk for
Chronic Low Self Esteem

---

*Number 5 above is a significant finding that can assist caregivers in understanding the dynamics of unresolved and maladaptive grief. It points out how essential it is for the nurse or some caregiver to promote an open environment where spouses can be honest with one another.

Comfort, Altered
Communication, Impaired Verbal
Community Coping, Ineffective
Confusion, Acute
Confusion, Chronic
Constipation
Decision Conflict (Specify)
Defensive Coping
Denial, Ineffective
Diarrhea
Dysfunctional Grieving
Family Coping, Compromised, Ineffective
Family Coping: Disabling, Ineffective
Family Coping: Potential for Growth
Family Process, Alcoholism, Altered
Family Processes, Altered
Fatigue
Fear
Grieving
Grieving, Anticipatory
Grieving, Dysfunctional
Growth and Development, Altered
Health Maintenance, Altered
Hopelessness
Individual Coping, Ineffective
Knowledge Deficit (Specify)
Loneliness, Risk for
Management of Therapeutic Regimen, Ineffective
Memory, Impaired
Noncompliance
Nutrition: Less than Body Requirements, Altered
Nutrition: More than Body Requirements, Altered
Nutrition: Potential for more than Body Requirements, Altered
Pain
Pain, Chronic
Parent/Infant/Child Attachments, Risk for Altered
Parental Role Conflict
Parenting, Altered
Parenting, Risk for Altered
Personal Identity Disturbance
Post-Trauma Response
Powerlessness
Protection, Altered
Role Performance, Altered
Self-Care Deficit
    Bathing/Hygiene
    Feeding

Dressing/Grooming
Toileting
Self-Esteem, Chronic Low
Self-Esteem, Situational Low
Self-Esteem, Disturbance
Self-Mutilation, Risk for
Sensory/Perceptual Alterations (Specify) (visual, auditory, kinesthetic, gustatory, tactile, olfactory)
Sexual Dysfunction
Sexuality Patterns, Altered
Situational Low Self-Esteem
Sleep Pattern Disturbance
Social Interactions, Impaired
Social Isolation
Spiritual Distress
Spiritual Well-Being, Potential for Enhanced
Suicide, High Risk for
Thought Processes, Altered

It is important for nurses to be able to recognize ineffective coping patterns in families during the early part of the patient's admission. When it is obvious that the family is not coping effectively and if this ineffective coping continues to occur, intervention should begin with the family. Intervention theory is outlined in Chapter 16. Unless the problem is severe, intervention can be appropriately carried out by the nurse. The information on therapeutic communication skills in Chapter 2 and crisis intervention in Chapter 16 can be used as a guide. If nursing intervention does not result in evidence of adaptation or effective coping, psychiatric consultation is recommended.

There are a few important points to keep in mind when working with family members who are experiencing anticipatory grief or bereavement. One is that the most helpful approach for some people is *talking*. Talking can allow the acceptance process to occur and unconscious blocks to be worked through. Chapter 2 explains helpful approaches with these family members. The subsection in this chapter on what to say to a dying patient can also be of assistance when discussing the actual or pending death of a loved one with family members.

Another important point is that some people do not want to talk. When a person resists your attempts to open the subject of the loved one's death, that person is giving you the message that he or she is not ready or willing to talk. If

the nurse persists, increased anxiety will result. The resistance of the family member can be gently tested every day or so. A person may be unable to talk because he or she is in the stage of denial, as described earlier in the chapter, or has a personality style that cannot tolerate interpersonal intimacy. Such personality styles are the aloof and uninvolved, suspicious, controlling, and superior types (see Chapter 15).

The attending physician should be included in the nursing care plan for the family. When the nurse articulates the observed problems and outlines the intervention approach that will be used, the physician will be more aware of the maladaptive process and may be able to provide extra support to the family.

NURSING INTERVENTION WITH THE DYING PATIENT

Care of the dying patient and family can be one of the greatest challenges in nursing. Sometimes it is difficult to know the "right" way to talk with these patients and their families. Many nurses worry that they will say or do something that will add to the patient's or family member's distress. It is important to remember one thing: there is no "right" way to work with a dying person.

Because the personality of every human is unique, there is a vast variety of interpersonal responses and styles of communication that are therapeutic. What one nurse would say to a dying person might be quite different than another nurse, yet both approaches can be equally therapeutic. In this section specific aspects of care of the dying person will be presented. The stress that nurses themselves experience in caring for the dying will also be discussed.

DISCUSSING DEATH WITH THE PATIENT

Although it may be difficult to acknowledge, the question about whether it is upsetting to a patient to talk about his or her own death may actually be a projection of the upset that caregivers may feel in talking to a dying patient about the subject. A study by Kubler-Ross (1975) reported that only 2% of dying patients did not want to talk about their deaths. Murray Bowen (1976), in his work with physically ill patients who were dying, as well as psychiatric patients who wanted to die, found that they were relieved to find someone they could talk with about dying; they felt better afterward.

The patient's physician is responsible for telling the patient and the family that the patient is dying. It is viewed as unethical to withhold information from the patient about his or her current condition or impending death. It is not uncommon, however, for the patient to deny the original discussion with the physician in which the person learns that he or she is dying. On occasion, nurses become angry with physicians whom they believe are not talking with dying patients or family members about the patient's terminal condition. Before making such a judgment, it is important for the nurse to talk with the physician about what he or she has told the patient. An individual's ego is on constant guard to protect from threatening or disturbing awarenesses. The dying patient's ego will maintain denial of unpleasant reality until its more mature defenses are able to cope with troubling thoughts and feelings about dying.

It can be helpful for the nurse to be present when the physician tells the patient the prognosis. Telling a patient that he or she has a terminal illness is difficult, and the physician understandably may choose to do this alone with the patient or the family. If the physician is willing to have the nurse present, the following benefits to the patient may occur:

1. The nurse will be present to support the patient emotionally when being told the threatening prognosis.
2. The nurse will be able to reinforce the information given to the patient by the physician.
3. The nurse knows exactly what the patient was told and will be in a position to assess the patient's response and plan appropriate interventions to promote adaptation.

APPROACHES WITH DENYING PATIENTS

If the patient's denial continues beyond a few days, it is important to begin to intervene gent-

ly to determine the strength of the denial. It is essential never to confront a denying patient directly with the reality he or she is struggling to avoid. The persistence of strong denial of more than a day or two indicates that the awareness of impending death is terrifying to him or her.

In order to understand the powerful effects of direct and forceful confrontation, think of the following analogy. The denial of such a patient can be compared to an eggshell. It appears hard, but it is brittle. A direct blow will cause it to fracture and the contents to spill out with no control. Similarly, direct confrontation could crack the patient's denial. The resulting inability to keep out the unbearable awareness could cause overwhelming anxiety.

A patient who is in denial can be compared to a person who is frightened and hides in a room for refuge; he shuts and locks the door to keep out the environment he fears. Can you understand how caregivers' or family members' direct confrontation of such a patient only results in a more disabling type of denial?

Because of the amount of time nurses spend with patients, they are often in a better position than the physician, who makes a brief, daily visit, to test denial gradually and gently in order to assess its strength. The answers patients formulate to nurses' questions can help in a gradual acceptance of the reality of their illness at their own pace. In the analogy of the frightened person hiding in the room described above, the patient is being allowed to open the door rather than the caregiver breaking it down. It is important to remember that the patient's "door" is closed because of his or her level of anxiety. The patient can be talked with through the "door" of denial by asking the following questions. These questions can be used with dying patients who are denying the severity of their illnesses or their family members who may be in denial.

QUESTIONS TO TEST THE STRENGTH OF DENIAL IN DYING PATIENTS

How are you feeling today?
How do you think you are doing?
How does your physician think you are doing?
How does your family feel about your being in the hospital?

What does your family think about your illness?

How much longer do you think you will be in the hospital?

These questions are usually not asked in a series; rather, they are interspersed in normal conversation with the patient. Similar questions can be asked each day so that the level of denial can be compared with that of previous days. If the answers indicate that the patient is continuing rigidly to deny awareness of his or her terminal status beyond a few days, the attending physician should be consulted. Specific examples of this strong denial can be discussed with a recommendation that the physician talk with the patient and family again.

If there is a clinical specialist (oncology, pulmonary, gerontology, or some other specialty) working with the dying patient, these concerns can be discussed. Specific recommendations can be requested of the clinical specialist. If, despite the assistance of these caregivers, the patient's or family member's denial persists, psychiatric liaison consultation should be considered and discussed with the patient's physician and specialist (O'Connor, 1991).

One important reason why a continuation of strong denial is maladaptive is that the psychic energy required to maintain the defense is both an emotional and physical drain. It causes the patient's openness as a person to be diminished. This guardedness has a serious effect on the quality of the patient's relationships with others (Carroll, 1993; Pickett, 1993; Pilkington, 1993; Wolfelt, 1991). The family, especially the spouse, may need to be able to talk to the patient, but the patient avoids any mention of his or her condition. Eventually, the patient's unyielding denial can undermine the effectiveness of the family system in coping with the impending death.

Another negative effect of strong denial is due to general system effects. The level of stress that results from constant psychic strain eventually causes the sympathetic nervous system to respond. This triggers a stress response in all of the other body systems (cardiovascular, pulmonary, gastrointestinal, and so on) (Gatti et al., 1993; Goldstein & Niaura, 1992; Temoshok & Dreher, 1993).

IMPORTANCE OF CONTROL IN THE DYING PROCESS

Kastenbaum (1978) reminds us that the anxiety-provoking aspects of working with dying patients frequently cause caregivers to need to control two aspects of the dying process:

Their own feelings about the patient's death.

The patient's feelings about his or her own death. (If the patient becomes out-of-control, the caregiver would feel inadequate in providing help.)

Caregivers, in their desire to give care, may indeed give good technical care but may become unaware of the way they remove the patient's control of his or her own dying process (May, 1993). The following poignant case example shows how this happens.

CASE EXAMPLE

Amos is a 53-year-old man with an 8-year history of chronic, obstructive pulmonary disease. His condition is terminal. He is not expected to live more than a few days. He has been a patient in the respiratory intensive care unit for 6 weeks. He is intubated by permanent tracheotomy. He is fully alert and very anxious. When his anxiety becomes acute, he has an order for a low dose of morphine. (Sedation of patients with advanced lung disease is usually avoided because it would compromise respiratory status.)

During his hospitalization, when he experienced respiratory distress despite the intubation, he asked for frequent "bagging." (Bagging is the extra breath of oxygen that can be given by attaching the oxygen to a semisolid plastic ball or bag, as it is called.) He asked for extra bagging three or four times an hour. He was very anxious before the bagging began and relaxed markedly when he received the extra oxygen. Eventually, he wanted to be bagged almost every 5 to 8 minutes. Recent x-ray studies, however, demonstrated that Amos's lung tissue was becoming dangerously dilated. There was danger that rupture of a segment of lung could occur with the extra pressure of bagging. Death would be the certain result.

His physicians abruptly ordered the cessation of all bagging. The patient was told of the decision. The nurses, who were at the patient's bedside almost constantly, cried because of their concern about the patient's emotional response to the loss of his only security in the unit. They also were crying because they had lost the only means they had to decrease his anxiety level and give him at least a small level of comfort. 🍎

What about the patient in this situation? Was he given any choice about the amount of medication he received? (A higher level could have given him a more comfortable emotional state and helped him to die more peacefully.) Was he given any choice in the bagging decision? What would you have wanted for yourself if you were the patient in this situation? If the patient were someone you loved?

The ultimate question of whether the care of this patient was the most supportive and allowed him any control of his own death is complicated by ethical questions. The ability to maintain life in sophisticated intensive care units often removes the chance to die naturally.

These are difficult issues. Many physicians in smaller hospitals and rural settings continue to maintain a high level of control over the patient's dying process. They believe it is their responsibility to make choices about how the patient will die. Neither a passive nor aggressive approach by a nurse will ever change such a physician's beliefs. Perhaps a gentle yet assertive approach on behalf of the patient or family will effect gradual change. The process can be slow, however, especially if the physician has been dealing with dying patients autocratically for many years. Intelligent study of these issues by hospital ethics committees made up of well-informed representatives of the caregiving professions can potentially provide guidelines to reduce the emotional distress caused by cases such as the one described above.

Maintaining the Patient's Choices

On some occasions, medical and nursing caregivers make choices for dying patients about treatment plans and use of analgesics, or make decisions regarding resuscitation in case of death. It is important to remember that this is the patient's life. If mentally competent, the patient should be presented with the options. For example, it may be a dying person's very important but unexpressed wish to be fully awake and alert as long as possible before death in order to interact with his or her family.

Well-meaning caregivers may decide that the patient's pain would be best controlled by a morphine drip that would maintain a constant analgesia but decrease alertness. They may have received approval from the family for this measure. Before caregivers assume that they know what is best for the patient, however, it is the alert patient's right to be a part of this decision-making process. The advantages and disadvantages of the possible alternatives can be described. Caregivers can strongly encourage particular approaches; usually the patient agrees. This patient, even when agreeing with caregivers' recommendations, will develop a deeper trust in the caregivers for having been given the opportunity to make the final decision. The lack of this approach may cause some caregivers to carry burdens of responsibility that they have taken on themselves.

WHERE TO DIE?

The staffing patterns and wards of general hospitals generally are not designed to provide the supportive and comfort-promoting measures that can contribute to a peaceful death. The main goal of general hospitals and caregivers is to save or maintain lives; death is not easily accepted there. Caregivers frequently consider the death of a patient to be a reflection on themselves and their care (Carroll, 1993; Cassem, 1991).

An alternative to care in the general hospital is a hospice. A *hospice* is a special institution for the dying that provides strong support to all people involved in the dying process: the patient, family, and caregivers. The hospice concept was begun in England and is being introduced in other countries in the form of hospice institutions as well as hospice home care programs run by visiting nurse agencies. In a hospice:

> [Care is] given by nurses who are able to accept their own feelings about death in order that they are able to listen compassionately and constructively to the fears of others. They

provide physical and psychological support that enables the patient to make the transition from life to death peacefully [Castles & Murray, 1979, p. 319].

A third alternative is to allow the dying person to remain at home. Before advocating one type of care over another, there are some important considerations. How is the patient coping with his or her impending death? How is the family coping with the patient's dying? If the patient and a majority of family members are coping by maintaining high levels of denial and there is virtually no openness in family communication, the patient would not do well at home until, and unless, the denial level in both the patient and the family is lowered. If a patient is discharged into a home where either the patient or family is maintaining a high level of denial, the potential for high anxiety and maladaptation because of the strained communications in the family system is inevitable.

Similarly, the patient and family who are grieving about the upcoming loss, have a very low level of defense, and are not coping well will, in some instances, be at further risk if they attempt to have the patient die at home. The family may need the extra support available in an institution, as well as the chance to be away from the patient for extended hours. Support is essential to this patient and family if the grieving is to proceed in an adaptive manner. A hospice environment would be ideal in helping them to work through these uncomfortable and overwhelming feelings.

Defense mechanisms cannot be willed into use. They are unconsciously set into action by protective emotional mechanisms. The external supportive environment provided by caring nurses in a hospice can avert a crisis until the temporarily overwhelmed egos resume their adaptive capabilities.

The home can be an ideal environment for a dying patient if the patient and most of the family members are coping well. "Coping well" means that while they may be experiencing the emotional upheaval of dying, their emotional responses are not stagnant. It is essential that the caregivers in the home receive support from others outside of the home. A prolonged illness in the home can result in family caregivers' emotional and physical exhaustion by the time their loved one dies. Home nursing services should be used in order to provide support. If a hospice approach to home nursing services is available, this can provide needed psychological support to the patient and family (Crawley, 1991; Miles, 1993; Nyatanga, 1993; Wolfelt, 1991).

PAIN MANAGEMENT

One day, while working with a staff that was greatly concerned about a dying patient who was experiencing severe pain, I suggested that nurses are in a prime position to monitor patients' pain and make recommendations for pain management. When I asked the nurses if they thought this might be so, they agreed unanimously. When I asked them why, they said, "Because we see how they suffer, and the physicians don't."

Pain management is an important instance of nurses being able to serve patients as advocates. (See Chapter 21 for a complete discussion of pain management.) Unless the physician is given specific examples of the patient's response to pain, he or she cannot make a decision regarding changes in pain medication. Nurses who have cared for many dying patients have had an opportunity to observe patients' responses to particular types of medications, doses, and time intervals. Nurses can and should make specific recommendations for medication management they believe would help the patient.

Usually, most physicians are receptive and frequently are willing to adopt all or part of nurses' recommendations for pain management in complex patients. If the physician chooses not to follow the nurse's suggestion, there often is an underlying reason why the change could further complicate the patient's physical condition. Without an opportunity for the physician to explain a rationale, the nurse may mistakenly believe that the physician is insensitive and uncaring.

The advantage of nurses being honest with physicians in these types of cases is that honesty promotes communication within the caregiving team at a time when the patient needs all members of the team to be working in his or her behalf. If conflict is present because nurses are angry at physicians' management of the patient, the patient's care becomes less than optimum.

Another important factor in the patient's ability to tolerate pain is the patient's ego defensive structure. A stoic patient is, in most cases, a person who has an internal locus of control (see Chapter 9) and usually uses a moderate level of denial in dealing with unpleasant external or internal stimuli. This person also frequently has a high level of differentiation between intellect and emotion; the patient's intellect is able to maintain control over the unpleasant feeling state associated with pain. This patient frequently may choose to remain "in control" of pain rather than to feel drugged. This person's perception of pain may indeed be at a level that is more tolerable than it would be for another patient with a similar disease.

At the other extreme is the patient who has always been highly dependent on others, has an external locus of control, and has a low level of denial in dealing with threatening perceptions. This patient often has a low pain threshold and chooses to be medicated as often and as much as possible, because otherwise he or she would feel out of control. This person's feelings often are at a low level of differentiation from his or her intellect; accordingly, the sensation of pain may quickly become overwhelming.

The final analysis of what nurses can do for dying patients in pain is to present the alternatives for the control of pain and then let the patient review the options to best support his or her needs. The nurse may become the liaison, if necessary, between patient and physician, so that the physician has the information necessary to order appropriate pain relief for the patient. Ongoing nursing assessment and evaluation of the patient's response to pain medication are essential if revisions in the physician's orders are necessary (Bouckoms & Hackett, 1991; Horsley, 1982).

In pediatric, geriatric, and intensive care settings, it is not uncommon for nurses to be asked by family members to medicate their loved ones. If this happens, but the nurse assesses that the patient is not in pain, it is helpful to sit and talk with the family members. They often are feeling helpless and guilty about their inability to do something to assist the loved one. With the opportunity to talk about these feelings, family members may become less insistent in their requests for pain medication that actually may not be necessary.

RELIGION AND THE DYING PATIENT

Most large hospitals employ chaplains. Hospital chaplains have prepared for their role with special counseling courses. In many instances they have completed pastoral counseling programs. They are aware of the effects of loss on the human spirit and are prepared to intervene with patients or family members. In many cases, patients and families have relationships with the clergy of the houses of worship to which they belong, and receive extra support from them during their time of crisis.

Nurses are usually the care coordinators of dying patients, and know what resources are available to them. It is important to offer the services of pastoral care to the dying patient and family. During this difficult period, it can be comforting for family members to speak with a clergyman. The emotions that people experience at such a time may cause them concern and guilt. Frequently, it is only by talking with an understanding clergyman that feelings of guilt can be relieved. Medical and nursing caregivers may be able to discuss these issues with them, but often they will only feel relief of their guilt by talking with a religious professional (Carpenito, 1993).

A frequent cause for concern in many dying patients and family members is their anger toward God for allowing the terminal illness to occur. These feelings arouse strong guilt (Carroll, 1993; Miles, 1993; Parkinson, 1992). Only when they are assured of the normality of these feelings, and their usually temporary status, does the feeling of guilt begin to diminish. Patients and family members also worry about their sins of omission and commission toward one another. Family members' feelings of ambivalence toward their dying member also arouse strong guilt feelings (Carroll, 1993; Miles, 1993; Parkinson, 1992). If you offer to call a chaplain and are refused, remember that later the patient or family member may be relieved by talking with a religious person. At appropriate intervals the availability of the hospital chaplain can continue to be offered to the patient.

WHAT CAN THE NURSE SAY?

In the physical care of patients, treatments are performed following somewhat rigid guidelines about how to carry out each step of the procedure. Many nurses experience self-expectations that they should be able to do something to help. Usually these self-expectations can be carried out in the physical care of the patient in the general hospital setting. There seems to be a never-ending list of medications to be given, treatments to be done, nursing care plans to be written, and so on. When caring for patients, nurses usually have a predetermined list of things to do. Their talking with patients usually falls into three categories:

1. Discussing the patient's physical and emotional response to the illness.
2. Formal teaching regarding hospital or home care protocols.
3. Superficial conversation about weather, news events, and so on.

When working with a long-term patient whose condition is terminal and who will be hospitalized until death, the usual discussion categories may be inappropriate, for several reasons:

1. Discussing the patient's responses to the illness may become taboo. Nurses may fear the patient's feelings and that they won't know how to respond to them.
2. Formal teaching is no longer needed by this patient because care has become supportive and palliative rather than restorative.
3. Superficial conversation may not be appropriate because the patient may be depressed, in pain, or both.

The consequence of nurses' loss of these normal communications usually causes some anxiety. This is a normal response. When there is uncertainty about how to act in a situation, anxiety is frequently experienced, and whenever possible, the situation is avoided as a way of reducing the anxiety.

Rather than being a situation to be avoided, working with dying patients can be one of the most rewarding aspects of nursing. In order to work comfortably with dying patients, caregivers must personally deal with some major personal philosophical issues that influence their comfort or discomfort with the dying patient. The issues are expressed in the following questions:

How do you feel about your own death?
What do you think happens after death?
To what emotional or physical degree should life be maintained?

These are questions that touch people at their core. They cannot be superficially answered; rather, they are pondered, sometimes for a lifetime.

When nurses are able to work through their own feelings and fears about their own deaths, they frequently find themselves more at ease with dying patients. Sometimes it is by working with dying people and learning from their dignity and peace that nurses' fears of death are decreased. Nurses who have thought about and resolved some of their concerns about death are able to be more open with dying patients. They are able to perceive accurately the emotional state of a dying person at a given time. By commenting to a patient, "You seem worried today" or "You seemed sad after your son left tonight," the patient feels understood. This is not an invasion of privacy.

If the nurse's perceptions are inaccurate or if the patient does not want to talk about feelings at that time, those intentions will be expressed, or lack of a verbal response will indicate the patient's unwillingness to enter into such a discussion. The dying person is responsible for his or her feelings; the chance that the nurse will suddenly trigger a strong emotional response is much less than the chance of triggering relief in allowing bottled-up feelings to be released. If the patient begins to cry, this can also be a relief. The nurse's concern can be supportive and can be demonstrated by sitting or staying with the patient or holding the patient's hand. Tears will subside and talking may occur. The patient may need someone to sit quietly with him or her. The patient's needs will be demonstrated verbally or nonverbally.

Many nurses worry that they will say something "wrong" to a dying patient. If a nurse genuinely cares about a patient, it is far more likely that her comments will tell the patient that he or she is understood. An important point to remember is that the nurse's presence and touch may be far more comforting to the patient than conversation; it is not essential to speak comforting words.

CAN NURSES SHOW EMOTION WHEN WORKING WITH DYING PATIENTS?

An issue that is rarely discussed is whether it is all right for nurses to show emotion when working with dying people and their families. Many nurses feel that it is not "professional" to be emotional with patients. They report that this belief came from their nursing education process. Accordingly, they judge themselves "unprofessional" if they are moved to tears by the tragedy of a stillbirth or the courage of a young dying father.

Stop and think for a moment. When you experienced a major disappointment or personal tragedy, was there someone you talked with whom you found very caring and supportive? Did that person stare at you without expression? Did that person rapidly shift the conversation to another, "safer" topic? Did that person occupy herself with busywork as a way of avoiding further awareness of your problem?

The answer is probably no. If she had done any of the things mentioned above, it is doubtful you would have considered her caring and supportive. Instead, she probably sat quietly and listened; she probably asked a few questions that let you know she understood. She most likely had an expression of caring and concern on her face. Her own eyes may have contained tears in response to your emotional pain. Which type of person described above is more aware of the feelings of others? Which type of person described above is more aware of her own feelings?

A common fear of all people is that they may become emotionally overwhelmed in a difficult circumstance. They really are not sure what is "OK" or "not OK" to feel. Because of this fear, they block their own emotional responses to some experiences. If a nurse is

moved to quiet tears with a patient, an apology is not necessary. In such an instance the patient will know that the nurse cares. Nursing peers will be able to understand; if not, it is their loss—and their patients'—that they have never shared such deep emotion with a patient. It also may help them to be able to allow such emotion in themselves.

If a nurse has known a patient and family during several admissions and cared for them on a daily basis, several hours a day, is it "unprofessional" to experience deep caring about them? Is it possible that by continually having to deny, repress, suppress, and avoid such feelings, nurses may diminish their own humanity as well as that of their patients and family members?

As the death of a patient approaches, particularly a tragic death, the nurse may occasionally cry on the way home from work or at home. The nurse may talk about the patient with a spouse or nonnursing friend and be moved to tears. All these responses are normal. They are part of the grief response. The nurse is, after all, losing someone who is special. The nurse may know the person more intimately than anyone else during the dying process. It is possible that the family members, because of a maladaptive response to the person's death, may have been unable to support him or her.

If a nurse is concerned about being overinvolved emotionally with a dying patient, it can be helpful to seek out a senior staff member or a clinical specialist who works with the dying. He or she can explore the possible causes of the strong feelings. Understanding the dynamics that cause attachment to a particular patient can help to reestablish an objective, empathetic posture.

Such a relationship with a patient does not occur frequently or with the majority of patients. After the patient dies, most nurses experience the normal bereavement process, but for a briefer period than one would experience with a family member or good friend. Again, it is important for nurses to acknowledge their sadness rather than try to stifle it or judge themselves "unprofessional" because of it. Many nurses, after this type of loss, find that they become more emotionally distant from their new patients for a time. Eventually, they are able to resume normal relationships with patients.

THE NURSE'S ROLE
AS PATIENT ADVOCATE

An important aspect of care of the dying person is the nurse's ability to assess the patient's needs for supportive care. On occasion, the physician's awareness of those needs may be different than that of nurses. Physicians may concentrate on the patient's biological rather than psychosocial and comfort needs. Many nurses express anger about what they consider to be physicians' insensitivity with dying patients. It is important to remember, however, that their orientation to patient care is different than nurses' orientation. Rather than being angry with physicians and lamenting the plight of the patient, the nurse can promote a holistic approach to the care of the dying patient.

The following is a case example of the powerful role that a nurse can play as the dying patient's advocate in a complex hospital care system.

CASE EXAMPLE

Jennifer was a bright, sophisticated, 22-year-old woman. At age 17 she attended a professional school in a South American city away from her family. Shortly after arriving in South America, she became fatigued, listless, and ill. Despite the persistence of symptoms, no laboratory work was done, and she was told that she had mononucleosis. When she returned to the United States 7 months later, she had several disquieting physical symptoms. A diagnostic medical workup revealed that her liver was permanently damaged from an undiagnosed and untreated case of hepatitis.

Despite aggressive medical treatment, her liver status continued to deteriorate. Her college education was consistently interrupted by her frequent illnesses and hospitalizations. It ultimately had to be abandoned. Her 22nd year was punctuated by acute medical emergencies and several episodes of cognitive mental disorder (CMD) caused by buildup of toxic wastes that the liver could not metabolize.

During her last admission, Jennifer was admitted to a medical teaching unit where her care was supervised by a large medical team who did not know her from previous admissions. At that time, Jennifer was hemorrhaging into all her body tissues because of the failure of two liver-produced clotting factors. She had severe ascites.

Her abdomen was swollen larger than the abdomen of a full-term pregnant woman. Her body was emaciated from metabolic wasting. On admission she was semicomatose because of liver-related encephalopathy. She became fully alert within 2 days. The chief medical resident and staff physicians were concerned about maintaining whatever liver function she had. They refused to order pain medication because they did not want to compromise the liver further with the metabolism of complex analgesics.

Her kidneys began to fail. It was obvious to nursing staff members who had cared for her on earlier admissions that death was near. The physicians remained committed to aggressive treatment. They refused to consider a no-resuscitation order in case of death because of her age. The nurses were upset because they believed that the patient had been through severe pain and should not have to experience the assault of a medical "rush" emergency.

The staff nurse caring for Jennifer approached the chief resident and gave him specific examples of Jennifer's excruciating pain in her abdomen, back, and legs. Jennifer whimpered when any part of her body was touched. Even when she temporarily lapsed into semiconsciousness, she cried out with pain when moved. With the nurses' examples, the chief resident quickly reversed the no-analgesic orders of the intern and other residents. The next day the head nurse approached him about reconsidering his order for an all-out resuscitation attempt in case of death. She emphasized that all the physical systems were in failure, that resuscitation, if effective, could not be maintained by Jennifer's body, that the patient had been through enough pain, and that both the patient and family had been through enough heartache and were prepared for her death. He then ordered that there be no resuscitation attempt and ordered that the patient's comfort level be maintained by adequate analgesics. Jennifer died peacefully 3 days later.

In this case the nurses did not aggressively confront the physicians, nor did they angrily or passively withdraw from their advocacy role. Instead, they continued to bring forward the aspects of the patient's care that they believed were important for consideration in order to ensure the patient the most peaceful and comfortable death possible.

REASONABLE LIMITS OF THE NURSE'S EMOTIONAL INVOLVEMENT WITH THE DYING PATIENT

Working with dying patients and their families is not easy. When done therapeutically, the caregiver's emotional investment can cause a drain on his or her emotions. Therapeutic involvement cannot occur unless the caregiver cares and gives. There are no shortcuts or ways to avoid it.

A nurse who cares very much about a dying patient may cry, laugh, and love him and his humanity. A nurse may feel committed to his well-being and may be the only person who is able to stay with him in his final days. Sister Madeleine Clemence Vaillot (1966, p. 504) advanced an existentialist explanation of commitment, in which she states:

> Commitment is the full, willing, and open-eyed acceptance of one's full share of life.... It is the acceptance of full responsibility for one's actions.... Lack of commitment, on the other hand, is a refusal: a refusal to use one's freedom to choose, to involve one's self with life's difficulties.

The reason why such an intense relationship does not happen routinely for a nurse with all dying patients is because of the protective functioning of the nurse's defense mechanisms. Even a healthy, mature ego would have difficulty resolving repetitive grief reactions to losses of innumerable patients in whom so much of the nurse's self was invested. Accordingly, the ego unconsciously uses the mechanisms of denial, repression, avoidance, and isolation as a way of coping with the stress of working with dying patients (Box 24-1).

Feeling such attachment to a patient is a rare gift for both the patient and the nurse. It goes beyond the normal nurse-patient relationship. In it there is an existential experience. *Existential* refers to the existence, the living process, of a human being (American Heritage College Dictionary, 1993). In an existential relationship, the two people share an encounter that is unique. There is full understanding and acceptance of the other. Both lives are permanently touched to their emotional depths, and sometimes to depths never before experienced (Clemence Vaillot, 1966; May, Binswanger, & Ellen-Berger, 1976). Some nurses may never experience such a relationship. Others experience this closeness at infrequent intervals during their professional lives, perhaps only once a year, once every 2 or 3 years, or once in a working lifetime.

Whether nurses experience an emotional commitment or maintain a mildly detached, yet still-involved, relationship with dying patients, it is important that they accept their own emotional reactions as normal. Some nurses experience anxiety in working with dying patients. Much of this anxiety appears to be caused by the nurse's discomfort with dying. In fact, in a study of staff nurses on general hospital units, nurses were asked to rank the most common stressors they experienced in their everyday work. The list of stressors included 25 items, such as too-frequent rotation of shifts, poor relationship with supervisors, lack of respect from subordinates, being overworked, inadequate staffing, and so on. The highest ranking stressor that staff nurses reported was working with dying patients. The second highest stressor reported by many nurses was having to deal with physicians who avoided discussions with dying patients or their family members.*

SUPPORT OF NURSES CARING FOR DYING PATIENTS

The most commonly recommended approach to support nurses caring for dying people is to provide them with a group in which they can discuss their reactions to working with dying patients (O'Connor, 1991). Such groups are

---

*Barry, P. (1981). Significant staff nurse stressors. Unpublished research.

BOX 24-1	Defense Mechanisms Normally Observed in Caregivers of Dying Patients	
	Denial	When the nurse cares for the dying patient, he or she engages in light banter, with no empathetic awareness of the patient's emotional reaction to dying.
	Repression	The nurse performs technical nursing care in an acceptable way. When unpleasant feelings such as sadness or hopelessness about the patient are initially experienced, they are excluded from conscious awareness by the ego.
	Avoidance (also called *withdrawl* or *professional distancing*)	When the dying process is coming to an end, the nurse may feel helpless and hopeless about the patient's condition. Rather than checking on the patient periodically, the nurse has many other tasks that keep him or her busy and away from the patient. The nurse responds to call lights of dying patients more slowly than to those of other patients.
	Isolation (also called *rationalization* or *intellectualization*)	The nurse is aware on an intellectual or superficial level of what the dying patient and family are experiencing. There is little or no affective or emotional component to this awareness, however. The nurse's discussion of the patient's response to dying has a cold, professional-sounding tone. The nurse is able to identify the patient's current response to impending death and is able to describe accurately the particular "stage" the patient is in.

usually led by psychiatrists, social workers, psychiatric nurse specialists, or psychiatric liaison nurse specialists. Whenever possible, the most appropriate leaders for this type of nurse group are psychiatric liaison nurse specialists. Their theoretical and clinical training is related to the stressful aspects of physical illness of all concerned: patients, families, and nurses. They are familiar with the interactive effects of these people within a complex hospital caregiving system.

Psychiatric or psychiatric liaison nurse group leaders are able to understand the specific issues of nurses that can contribute to the stress of working with dying patients. Some of these issues are the socialization process of the nursing student, which may have encouraged repression of unpleasant affects such as sadness, anger, and guilt about dying patients; the type of stress involved in long, unbroken hours of nursing care, as opposed to the much briefer contacts of nonnursing caregivers; and, most important, the philosophy of nursing, which is strongly psychosocially oriented when compared to the more predominant interest of medical caregivers in the patients' biological processes.

It is important for nurses working with dying patients to be aware of their own feelings about their patients. Without an opportunity to vent this emotion, it remains trapped within.

SUPPORT OF THE STUDENT NURSE WORKING WITH DYING PATIENTS

In addition to such a group for graduate nurses, it is important that nursing educators review the philosophy of their curricula, as well as their own convictions, about what types of responses of students to dying patients are acceptable. One of the strong contributing factors to nursing students' repression of unpleasant emotion can be concern about the grade they will receive in their clinical settings. Students frequently fear that their grades will be affected if they display more than a mild emotional response to the death of a patient.

One way of avoiding this problem is to consider an ongoing group experience for students. The group can be led by a member of the faculty who is a psychiatric liaison or psychiatric clinical specialist. Such a group can have a positive outcome with an every-other-week meeting. The focus of the group could be discussion of the students' feelings about specific patients and of psychosocial care problems of specific patients. There should be no grading involved in this group experience, and confidentiality of the group should be maintained.

The adaptive mind will not allow an intolerable amount of emotion to accumulate. In its adaptation attempt, it will either repress the painful emotion or not allow it to be experienced. Repression can be an adaptive response in nurses in the care of acutely ill patients. However, repeated episodes of unpleasant emotion or deep, continued repression that occur with patient encounters are not conducive to positive adaptation; rather, they may cause nurses to "shut down." They may no longer be able to be as open or responsive to their patients.

CONCLUSION

This chapter has discussed responses that can be observed when working with dying patients and their families, and appropriate nursing interventions in caring for these patients and families. This information can also be generalized and used when caring for *any* patient who is experiencing a major loss as the result of an illness that will have an ongoing effect on his or her life. The patient may have undergone coronary artery bypass surgery or amputation of a limb, or have been diagnosed with a chronic, degenerative, and ultimately terminal illness. In all of these cases, the patient and family will respond with the same emotions and process as the dying patient and family, although probably to a lesser degree.

This chapter has also addressed nurses' reactions to working with dying patients. By understanding common concerns, nurses can gain insight into their own emotional responses to dying patients, as well as those of the patient, family, and other caregivers.

BIBLIOGRAPHY

Aguilera, D. C. (1994). *Crisis intervention: Theory and methodology* (7th ed.). St. Louis: C. V. Mosby.

Aldrich, C. K. (1974). Some dynamics of anticipatory grief. In B. Schoenberg, A. Can & A. Kutscher (Eds.), *Anticipatory grief.* New York: Columbia University Press.

American Heritage college dictionary (3rd ed.). (1993). Boston: Houghton-Mifflin.

Bahnson, C. (1981). Stress and cancer. II: The state of the art. *Psychosomatics, 22*(3), 207–220.

Baile, W. F., DiMaggion, J. R., Schapira, D. V., & Janofsky, J. S. (1993). The request for assistance in dying. The need for psychiatric consultation. *Cancer, 72*(9), 2786–2791.

Baum, M., & Page, M. (1991). Caregiving and multigenerational families. *Gerontologist, 31*(6), 762–769.

Binger, C., Ablin, A., & Feuerstein, R. (1969). Childhood leukemia: Emotional impact on patient and family. *New England Journal of Medicine, 280*(8), 414–418.

Bouckoms, A., & Hackett, T. P. (1991). The pain patient: Evaluation and treatment. In N. H. Cassem (Ed.), *Massachusetts General Hospital handbook of general hospital psychiatry* (3rd ed.). St. Louis: Mosby-Year Book.

Bowen, M. (1976). Family reaction to death. In P. Guerin (Ed.), *Family therapy: Theory and practice.* New York: Gardner Press.

Bowlby, J. (1980). *Attachment and loss, Vol. 3: Sadness and depression.* New York: Basic Books.

Brotzman, G. L., & Butler, D. J. (1991). Cross-cultural issues in the disclosure of a terminal diagnosis. A case report. *Journal of Family Practice, 32*(4), 426–427.

Campbell, R. J. (1989). *Psychiatric dictionary* (6th ed.). New York: Oxford University Press.

Carpenito, L. (1993). *Nursing diagnosis: Application and clinical practice.* Philadelphia: J. B. Lippincott.

Carroll, R. (1993). Mourning: A concern for medical-surgical nurses. *Medical-Surgical Nursing, 2*(4), 301–303, 338.

Cassem, N. H. (1991). The dying patient. In N. H. Cassem (Ed.), *Massachusetts General Hospital handbook of general hospital psychiatry* (3rd ed.). St. Louis: Mosby-Year Book.

Cassem, N. H., & Barsky, A. J. (1991). Functional somatic symptoms and somatoform disorders. In N. H. Cassem (Ed.), *Massachusetts General Hospital handbook of general hospital psychiatry* (3rd ed.). St. Louis: Mosby-Year Book.

Castles, M., & Murray, R. (1979). *Dying in an institution.* New York: Appleton-Century-Crofts.

Claxton, J. W. (1993). Paving the way to acceptance. Psychological adaptation to death and dying in cancer. *Professional Nurse, 8*(4), 206–211.

Clemence Vaillot, M. (1966). Existentialism: A philosophy of commitment. *American Journal of Nursing, 66*(3), 500–505.

Couldrick, A. (1991). Optimising bereavement outcome: Reading the road ahead. *Recent Results in Cancer Research, 121*, 432–436.

Crawley, P. (1991). The pain of grief. *Queensland Nurse, 10*(3), 24.

Creagan, E. T. (1993). Psychosocial issues in oncologic practice. *Mayo Clinic Proceedings, 68*(2), 161–167.

Davidhizar, R., & Kirk, B. (1993). Emergency room nurses: Helping families cope with sudden death. *Journal of Practical Nursing, 43*(2), 14–19.

Davies, B. (1993). Sibling bereavement: Research-based guidelines for nurses. *Seminars in Oncology Nursing, 9*(2), 107–113.

de Vries, B., Bluck, S., & Birren, J. E. (1993). The understanding of death and dying in a life-span perspective. *Gerontologist, 33*(3), 366–372.

Engel, G. (1961). Is grief a disease? A challenge for medical research. *Psychosomatic Medicine, 23*, 18.

Engel, G. (1975). Reactions to the death of a twin. *Rochester Review*, Fall, 4–12.

Funk, M. (1992). Caring. *Image: The Journal of Nursing Scholarship, 24*(2), 159.

Gatti, G., Masera, R., Pallavicini, L., Sartori, M., Staurenghi, A., Orlandi, F., & Angeli, A. (1993). Interplay in vitro between ACTH, beta-endorphin, and glucocorticoids in the modulation of spontaneous and lymphokine-inducible human natural killer (NK) cell activity. *Brain, Behavior, and Immunity, 7*(1), 16-28.

Goldstein, M. G., & Niaura, R. (1992). Psychological factors affecting physical condition. Cardiovascular disease literature review. Part I: Coronary artery disease and sudden death. *Psychosomatics, 33*(2),134–145.

Greenberg, I. (1965). Studies of attitudes toward death. In Group for Advancement of Psychiatry, *Death and dying: Attitudes of patient and doctor, Vol. 5, Symposium 11*. New York: Mental Health Materials Center.

Hansen, J. (Ed.). (1984). *Death and grief in the family*. Rockville, MD: Aspen Systems Corp.

Hardy, J., Wolff, H., & Goodell, H. (1940). Studies on pain. A new method for measuring pain threshold: Observations on spatial summation of pain. *Journal of Clinical Investigation, 19*, 649.

Harris, J. M. (1991). Death and bereavement. *Problems in Veterinary Medicine, 3*(1), 111–117.

Harrison, D. S., & Cole, C. D. (1991). Family dynamics and caregiver burden in home health care. *Clinics in Geriatric Medicine, 7*(4), 817–829.

Herth, K. (1993). Hope in the family caregiver of terminally ill people. *Journal of Advanced Nursing, 18*(4), 538–548.

Horsley, J. (1982). *Pain: Deliberative nursing interventions/ CURN project*. New York: Grune & Stratton.

Hover, M. (1993). The ministry of caring, Part 3. *North Carolina Medical Journal, 54*(2), 105.

Jagger, C., & Sutton, C. J. (1991). Death after mental bereavement—is the risk increased? *Statistics in Medicine, 10*(3), 395–404.

Kaplan, H. I., & Sadock, B. J. (1994). *Synopsis of psychiatry: Behavioral sciences, clinical psychiatry* (7th ed.). Baltimore: Williams & Wilkins.

Kaplan, H. I., & Sadock, B. J. (1995). *Comprehensive textbook of psychiatry/VI* (6th ed.). Baltimore: Williams & Wilkins.

Kastenbaum, R. (1978). In control. In Garfield, C. (Ed.), *Psychosocial care of the dying patient*. New York: McgrawHill.

Kelner, M. J., & Bourgeault, I. L. (1993). Patient control over dying: Responses of health care professionals. *Social Science and Medicine, 36*(6), 757–765.

Kubler-Ross, E. (1975). *Death: The final stage of growth*. Englewood Cliffs, NJ: Prentice-Hall.

Kubler-Ross, E. (1981). *Death: The final stage of growth*. Englewood Cliffs, NJ: Prentice-Hall.

Levine, J., Rudy, T., & Kerns, R. (1994). A two factor model of denial of illness: A confirmatory factor analysis. *Journal of Psychosomatic Research, 38*(2), 99–110.

Maddison, D. (1968). The health of widows in the year following bereavement. *Journal of Psychosomatic Research, 12*, 297.

Maddison, D., Viola, A., & Walker, W. (1969). Further studies in conjugal bereavement. *British Journal of Psychiatry, 113*, 1057.

Martinson, I. M., Chang, G. Q., & Liang, Y. H. (1993). Chinese families after the death of a child from cancer. *European Journal of Cancer Care (England), 2*(4), 169–173.

May, C. (1993). Disclosure of terminal prognoses in a general hospital: The nurse's view. *Journal of Advanced Nursing, 18*(9), 1362–1368.

May, R., Binswanger, L., & Ellen-Berger, H. (1976). Existential psychotherapy and dasein analysis. In W. Sahakian (Ed.), *Psychotherapy and counseling* (2nd ed.). Chicago: Rand McNally.

McCaffery, M. (1968). *Cognition, bodily pain, and man-environment interactions*. Los Angeles: University of California Student Store.

McCallum, M., Piper, W. E., & Morin, H. (1993). Affect and outcome in short-term group therapy for loss. *International Journal of Group Psychotherapy, 43*(3), 303–319.

McCarthy, J. (1980). *Death anxiety: The loss of the self*. New York: Gardner Press.

Miles, A. (1993). Caring for the family left behind. *American Journal of Nursing, 93*(12), 34–36.

Nagy, M. (1959). The child's view of death. In H. Feifel (Ed.), *The meaning of death*. New York: McGraw-Hill.

Nilchaikovit, T., Hill, J. M., & Holland, J. C. (1993). The effects of culture on illness behavior and medical care. Asian and American differences. *General Hospital Psychiatry, 15*(1), 41–50.

Nuland, S. B. (1994). *How we die: Reflections on life's final chapter*. New York: Alfred A. Knopf.

Nyatanga, B. (1993). Emotional pain in terminal illness: A dilemma for nurses. *Senior Nurse, 13*(3), 46–48.

O'Connor, S. (1991). Psychiatry liaison nursing in a changing health care system. In N. H. Cassem (Ed.), *Massachusetts General Hospital handbook of general hospital psychiatry* (3rd ed.). St. Louis: Mosby-Year Book.

Parad, H., & Caplan, G. (1965). A framework for studying families in crisis. In H. Parad (Ed.), *Crisis intervention: Selected readings*. New York: Family Service Association of America.

Parkes, C. (1972). *Bereavement: Studies of grief in adult life*. New York: International Universities Press.

Parkinson, P. (1992). Terminal care: Coping with dying and bereavement. *Nursing Standard, 6*(17), 36–38.

Pattison, E. (1978). The living-dying process. In C. Garfield (Ed.), *Psychosocial care of the dying patient*. New York: McGraw Hill.

Piaget, J., & Inhelder, B. (1969). *Psychology of the child*. New York: Basic Books.

Pickett, M. (1993). Cultural awareness in the context of terminal illness. *Cancer Nursing, 16*(2), 102–106.

Pilkington, F. B. (1993). The lived experience of grieving the loss of an important other. *Nursing Science Quarterly, 6*(3), 130–139.

Psychological Work Group of the International Work Group on Death, Dying, and Bereavement. A statement of assumptions and principles concerning psychological care of dying persons and their families. *Journal of Palliative Care, 9*(3), 29–32.

Rees, W., & Lutkins, S. (1967). Mortality of bereavement. *British Medical Journal, 4*, 13.

Robinson, K. R. (1993). Denial: An adaptive response. *Dimensions of Critical Care Nursing, 12*(2), 102–106.

Rosenbaum, J. (1981). Widows and widowers and their medication use: Nursing implications. *Journal of Psychiatric Nursing, 19,* 17.

Schneider, J. (1984). *Stress, loss, and grief: Understanding their origins and growth potential.* Baltimore: University Park Press.

Schwab, J. (1968). *Handbook of psychiatric consultation.* New York: Appleton-Century-Crofts.

Shuchter, S. (1986). *Dimensions of grief: Adjusting to the death of a spouse.* San Francisco: Jossey-Bass.

Simpson, C. (1993). A process of dying by default. *Australian Family Physician, 22*(7), 1279–1281, 1283.

Smith, N., & Regnard, C. (1993). Managing family problems in advanced disease—a flow diagram. *Palliative Medicine, 7*(1), 47–58.

Stein, M., Miller, A., & Trestman, R. Depression and the immune system. In R. Ader, D. L. Felten, & N. Cohen (Eds.), *Psychoneuroimmunology* (2nd ed.). New York: Academic Press.

Steinmetz, D., Walsh, M., Gabel, L. L., & Williams, P. T. (1993). Family physicians' involvement with dying patients and their families. Attitudes, difficulties, and strategies. *Archives of Family Medicine, 2*(7), 753–760.

Temoshok, L., & Dreher, H. (1993). *The Type-C connection: The mind-body link to cancer and your health.* New York: New American Library.

Thomas, C. L. (Ed.). (1993). *Taber's cyclopedic medical dictionary* (17th ed.). Philadelphia: F. A. Davis.

Thompson, D. G. (1992). Support for the grieving family: A case study. *Neonatal Network, 11*(6), 73–75.

Tradimus. (1991). Grieving: Confronting death. *Nursing Standard, 6*(11), 55.

Ufema, J. (1991). Helping loved ones say good-bye. *Nursing, 21*(10), 42–43.

Waltman, N. L., & Zimmerman, L. (1991). Variations among nurses in behavioral intentions toward the dying. *Hospital Journal, 7*(4), 37–49.

Widdrington, C. (1992). Preparing for loss. *Nursing Times, 88*(49), 26–28.

Wolfelt, A. D. (1991). Toward an understanding of complicated grief: A comprehensive overview. *American Journal of Hospital Palliative Care, 8*(2), 28–30.

Woodward, C. A., & King, B. (1993). Survivor focus groups: A quality assurance technique. *Palliative Medicine, 7*(3), 229–234.

Zisook, S., Schuchter, S. R., Sledge, P., & Mulvihill, M. (1993). Aging and bereavement. *Journal of Geriatric Psychiatry and Neurology, 6*(3), 137–143.

PART V

PSYCHOSOCIAL INTERVENTIONS FOR SPECIFIC AGE GROUPS AND CLINICAL SETTINGS

The following section addresses specific issues that arise when working with patients throughout the life span—infants, children and adolescents, the maternity patient, and older adults—and/or in specific clinical settings—the emergency room or the home care setting. Patients who are distressed by physical illness experience different types of coping challenges. A child's understanding, fears, and coping mechanisms will differ from those of a young adult or a senior citizen. This section provides tools to help nurses assess these patients and tailor nursing care plans and interventions to patients in all these age groups.

Clinical settings can also create coping challenges for the patient. Both the emergency room and the home care setting present unique stresses that impact the patient and family. As the medical system and patient care change, more patients are at risk of ineffectively coping with these stresses. With the practical recommendations in this section, nurses will be able to guide patients and families towards effective coping, full use of the positive potential of these care settings, and adaptive outcomes.

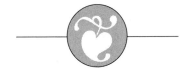

CHAPTER 25

Psychosocial Intervention in the Emergency Department

Marcy Bartolovic

Nursing has been described as an art and a science. The study of nursing as a science has great merit in developing the profession along a more technical, scientific pathway. This is essential given the rapid expansion of technology in health care today. On the other hand, to speak of nursing as an art allows for a more open dialogue and a greater capacity to explore and describe its impact and potential as a discipline. In this way, nursing can be seen as a discipline involving many talents. Perhaps the atmosphere where both of these elements converge so colorfully, allowing nurses to demonstrate their greatest art and knowledge of science, is in the setting of an emergency room, also referred to as an emergency department (ED).

The function of an emergency department has evolved over the past three decades. As a specific service, the emergency department provides a means for an unrestricted population to access health care continuously. The name implies that all who seek services in this setting will be experiencing emergencies. This may be true in many cases. However, the general public has increasingly looked upon the emergency room as an alternative point of entry into the health care system. According to the American Hospital Association (1992), there were 93,469,930 outpatient visits to emergency departments in more than 6,500 hospitals surveyed in 1991. This represents an increased patient volume of more than 6 million since 1989. In fact, the number of ED visits has increased steadily since 1983 (Aghababian, Peterson, & Gans, 1992).

EMERGENCY DEPARTMENT POPULATION AND TRENDS

Several events have influenced the growing number of patients seen in the emergency department. Legislative changes in the 1960s, the advanced management of emergency care, and our current socioeconomic climate have contributed to this growth (MacPhail, 1992).

Patricia Barry: *Psychosocial Nursing: Care of Physically Ill Patients and Their Families,* 3rd ed.
© 1996 Lippincott–Raven Publishers

There are currently 37 million uninsured people in the United States, with thousands more considered underinsured. Statistics show that low-income patients make 64% more use of emergency services than do those with insurance coverage. Shorter hospital stays are also part of the changing health care environment. Patients with acute medical problems are being discharged from the hospital sooner. Consequently, these patients are becoming frequent visitors to the emergency department for completion of their care (Aghababian, Peterson, & Gans, 1992).

These trends add to an already diverse patient population in the ED. This specialized health care setting has developed into a treatment resource for a much broader patient population, beyond the traditional medical emergencies. Consequently, the needs of patients in the emergency department have become more complex and specialized. Hess and Ruster (1990) discuss studies which support the notion that a large portion of emergency department patients present with nontraditional emergencies. Specifically, there is an increase in patients who present with nonmedical and secondary psychosocial problems and/or primary problems that are psychological in nature. Hess and Ruster (1990) note the severity of these psychosocial problems, including attempted suicides, family violence, child abuse, rape, and injuries resulting from criminal involvement.

HEALTH AND ILLNESS IN THE ED: A DIFFERENT PERSPECTIVE

As noted above, there are countless reasons why people utilize an emergency department. However, a central point is common to all cases. At the most basic level, emergency departments service individuals who have experienced an interruption in their health. This interruption may occur as a result of illness, injury, or trauma, which affects the patient's physical and emotional health.

Our bodies are so dynamic that when a person experiences an interruption in health, the body's built-in compensatory mechanisms take over. The patient's body immediately attempts to reestablish its own homeostasis. A simultaneous chain reaction of unconscious, involuntary phenomena takes place within a person to help the person achieve physical, emotional, and psychological adaptation to interruptions of health. The essence of this chapter lies within this naturally occurring response to illness.

At times, depending on the nature and severity of the illness, injury, or trauma, the body's adaptive mechanisms can become too compromised to function effectively. Most individuals intuitively know when a situation overloads their bodies' adaptive functioning. Generally, this maladaptation causes individuals to seek the kind of health care that can assist them in stabilizing their health. It can be assumed, then, that patients presenting to the emergency room are experiencing a maladaptation in their health in a way that causes an extreme imbalance in several aspects of their lives. Accordingly, the type of nursing care provided in the emergency department must go beyond treating the presenting problem to include interventions which will increase patients' coping with, and adaptation to, the presenting problem.

The care of patients in an ED setting will be discussed from a biopsychosocial perspective. To care for patients in an ED means, potentially, to intervene with the immediate health problem while assessing for factors which may impede patients' healing and recovery processes. Nursing actions will be discussed relative to the enhancement and mobilization of those psychosocial factors that assist the patient in coping with changes caused by illness or injury. Psychosocial assessment and intervention will be reviewed for patients experiencing an acute physical illness, an acute physical trauma, a psychiatric emergency, and a chronic mental illness within the context of being homeless.

HEALTH, ILLNESS, AND ADAPTATION

A BIOPSYCHOSOCIAL FRAMEWORK

A biopsychosocial framework applied to health, illness, and adaptation provides nursing with a means of understanding, and a way of organizing, an individual's many responses to the actual or potential health problem causing him or her to seek emergency services. The nurse should provide care to patients based on three dimensions: physical, psychological, and social.

The patient's *physical* dimension consists of the body's physiological response to illness, injury, or stressful events. The physical dimension involves adaptation, or coping, at the biological level. The *psychological* dimension consists of a person's emotional, cognitive, and behavioral response to illness or injury. Generally, these reactions are determined by intrapersonal dynamics. Here, an individual's adaptation, or coping, is influenced internally by factors of human development, especially those factors involved in a child's maturation to adulthood. The *social* dimension refers to the social forces influencing a person's emotional and cognitive state, as well as his or her behavior. These social forces encompass the family and community (Abraham, Fox, & Cohen, 1992). This dynamic collection of adaptive responses to illness can be viewed broadly as a process for coping with a stressful event.

STRESS THEORY

When discussing the concept of stress, three terms are generally identified: stress, stressors, and stress reactions. Thompson (1992) provides a helpful review of these terms.

Contrary to what many people believe, *stress* is not a three-dimensional object existing in the world. It is the reaction of an organism to events in the environment. These events are viewed as *stressors* and are defined as "things that cause harm to an organism" (Thompson, 1992, p. 148). *Stress reactions* are an organism's various physiological and psychological responses when it encounters a stressor. The following paragraph applies these concepts in the emergency room setting.

In the ED, an event can be interpreted as the presenting problem or reason causing a patient and family to seek emergency services. If events in the world are described as stressors, one can understand the presenting problem as a stressor for the patient who, according to the above

description, will experience a stress reaction to this stressor. This stress reaction will result in responses, or behaviors, revealing how the person is coping at the physiological, psychological, and social levels. Examples of coping responses include abnormal vital signs (physical), anxiety (psychological), or withdrawn behavior (social). Generally speaking, when an individual's stress level increases, coping behaviors decrease or become maladaptive, resulting in an interrupted level of functioning.

Coping and Crisis: An Overview

The combination of these events creates the *potential* for a person to become prone to a crisis state. Roberts (1990) cites the definition of a crisis as described by Bard and Ellison (1974, p. 68) as "a subjective reaction to a stressful life experience, one so affecting the stability of the individual that the ability to cope or function may be seriously compromised" (p. 8). Applying this definition to the ED, there is potential for a patient to experience an illness as a crisis if the patient perceives the illness as leading to an acute disruption or imbalance in life and is unable to resolve the disruption by previously used coping methods.

Roberts (1990) explains how an individual's perceptions are formed during the development of a crisis, as described by Naomi Golan (1978, p. 8). "The person 'may perceive the initial and subsequent stressful events primarily as a threat, either to his instinctual needs or to his sense of autonomy and well being; as a *loss* of a person, an ability, or a capacity; or a *challenge* to survival, growth or mastery'" (p. 10). Therefore, a crisis is not a situation by itself. Rather, it is the perception of or meaning a person gives to a situation, as well as the person's response to it, that constitutes a crisis.

ACUTE PHYSICAL ILLNESS

COPING AND CRISIS IN THE ED

Applying this concept to the emergency department, it is unlikely that a patient will directly view or report an illness as a crisis. The person is more likely to *show* the nurse how significant or potentially significant the illness has become. In other words, if a man perceives his current physical condition as seriously impacting his current lifestyle, the probability is high that he will display many maladaptive coping behaviors. These behaviors can be thought of as the man's way of communicating to caregivers that he is scared and unable to cope with the situation at hand. He may not even understand what is happening to him; consequently, he may not be able to verbalize such feelings.

The nurse can interpret an increase in maladaptive coping as the *beginning* of a potential crisis. That is to say, the potential is great for the patient to experience illness as a crisis if psychosocial nursing interventions are not directed at uncovering and supporting the patient's current psychological and social coping mechanisms.

For example, a patient who has not stopped smoking since being diagnosed with the illness may present with respiratory distress related to the illness. Rather than identifying psychosocial factors (i.e., 20 years of smoking) that led to the patient's development of emphysema, the nurse should recognize and focus on those psychosocial factors that may serve as barriers to the patient's ability to recover from attacks of respiratory distress. In other words, the nurse should identify which factors have the greatest influence on the patient's inability to stop smoking. Several psychosocial factors may be involved; for example, the patient may have a lack of social support, or may live alone and see smoking as a way to deal with boredom. The point is that cessation of smoking is critical to the patient's recovery process from the effects of emphysema. If the nurse assesses for these factors, suggestions and recommendations can be made that can enhance the patient's recovery and adaptation to altered respiratory status. This example illustrates the key to effective psychosocial interventions in the emergency department.

COMMON PSYCHOSOCIAL COPING BEHAVIORS

Nurses must be able to understand the normative reactions that characterize potential crises. Common psychological reactions to a crisis can be categorized as emotional, cognitive, and behavioral.

Common *emotional* responses to a crisis are anxiety, fear, panic, despair, shock, denial, insecurity, grief, survivor guilt, numbness, frustration, anger, and irritability. From a *cognitive* perspective, common reactions include a sense of confusion, limited attention span, inability to concentrate, and poor short-term memory, as well as an inability to trust. Common *behavioral* responses include withdrawal from others, interrupted sleep, angry outbursts, changes in appetite and activity level, increased tiredness, crying, an expressed anger toward God, and substance abuse (Greenstone & Leviton, 1993).

It is equally important for a nurse to understand the role that social support plays in a patient's ability to adapt to illness. Flannery (1990) notes several studies which describe the nature of social interactions or social support that influence a person's health and adaptation. Increasing empirical support suggests that four types of social interchange appear to be adaptive in modifying the impact of life's stress (Box 25-1).

As Box 25-1 indicates, the first type of social interaction that supports effective coping is *emotional support,* characterized as the sharing of feelings with others who are able to listen with a sympathetic ear. The second social interaction deals with *information,* in the form of specific facts, provided to the person under stress; the purpose is to aid in resolution of the stressor. The nurse can take on this role while providing care in the ER. The third type of interaction, *social companionship,* includes the presence of others, which can potentially reduce a person's sense of aloneness, helplessness, and vulnerability. This type of companionship also provides meaning to the events of everyday life. The last social interaction involves the exchange of money or tangible goods. This category is termed *instrumental support.*

The common theme of the above four social groupings is their enhancement of personal mastery over stress by increasing coping resources (Flannery, 1990). However, not all social interchanges positively impact on a person's coping. Flannery (1990) also describes social interactions, identified in the research literature

BOX 25-1	Social Interchanges That Support Effective Coping
	1. Emotional support: the sharing of feelings with others 2. Providing information: the receiving of specific facts from others 3. Social companionship: the presence of others 4. Instrumental support: the exchange of money or tangible goods Source: Flannery, 1990

and shown in Box 25-2, which increase the probability of negative health outcomes.

Even though a patient may not view a physical illness as a crisis, the potential is there for one to develop. An astute and sensitive nurse will take a proactive, psychosocial approach to planning care for this patient. Nursing assessment and intervention should focus on helping to mobilize the patient's existing psychosocial coping methods, to prevent maladaptation to illness and ineffective coping.

ENVIRONMENTAL INFLUENCES

Helping to mobilize a patient's coping skills may seem like an easy, straightforward task. However, in the midst of an unpredictable, time-intensive, often hectic environment, this type of holistic assessment is anything but easy, even for the skilled nurse. Being able to maintain such a global approach in caring for patients, when the ED environment is structured to service very specific needs of individuals and families, presents a unique professional challenge for the nurse.

In this setting, where critical factors of life and death are a common, everyday experience, the nurse's attention is naturally drawn to highly focused issues, where the priority of care is based on the patient's physical well-being. This type of environment does not readily foster a holistic nursing care approach. Consequently, there is a great potential to focus only on the patient's physical needs, while psychosocial needs are overlooked.

If this were to occur, the true meaning of nursing might be abandoned. More importantly, there is an increased likelihood that the patient's and family's potential for health and adaptation would not be fully realized. Therefore, understanding the patient's acute physical illness and the family's involvement from a biopsychosocial framework enables the ED nurse to provide care to the total person, including the family.

ASSESSMENT PROCESS FOR ACUTE PHYSICAL ILLNESS

Primary, Secondary, and Focused Assessments

To help the nurse meet this challenge, the Emergency Nursing Core Curriculum outlines a systematized assessment and priority process that helps the nurse in the ER address the patient's and family's health using a holistic approach (Blair & Hall, 1994). This process involves primary, secondary, and focused assessments.

The *primary assessment/resuscitation phase* involves assessing those critical factors where any significant deviation from the norm requires immediate intervention. Such factors include the patient's airway, pulmonary and cardiac functions. Primary assessment should also include a brief neurological evaluation. This type of assessment is performed rapidly, while simultaneously evaluating and intervening with life-threatening injuries (Blair & Hall, 1994; Jutzi-Kosmos, 1990). Nursing interventions focusing on the patient's physical well-being are paramount at this point.

BOX 25-2	Social Interchanges That Reduce Effective Coping
	1. Value conflicts 2. Emotional demandingness 3. Emotional overinvolvement 4. Poor interpersonal skills Source: Flannery, 1990

Once the above factors no longer present a life-threatening risk to the patient, the *secondary assessment* follows. It is generally brief. During this phase the patient's general appearance is observed during a brief, head-to-toe assessment, to determine significant deviation from the norm. Additional subjective data is collected as well, including the patient's report of the history of the present illness or injury; past medical history; and social, psychological, and environmental factors. It is at this stage that the psychosocial assessment is conducted.

The *focused assessment* is more detailed than the previous assessments. It centers on the patient's presenting problem, and is guided by the subjective and objective data collected in the previous assessments (Blair & Hall, 1994).

Psychosocial Assessment: An Overview

The patient's report of how an illness or injury came about, the related symptoms, and the patient's past medical history may be fairly easy and straightforward for the patient to explain and for the nurse to gather. However, collecting data associated with the social, psychological, and environmental factors influencing the patient's presentation to the ED may not come as easily.

Time constraints as well as broad questions about the patient's personal life may cause this subjective part of the secondary assessment to be difficult to obtain. The nurse must be aware that the patient may have greater difficulty talking about these factors, which may require reflection and time on the patient's part. Some patients may not be prepared to explore, or may not be interested in exploring, these areas with a nurse.

Think back to a time when you were thrown in a situation unexpectedly, or perhaps even found yourself in an ED because of an illness or injury. Probably your foremost thought was for someone to take away the pain and fix the problem. The ED patient is no different. Psychologically, people in the ED are preoccupied with the event at hand; it can be assumed that they had little or no time to prepare for this situation. This often leaves the patient feeling helpless, scared, and frustrated.

A strong element of uncertainty and fear of the unknown is present with the ED patient. Added to this can be increasing levels of tension caused by the long waiting periods common in today's emergency departments. Therefore, before the nurse delves into the psychosocial area of an assessment, preparation will need to take place to set the stage. This is necessary if the nurse is to obtain and utilize accurate information about the patient's psychosocial dimension, in a way that enhances the patient's recovery from illness.

PREPARING FOR THE PSYCHOSOCIAL ASSESSMENT

Preparing the Setting

The nurse must first prepare the setting. When possible, it is beneficial to create an environment of privacy, the best one can in such a public forum as an emergency department. Sitting with the patient is ideal; however, standing near the patient and maintaining a body posture that conveys a sense of support, concern, and understanding will work as well. Keeping interruptions to a minimum adds to the therapeutic nature of the assessment. Active listening (see Chapter 2) is another key therapeutic tool. Listening skills are as significant as the nurse's visual and technical skills were during the primary assessment phase. The key is not to appear hurried or to rush the patient through the interview.

Patient Preparation

Next, the nurse should prepare the patient for this part of the assessment. Explain that the first priority of care involved ensuring the patient's stability when he or she entered the ED. The patient can be reassured that the care received up to this point has reduced immediate danger. If continued monitoring and physical care will be required in the ED, explain that also.

Letting the patient know what has just happened and what still needs to occur will usually decrease anxiety about the ED experience. You may notice subtle changes in the patient's nonverbal behavior, indicating that anxiety has decreased. These changes may include a more relaxed facial expression and better eye contact; other behaviors may also be exhibited. At this point the nurse can explain that other areas of life will be explored and that, while the patient may not think these questions are related to the situation that brought him or her to the ED, they are equally important.

Preparing the patient for this sometimes personal, probing, and complex assessment increases the chances that the patient will be more open to talk about these areas.

Nurse Preparation

Review the earlier discussion on stress theory in this chapter and in Chapter 6. Remember that physical illness serves as a stressor for the patient. Within this perspective, it is helpful for the nurse consciously to reframe his or her understanding of acute physical illness from a medical model to a psychosocial one.

The psychosocial model provides the nurse with a means of uncovering information about the patient's level of adaptation to physical illness. Conducting this important assessment enables the nurse to view emotional, behavioral, and social changes, secondary to physical illness, as the person's attempt (not the body's attempt) to adapt to changes in physical well-being. The above preparations are important for increasing chances that the nurse will collect valuable data so that the best plan of care can be implemented.

PSYCHOSOCIAL ASSESSMENT, INTERVENTION, AND INTERVIEWING STYLES

A nurse's interviewing style will greatly influence the amount and quality of information obtained from a patient regarding adaptation and coping with an illness. The nurse must remember that the patient may not be aware of some of these coping responses, and may even feel frightened or embarrassed to talk about them. To convey a sense that changes from normal functioning during a time of illness are normal and alright to talk about, the following approach can be used.

Sometimes, when a person becomes sick or unexpectedly ill, it can be a scary experience. It's normal, and even common, for people to think about how their life might be affected as a result of their illness. Some people say they notice themselves acting and feeling differently. Comments like, "I haven't felt like myself since I got sick" are common. Have you been experiencing similar changes since the onset of this illness? If so, tell me about them.

After introducing the subject, the nurse must be patient enough to sit back and listen actively. It is important to let the patient talk about his or her experience with the illness thus far. The nurse can listen specifically for those common emotional, cognitive, and behavioral coping responses previously described. It is useful also to listen for statements like "I'm scared," "I've never felt this way," "I feel stuck," "Nothing can help me," "I need help now." Statements such as these are signs that the patient is beginning to feel that life, as he or she perceives it, is out of control (Greenstone & Leviton, 1993). The nurse should view a patient who is making such remarks as having a strong potential for poorly adapting to the illness, and therefore prone to experiencing the illness as a crisis.

Assessing the patient's level of social support can help the nurse further determine the patient's ability to adapt to illness. Remember that the available type of social support can impact a person's ability to adapt to stress or illness. Social support can come from a variety of sources including family, friends, social agencies, religious affiliation, and others. The nurse can be a temporary source of social support to the patient as well.

The patient's social supports can be identified by asking the patient who he or she can count on when things get rough, and who is available to help the patient through the current situation. The nurse should evaluate the adequacy of the reported level of social support against the amount of meaning the patient places on his or her current condition.

During this time the nurse can show support through nonverbal behaviors, such as by gently leaning toward the patient, maintaining eye contact, and nodding in understanding. Simple utterances such as "uh-huh" or "go on" can effectively encourage the patient to continue talking. Such behaviors will help increase the patient's level of trust in the nurse and decrease the general anxiety the psychosocial assessment tends to create. With the patient feeling calmer and probably safer, he or she is likely to be more open about the effect of physical illness on daily life.

Having assessed the patient's capacity to cope with the newly created stress of the current illness or injury, the nurse can now focus interventions on helping the patient mobilize previously held psychosocial coping methods, to prevent maladaptation to illness.

FAMILIES OF PHYSICALLY ILL PATIENTS

In keeping with a holistic approach to care in the ED, the nurse needs to understand the patient in a family context. The nurse must include the patient's family as part of the care provided to the patient.

Family members go through their own process of adaptation to the patient's arrival in the ED. Just as the patient may not have had time to prepare for the urgent situation bringing him or her to the ED, the family also may be unprepared. This may leave family members feeling helpless, frustrated, and unsure of what the next few hours might bring. The nurse can involve the family by addressing their concerns and questions.

Several studies have been conducted to identify the needs of families in critical care areas. While emergency departments were not part of the sampling, the setting of an ED is very similar to these areas. Therefore, their findings are of use to the nurse caring for families in the ED (Box 25-3).

Hickey (1990) reviewed eight separate studies of family needs in critical care environments and identified recurrent themes within the studies. The most important issue for families centered around *information*. Specifically, families expressed a need to have their questions answered honestly and to know specific facts about the condition and progress of their family member. Other important issues involved the need for reassurance that things would be alright, and the need for convenience in the form of phone availability near a waiting room. Other needs were also identi-

fied; Box 25-3 lists them in descending order of importance.

Families are interested in outcomes and the patient's chance for recovery. In addition, they like to be notified if the patient's condition changes and want to receive information that is understandable. Families in the studies Hickey reviewed also expressed a need to have hope, to believe that hospital personnel care about their loved one, to be reassured that the best possible care is being given, to know exactly what is being done for the patient, and to see the patient frequently.

Nurses are in a key position to be able to help families work through their own complex reactions to the unexpected physical illness of a family member. The above family needs can be a useful reference to the nurse when providing care to families in the ED.

PHYSICAL TRAUMA IN THE ED

In many situations seen in the ED, the consequence of a patient's physical condition significantly compromises that patient's psychological condition. Nowhere is this more evident than when an individual becomes the victim of physical trauma. Not only is stabilization of the patient's physical well-being a priority, so are the patient's and family's psychological well-being. In fact, trauma is viewed as one of the major health and social problems facing the country today (Jutzi-Kosmos, 1990). Therefore, to meet the many needs of the trauma victim and family effectively, the nurse must possess a broad practice framework in order to be able to understand and interpret the changes taking place with a trauma victim.

TRAUMA AND TRAUMATIC STRESS

Physical trauma is an event experienced by victim and family that is unexpected, unplanned, and frequently unpredictable. Such an event creates tremendous upheaval in a person's physical, emotional, and social well-being. Being placed in a situation where one's physical state

BOX 25-3	Needs of Families
	1. Information and answers
	2. Reassurance
	3. Convenient waiting accommodations
	4. Chances for recovery
	5. Notification of condition changes
	6. Hope
	7. Caring staff attitude
	8. Frequent contact with patient
	Source: Hickey, 1990

is unexpectedly traumatized and where the person's ability to prepare for the event is irreclaimable places an individual in a position to experience traumatic stress (Kleber & Brom, 1992).

The concepts of *stress* and *trauma* are not independent of one another, but rather have overlapping qualities. This phenomenon was talked about as early as the 1950s by Bastiaans (1957) when studying concentration camp survivors. In Bastiaans' study, concepts of homeostasis, adaptation, defense, and traumatization were grouped around Selye's concept of stress. "According to Bastiaans, traumatizing stress is a special form of stress, one with more emphasis on shock, alarm and exhaustion than normal stress situations" (Kleber & Brom, 1992, p. 22). Traumatic stress occurs after an extreme life event.

Such extreme circumstances provide no warning that the event is going to take place, and therefore no preparation is taken by individuals to protect themselves. A normal, everyday event is transposed to a catastrophe which changes one's view of self in the world, as well as the predictability and benevolence of life as a whole (Kleber & Brom, 1992).

REACTIONS TO TRAUMATIC EVENTS

Kleber and Brom (1992) describe extreme life events as situations where serious human suffering is experienced or witnessed, with no means to prevent the event from occurring. Being confronted with death and violence also plays an important role in the description

of an extreme life event. Some examples include natural disasters, crimes of violence, acts of war, accidents, and the sudden loss of a loved one. Kleber and Brom (1992) also describe three characteristics experienced by an individual in an extreme situation or traumatic event. These include powerlessness, acute disruption of one's existence, and extreme discomfort.

Powerlessness results from a lack of warning about an event, causing the person to have little influence upon the occurrence and development of the event. Powerlessness is seen in acts of war, natural disasters, accidents, and sudden death. The unavoidable, unpredictable nature of some of these events renders a person completely overwhelmed and helpless.

Acute disruption of one's existence refers to the abrupt shift in the individual's and family's life created by the extreme event of physical trauma. Individuals find themselves in a situation that drastically interrupts their course of living. Their world suddenly looks different. The predictable, preconceived daily life existence once known by the person and family is destroyed. Here, disruptions of self-image and identity are experienced.

Finally, the concept of extreme discomfort does not necessarily refer to the physical pain associated with trauma, but rather the extreme, unpleasant life change which physical trauma creates for individuals and families.

NURSING IMPLICATIONS

Traumatic stress and physical trauma have implications for nurses in the ED. The nurse needs to know that physical trauma, because it is an extreme life event, has the potential to create traumatic stress. In this unbalanced state, the patient will consciously and unconsciously go through a process of psychological adaptation and coping, in an attempt to regain order and equilibrium in his or her life. Therefore, the nurse should assess the patient's coping response to such stress. Kleber and Brom (1992) describe a stress response syndrome, introduced by Horowitz and Kaltreider (1980), as a way of understanding an individual's pattern of coping with traumatic stress.

THE PROCESS OF COPING
WITH TRAUMA

Early Symptoms

The process of coping with a traumatic event begins at the onset of the trauma. Before experiencing the specific symptomatology of denial, the patient may first experience a feeling of bewilderment and disbelief, sometimes accompanied by crying or screaming. These behaviors serve as a psychological protection, of sorts, from the potential catastrophic implications of the event.

Denial and Intrusion

The next step is for the patient to go through an alternating pattern of denial and intrusion. These internal responses manifest specific symptomatology (Kleber & Brom, 1992).

According to Kleber and Brom (1992), when the patient copes through the use of *denial,* he or she is essentially denying the implications of the traumatic event. At this stage the patient may experience emotional numbness and wants to avoid thinking about the traumatic event, and avoid activities that serve as a reminder of the trauma. The patient also experiences a lost sense of reality at this point. Other manifestations of denial include an inability to concentrate, amnesia, an excessive preoccupation with how things could have happened differently, a sense of denial that anything has changed, or preoccupation with other matters not related to the trauma.

The other internal coping response displayed by the patient is that of *intrusion.* Here, the patient experiences repeated surges of emotions and images, implying a reexperience of the traumatic event. At this stage the patient may describe feelings of being back in the traumatic event and may display an increased startle response, as well as hypervigilant behavior. Other behaviors experienced at this stage, but unlikely to be seen during treatment in the ED, include nightmares, recurring thoughts about the event while sleeping.

This alternating pattern of psychological adaptation allows the patient to begin slowly to integrate what has just occurred until he or she is able to deal with the impact of the situation.

It also allows the patient to move further along the continuum of coping, to the working-through or integration phase.

Integration

During the *integration* phase, the patient experiences a decrease in the intensity of emotion connected with the event, along with an increased sense of reality about the event. Eventually the patient's mood stabilizes and the patient begins to be able to come to terms with the event's significance. At this point the patient is in the final phase of the coping process (Kleber & Brom, 1992).

The process of coping seen with trauma is a normal, predictable pattern of reactions to a serious life event. However, when this process is delayed, blocked, or becomes too intense, ineffective coping patterns are established that can lead to pathology. Maladaptive responses to the stress associated with a traumatic event can lead to other stress-related disorders, such as post-traumatic stress disorder (PTSD), adjustment disorder, brief reactive psychosis, major depression, and dissociative disorder (Kleber & Brom, 1992).

PSYCHOSOCIAL ASSESSMENT
AND INTERVENTION WITH
TRAUMA PATIENTS

The above framework adds tremendous value to the nurse's psychosocial assessment and intervention with the trauma victim and family in the emergency department. During the secondary assessment phase described above, the nurse should observe and understand the patient's behavior in the ED in relation to the coping framework.

Once the patient's physical condition has stabilized after entry into the ED, the nurse can provide interventions that enhance self-control and mastery. Because powerlessness is a characteristic of traumatic stress, consider nursing interventions aimed at increasing the patient's sense of control. Examples include giving the patient choices in care and allowing family members to be present whenever possible.

From an assessment perspective, the nurse will collect additional data that involves understanding how the event happened. Let the patient tell his or her story and actively listen for how the event was experienced. The nurse should also use this as an opportunity to explore the patient's early signs of coping, since it is reasonable to assume that the patient will begin to cope actively from the very moment of injury. Active assessment for symptoms described in the coping process is recommended.

This assessment can be achieved by asking what the patient did immediately following the event. This is different than asking for an account of the event. What is being established here is the patient's initial focus of activity or goal after the accident. The answer will help the nurse understand what is most important to the patient and will enhance the effectiveness of nursing interventions in the ED.

For example, the nurse can assess for cues that reflect whether the patient displayed behavior that illustrates a preservation of human dignity, perhaps by covering part of his or her exposed body. Other cues reflect the importance of preserving communication; examples include an attempt by the patient to talk or make eye contact with rescue workers. Perhaps the patient's efforts focused on taking direct action to reverse the incident, such as looking for someone or trying to seek help. The patient may also describe efforts to preserve identity and social contact, such as searching for his or her wallet or other forms of identification. Other behaviors immediately following an incident may focus on concern for family members, as in the case of a mother who would not permit her daughter to learn of the mother's accident until after an important awards ceremony had taken place the same night (Shalev, Schreiber, & Galai, 1993).

Depending on how long it took to transport the patient to the ED and/or how long the patient must stay in the ED before being admitted, the nurse should be prepared for other psychosocial interventions. For example, the initial shock of the event may dissipate while the patient is in the ED and the patient may begin recognizing the acute disruption the event poses. At the scene of the event the patient may have taken on the role of survivor while waiting for help to arrive. Now that he or she is being cared for in the ED, the patient's attention may shift to the role of suffering patient and all that this means to identity.

Here, secondary stressors become evident. These stressors may include uncontrollable pain, unknown outcomes of the injury, potential loss of control over body functions, and inability to monitor contacts with the environment. Nursing interventions at this point should focus on helping the patient to manage the stressors, offering support in the changing circumstances, and helping the patient to reestablish boundaries. The nurse can achieve these goals by being nonintrusive, showing acceptance, and maintaining an open expression of concern (Shalev, Schreiber, & Galai, 1993).

The nurse should also understand that the person's emotional recovery process from trauma will extend beyond the care provided in the ED. Consideration should be given to planning for the patient's needs throughout hospitalization. For example, depending on the severity of the traumatic event or the person's coping ability, the nurse can request the involvement of the psychiatric liaison consultants to provide further support and enhance the healing process during the patient's hospital stay. If several patients are involved in the same traumatic event, the nurse may want to suggest admitting the patients on the same unit. Studies have shown that mutual support by other trauma survivors may enhance the patient's recovery process (Shalev, Schreiber, & Galai, 1993).

FAMILIES OF TRAUMA PATIENTS

Psychosocial care of the trauma victim in the ED would not be complete without involving the family. Families are also victims of trauma. They may not be physically shattered, but they can be emotionally shattered. Consequently, they may engage in behavior that is not necessarily characteristic of the family under more normal circumstances.

Family members' behaviors can be viewed as reactions to several factors related to the trauma, as described by Solursh (1990). Due to the sudden and unpredictable nature of trauma, the family experiences a crisis. Family members will initially display coping responses in the form of shock, disbelief, numbness, and a lost sense of reality. Displays of anger and guilt may follow. This highly charged experience has the potential to cause family members to display their emotions in irrational ways. The relationship a particular family member has with the trauma victim has an impact on that member's response to the event as well.

When confronted with an angry family member, the nurse should not take it personally. Instead, the behavior should be recognized as a necessary step in the grieving process (Solursh, 1990).

As family members continue to try to make sense of their disrupted lives, they may experience a crisis with their faith, with changed family roles, and with their finances. As the family members try to regain a balance in many areas of their lives, the nurse will be in a key position to foster their adaptation to traumatic events.

Nursing Interventions

The nurse needs to be aware of the above factors when working with families of trauma in the emergency department. Families require as much support as the trauma victim in the ED.

A nurse can provide psychosocial support to family members in several ways. Keeping them frequently informed about the patient's status will help keep their anxiety about the unknown at manageable levels. Providing a quiet room where they can collect themselves and begin planning for the next few days shows support and respect for what they are going through. During this time, the nurse should assess the family's ability to cope with the situation. The nurse should also explain that what the family is experiencing emotionally is normal coping behavior for such extreme circumstances. At a point when the family displays somewhat calmer and more rational behavior and when anxiety levels have decreased, the nurse can begin to educate members about the normal coping responses and behaviors trauma victims display, using the coping framework described above.

At times a trauma victim presents to the ED in an unconscious state, requiring cardiopulmonary resuscitation. One ED program has had great success in permitting the family to become part of the resuscitation team by providing support to the patient during controlled periods of treatment. This effort has been found to facilitate the family's acceptance of death and the process of grieving in the ED (Hanson & Strawser, 1992). Emergency department nurses may want to explore the possibility of starting such a program where they work.

CARE OF THE PSYCHIATRICALLY ILL PERSON

Even though emergency departments are set up to treat general medical conditions, it is becoming increasingly obvious that no physical illness comes in a neat package. When people become physically ill, an entwined set of events challenges them physically, psychologically, and socially. Similar challenges are also present when people become psychiatrically ill. Rather than experiencing a medical crisis, these patients are experiencing an emotional crisis.

The term *psychiatric* is used to describe conditions attributed to the presence of mental illness. The patient with a psychiatric emergency presents to the ED with a severe dysfunction of behavior, mood, thinking, or perception. In the absence of appropriate interventions, such dysfunctional behavior could create a threat to life, adequate functioning, or psychological integrity (Steele & Grover, 1992).

Perhaps no other mental illness creates such acute psychological trauma for a person as those illnesses such as chronic schizophrenia that yield psychotic features or psychosis.

PSYCHOSIS: AN OVERVIEW

Hillard (1990) describes acute psychosis as "one of the most serious psychiatric emergencies. Patients with chronic psychotic disorders are one of the largest and most important subpopulations of psychiatric emergency patients" (p. 229). Psychosis causes individuals to experience a loss of contact with reality. They lose their ability to understand circumstances rationally. There is a loss of rational control. Consequently, the psychotic patient may behave in a frightened, terrified manner.

The patient's ability to understand and respond to the nurse in a rational way is diminished. This creates a scenario where the patient easily may become threatened by simple comments or physical contact, increasing the potential that the patient will act out verbally and/or physically. A person with acute psychosis must generally be regarded as at increased risk for suicide and other disruptive behaviors (Hillard, 1990).

"Acting out" behavior in a psychotic individual can be interpreted as the person's attempt to regain control of his or her perceived reality. It is helpful to remember that the person's perceptual ability is altered to such a degree that the person is struggling with what is real and what is not real. This altered mental state does not enable the person to trust what he or she sees, feels, or hears. The result is a sense of confusion, fear, and distrust. The nurse can ease the patient's experience of this phenomenon by providing interventions that take into consideration the lost ability to be rational.

Most nurses believe that patients experiencing psychosis are not good historians. It is important to realize, however, that on some level these patients intuitively know that something is seriously wrong but lack the ability to articulate that fact.

The nurse is cautioned not to link psychosis exclusively with mental illness. A person can experience psychosis as a result of many factors. Psychosis can be broadly categorized as a *new onset* or a *chronic* condition. The nurse caring for a patient who is psychotic can use this as a reference point when beginning an assessment of this phenomenon.

NURSING ASSESSMENT AND INTERVENTION WITH NEW ONSET PSYCHOSIS

If the patient's past history with psychosis is not known to the ED personnel, steps must be taken to determine the cause of the psychotic behavior. New onset psychosis can be caused by substance use, organic causes, or hysteria. It is important that the nurse assess for each of these factors, in order to understand the etiology of the psychosis and provide interventions accordingly.

Substance Abuse

The nurse should ask the patient about any recent substance use or abuse. Substances such as lysergic acid diethylamide (LCD), phencyclidine (PCP), cocaine, and amphetamines can produce psychotic symptoms. Withdrawal from sedatives and hypnotics will yield similar results. When substance abuse is believed to be the cause of the current psychotic state, the nurse can anticipate and plan for several hours of observation to monitor the patient's behavior. A toxicology profile is often ordered by the physician to confirm the suspected ingestion of drugs (Hillard, 1990).

Organic Psychosis

If substance abuse has been ruled out, the nurse can begin to assess for an organic cause of the psychosis. Hillard (1990) notes that "any illness that can cause delirium can cause psychosis in the sense of a loss of contact with reality" (p. 231).

The nurse must rely on medical assessment skills and perform a focused physical assessment. The nurse should specifically assess for abnormal vital signs; decreased level of consciousness; disorientation to time, place, or person; the presence of medical symptoms that are closely related to the onset of psychiatric symptoms; the start and/or stopping of new medications around the same time that the psychiatric symptoms appeared; and the rapid onset of symptoms without a prodromal period. Such manifestations suggest that the psychosis has an organic etiology (Hillard, 1990).

Hallucinations are also suggestive of an organic origin to psychosis. While visual hallucinations may be seen in psychiatric disorders such as schizophrenia, they are more characteristic of organic brain syndrome, as are tactile (touch), olfactory (smell), and gustatory (taste) hallucinations (Hillard, 1990).

The nurse who assesses a patient as having organic psychosis should develop nursing interventions that focus on the patient's safety, further assessment, and medication therapy. The use of antipsychotic medications with this type of patient should be kept to a minimum in the ED, as such medications interfere with further diagnostic workup. The approach in intervening with organic psychosis is the same as functional psychosis. Hospitalization is generally required.

Factitious and Hysterical Psychosis

Sometimes, for conscious or unconscious reasons, patients may act psychotic when in fact they are not. This presentation is described as *factitious, malingered,* or *hysterical* psychosis. The nurse can begin to assess for this category of psychosis by looking for other characteristic symptomatology. These symptoms include a normal range of affect with little variation when responding to delusions, and unusual hallucinations. An obvious secondary gain, such as avoiding jail, is another telling sign of this psychosis, as well as the patient's eager admission to almost any psychotic symptom suggested by the nurse. Even though factitious and hysterical psychosis are not commonly seen, the nurse should be aware of the presentation (Hillard, 1990).

CHRONIC PSYCHOSIS

An Overview

Over the past several years there has been a movement to integrate the chronic mentally ill back into communities and out of long-term, state psychiatric facilities. Even though many new and innovative community programs have been developed to sustain this shift in treatment, support to individuals is often intermittent. Because this population characteristically has poor social and coping skills, the patient and family alike can become overly stressed. The result may be a crisis, with the ED serving as a natural safe haven, or intermediary, when problems arise.

The most frequent ED presentation of a chronically and persistently mentally ill person is after a period of discontinuing medication, which results in decompensating behavior. Psychosis is commonly seen with this type of decompensation (Hillard, 1990). Inherent in the psychiatric illness of chronic schizophrenia, for example, are sporadic attempts by the patient to discontinue medications. The pa-

tient may have difficulty understanding that medications are needed even when he or she is feeling good. Consequently, when the patient feels more stable medications may be curtailed, only to cause a relapse.

Each patient displays a unique pattern of symptoms during the relapse phases of chronic psychosis. These include the decompensation phase, the postpsychotic phase, and the adaptive plateau phase. The nurse can structure assessment according to these three phases.

Nursing Assessment and Intervention With Phases of Chronic Psychosis

Decompensation Phase

Common signs and symptoms during the decompensation phase include hallucinations, suspiciousness, changes in sleep, increased anxiety, and angry outbursts leading to increased disruptive behavior. The presence of a thought disorder and depressive symptoms are also common (Hillard, 1990). After the nurse assesses the patient for signs and symptoms of decompensation, it is important to assess the patient's medication regime and related compliance. The nurse should try to learn if the onset of the symptoms is associated with any medication changes.

Before nursing interventions are planned and implemented, the nurse should remember that the psychotic patient has a distorted sense of reality. Because the patient's ability to process stimuli is decreased, it is helpful to ask questions and make remarks in a simple, clear, and concise fashion. It is helpful also to inform the patient briefly about the nurse's role in care and what can be expected in the ED, before beginning the assessment. The patient can be reassured that safety is a major concern and that he or she will be protected from harm. The nurse should focus interventions on providing safety, developing trust, and decreasing the patient's fear and anxiety.

Postpsychotic Phase

This type of relapse may be a function of the patient's stage of illness. For example, when the patient is discharged home after being treated for a psychotic episode, a period of reintegration takes place. A reintegration into the family and community occurs but can be a frequent cause of conflict as this process unfolds. As noted previously, patients with a chronic psychiatric illness inherently have poor coping and social skills. The smallest conflict or frustration may be enough to cause the patient to experience more stress. For the patient with poor coping skills, this situation may be enough to cause maladaptive coping, which may result in the patient experiencing a relapse.

Psychosis seen as result of this circumstance is known as the *postpsychotic phase* (Hillard, 1990). Nursing interventions during this transitional period consist of helping the patient to identify strengths and adaptive coping behaviors. The nurse should educate the patient about this phase of recovery after a psychotic episode and talk about the normal period of adaptation that is taking place. The nurse should also provide reassurance to the patient and ensure that enough social support, including family and professional support, is in place to help the patient successfully manage this stage.

Adaptive Plateau Phase
As the patient continues on the path of recovery and reintegration into the community and family, an *adaptive plateau phase* may be reached (Hillard, 1990). At this stage the patient is relatively asymptomatic when presenting to the ED, but sees the ED as a place of safety. The dynamics behind the patient seeking this type of support are likely to be connected to progress or movement toward restabilization in the outpatient program.

The patient at this stage will show signs of motivation in complying with his or her outpatient treatment goals. These goals may include a reduction of medication, involvement with vocational rehabilitation, and movement of the patient toward independent living. This progress, although positive, may be unsettling for the patient. Consequently, maladaptive behaviors related to regression may be displayed; they serve as the catalyst for the patient to seek out the ED services as a safe haven.

Nursing intervention for a patient at this phase involves listening to the patient's fears and concerns. Once again, the patient's posthospitalization accomplishments and posi-

tive adaptations can be reviewed. Talking with the patient's family and outpatient therapist about the patient's presentation to the ED is also beneficial in supporting this adaptive process.

It is important for the nurse to assess the symptoms seen and reported in each phase against the patient's baseline behavior or normal level of functioning. The nurse must distinguish between which symptoms are part of the patient's daily life and which are attributed to the current relapse. Because making this distinction is a key feature in being able to plan for the most appropriate care, it is beneficial for the nurse to document, in the medical record, a detailed description of the patient's current behavior. This is easily done by conducting a mental status examination of the patient. It is also helpful to establish and document how this behavior differs from the patient's norm. This detailed description in the chart will be a useful future reference for the nurse caring for the chronic mentally ill patient in the ED, since this type of patient may not always be able to give a detailed account of the current relapse.

Family Involvement

Throughout these phases, the family will be a prime resource to the nurse. Generally, the family knows the mentally ill patient best and is often a good resource for establishing how the patient responds when functioning at an optimum level. The nurse should also recognize the family as presumably the patient's main social support in the community. The family may be equally stressed by shouldering the burden of caring for a loved one with a chronic mental illness and by being part of their network of social support.

The family may not recognize its own stress response to the situation. The nurse should take the opportunity while talking with family members, over the phone if necessary, to establish how they are coping with the patient's process of adaptation in the community and at home. The nurse can help them understand the different phases described above, explain the normal behavior seen in each phase, and provide support by letting family members know it is alright to take time for themselves. The nurse can explain that this type of self-care indirectly helps the patient adapt to community living. Many support groups for families of the chronic mentally ill have been established. The nurse may suggest and support the family's involvement in such a group as perhaps the family's first step in taking care of themselves.

Nurses are, indeed, in a privileged role to be able to influence and facilitate healthier adaptation by patients and families alike. Whether one is challenged physically or psychiatrically, the nurse is in a key position to help those facing such challenges.

Out of the many diverse populations treated in the ED, perhaps no other group faces as great a challenge as those who are mentally ill and homeless.

THE HOMELESS MENTALLY ILL

The homeless, mentally ill population has increased as a result of the deinstitutionalization movement over the past several years, coupled with inadequate community supports. In addition, more and more young adults are at risk for developing a mental illness (Barker, 1990). Schizophrenia, psychotic disorders, and affective disorders are among the major mental illnesses seen among the homeless population. According to Jones and Katz (1992), approximately one-third of the single, homeless population is mentally ill.

Contributing Factors and Characteristics

Several factors contribute to homelessness among the mentally ill. These include lack of housing, being dually diagnosed with mental illness and substance abuse, limited commitment laws, the lack of service integration in the mental health delivery system, and the presence of mental illness itself (Lamb & Lamb, 1990).

A study conducted by Lamb and Lamb (1990) identified how various aspects of mental illness may contribute to homelessness. Three general aspects are noted: the disorganization and poor problem-solving abilities inherent in mental illness, severe paranoia, and depression. Paranoia was found to be an influ-

encing factor in preventing the person from accepting assistance. Depression left individuals unable to mobilize themselves to seek care and assistance needed to reverse their homeless situation. The study also noted that mental illness symptoms are exacerbated by the stress of homelessness.

Barker (1990) provides a portrait of the homeless, mentally ill patient. This person is male, between the ages of 30 and 50, and has been an area resident for some time. He sleeps in a variety of shelters and has a history of evictions, secondary to conflicts related to his behavior. He fears personal assault or robbery; however, the majority of homeless individuals have limited-to-no finances.

With the homeless mentally ill enduring the challenge of daily survival on many levels, the adverse impact on their physical and mental well-being is severe. These individuals are at risk for developing maladaptive behaviors which place their physical, psychological, and social selves in jeopardy.

A Biopsychosocial Perspective

Those who are homeless utilize the ED almost exclusively for whatever medical care they can receive (Aghababian, Peterson, & Gans, 1992). According to Barker (1990), "at least one in four homeless persons presenting in an emergency room will have a medical illness requiring treatment" (p. 355). Because members of the mentally ill, homeless population exhibit the most severe forms of mental illness, they are particularly at risk for medical problems related to exposure, alcohol and substance abuse, violence, contagious diseases, and inadequate nutrition (Barker, 1990). They are also at risk for developing further psychological and social problems. In fact, some studies view homelessness as a psychological trauma (Goodman, Saxe, & Harvey, 1991).

A wide range of psychological conditions, some of which have been discussed in this chapter, have been associated with psychological trauma. According to Goodman, Saxe, and Harvey (1991), "at least two commonly reported symptoms of psychological trauma—social disaffiliation and learned helplessness—are highly prevalent among homeless individuals and families" (p. 1220).

Social Disaffiliation

Social disaffiliation is a key feature of psychological trauma. Goodman, Saxe, and Harvey (1991), describing the work done by Van der Kolk (1987), note "that the essence of psychological trauma is the perceived severance of secure affiliative bonds, which damages the psychological sense of trust, safety and security" (p. 1220).

Becoming homeless creates a situation where relationships become disbanded. Consequently, homeless individuals may display maladaptive behaviors of distrust and hypervigilance. Such behaviors may also be exaggerated by the presence of a paranoid disorder or by the development of a learned response to a hostile world (Barker, 1990). Patients can demonstrate this type of behavior by refusing to provide historical information, including their name. They may be hesitant to tell others where they sleep.

An inability to feel safe or to trust is often compounded by the failure of social support networks or by the withdrawing of current support systems (Goodman, Saxe, & Harvey 1991). The incidence of substance abuse among this population also influences their receding social networks. Many families do not welcome the substance-abusing family member into their home, and most community residential facilities do not tolerate residents using drugs or alcohol (Lamb & Lamb, 1990). Consequently, the homeless, mentally ill person often has no choice but to return to the streets.

Becoming homeless also deprives an individual of the social roles he or she once maintained in the family, community, and society. In essence, the homeless, mentally ill person has lost the ability to perform accustomed social roles. Eventually, lost identity causes these individuals to lack confidence in their ability to provide self-care; they also develop a belief that others do not want to help them (Goodman, Saxe, & Harvey, 1991). These experiences draw the homeless mentally ill further away from social support.

Learned Helplessness

Homelessness also renders people unable to control their daily lives. Their sense of personal control is diminished or nonexistent. Living in this helpless state leads to the phenomenon of *learned helplessness*. Seligman (1975) describes learned helplessness as occurring when a person ceases to believe they have the ability to make a difference in the course of their lives. It is often accompanied by profound depression. This cognitive distortion sets the stage for maladaptation. For example, a high rate of depression that stems from the ongoing experience of helplessness, as well as a generalized passivity, is seen with learned helplessness. This, in turn, may cause the person to display further maladaptive behaviors involving indifferent attitudes and issues of dependency.

Nursing Assessment and Intervention With the Homeless Mentally Ill

Nurses are cautioned not to have a preconceived notion that the homeless individual caused his or her circumstances. It is essential for the nurse to view this person as unique, with his or her own history and perspective. Accordingly, the nurse should provide psychosocial interventions using an optimistic, creative, and active approach based on the patient's life experience.

Homeless, mentally ill persons may present to the emergency department for a variety of reasons. They may be there voluntarily or involuntarily. Whatever the cause, a key to planning any psychosocial intervention must be an understanding of the patient's strong level of distrust. The patient's inability to trust others will influence how he or she responds and interacts with ED personnel. More importantly, it will influence the outcome of care provided in the ED.

The nurse should focus interventions toward developing trust. If this is not the nurse's initial goal, all subsequent interactions with the patient will most likely be ineffective. Since this patient's presentation is similar to behavior of the psychiatrically ill person, review the interventions outlined above.

The nurse can establish trust by effectively engaging the homeless, mentally ill patient. Engagement is a process that happens over time with this individual. It is derived from the patient's having a positive experience with others, as well as receiving concrete and appropriate services. Being knowledgeable about this type of population and employing a flexible attitude are strategies that will increase the nurse's ability to engage the patient effectively (Barker, 1990). Talking about subjects that are important and significant to him or her is also effective. Barker (1990) notes that the homeless mental health consumer is concerned with problems related to lack of material resources, employment opportunities, privacy, and protection.

Once some level of trust has been established, and after the patient's chief complaint is explored, the following areas also need to be assessed. The nurse will want to do a focused assessment of the signs and symptoms of depression and substance abuse, problems that are prevalent among this population. Suicidal or homicidal plans should also be evaluated. If the patient's safety in the ED is not a concern, the nurse can focus on allowing the patient to have as much control of choices regarding care as possible. However, because this patient may approach life with a generalized passivity, the nurse must be cognizant that the patient may not report symptoms of an illness accurately or completely. Therefore, the nurse may want to put more emphasis on the objective part of the assessment, since the subjective part may not yield reliable information.

Undoubtedly, the nurse will feel challenged by this patient's display of maladaptive behaviors. The nurse may feel frustrated by the patient's indifference to and possibly refusal of care. A painful awareness of the lack of services available to this population may occur as care plans are developed. However, challenges like these empower nurses to create their greatest work of art. The challenge can be confronted.

CONCLUSION

Patients presenting to the ED are experiencing various challenges in adaptation. They bring unique personalities, backgrounds, histories, stressors, and coping abilities. Just as the patient is presenting with many challenges, the nurse is equally challenged. For it is the nurse, through the art of nursing, who must use his or her knowledge, skills and tools like an artist, to recognize, uncover and identify the challenges facing the patient. Ultimately, these challenges will have the greatest impact on the patient's recovery.

BIBLIOGRAPHY

Abraham, I. L., Fox, J. C., & Cohen, B. T. (1992). Integrating the bio into the biopsychosocial: Understanding and treating biological phenomena in psychiatric-mental health nursing. *Archives of Psychiatric Nursing*, 6(5), 296–305.

Aghababian, R., Peterson, L., & Gans, L. (1992). Utilization of emergency services: The nineties. In G. R. Schwartz, C. G. Cayten, M. A. Mangelsen, T. A. Mayer, & B. K. Hanke (Eds.), *Principles and practices of emergency medicine: Vol. II* (3rd ed.). Philadelphia: Lea & Febiger.

Aguilera, D. C. (1990). *Crisis intervention: Theory and methodology* (6th ed.). St. Louis: C. V. Mosby.

American Hospital Association. (1992). *American Hospital Association hospital statistics.* Chicago: American Hospital Association.

Bard, M., & Ellison, K. (1974). Crisis intervention and investigation of forcible rape. *The Police Chief*, 41, 68–73.

Barker, G. A. (1990). The homeless mentally ill. In J.R. Hillard (Ed.), *Manual of clinical emergency psychiatry.* Washington, DC: American Psychiatric Press, Inc.

Bastiaans, J. (1957). *Psychosomatische gevolgen van onderdrukking en verzet.* Amsterdam: Noord-Hollandse Uitgevers Maatschappij.

Blair, F. A., & Hall, M. M. (1994). The nursing process: Assessment and priority setting. In A. R. Klein, G. Lee, A. Manton, & J. G. Parker (Eds.), *Emergency nursing core curriculum* (4th ed.). Philadelphia: W. B. Saunders.

Flannery, R. B., Jr. (1990). Social support and psychological trauma: A methodological approach. *Journal of Traumatic Stress, 3*(4), 593–611.

Flannery, R. B., Jr., & Harvey, M. R. (1991). Psychological trauma and learned helplessness: Seligman's paradigm reconsidered. *Psychotherapy, 28*(2), 374–378.

Fought, S. G., & Throwe, A. N. (1994). Psychological emergencies. In A. R. Klein, G. Lee, A. Manton, & J. G. Parker (Eds.), *Emergency nursing core curriculum* (4th ed.). Philadelphia: W. B. Saunders.

Golan, N. (1978). *Treatment in crisis situations.* New York: Free Press.

Goodman, L., Saxe, L., & Harvey, M. (1991). Homelessness as psychological trauma. *American Psychologist, 46*(11), 1219–1225.

Greenstone, J. L., & Leviton, S. C. (1993). *Elements of crisis intervention: Crises and how to respond to them.* Pacific Grove: Brooks/Cole Publishing.

Grover, N. H., & Steele, T. W. (1992). Psychiatric emergencies: Biopsychosocial stressors. In S.B. Sheehy (Ed.), *Emergency nursing: Principles and practice* (3rd ed.). St. Louis: Mosby Year Book.

Hanson, C., & Strawser, D. (1992). Family presence during cardiopulmonary resuscitation: Foote Hospital emergency department's nine-year perspective. *Journal of Emergency Nursing, 18*(2), 104–106.

Hess, H. J., & Ruster, P. L. (1990). Assessment and crisis intervention with clients in a hospital emergency room. In A. R. Roberts (Ed.), *Crisis intervention handbook: Assessment, treatment and research.* Belmont: Wadsworth Publishing.

Hickey, M. (1990). What are the needs of families of critically ill patients? A review of the literature since 1976. *Heart & Lung, 19*(4), 401–415.

Hillard, J. R. (1990). Psychosis: Acute and chronic. In J. R. Hillard (Ed.), *Manual of clinical emergency psychiatry.* Washington, DC: American Psychiatric Press, Inc.

Horowitz, M. J., & Kaltreider, N. B. (1980). Brief psychotherapy of stress response syndromes. In T. Karasu & L. Bellak (Eds.), *Specialized techniques in individual psychotherapy.* New York: Brunner/Mazel.

Jones, B. E., & Katz, N. D. (1992). Evaluating recent research on the homeless mentally ill. *Psychiatric Quarterly, 63*(1), 41–50.

Jutzi-Kosmos, C. (1990). Assessment of multiple trauma and thoracic trauma. In S. Kitt & J. Kaiser (Eds.), *Emergency nursing: A physiologic and clinical perspective.* Philadelphia: W. B. Saunders.

Kleber, R. J., & Brom, D. (1992). *Coping with trauma: Theory, prevention and treatment.* Amsterdam: Swets & Zeitlinger.

Lamb, H. R., & Lamb, D. M. (1990). Factors contributing to homelessness among the chronically and severely mentally ill. *Hospital and Community Psychiatry, 41*(3), 301–305.

MacPhail, E. R. (1992). Overview of emergency nursing and emergency care. In S.B. Sheehy (Ed.), *Emergency nursing: Principles and practice* (3rd ed.). St. Louis: Mosby Year Book.

Moore, K. W., & Schwartz, K. S. (1993). Psychosocial support of trauma patients in the emergency department by nurses, as indicated by communication. *Journal of Emergency Nursing, 19*(4), 297–302.

Motto, J. A. (1992). Psychiatric emergencies. In C. E. Saunders & M. T. Ho (Eds.), *Current emergency diagnosis and treatment* (4th ed.). Norwalk: Appleton & Lange.

Roberts, A. R. (1990). An overview of crisis theory and crisis intervention. In A. R. Roberts (Ed.), *Crisis intervention handbook: Assessment, treatment and research.* Belmont: Wadsworth Publishing.

Schwartz, G. R. (1992). The work environment. In G. R. Schwartz, C. G. Cayten, M. A. Mangelsen, T. A. Mayer, & B. K. Hanke (Eds.), *Principles and practices of emergency medicine: Vol. II* (3rd ed.). Philadelphia: Lea & Febiger.

Seligman, M. E. P. (1975). *Helplessness: On depression, development and death.* San Francisco: Freeman.

Shalev, A. Y., Schreiber, S., & Galai, T. (1993). Early psychological responses to traumatic injury. *Journal of Traumatic Stress, 6*(4), 441–450.

Solursh, D. S. (1990). The family of the trauma victim. *Nursing Clinics of North America, 25*(1), 155–162.

Steele, T. W., & Grover, N. H. (1992). Psychosocial and mental health assessment. In S. B. Sheehy (Ed.), *Emergency nursing: Principles and practice* (3rd ed.). St. Louis: Mosby Year Book.

Thompson, J. (1992). Stress theory and therapeutic practice. *Stress Medicine, 8,* 147–150.

Van der Kolk, B. A. (1987). The psychological consequences of overwhelming life experiences. In B. A. Van der Kolk (Ed.), *Psychological trauma.* Washington, DC: American Psychiatric Press.

CHAPTER 26

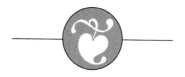

Psychosocial Assessment and Intervention in Maternal/Child Health

Lori Clark

The psychological aspects of pregnancy are of interest to health care providers for a variety of reasons. First, pregnancy and motherhood are significant markers in a woman's life, a time when her existing identity is reconfigured to accommodate her new maternal role. This occurs whether the woman is pregnant for the first time or is already a mother. Second, pregnancy is an interrelated physical and social experience which has psychological ramifications. In order to effectively interact with a woman during the perinatal period, health care workers must be knowledgeable about the unique psychosocial aspects of pregnancy and their impact on the health of not only the mother, but the entire family constellation.

PSYCHOSOCIAL AND CULTURAL ADAPTATION TO PREGNANCY

CHANGES IN FAMILY STRUCTURE

The American family has undergone unparalleled change in the past two decades. Histori-cally, families both worked and played together; the family unit was the center of most activity and members lived according to rigid societal and moral rules. In contrast, the family of the late 20th century is more individualized and less family-centered. This is a direct result of relatively recent social changes which have influenced family structure and function. The following social trends have been identified as having a profound impact on the family (Auvenshire & Enriquez, 1990).

1. Decrease in the average size of the family primarily resulting from a decline in families with five or more children. Childlessness has remained at approximately 8% to 10% of marriages; one-child families remain at 10%.
2. Decline in marriage rates, which has been accompanied by an increase in unwed teenage motherhood.
3. Marked increase in the divorce rate and the rate of remarriage.

Patricia Barry: *Psychosocial Nursing: Care of Physically Ill Patients and Their Families*, 3rd ed.
© 1996 Lippincott–Raven Publishers

4. An increase in the numbers of households comprised of single adults, aged adults, unrelated adults, newly married adults, and single parents and their children.
5. Escalation of women's status both in and out of the family setting via increased education and career opportunities.

DEVELOPMENT OF MATERNAL IDENTITY

As noted earlier, pregnancy is a significant life event which has the potential to contribute to a woman's personal growth. Becoming pregnant and the subsequent development of a maternal identity involve a complete rethinking and redefining of self. This is a complex, active process that occurs over time, beginning at the discovery of pregnancy and continuing throughout the first year after birth. The pregnancy experience itself facilitates incorporation of this new dimension into a mother's existing self. Interpersonal and intrapersonal experiences of pregnancy, childbearing, and childrearing can either foster or inhibit the process.

Rubin (1975) described four developmental stages though which a pregnant woman becomes ready for mothering.

1. Seeking safe passage for herself and her child throughout pregnancy, labor, and birth.
2. Ensuring the acceptance of her child by the significant persons in her life.
3. Binding-in to her child.
4. Learning to give of herself.

Each woman's journey in completing these developmental tasks is unique, based on her individual strengths and weaknesses and her past and present life circumstances. A woman who believes she will deliver her infant without any significant problems, whose motherhood is accepted by the people who are important to her, and who feels she is able to give of herself to the newborn baby whom she values as a separate being, enters motherhood with few, if any, psychological burdens. Unfinished tasks can be psychologically draining, making less energy available to her in her new mothering endeavors.

Seeking Safe Passage

Seeking safe passage involves both the woman's and infant's intact or "safe" completion of pregnancy and childbirth. To gain relevant information, multiple sources of information are sought. These sources may include books, prenatal classes, health care providers, other pregnant women, friends, and family. Information about the probable course of pregnancy, potential risks, and measures to avoid or counteract these risks, is sought and discussed at length. Great credence is given to the personal stories and experiences of friends and other pregnant women.

The task of ensuring safe passage requires women to identify and address their fears. The anxiety caused by this fear is modulated to some degree by a woman choosing or not choosing to seek information about an aspect of pregnancy. Until a woman is ready to receive information, providing it will be futile.

Primigravidas and multigravidas differ in the process of seeking safe passage. Multigravidas draw on their own previous experiences which, depending on the outcome, can facilitate or hinder this developmental task. Multigravid women should be asked to recount past childbearing experiences to identify areas of concern. In contrast, the lack of childbearing experience creates a diffuse focus and fears for many first-time mothers. Factual information about the pregnancy, delivery, and childbearing options is generally well-received. Women who experience medical problems during pregnancy have difficulty completing this task as the passage is no longer viewed as safe.

Acceptance by Others

Acceptance of the unborn infant by significant persons in the mother's life involves opening and restructuring existing relationships to accommodate the coming baby. This change is most significant for the father. The partner's willingness to alter his current role to incorporate the infant into the family is strongly correlated with the mother's positive adjustment.

Health care workers can support the mother's efforts to complete this task by encouraging discussions with her partner about how their relationship will be altered and the subsequent need to reorganize responsibilities. They can also suggest age-appropriate ways to include other children in the pregnancy in anticipation of a new sibling. Anticipatory guidance should also include discussions of the losses that will inevitably accompany the gains.

Binding-in

Binding-in is the process by which the mother comes to accept the pregnancy and feels a loving, emotional bond to the unborn baby. The circumstances under which the pregnancy was conceived greatly influence this developmental task. An unplanned pregnancy with an absent partner holds different meaning than a long-awaited pregnancy in the context of a stable, loving relationship. Although the binding-in process refers to the dynamic between a mother and her fetus, the external environment created by the degree to which others accept the pregnancy either eases or restricts a mother's ability to develop a relationship with her unborn child.

The signals provided by the fetus influence the binding-in process. Ultrasonography and fetal movement aid in creating the maternal-fetal bond. The task, however, is not linear. Obstetrical complications can delay binding-in. Additional emotional support is needed to allow a mother who is uncertain about the outcome of her pregnancy the ability to invest in an antenatal relationship with her unborn child.

Giving of Oneself

In order to give of oneself, the pregnant mother must define the essential components of giving. Caring, involvement, and some degree of self-deprivation are encompassed in giving. Pregnancy and mothering require self-denial and delayed gratification for the benefit of the child. Giving, therefore, necessitates self-esteem. In order to give without awareness of the self-sacrifice involved, a woman must have something inside to give, which generally results from having received sufficiently. Health care providers can help a woman feel replenished by providing personal attention and relief from uncertainty or anxiety. These measures serve to bolster a woman's self-esteem and respect so she is able to give.

PRIMIPAROUS MOTHER

Maternal adaptation to pregnancy is accomplished via preparation throughout pregnancy for labor, birth and becoming a new mother. First-time mothers generally have a greater need for information.

In a study comparing patient and provider perceptions of what pregnant women want to know, the interests of primiparous women differed significantly from those of multiparous women (Freda et al., 1993). First-time mothers expressed higher levels of interest in all topics. A majority of primiparous women was interested in 89% of the suggested 38 subjects, indicating a desire for information on a variety of subjects during pregnancy. The topics of greatest interest were fetal development, nutrition, vitamins, and danger signs of pregnancy.

It is important to note that health care provider interests did not parallel pregnant women's responses in the study. To be most effective, teaching plans should begin with what the mother wants to know, even if providers believe that information is not the most important. Health care providers, particularly nurses, should be attuned to the increased need for information on a broad spectrum of topics. This need for information has been institutionalized to some extent by childbirth preparation classes.

A woman typically has fears about the process of labor and birth. The primipara who has not experienced the process of childbirth fears the unknown. Common fears include how she will respond to the pain of labor, losing control emotionally, and the outcome for herself and her infant. While information and reassurance from her providers and partner can resolve some of the fears, each woman must cope with her fear individually. Rehearsing labor techniques with a partner can be an effective strategy for reducing fear.

Recent statistics suggest a significant increase in the number of primiparas who are 35 years of age or older. Generally, women who delay parenthood are better educated and have achieved higher occupational levels than their younger counterparts (Reece, 1993). The pregnancy experience of this subgroup is unique in that the women are socialized to believe they are at higher risk medically while, in fact, research findings are inconsistent (Harker & Thorpe, 1992). This labelling leads to heightened anxiety as these primiparas perceive that if the current pregnancy has a negative outcome, they will have little time to conceive another child.

As a result of their generally higher educational status in combination with heightened anxiety, elderly primiparas often desire great quantities of information from providers. The disproportionate number of these women in childbirth preparation classes is evidence of this phenomenon. Despite the stressors created by their maternal age, older primiparas are reported to have greater motivation for motherhood, stronger maternal-fetal relationship, and an increased maternal role conceptualization than earlier childbearers (Gottesman, 1992).

MULTIPAROUS MOTHER

Nursing research has identified some important differences between primiparous and multiparous pregnancies. The multipara experiences all of the physical and psychosocial changes associated with pregnancy. In addition, she must manage the needs of her other children and begin to prepare them for the change associated with the addition of a sibling.

Multiparas may have specific concerns or preconceived notions based on their previous birth experience. Many times, obstetrical visits for a multipara is briefer as she typically does not appear to need information. This can be perceived as a lack of support or, worse yet, a lack of interest in the woman's current pregnancy.

Time should be allocated during a health care encounter to review not only the medical data but the emotional experience of past pregnancies, with particular attention focused on residual fears. Anticipatory guidance should also include assistance in preparing older children for the arrival of the newborn and planning for additional assistance immediately after the birth to ensure rest and time with the new baby. It is important that the multiparous mother feels supported by the health care system since, traditionally, society withdraws visible support (such as showers and gifts) with subsequent pregnancies.

THE SINGLE MOTHER

The single-parent family is the most common variation of the normative two-parent family structure. The number of single-parent families with children under the age of 18 rose from 3.8 million in 1970 to 9.7 million in 1990 (U.S. Bureau of the Census, 1990). This trend is expected to continue into the next century.

The vast majority of single-parent homes are headed by women who are lone mothers and, consequently, represent the poorest of all demographic groups. Sixty percent of children living in mother-only families are impoverished, in stark contrast to only 11% in two-parent families (Kamerman & Kahn, 1988). Regardless of income level, single mothers have higher rates of stress than their married counterparts. Financial concerns create the greatest amount of stress, as evidenced by higher levels of anxiety, depression, and health-related problems among single mothers (Olson & Banyard, 1993).

Effect on Pregnancy

Stress may affect a pregnancy in several ways. First, it can divert a woman's attention away from pregnancy-related issues. As a result, a woman may have a decreased recognition of pregnancy risks or problems and may delay or decrease compliance with care. Second, a woman may adapt unhealthy coping mechanisms to deal with the stress, including smoking, drinking, substance use, and excessive work. Finally, stress can negatively impact interpersonal relations, thereby limiting the amount of support available to a single, pregnant woman (Culpepper & Jack, 1993).

In prenatal care and other contacts with the health care system, health care workers systematically need to assess a single pregnant woman's stressors and identify coping mechanisms, both adaptive and maladaptive. Discussion should support continuation of adaptive behaviors (for example, exercising) and strategies to minimize maladaptive behaviors (for example, a smoking cessation or drug treatment program) throughout the duration of pregnancy. Women who report and/or demonstrate high levels of stress should be referred to social services or some additional form of mental health support.

Social support is thought to mitigate the negative effects of stress. Support has been operationalized in the literature as emotional support (expressions of caring and esteem), informational support (advice or guidance), and instrumental support (tangible goods or assistance with tasks) (Pakizegi, 1990; Richardson, Barbour & Bubenzer, 1991). The stress-buffering effect of social support is contingent on the amount of support *received,* not the amount of support available. Results of a recent study indicated that women who received more support had better labor progress, were at lower risk for depression, and had infants with higher Apgar scores. Moreover, higher-quality support and a larger support network were associated with better infant outcomes (Collins et al., 1993). It appears that it is not living alone, per se, that places single mothers at risk, but rather the lack of social support that often accompanies single status.

Throughout the course of prenatal care, all aspects of social support should be explored. The mother's current relationship with the baby' father should be assessed to identify if she perceives him as a stressor or a support. Health care workers can be instrumental in providing emotional support via expressions of caring and warmth, providing anticipatory guidance, and meeting the need for safe shelter, food, and finances. These measures increase the amount of support received, thereby reducing stress and its associated negative outcomes.

Single women are also more likely to have an unwanted pregnancy than are married women. Recent estimates report that 10% of pregnancies were unwanted for married women and 25% for single mothers (Williams & Pratt, 1990). Unwanted pregnancies have been associated with a delay in seeking prenatal care, continued adverse health behaviors such as smoking and use of alcohol, and poorer infant outcomes (a higher incidence of low birth weight). Unplanned children are also at greater risk of being abused. This data warrants exploring, at the first prenatal visit, circumstances surrounding the conception of the pregnancy. Comments suggesting an unplanned and unwanted pregnancy should generate a referral to a mental health worker.

Effect on Parenting

The multiple demands involved in single parenting increase the mother's vulnerability to anxiety and depression. Literature suggests that much of the strain and psychological distress associated with single parenthood results from oppressive life conditions rather than episodic, stressful life events. Conditions identified as emotionally distressing include ongoing financial worries, parenting problems, and inadequate and/or dangerous living arrangements and intimate relationships (Makosky, 1982; Olson & Banyard, 1993). In one recent study, mothers reported incidents of child misbehavior as the most stressful ongoing event. Behavior was most apt to be managed with a punitive response involving threatening punishment or actually punishing the child (Olson & Banyard, 1993).

These findings have implications for supportive intervention with single mothers of young children. As caregiving issues are the most consistent sources of stress in a single mother's life, assistance in locating childcare resources should be provided and the mother's interactions with her children restructured to lessen the frequency of coercive parent-child interactions. Less obvious but equally important is assisting single mothers to mobilize and sustain supportive relationships with other adults.

Single Mothers by Choice

Single mothers by choice represent a select group of single women who choose to have children outside of marriage or in the absence of a long-term partner (Pakizegi, 1990). They span a wide age range and, on the whole, appear to be more educated and hold a better job than the average woman nationally. Despite these advantages, there is some evidence that the social class of single mothers by choice is still lower than that of two-parent families.

The conscious decision to have a child appears to mitigate the characteristic anxiety and depression noted in single-parent households (Olson & Haynes, 1993). In a study comparing single mothers by choice and married mothers, no significant differences were found in availability of emotional and informational support, or in levels of anxiety and depression. However, single mothers by choice experienced more negative life stresses, including limited finances and job mobility, and had access to lower levels of tangible support (Tilden, 1984).

Although research on single mothers by choice does not directly address motivation for parenthood, findings in one study indicate that at least 60% of the single mothers by choice either had a previous pregnancy which had been aborted or had placed the child up for adoption (Mechanek, Klein, & Kuppersmith, 1988). Clinicians should explore previous pregnancy histories and discuss any unresolved feelings of grief. Due to inconsistent societal support for single parenthood, doctors and nurses are the people to whom most single mothers by choice who seek support turn for advice. These opportunities should be used for discussing previous reproductive history, identifying the stressors of single parenting, and problem solving to develop a supportive network.

Adolescent Pregnancy

Recent statistics indicate that the United States exceeds all other western industrial countries in its birthrate for adolescents. In contrast to prior decades in which pregnant teens frequently wed, most teenage mothers today are single parents. The consequences of teenage pregnancy include low educational and occupational achievement, low self-esteem, isolation from peers, and an increased incidence of developmental delays among offspring.

Research suggests that the extent to which a teen mother is at risk for psychological problems and to which her infant is at risk for developmental problems is, to a large degree, a function of the social support received (Nath et al., 1991). A teenager's family and peers provide the greatest amount of support, including emotional support during and after pregnancy. Peers tend to provide emotional support, while the family provides tangible assistance.

The unique developmental circumstances of adolescent parenthood create conflict in the family relationship. While teenage mothers receive considerable support from their families, they also experience interference as they try to assert their independence (Richardson, Barbour, & Bubenzer, 1991). Given this bittersweet connection, clinicians should not assume that increasing family support will improve the teenage mother's stress. It may actually increase it. In order to master the developmental task of adolescence, teenage mothers must be allowed to achieve autonomy from their own parents.

Childbirth preparation classes also need to be tailored to the developmental abilities and desires of this population. In a recent study evaluating the use of a modified childbirth curriculum which included a wide spectrum of topics, adolescents were most interested in fetal development. A skilled instructor can incorporate discussions of family planning and avoidance of substance use under the broader topic of fetal development. Relaxation breathing techniques and breastfeeding were also of interest (Carrington et al., 1994).

Interventions targeted at pregnant and parenting teens must incorporate all of the complex issues and needs of single parenting, in addition to the developmental needs of adolescence. Concerns about body image (Stenberg & Blinn, 1993) and altered relationships with the baby's father and with friends should be central to any adolescent pregnancy program.

CULTURAL ADAPTATIONS TO PREGNANCY

Culture is especially significant in the childbearing process because it defines the meaning of the experience and guides how those involved react to the events. As individuals and families leave their countries of origin and come to the United States, traditional practices and practices of American society blend, conflict, or coexist.

African Americans, Hispanics, and Asian Americans constitute three major ethnic groups in the United States (Brooks, 1991; Harrison et al., 1990). The following is a brief discussion of practices related to pregnancy and parenting among these ethnic groups. A section on Southeast Asians is included because this subgroup has distinct birthing practices and has increased in numbers in the past decade. The practices described represent generalizations that do not apply to all persons. Each individual's experience of a culture is unique based on his or her understanding, value of, and experiences within that culture. Knowledge of traditional practices allows clinicians to better explore and support cultural variation in childbearing.

African Americans

In African American culture, pregnancy is viewed as a normal, healthy state. Socioeconomic status, more than traditional African culture, may seriously influence the pregnancy experience. African American women are more likely than any other ethnic group to receive inadequate prenatal care, resulting in poorer infant outcomes.

African American families are characterized by their role flexibility (Dore & Dumois, 1990). Although single motherhood is not desired, single mothers and their children are not stigmatized. Extended family members and friends often play a central role in health care decision making and mobilize to support a pregnant woman in time of need. Strong value is placed on loyalty and responsibility to others. This concept is embodied in the African American proverb, "It takes a village to raise a child" (Hines et al., 1992). African American families typically share one another's joy, pain, frustration, and shame. The African American church plays a strong unifying role within this community (Corrine et al., 1992). Spirituality provides strength to cope with daily struggles. Adversity, whether social or medical, is often met with increased spiritual activity.

Hispanics

The Hispanic population is comprised of persons from Mexico, Puerto Rico, the Dominican Republic, Cuba, and Central and South American countries. Mexican Americans comprise about 60% of the Hispanic population. Hispanic mothers as a group are younger, have less education, and are poorer than their ethnic counterparts (Caudle, 1993). Furthermore, Hispanic women are often medically uninsured, do not receive early prenatal care, and have short intervals between births of their children. Many Hispanics begin to bear children in their teen years and, as a result, have one of the highest parity rates of ethnic women (Zayas & Busch-Rassnagel, 1992). A strong belief in Catholicism contributes to large families.

Familialism is a key cultural value among Hispanics. Decision making about health and, therefore, pregnancy is a family, not an individual, decision. Partners are expected to be present at labor, but not to participate actively (Khazoyan & Anderson, 1994). Families are patriarchal in structure but the mother is responsible for caring for members of the family. The role of motherhood has high social value in Hispanic culture (Dore & Dumois, 1990; Hines et al., 1992).

Childbearing rules include a series of prescriptions and taboos. Women may wear a steel object or red underwear as protection, may avoid drinking milk, and may stay physically active to prevent the development of a large baby and a difficult delivery. Sexual activity is often continued to lubricate the birth canal (Khazoyan & Anderson, 1994).

Many Hispanics believe in the use of "cold" remedies for "hot" diseases and "hot" remedies for "cold" diseases. The postpartum period is considered a "cold" time in which "hot" foods should be served. Consequently, Hispanic women may refuse fruits and vegetables (Caudle, 1993). The infant's umbilicus may be bound to prevent bad air from entering. Women should be taught to change the binding frequently to prevent infection.

Southeast Asians

The Southeast Asian immigrant population consists of Vietnamese, Cambodian, Laotian, and Hmong people. Most women entering the United States from Southeast Asia are in their childbearing years. Consequently, prenatal care is often the first contact with the health care system.

Prenatal care is not the norm in Southeast Asia; therefore, most women ascribe to traditional beliefs during pregnancy. Heavy lifting and strenuous work are not permitted. Myths regarding childbearing are common. It is believed that raising the arms over the head can cause the placenta to pull away. Sexual activity is often avoided as vernix is considered to be accumulated sperm (D'Avanzo, 1992).

Family structure is patriarchal, with high value placed on extended family relationships, loyalty, and respect for authority. These values are depicted by the lack of eye contact and the stoic management of the labor experience. The role of the partner varies at childbirth. Regardless of his role, it is considered shameful to demonstrate pain in front of a man. As modesty is highly valued, female interpreters and practitioners are preferred. Squatting is the preferred birthing position. Since an individual's head is considered sacred, it is inappropriate to touch the laboring Southeast Asian woman's head during labor. It is equally inappropriate to caress the newborn infant's head (D'Avanzo, 1992).

Most Southeast Asian women follow the traditional practice of yin (hot) and yang (cold). Pregnancy is a cold state. Women are encouraged to conserve heat by not bathing and by eating "hot" foods. During the first 40 to 60 days postpartum, extended family provide virtually all care to the newborn child as this is a period of restricted activity for the mother.

Asian Americans

Asian American families represent immigrants from China, Japan, and Korea. Of any minority group in the United States to date, Asian Americans have attained the highest median income and educational level. Cultural norms are similar to those of Southeast Asians, where high value is placed on loyalty to the family, conformity, and emotional reserve. As these Asian countries, particularly China, became overpopulated, small families were encouraged. Both historically and currently, a male child has been preferred and confers high status on the mother.

Childbearing practices are consistent with those of Southeast Asians. This is particularly true for the postpartum period during which the balance between yin and yang is observed during a 40-day period of rest.

PSYCHOSOCIAL IMPLICATIONS OF HIGH-RISK PREGNANCY

The experience of pregnancy is an interwoven biological and psychosocial process oriented toward the delivery of a healthy newborn by a well woman who has the ability and the desire to mother the infant. Advances in reproductive technology during the past decade have changed the profile of the maternity population, creating a new high-risk subgroup. Approximately 30% of all pregnancies are now labeled high-risk (Wall, 1988). The psychosocial experience of the high-risk mother has inevitably been altered by these scientific developments.

ALTERED MATERNAL-INFANT ATTACHMENT

As outlined earlier, Rubin (1975) described four developmental stages through which a pregnant woman develops readiness for mothering: seeking safe passage; securing and assuring acceptance of the child by significant others; binding-in to the child; and giving of oneself. During low-risk pregnancies, mothers complete these developmental tasks resulting in assimilation of the motherhood role. In a high-risk pregnancy, motherhood is uncertain as continuation of the pregnancy is often tenuous. The elements of the developmental tasks of pregnancy are altered based on this high-risk perinatal experience (Stainton, McNeil, & Harvey, 1992).

Seeking Safe Passage

Not surprisingly, a woman experiencing difficulties in her pregnancy is concerned about safety both for herself and her unborn infant. Seeking information represents a desperate search for meaning in an unfamiliar and frightening situation. Typically, pregnant women do not know what questions to ask. Furthermore, the answer is often presented in medical terminology based on medical condition rather than on the woman's situation. Parents attempt to adapt by becoming fluent in medical language so they can converse with their providers. Frequently, a distorted reliance on technical information, such as fetal heart rate or oxygenation levels, develops as a mother's means of assessing her own and her unborn infant's safety.

Health care providers should be sensitive to the need for additional information. Understandable language and common terms should be used to describe situations or treatment options. Data should provide all known information on the effects of a diagnosis or proposed treatment option for not only the mother, but also the unborn infant.

Seeking Acceptance by Others

As a result of a high-risk pregnancy, the roles of significant members of the family are altered, potentially jeopardizing their acceptance of the infant. Restrictions required of the woman may involve changes in eating, sleeping, childrearing, homemaking, and social and recreational activities. Many women require bedrest and are hospitalized. A domino effect is seen. Changes in the mother's lifestyle necessitates change in the living patterns of other members. The father is required to assume additional responsibilities, which can stress the marital or couple's relationship. This, in turn, can be perceived as jeopardizing the father's acceptance of his unborn child.

A recent study evaluating the impact of maternal activity restriction on the expectant father, to minimize the risk of preterm labor, reported high levels of worry immediately after the high-risk diagnosis (May, 1994). Later, fathers reported stress related to responsibilities for child-care, household management, and maintaining a supportive environment for their partners. Fathers reported few sources of personal support and little or no contact with health professionals during their partner's activity restriction. Fathers are deeply affected by antenatal hospitalization. In another study, almost 30% of fathers reported levels of depression (Mercer & Ferketich, 1988).

Systematic and ongoing appraisal of the family's situation and its ability to cope with the stressors of a high-risk pregnancy should be conducted during the family's encounters with the health care system to mitigate the emotional distress and disruption reported by fathers. Appropriate health care interventions might include anticipatory guidance, problem solving to identify additional supports, referrals for home care and/or homemaker services, and an opportunity for the family to share frustrations with a competent individual.

The expectant mother's relationship with her mother can also be altered. Many women become closer with their own mothers during pregnancy as the older women share their childbirth experiences. During a high-risk pregnancy, this ability to share is altered because the expectant mother often requires information and explanations from health care workers about treatments and procedures (Stainton, 1994). If geographically available, the expectant mother's mother is frequently asked to assume caretaker responsibilities. This can result in intergenerational and territorial tensions concerning child-care and household management. Again, this potentially can alter excitement and acceptance of the coming grandchild.

The uncertainty of a high-risk pregnancy heightens the mother's need for acceptance, a need which typically extends far beyond the extended family. Women seek acceptance from caregivers who become greatly involved in the mother's life. A wide range of attitudes and behaviors is adopted to ensure acceptance. These may range from strongly assertive, almost aggressive, actions, to passive compliance.

Multigravid women are in a double-bind situation. They desire the new baby to be accepted by its siblings, but want to protect the older children in case of pregnancy loss. The children's future relationship with their new sibling is further jeopardized by the absence of the mother from the home or by her activity restriction. Resentment can easily develop. Health care workers need to help the mother spend quality time with her other children. Sedentary activities for the mother and child, such as painting or reading together, can be arranged in either the hospital or the home.

Binding-in

Women who have a high-risk pregnancy experience a wide range of responses to creating antenatal ties or "binding-in" to the infant. The nature of the medical problem and a woman's individual life experiences influence the response (Stainton, 1990). Women who have had a perinatal loss often attempt to protect themselves from the pain of loss by avoiding binding-in behaviors such as choosing names or arranging the nursery. As the pregnancy continues, it is increasingly difficult to continue this protective wall. Fetal movement draws a mother into a relationship and serves as an indicator amidst the uncertainty that the unborn infant is alive and all right. In most circumstances, delivery, even if the infant requires hospitalization in the Neonatal Intensive Care Unit, liberates the mother by ending the uncertainty of the pregnancy.

Giving of Oneself

Giving of oneself in a high-risk situation is intensified. Women describe tending to focus on "getting through" the situation and rearranging family functioning to support this outcome. Women report a sense of personal responsibility for navigating the high-risk pregnancy. As the center of the family structure, this is difficult. It often requires a woman to change her lifestyle and give up social events and independence to preserve the unborn child. Women on bedrest often try to assume responsibility for coordinating household management from a remote location in relative social isolation. Provision of nursing care by a care group of staff (primary nursing) and the use of social services during inpatient hospitalization is warranted to assist with problem-solving and to provide emotional support to the mother.

THE PSYCHOSOCIAL EXPERIENCE OF HIGH-RISK PREGNANCY

Another complex aspect of high-risk pregnancy is a change in pregnancy status from a well to an illness perspective. The sick role is imposed and the mother becomes a patient. This philosophical change alone has been documented as a major stressor (Maloni & Kasper, 1991).

Treatment for high-risk pregnancy usually requires a significant change in lifestyle for the woman and her family and often requires bedrest. Women on bedrest score significantly higher on anxiety, depression, and somatic complaints. Bedrest also disrupts family life, particularly if there are children at home. It can also result in extra expenses which may add to the stress of the high-risk pregnancy (Crowther et al., 1990; Curtis, 1986).

One recent study described the experience of high-risk pregnancy from the perspectives of both mothers and fathers (McCain & Deatrick, 1994). Three emotional responses to the high-risk pregnancy were documented:

1. *Vulnerability*: the realization that the pregnancy outcome was at risk
2. *Heightened anxiety*: the transition from normal activities to bedrest and hospitalization
3. *Inevitability*: the premature delivery of an infant with a guarded diagnosis.

Vulnerability was successfully managed by seeking medical care and searching for causes of the symptoms. Anxiety was diffused by compliance with treatment and accepting support. Assimilating information from health care providers during delivery, in combination with seeing and touching the newborn, dissipated negative feelings associated with the inevitability of the birth.

This study and other relevant literature indicate that positive psychosocial resolution is possible in a high-risk pregnancy (May, 1994; Stainton, Harvey & McNeil, 1992; Stainton, 1994). Therapeutic interventions include providing emotional support and physical presence during antenatal admissions, being respectful of the woman's need to balance her concerns for the unborn child versus her other children, supporting the partner's presence and contribution during antenatal hospitalization, accepting the search for causes, and allowing for hope of a successful pregnancy outcome in lieu of serious medical complications.

There is no consensus on whether women requiring bedrest are best managed in the hospital or in the home. While antepartum admission is disruptive, it represents the mobilization of professional health care resources. In contrast, home management is superficially less disruptive, but may be more isolating with intermittent contact with health professionals. Generally, minimal, if any, home assistance is available to families outside their own support network. Prescribed activity restriction can generate stress in family relationships as a woman must relinquish important and usually satisfying roles to her partner. Thoughtful individual assessment of the woman's medical condition, family requirements, and support structure should determine the location for high-risk pregnancy management.

PSYCHOSOCIAL RESPONSES TO CHILDBIRTH

NATURAL CHILDBIRTH

The experiences of pregnancy and childbirth impact the mother's and father's adjustment to their parental roles. The nature of the childbirth experience is believed to be influenced by childbirth preparation. Spousal support during labor for Lamaze-prepared parents has been associated with both increased maternal and paternal satisfaction with the childbirth experience (Pridham et al., 1991).

Childbirth preparation is aimed at providing factual information to expectant mothers, thereby reducing the negative preconceptions women have about labor. This is accomplished by education and the formation of newly conditioned reflexes in response to uterine contractions. Selective breathing and active relaxation techniques are used to produce this response. Relaxation has been shown to be an effective tool in reducing the stress response. In combination with specific information about labor which diminishes the fear of the unknown, the laboring woman can better respond to the sensations of labor (Shrock, 1988). A clinical study of labor pain suggests that a woman's confidence in her ability to cope with labor contributes significantly to her perception of pain during labor (Lowe, 1991).

Some women are choosing to express their preferences for care in the form of a birth plan. Creation of such a plan reflects a woman's desire to have some control over the care she receives. Therefore, birth plans represent a shift from a passive patient to an active participant. The birth plan can be used as an educational tool as it provides an opportunity to discuss expectations. The uncertainty inherent in childbirth and the necessity for medical intervention in an obstetrical crisis should be discussed at length to avoid unreal and unsafe expectations.

Almost all childbirth preparation methods advocate using a prepared support person during labor. The physical presence of this person provides psychological support. Fathers who attended childbirth preparation classes and participated in the labor and birth with their partner also reported a more positive experience (Nichols, 1993). From their perspective, four categories of activity were helpful to their wives during labor and delivery. These measures included, in descending order of importance, comfort and physical measures ("scratching her back" or "helping her focus"); psychological support ("reassurance" or "encouragement"); presence ("just being there"); and communication ("talking to my wife" or "listening to her").

Of all health professionals, nurses have the most contact with a couple during childbirth. In several studies, women have identified specific nursing behaviors as supportive during labor. Positive behaviors included participation in the labor process; acceptance of individual style and coping; provision of information, encouragement, and presence based on need and demonstrated competence (Bryanton, Fraser-Davey, & Sullivan, 1994; Mackey & Stepans, 1994). Behaviors in the emotional support category were the most helpful (Bryanton, Fraser-Davey, & Sullivan, 1994).

MEDICATION-ASSISTED CHILDBIRTH

Some women who desired a natural childbirth may require medication. The change in birth plan can be disappointing and threatening for a woman, as it represents a loss of control. Nursing care at this time should focus on supporting the decision or need for medical intervention, acknowledging the mother's feelings of failure, and recreating a sense of control by outlining other choices that are within the mother's control.

In contrast, some women may desire or request medication-assisted childbirth, particularly epidural anesthesia. The use of medication can reduce stress for some women who feel they are losing control. It can preserve the mental strength or psyche required to complete labor. Nursing care at this juncture should support the woman's decision and ensure that the woman is aware of all medication options so she can make an informed choice.

CESAREAN SECTION

One in four births in the United States occurs via cesarean delivery, making the cesarean section the most common hospital surgical procedure (Stafford, 1990). The normal birth process is stressful for parents; cesarean section adds the stress of surgery. Women who have experienced cesarean delivery have reported feelings of depression, anxiety, guilt, less satisfaction with the birth experience, loss of control, and loss of self-esteem. Unplanned or emergency cesarean delivery is especially problematic as the events occur in rapid succession, straining a woman's ability to assimilate the experience (Fawcett, Pollio, & Tully, 1992). Not surprisingly, women who have an unplanned cesarean section express more negative perceptions of the birth experience than those who have planned cesarean deliveries.

Nursing care during a crisis should provide support by acknowledging the woman's feelings of fear, giving anticipatory guidance about the impending surgical procedure, and keeping the woman apprised of the health status of both herself and her infant with simple explanations. False assurances should be avoided, as they are perceived as insincere and dissolve a trusting relationship with the patient. Women with anticipated cesarean delivery should be educated prenatally about the procedure, anesthesia options, and anticipated postoperative recovery. A recent study indicated that women who selected regional anesthesia had a more positive perception of the experience than those mothers who had general anesthesia (Reichert, Baron, & Fawcett, 1993).

Women experience a number of physiological, psychological, and lifestyle concerns after cesarean delivery. Mothers need an opportunity to review the events of the cesarean birth, particularly if they had an unplanned procedure or general anesthesia. In one study, physical concerns decreased after the second week postdelivery, whereas psychological and lifestyle concerns did not (Miovech et al., 1994). The most prevalent concerns 8 weeks after delivery were changes in activity (being housebound, taking longer to do things), body image changes (weight gain, stretch marks), and concerns with family interactions (perceived lack of support by partners, separations).

Early discharge potentially compromises the ability to give comprehensive care. Ideally, information relevant to the discharge plan should be gathered in the prenatal period. Specific information about incisional pain, body image changes, and changes in activity or family interactions should be given prior to going home. Discharge planning should also include helping parents make arrangements for obtaining help from friends and family to reduce fatigue.

PERINATAL LOSS AND GRIEF

OVERVIEW

Some infants are born to death, a disheartening fact that all obstetrical nurses eventually confront. The impact of these ended beginnings is tremendous both for families and for health care providers. Perinatal loss is different from other types of loss in that it strikes the young, the inexperienced, and the unprepared. As Bourne (1979) poignantly stated, "It is one of nature's obscenities" (p. 104).

Each year, up to 15% to 30% of all pregnancies end in miscarriage (Wilcox, Weinberg & O'Connor, 1988), and approximately 1% in stillbirth, and 1% in neonatal death (Ewton, 1993). Although the statistics reflect the numerical magnitude of the problem, they tell nothing about the tears, regrets, feelings of guilt and isolation, and the long process of rebuilding hope.

The 20th century is a death-denying, emotion-repressing culture (Kubler-Ross, 1969). The concept of fetal or infant death is, in fact, quite alien. The death of an infant is particularly unsettling because it is in stark discord with the typical chronology of life. An unspoken notion exists that children are not supposed to die, certainly not before their parents. Perinatal death defies the natural order of things and forces the most rigid of individuals to confront the uncertainty and frailty of human existence.

The grief experienced by parents is unparalleled. Children represent the future, the beginning of life and, in a sense, immortality. When a child dies, not only is an extended part of the mother's identity connected with future hopes and aspirations lost, but the societal rite of passage associated with parenthood is denied. The problem is further compounded by a lack of ritual to recognize the loss of the infant or fetus. As a rule, a private graveside service and an epitaph reading "daughter of" or "son of" will mark the infant's brief life.

Resolution of the loss is hindered by the absence of a rich storehouse of memories which serve as a vehicle for resolution in the grief process. The loss of an unborn child is the loss of future dreams, future relationships, and future fantasies which have not yet been experienced and, therefore, are not able to be placed within the context of a rational discussion. This lack of identity or history creates an additional barrier for significant others to relate to parents meaningfully. Although most friends and family members are initially supportive, they had no opportunity to know the infant and are eager to proceed with life beyond the loss. For the mother, the depth and breadth of her grief goes largely unacknowledged and consequently potentially unresolved (Brost & Kenney, 1992).

The effects of fetal and infant death touch not only the family, but also the professionals involved. Death symbolizes failure in an era of intricate technology. On units that typically celebrate new life, fetal and infant death is an unwelcome intruder. In spite of the frequency of the event, health care professionals are often unprepared to support the grieving parents adequately, as they are unable to deal with their own emotions. If strategies are not implemented to educate professional staff about appropriate responses and care, the parents may perceive an overall lack of support and be further at risk for dysfunctional grieving.

PRENATAL MATERNAL ATTACHMENT

A common misperception exists throughout the community and health care profession that the grief experienced by bereaved parents is directly proportional to the length of gestation or age of the infant; somehow, the amount of grief is related to the amount of time parents spent with the infant. Several studies contradict this widely held notion.

Klaus and Kennell (1982) described the intense emotional attachment that develops between a mother and her baby as a process that begins long before birth. As a result of a young girl's socialization, she may begin to integrate the societal roles of wife and mother through her fantasies of marriage and motherhood. After conception, the maternal-infant bond intensifies. Prior to the detection of fetal movement, a woman incorporates the fetus as part of herself. The experience of fetal movement allows the mother to conceptualize the fetus as a separate person. Often, the prospective mother will begin to fantasize about the baby's appearance and sex, evidenced by name selection. Long before delivery, a woman subconsciously makes plans for this baby's childhood, adolescence, and adult life.

The expression of grief after perinatal death is viewed as evidence of maternal-infant attachment (Bowlby, 1979). This expression of maternal grief has been demonstrated regardless of a woman's pleasure with being pregnant, the extent to which parent-infant contact occurred after delivery, and the duration of her pregnancy. Kennell, Slyter, and Klaus (1970) found that all women they interviewed after a neonatal death experienced some degree of grief whether or not they had ever touched their infant and whether or not they were mourning an unplanned pregnancy. Other findings support the notion of prenatal maternal-infant attachment. Benfield, Lieb, and Vollman (1978) interviewed 50 couples whose newborn had died. Again, a grief response was present regardless of infant birthweight, duration of life, or extent of physical contact prior to infant death.

More recently, Peppers and Knapp (1980) compared the reactions of 67 women who had experienced a miscarriage, stillbirth, or neonatal death. No differences were found based on the particular type of perinatal loss. These studies suggest that even a woman who miscarries an unwanted pregnancy, a fetus with whom she has no physical contact, experiences grief, demonstrating prenatal maternal-infant attachment.

MODELS OF PERINATAL GRIEF AND MOURNING

Mourning is described as the process by which an individual recognizes and adapts to the death of a loved one. The emotion that dominates this process is *grief.* While each perinatal death and its subsequent effects on the family are unique, specific responses appear to be in common to all bereaved parents. Furthermore, these responses tend to follow a somewhat predictable pattern (Lindemann, 1944; Miles, 1985; Parkes, 1972). Although descriptions differ among authors slightly, the process involves four fundamental phases:

1. Shock and disbelief
2. Yearning, searching, and anxiety
3. Disorganization, despair, and depression
4. Reorganization

Transition from one stage to another is rarely a distinct process. The feelings, symptoms, and/or behaviors may occur individually or simultaneously and may recur at any time. The process may be envisioned as a wheel of reactions (Fig. 26-1).

Shock and Disbelief

The phase of shock and disbelief is characterized by a period of denial, which generally lasts from a few hours up to two weeks. Feelings of emptiness, numbness, apathy, and an unexpected calm are typical, resulting in impaired concentration and decision-making abilities. Common responses include "there must be a mistake" or "this can't be happening." The initial denial and inability to react serve as an adaptive defense mechanism, protecting the parents until they can cope with reality. These intense feelings usually subside after the first few weeks. Shock and denial that persist may indicate an abnormal response, suggesting the need for mental health intervention.

Yearning, Searching, and Anxiety

After the initial shock subsides, an acute period of yearning, searching, and anxiety begins. Behavior during this time reflects an underlying urge to recover the deceased infant. Physical symptoms and behavioral changes such as tears, insomnia, anorexia, loneliness, and preoccupation with the deceased—specifically, an intense desire to physically hold, touch, or see the infant again—are common. Feelings of helplessness arise which come "primarily from the fact that, as protector of the child, the parents could do nothing to prevent the death" (Miles, 1985, p. 226). Helplessness, in turn, produces feelings of anger, guilt, and fear. An intense need to affix blame emerges as a way of diffusing the impact of these intense emotions. Blame may be directed at the deceased, the significant other, health care professionals, or, not uncommonly, the mother herself.

Due to the intense nature of these emotions, normal patterns of behavior are disrupted, resulting in profound personality changes. The period between the second week and fourth or fifth month after the loss are most characteristic of this phase.

Disorganization, Despair, and Depression

Disorganization, despair, and depression follow the period of yearning and searching, and reflect the emotions associated with comprehension of the reality of the death. Although acute grieving is less pronounced, feelings of listlessness, aimlessness, futility, anorexia, malaise, and insomnia predominate, often resulting in social withdrawal. This phase is most intense 4 to 6 months after the death and usually lasts several months. The physical symptoms associated

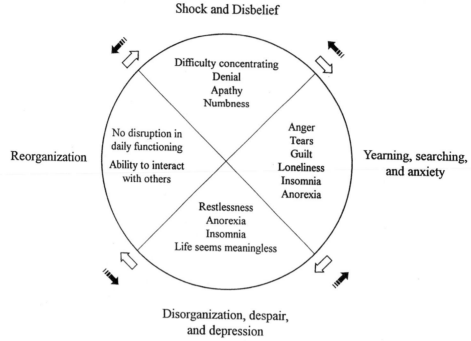

FIGURE 26–1. Wheel of reactions.

with the depression often prompt a mother to contact her physician for medical treatment, providing an opportunity for not only medical but also psychosocial intervention.

Reorganization

Reorganization, the final stage, is characterized by a gradual acceptance and adaptation to the death. As the mourner is emancipated from the oppressive emotions of the above three stages, he or she describes feelings of renewed energy, greater ease in decision-making and problem-solving, and a gradual return to normal daily life (including usual sleep and eating patterns). There can be an intensification of profound feelings of loss as the 1-year anniversary of the death approaches. Full resolution often encompasses a period of up to 2 years.

Following the second anniversary, memories of the deceased are not absent, but rather may be recalled with feelings of sadness that do not disrupt daily functioning. As Stack and

Barnas (1987) succinctly stated, "The end point of the grieving process is not to forget the lost loved one but to remember without feeling so much pain" (p. 120).

HEALTH CARE WORKERS' ASSESSMENT AND INTERVENTION

In order for staff, physicians, nurses, and social workers to intervene effectively with families experiencing perinatal loss, they need to be aware of their own feelings and attitudes. Literature refers to perinatal loss as a "professional blindspot." Parents often depend on physicians and other health care workers to provide support denied by the community. Although professional staff are in the best position to assuage maternal guilt or self-blame, they often withdraw as a result of a personal sense of failure or inadequacy. Not surprisingly, many families identify another parent or couple who has lost a child as the preferred source of grief support.

Specific behaviors of health care workers have been identified by parents as supportive or damaging (Benfield, Lieb, & Vollman, 1978; Estok & Lehman, 1983; Yoder, 1994). *Damaging* caretaker behaviors include:

- Lack of touch (physical distancing) by caregivers
- A delay in announcement of infant death by physicians
- The use of magical thinking by the caregivers ("you can always have another baby")
- Avoidance of conversation about death

In contrast, *supportive* measures include:

- Providing an opportunity to sit and discuss the death with the staff
- Granting verbal and tactile permission to grieve
- Helping a mother verbalize feelings of guilt or self-blame
- Creating a memory to mourn (providing an opportunity to see and hold the baby)
- Enhancing the reality of death by use of photographs, baby blanket, lock of hair, and/or discussions of a funeral or memorial service
- Assisting family involvement by extending visiting hours and by inclusion in discharge planning
- Anticipatory guidance and problem-solving regarding potential difficulties following discharge (what to tell friends or children about the death and what to say in awkward situations)
- Appropriate referral to a community support group and postdischarge follow-up (phone call or home visit within the first week, and a 2- to 3-week postpartum visit in contrast to the conventional 6-week visit)

Two additional supportive measures can be easily instituted. First, caregivers should utilize a flexible policy of room and roommate assignment, offering alternatives. This allows the mother to determine her own need for privacy and seclusion from other mothers. Second, caregivers should avoid or limit administration of mood-altering agents that may suppress the acute grief response. Above all, staff must respect and support the individual differences of mourning and grief.

CULTURAL INFLUENCES ON PERINATAL LOSS

Although expression of grief is individual, the process almost always is influenced by a person's cultural background. Culture influences the meaning of the death for a family, customs surrounding death and funerals, family-life patterns (lines of authority and help available), and families' expectations of health care professionals during that time (Lawson, 1990). A parent's identification with a cultural group not only influences their expressions of grief but may also become more intense in times of crisis.

Health care professionals must balance their knowledge of a particular cultural group with the tendency to stereotype members of a particular culture. In all cases, individual feelings should be explored with open-ended, non-judgmental questions: "What do you think caused this death?" "Since the death, what has been happening to you and your family?" "What do you think might help you?"

Native Americans

Native American families, encompassing many tribal groups, consider children of great value. Infant death, therefore, is perceived as a significant loss. The concept of family extends far beyond the nuclear concept including the entire community. All members assume roles in the grieving process. Expressions range from quiet and stoic to dramatic and hysterical. Among Native Americans, the grieving or healing process and religion are inseparable. Native ceremonies tend to focus on restoring harmony in nature. They may include somber wakes where food and memorial gifts are distributed. Some tribes hold a memorial service at the first anniversary of the death.

African Americans

Although African American women, particularly inner-city women, disproportionately comprise infant loss statistics, little information is available in the literature about the experience of perinatal loss in the African American community. Anecdotal clinical experience and interviews with community members provided the data for this subsection.

The African American church plays a central role following infant loss. The focus during death, including infant death, is the deceased's passage to be with God in the afterlife. Funeral services, therefore, are a time of celebration. Burial rather than cremation is the norm. Importance is placed on the physical appearance of the deceased for viewing. Ornate coffins made of high quality fabrics and materials are desirable.

The extended family and friends mobilize to provide emotional support to a bereaved woman. Members of the African-American community report that trust is difficult to establish outside of their community due to the historical experience of slavery and the ongoing experience of discrimination. Therefore, support groups are rarely used. The network of family and friends usually include someone who has experienced a perinatal loss. This person serves as an informal support group for the woman within the "safe" context of the African-American community.

Hispanics

Hispanic families also consider children essential components of the family. Although the family is patriarchal in structure, extended family and close friends are the primary source of social support and tangible aid. Relevant information and social services should be directed toward the entire family. Women who are separated from their extended family may feel unusual isolation. Health, viewed as a harmonious relationship between social and spiritual realms, is a combination of both folk and biomedical models. Death and the belief in the afterlife are deeply rooted in Roman Catholicism.

Asians and Southeast Asians

Asians and Southeast Asians include people of many nations, ethnic groups, and religions. Despite these differences, the family unit is the core of society, with value placed on large families with many children. The structure is patriarchal, with the oldest male typically making decisions about health care; therefore, interventions need to be addressed to this individual. Guided by the religions of Buddhism, Taoism, and Confucianism, elaborate funeral ceremonies mark a soul's passage to the afterlife. White clothing and headbands may be worn by mourners. Vietnamese and Hmong tend to bury their dead while Cambodians and Laotians prefer cremation. Since mental illness is considered a family disgrace, Asian and Southeast Asian mourners may report somatic complaints as signs of depression and grief.

Understanding a grieving woman's culture allows a health care professional to advocate better for the family in terms of the traditions important to them. It also allows health care professionals to assist in identifying supports and resources within the woman's own family and in her community.

PATHOLOGICAL GRIEF REACTIONS

When the normal process of grieving is blocked or suppressed, pathologic grief sequelae may arise. Recent long-term studies have shown that the mother suffered a poor outcome in approximately one-third of perinatal deaths (Kirkley-Best & Kellner, 1982; Rowe et al., 1978). There are three occasions when the mother seems most vulnerable:

1. When she tries to confirm perceptually who died. A lack of tangible evidence that the baby existed blocks a woman's attempt to appreciate the reality of the death. Creation of a memory via photographs, mementos, and an opportunity to hold the deceased infant helps to confirm the infant's life and death.
2. When she tries to get emotional support. The mother's need for emotional support from friends and family is often unmet as discussions of her pregnancy, delivery, and the baby are avoided.
3. When she compares her feelings with those of others. Well-meaning family and friends who do address the death often minimize the event.

These unique features surrounding perinatal death create a high-risk environment for pathologic grief reactions.

Pathological grief manifests itself in two ways: the absence of grief, and/or prolonged grief. Women often report recurring somatic symptoms or abnormal behaviors such as an unwillingness to remove nursery furnishings; constant verbalization about other losses; feelings of worthlessness and need for punishment; thoughts of suicide; sudden, radical change in lifestyle; and/or repression of hostility (Ewton, 1993). Two groups of women appear to be at particular risk for pathological reactions: women whose subsequent pregnancy occurs within less than 6 months after the death, and women whose pregnancy involved a surviving twin (Rowe et al., 1978).

Counseling at the time of the loss can include recommendations about waiting 6 months for a subsequent pregnancy, to allow for the beginning of grief resolution and to minimize the risk of pathological grief. Women in these high-risk subgroups, in addition to women who demonstrate symptoms of pathological grief, need a referral to an appropriate mental health professional for assistance in grief resolution.

FATHERS' GRIEF

Frequently, following a perinatal loss, fathers are put in the position of being a care provider rather than a recipient of support themselves. The father has been described as the forgotten mourner. Another obstacle to paternal grief work is society's expectation that men demonstrate courage and show no emotion.

There is some evidence that men and women grieve differently. Stinson, Lasker, Tohmann, and Toedter (1992) compared mothers' and fathers' grief following a pregnancy loss. While women scored significantly higher on active grief measures, women and men did not differ significantly in their experience of despair. Active grief reflects feeling sad or missing the baby—an open expression of grief. For women, this is considered socially acceptable behavior. Despair reflects feelings of worthlessness, guilt, and vulnerability. It also indicates risk for chronic grief. These data suggest that men do grieve intensely but may internalize these feelings of loss, which is more acceptable in the male cultural norm.

The differences in expression of grief increase the chance of conflict between the father and mother. In one study, one-third of women reported marital difficulties (Cullberg, 1972). The marital conflict evolves from the disparity in grieving styles, which represents a significant communication problem. Routine referral for short-term counseling (approximately six sessions) can be helpful in preserving the couple's relationship by normalizing each person's grief response. During therapy, counselors can model appropriate responses to each partner. Therapy is most effective 3 to 6 months after the loss. Within this time frame the initial shock and disbelief have subsided, and couples often are open to additional information to dissipate feelings of anger and depression. Counseling also provides an opportunity to assess for early signs of pathological grief and to intervene accordingly.

SIBLINGS' GRIEF

Many parents experiencing perinatal death have children. Brief, honest information geared to a child's level of understanding needs to be given to siblings. Children aged 3 to 5 have difficulty understanding that death is a final process, while children aged 5 to 9 understand the finality of death but do not understand that eventually they will die too. Children over 9 usually understand the inevitability of death. The child's cognitive abilities are often reflected in seemingly inappropriate questions which can be disturbing to the parents (i.e., "When is the baby coming home?").

Siblings also need to be reassured about their own and their mother's well-being. Parents should have an open discussion and explain that no one is to blame for the loss nor is anyone going to die because of this pregnancy loss. Children should be given the opportunity to express their feelings verbally, artistically, and through play. Common grief reactions in children include regression, physical complaints, anger, guilt, fear, and problems in school. Readers can find more information on sibling responses in Chapter 27.

SUBSEQUENT PREGNANCY

Parents are encouraged to resolve their grief before embarking on the next pregnancy—a time frame that is determined individually. Clinicians generally recommend deferring subsequent pregnancy for at least 6 months after a perinatal loss to allow for grief resolution and to minimize the risk of a pathological grief reaction. The decision to attempt another pregnancy is usually accompanied by strong ambivalence. Understandably, heightened anxiety often accompanies the subsequent pregnancy (Brost & Kenney, 1992).

Prenatal care providers need to encourage the mother to verbalize her concerns and fears about this pregnancy. Relevant anticipatory guidance should be provided based on the mother's response. As a therapeutic relationship is established, the meaning of the previous loss can and should be explored in an effort to help couples integrate their previous loss into their lives. Parents should be encouraged to use a support network. It is important for professionals to provide factual information to the support network about the risks of a subsequent pregnancy, to dispel myths which often impede the therapeutic effect of support persons.

SPONTANEOUS ABORTION

A spontaneous abortion or miscarriage experience will become part of the life history of a substantial number of women. The exact number is difficult to estimate as some women early in gestation abort privately and do not seek follow-up health care. According to best estimates, miscarriage occurs in up to one-third of all pregnancies (Wilcox, Weinberg, & O'Connor, 1988).

Contrary to public opinion, the woman who experiences a miscarriage grieves in the same manner as a woman who has a stillbirth or neonatal death. Women report intense feelings of anger, guilt, and depression. Despite a documented need for emotional support following a miscarriage, literature consistently reports that women experiencing a miscarriage perceive health care workers as cold and indifferent to their situation.

A recent study surveyed obstetrical nurses who provided care to women who had experienced a miscarriage or stillbirth. Both the gestational age and whether the pregnancy was planned or unplanned had a significant effect on the nurse's perception of the event's emotional seriousness and the priority of care (i.e., time spent with the patient) the nurse gave the patient (Reed, 1992). Nurses felt that a woman who was further along in gestation when she experienced a loss or who was grieving a planned pregnancy was a higher priority for care and perceived the event as more serious emotionally.

Because previous studies contradict this notion, the Reed study raises serious concerns about the quality of care currently received by women experiencing a miscarriage (Klaus & Kennell, 1982; Kennell, Slyter & Klaus, 1970; Benfield, Lieb & Vollman, 1978; Peppers & Knapp, 1980). The grief reaction is based not on the duration of the pregnancy but on the degree of attachment to the fetus. The technological development of ultrasonography has facilitated an earlier, more intense investment in the pregnancy. Miscarriage is viewed by most women as a major life event (Bansen & Stevens, 1992).

In the context of perinatal loss, several aspects of the miscarriage experience are unique. Physically, women describe their experience as painful, with heavy bleeding; moreover, many women report a fear of dying (Bansen & Stevens, 1992). Neither health care providers nor the lay public considers miscarriage to be a painful or life-threatening event. Based on feedback from women who have experienced a miscarriage, greater physical attention, provision of information, and emotional support are warranted.

Women have also noted that the grieving process following a miscarriage is difficult because of a lack of tangible evidence of the pregnancy. Since most women do not see the fetus or products of conception, it is difficult to confirm the reality of the pregnancy and the subsequent loss (Keye, 1994). Because miscarriage occurs primarily in the first trimester, before outward signs of pregnancy are evident, the loss is compounded by a lack of recognition by friends and family who may not have been aware of the pregnancy. Women report experiencing a "conspiracy of silence." Health care professionals should provide anticipatory guidance and role-play difficult social situations with the woman.

Women who experience multiple pregnancy losses are particularly at risk for pathological grief reaction, since the grief response may be cumulative. They may experience general feelings of depression and unhappiness, as well as increased ambivalence about each pregnancy. There frequently is a sense of loss of control over reproductive options. This scenario is particularly common in women who have undergone treatment for infertility.

Couples who have experienced multiple pregnancy losses often protect themselves by restricting the news of the pregnancy to a select group of people and avoiding preparation activities for the infant (for example, purchasing toys or a crib), in anticipation of another pregnancy loss. This phenomenon has been described as "waiting to lose" (Harris, Sandelowski, & Holditch-Davis, 1991, p. 218). Health care providers should assess and acknowledge fertility history, provide detailed information about the plan of care, support the couple during vulnerable times (previous loss markers), and assist with referrals for unresolved grief.

Despite the overwhelming sense of loss, many women, particularly previously infertile women, express positive gains from the miscarriage. Positive outcomes include knowing that pregnancy was possible, having a diminished sense of further risk, knowing they could make a normal baby, and/or being assured they did not lose a normal baby (Harris, Sandelowski, & Holditch-Davis, 1991). Even for women who can identify a positive outcome following a miscarriage, the gain is never the predominant theme.

STILLBIRTH

The concept of prenatal maternal attachment is well-documented in literature. By definition, stillbirth occurs after the fetus is viable (20 weeks gestation), at which time the mother has recognized the fetus as a separate entity, usually via fetal movement. It is the absence of this fetal movement that often prompts a mother to contact her health care provider for reassurance. Generally, stillbirth is unexpected and, consequently, couples are physically and emotionally unprepared for the loss. The majority of stillbirths are of unknown etiology, which can inhibit grief resolution as the mother is unsure to what she should attribute the loss.

The delivery of the infant is accomplished by either induction of labor or spontaneous labor. A woman laboring with a stillborn infant should have a specific nurse assigned only to her care and management of labor. Nurses should provide as much pain relief as is safely possible, clarify misperceptions, provide information, encourage verbalization of feelings, and prepare the woman for delivery of a still, pale or reddish infant with peeling skin and a markedly molded head.

Silence and tension are common at the discovery of a stillbirth. The absence of a fetal heart rate is often rationalized by health care professionals as "positional" or a "defective fetoscope." Well-meaning staff continue to search repeatedly for a fetal heartbeat, often soliciting the help of peers. This action heightens a woman's anxiety, with feelings of impending doom. If a woman presents to a labor and delivery unit without a fetal heartbeat, resource staff should be notified immediately and the diagnosis confirmed by ultrasound. The provider with whom the patient has the strongest relationship should remain with the woman to provide information and give emotional support.

Overwhelming feelings of guilt characterize women experiencing a stillbirth. An autopsy can provide concrete information absolving the mother from responsibility. When no cause is determined (approximately 50% of the time), the normality of the child and the low risk of recurrence should be stressed.

One important aspect of the grieving process is confirming perceptually who died. Historically, women who delivered a stillborn infant lacked concrete remembrances of the infant. The simplest way to help parents confirm who died is to let them see the baby (Bourne, 1979). Most parents choose to hold the baby (Kellner, Donnelly, & Gould, 1984) and should be given time to do so. The decision to have the health care worker present or absent should be the parents' choice. Naming the baby further acknowledges his or her existence and facilitates discussion about the infant (Kellner, Donnelly, & Gould, 1984). Tangible evidence such as footprints, photographs, identification bracelets, and locks of hair are appreciated by parents. These mementos create remembrances of the stillborn infant that can be referred to in the future or shared with relatives and friends.

SUPPORTING ADJUSTMENT TO A CHILD WITH BIRTH ANOMALIES

Childbirth is considered a time of celebration filled with parental pride for the new infant. After months, possibly years, of hoping and planning, the birth of a child with an anomaly shatters dreams and expectations and creates tremendous anxiety, feelings of helplessness, and an overwhelming sense of guilt.

A child born with a congenital anomaly represents another type of perinatal loss—the loss of the wanted or perfect child. Mothers and fathers experience a grief reaction similar to that described for a stillbirth or miscarriage. Within the context of the grief process, the guilt experienced by parents is profound. Parents may believe consciously or unconsciously that the child is a result of something they either did or failed to do (Kennell & Trause, 1978). Parents are at greater risk for overwhelming or pathological feelings of guilt if the anomaly is the result of a genetic or inherited disorder.

PSYCHOSOCIAL ISSUES

Congenital abnormalities have varying degrees of associated medical risk and significance for the family. Ekwo, Kim, and Gosselink (1987) examined parental perceptions of the burden associated with a child who had a genetic disease. Genetic conditions relating to physical handicap or facial abnormalities (i.e., cleft palate) were perceived as the least serious, whereas congenital anomalies leading to prolonged illness or early death (i.e., cystic fi-

brosis) were considered the most serious or problematic. Genetic factors causing mental retardation, such as Down syndrome, fell somewhere between the extremes.

Despite these findings, each family's response and experience following the birth of a child with a congenital anomaly is unique. Family A, who has a newborn with a surgically correctable cleft palate, may be more distressed and dysfunctional than Family B, who is facing the long-term care of a child with Down syndrome.

HEALTH CARE INTERVENTION

The meaning ascribed to the birth, and its immediate and long-term effect on the entire family, should be assessed systematically by multidisciplinary members of a health care team. Prior to the birth of a child with an anomaly, most parents have had no experience with individuals with disabilities, and may be unaware of the impact the birth will have on their lives. Potential problem areas in families include unresolved feelings of guilt and feelings of inadequacy as individuals and parents, a tendency to overfocus on and overprotect the affected child, propensity for marital discord and distress, and dysfunctional interactions with other family members. Support groups with other families who have children with similar disorders can be invaluable.

Historically, the birth of a child with an anomaly was an unexpected event. With the advent of ultrasonography and genetic testing, diagnosis frequently is made prenatally. Parents' perceptions of the manner in which they were informed of the diagnosis have a major impact on how they later define the experience and their future interactions with the child (Van Riper, Pridham, & Ryff, 1992). Because this is a time of crisis for parents and assimilation of new information is difficult, a provider with whom the parents have an established relationship should be present to provide simple explanations. Merely a decision to continue the pregnancy does not represent resolution of the grief nor acceptance of the child.

After delivery, parents should be encouraged to interact with their newborn. This can be achieved by health care workers depicting positive aspects of the child and assuring parents that this is still a time for celebration. Parental cues of readiness to interact with their newborn should be respected, as parents who are forced to interact with their infant before they are emotionally ready may develop feelings of disappointment, guilt, inadequacy, uselessness, and profound sadness (Edwards & Saunders, 1990).

Persistent inability to interact with the newborn is pathological and places the child at risk for neglect. If noninteractive behaviors are observed after the initial birth period, referrals to appropriate mental health services should be made. All parents who give birth to a child with a congenital anomaly should be referred to a mental health worker prior to discharge for assistance in the grief process and linkage to community resources.

PSYCHOSOCIAL ISSUES CONNECTED WITH THERAPEUTIC ABORTION

Approximately 1.5 million therapeutic abortions are performed in the United States annually, involving 27.4 of every 1000 women between the ages of 15 and 44 (Dagg, 1991). Despite the frequency of this medical procedure, relatively little research has focused on the psychological effects of therapeutic or elective abortion.

ADOLESCENT ABORTION

Teenagers disproportionately comprise abortion statistics. While women under 20 account for 13% of all U.S. births, they comprise 26% of all abortions (Henshaw & Van Vort, 1989; Greydanus & Railsback, 1985).

Unfortunately, sexual activity is a prime opportunity for adolescents to express their autonomy. Whether adolescent girls are unaware of the likelihood of pregnancy or choose to ignore the consequences of their behavior (Alan Guttmacher Institute, 1981), pregnancy often results from this increased sexual activity. Cognitive limitations relating to the consequences of their actions are also

seen in delayed decision making once pregnancy has occurred. Teenage women disproportionately represent the number of second trimester abortions (Trad, 1993). This suggests that many adolescent girls delay confronting pregnancy and the difficult decision to carry to term or abort.

Counseling Prior to Procedure

In order to make an informed choice about pregnancy options, adolescents should be referred for counseling prior to the abortion procedure. Motivation for seeking an abortion should be explored. Parents have a major influence on their teenager's pregnancy decisions (Lewis, 1987). Most adolescents have discussed the issue with their mother and do not appear to be influenced by peers (Lewis, 1980).

Trad (1993) encourages the use of a mental health therapeutic technique, *previewing*, through which adolescents can better envision the long-term consequences of each decision. Previewing is a strategy that uses imagery to create an upcoming situation so that future responses can be explored and predicted.

Health care workers who morally object to abortion are professionally obligated to refer a patient to a competent colleague for counseling.

Counseling and Intervention after Procedure

Most adolescents fare well psychologically following an abortion when both pre- and postabortion counseling is provided (Greydanus & Railsback, 1985). In most cases, a feeling of malaise after the procedure appears to be replaced by a feeling of relief.

Regardless of the long-term resolution, the adolescent's decision to abort is difficult. Some reports indicate that, from a psychological standpoint, abortion may be more difficult for adolescents than for adult women (Greydanus & Railsback, 1985). This may reflect the adolescent's limited cognitive abilities in processing the grief after the procedure.

Known negative psychological sequelae of abortion include depression, guilt, unhappiness, regret, and anxiety. Several precipitating factors have been associated with these negative responses including preexisting psychiatric disorder, fanatical or dogmatic religious beliefs, weak family support, poor counseling, ineffective coping skills, and late gestational abortions (Trad, 1993; Greydanus, 1983). Negative reactions are diminished with appropriate counseling.

ELECTIVE TERMINATIONS

Counseling

Women who desire an elective or therapeutic pregnancy termination should be afforded the same mental health counseling recommended for adolescents. The confidential nature of all discussion should be reiterated since fear of disclosure dissuades some women from seeking assistance. Literature suggests that, for the great majority of women, a decision about abortion, although difficult, does not involve a great deal of conscious ambivalence (Dagg, 1991).

Counseling and Intervention after Procedure

Risk factors for negative sequelae identified for adolescents following an elective termination hold true for women of all ages. The presence of support or, more accurately, perceived degree of support has been associated with a positive, initial psychological response. This notion is further supported by documentation that unmarried women are more prone to negative outcomes than are married women, which may be due to a lack of emotional support (Adler, 1975). More recently, however, Major, Mueller, and Hildebrandt (1985) reported that women whose partners accompanied them to the clinic experienced greater depression and more physical complaints. A strong relationship with her partner was correlated with greater regret one year after the procedure.

Regardless of the circumstances surrounding the elective abortion, most women report symptoms of distress and dysphoria immediately after the procedure. These symptoms seem to be continuations of symptoms that

predated the abortion and actually reflect the circumstances surrounding the abortion, not the procedure itself (Dagg, 1991). Long-term studies indicate that the majority of women report positive feelings about their decision; a small minority express regrets (Dagg, 1991).

It is reported that women who have undergone an abortion, while feeling justified that abortion was the most acceptable choice at the time, may carry forward a deep feeling of loss, regret, and guilt (Dagg, 1991). A therapeutic process can assist women to work through some of these feelings. Near the anniversary date of the abortion, these feelings may become more active. One therapeutic intervention involves the mother writing a letter to the aborted baby explaining the decision and subsequent thoughts and feelings. Often, the writer will describe sorrow and sense of regret and ask the baby for forgiveness.

GENETIC TERMINATIONS

Counseling

The decision to engage in genetic counseling should include discussions of not only testing procedures and their associated risks, but also the possibility that a couple with positive test results will be faced with a decision about an elective abortion. Most counselors rarely discuss this prior to the test and diagnosis. In counseling sessions, a couple rarely asks questions about abortion due to ignorance about what questions to ask.

Furthermore, few women are knowledgeable about the differences between first and second trimester abortions (Kolker & Burke, 1993). This information is critical since women face diagnostic choices. Chorionic villus sampling (CVS), with a higher procedural risk of miscarriage, is completed in the first trimester, while amniocentesis, with lower associated risk and greater accuracy, is performed in the second trimester (Boss, 1994).

Lack of information about the implications of genetic testing on abortion inhibits an informed choice and leaves couples unprepared and at risk for pathological grief responses if it is necessary to terminate the pregnancy. Although no religions favor abortion, some tolerate it early in pregnancy under special circumstances. For traditionally observant Moslem and Jewish women, for instance, an amniocentesis, performed in the second trimester, provides data too late for an abortion to be acceptable since the procedure is performed after the fetus is viable. Chorionic villus sampling provides genetic knowledge in the first trimester, a time frame that is more acceptable if termination is desired (Kolker & Burke, 1993).

Counseling and Intervention after the Procedure

The response to genetic abortion is akin to the grief response for perinatal loss. Multiple studies have demonstrated that the medical or genetic indications for terminating a pregnancy increase the risk of adverse psychological sequelae in the mothers. As most genetic terminations are currently done in the second trimester, mothers have already experienced fetal movement, which is associated with greater maternal-infant attachment. However, unlike a stillbirth, where the loss is passive, genetic terminations require deliberate choice. Women must choose between giving birth to an affected child or to abort. This decision appears to complicate the grieving process.

Not surprisingly, women report overwhelming feelings of guilt. Blumberg, Golbus, and Hanson (1975) report an incidence of depression and marital disruption following a genetic termination as high as 92% among women and 82% among men. All women who undergo a genetic termination should be encouraged to engage in short-term (approximately six sessions) couples counseling and to explore a support group.

The same support measures recommended after a stillbirth apply to a genetic termination. Specifically, women should be encouraged to see and hold the infant (Mueller, 1991). Normal aspects of the infant should be highlighted in photographs taken for the mother by staff. Other remembrances should also be provided. Long-term counseling is critical as it affords the opportunity to discuss subsequent pregnancies, the need for genetic counseling, and the risk of disease recurrence.

SUBSEQUENT PREGNANCIES

Women who have historically elected to abort may choose to continue a pregnancy in the future. Unresolved feelings of grief, particularly guilt, may arise at that time. Standard obstetrical intake data provides the relevant historical information. In a nonjudgmental manner, circumstances surrounding the event and residual feelings should be explored. Questions may include:

- Was a first or second trimester procedure done?
- Was it an elective termination or a selective termination for genetic reasons?
- What are your thoughts about this pregnancy?

If a woman reports overwhelming feelings of sadness, depression, or guilt, a referral to mental health services should be initiated. Unresolved grief from a previous termination can interfere with the current maternal-infant attachment process, placing the unborn infant at risk.

Women who have difficulty conceiving or who miscarry after an elective abortion may suffer intense feelings of grief, often in isolation. Feelings of guilt and responsibility for current losses by somehow injuring her reproductive organs during the induced abortion are common. Furthermore, many women choose not to inform their partner of the previous pregnancy and termination and, therefore, cannot benefit from the partner's support. Again, persistent or unresolved feelings of depression or guilt warrant a mental health referral.

CONCLUSION

Pregnancy is a significant developmental marker for a woman. The multiple physical, psychosocial, and environmental factors to which a woman is exposed during pregnancy greatly influence her acquisition of the maternal role and identity, the developmental task of pregnancy. Assessment of risk during pregnancy, particularly psychosocial risk, and referral to appropriate mental health services is vital to the health of not only the mother, but the entire family constellation.

BIBLIOGRAPHY

Adler, N. F. (1975). Emotional responses to women following a therapeutic abortion. *American Journal of Orthopsychiatry, 45*, 446–454.

Alan Guttmacher Institute. (1981). Teenage pregnancy: The problem that hasn't gone away. Section 8. *Abortion Services*, 50–57.

Auvenshire, M. A., & Enriquez, M. G. (1990). *Comprehensive maternity nursing: Perinatal and women's health* (2nd ed.). Boston: Jones and Bartlett Publisher, Inc.

Bansen, S. S., & Stevens, H. A. (1992). Women's experiences of miscarriage in early pregnancy. *Journal of Nurse Midwifery, 37*(2), 84–88.

Benfield, D. G., Lieb, S. A., & Vollman, J. H. (1978). Grief response of parents to neonatal death and parent participation in deciding care. *Pediatrics, 62*(2), 171–177.

Blumberg, R. B., Golbus, M. S., & Hanson, K. H. (1975). The psychological sequelae of abortion performed for a genetic indication. *American Journal of Obstetrics and Gynecology, 122*, 799–808.

Boss, J. (1994). First trimester prenatal diagnoses: Earlier is not necessarily better. *Journal of Medical Ethics, 20*, 146–151.

Bourne, S. (1979). Coping with perinatal death. *Midwife Health Visitor Community Nurse, 15*, 89–95.

Bowlby, J. (1979). *Attachment and loss*. New York: Basic Books.

Brooks, J. B. (1991). *The process of parenting*. Toronto: Mayfield Publishing.

Brost, L., & Kenney, J. W. (1992). Pregnancy after perinatal loss: Parental reactions and nursing interventions. *Journal of Obstetric, Gynecologic, and Neonatal Nursing, 21*(6), 457–463.

Bryanton, J., Fraser-Davey, H., and Sullivan, P. (1994). Women's perceptions of nursing support during labor. *Journal of Obstetric, Gynecologic, and Neonatal Nursing, 23*(8), 638–644.

Carrington, B. W., Loftman, P. O., Boucher, E., Irish, G., Piniaz, D. K., & Mitchell, J. (1994). Modifying a childbirth education curriculum for two specific populations: Inner-city adolescents and substance-using women. *Journal of Nurse Midwifery, 39*(5), 312–320.

Caudle, P. (1993). Providing culturally sensitive health care to Hispanic clients. *Nurse Practitioner, 18*(12), 40, 43–44, 46, 50–51.

Collins, N. L., Dunkel-Schetter C., Lobel, M., & Scrimshaw, S. (1993). Social support in pregnancy: Psychosocial correlates of birth outcomes and postpartum depression. *Journal of Personality and Social Psychology, 65*(6), 1243–1258.

Corrine, L., Bailey, V., Valentin, M., Morantes, E., & Shirley, L. (1992). The unheard voices of women: Spiritual interventions in maternal-child health. *Maternal Child Nursing, 17*, 141–145.

Crowther, C., Verkieyl, D., Neilson, J., Bannerman, C., and Ashurst, H. (1990). The effects of hospitalization for rest on fetal growth, neonatal morbidity and length of gestation in twin pregnancy. *British Journal of Obstetrics and Gynecology, 97*, 872–877.

Cullberg, J. (1972). Mental reactions of women to perinatal death. *Psychosomatic Medicine in Obstetrics and Gynecology: Proceedings of the Third International Congress*, 326–329. Basel: Karger.

Culpepper, L., & Jack, B. (1993). Psychosocial issues in pregnancy. *Primary Care, 20*(3), 599–619.

Curtis, K. (1986). *The psycho-physiologic effects of bedrest on at risk pregnant women: A pilot study*. Unpublished masters thesis. Madison, WI: University of Wisconsin.

Dagg, P. K. (1991). The psychological sequelae of therapeutic abortion—denied and completed. *American Journal of Psychiatry, 148*(5), 578–585.

D'Avanzo, C. E. (1992). Bridging the cultural gap with Southeast Asians. *Maternal Child Nursing, 17*, 204–208.

Dore, M. M., & Dumois, A. O. (1990). Cultural differences in the meaning of adolescent pregnancy. *Families in Society: The Journal of Contemporary Human Services, 71*, 93–101.

Edwards, L., & Saunders, R. (1990). Symbolic interactionism: A framework for the care of parents of pre-term infants. *Journal of Pediatric Nursing, 5*, 123–128.

Ekwo, E. E., Kim, J., & Gosselink, C. A. (1987). Parental perceptions of the burden of genetic diseases. *American Journal of Medical Genetics, 28*, 955–963.

Estok, P., and Lehman, A. (1983). Perinatal death: Grief support for families. *Birth, 10*(1), 17–25.

Ewton, D. S. (1993). A perinatal loss follow-up guide for primary care. *Nurse Practitioner, 18*(12), 30–36.

Fawcett, J., Pollio, N., & Tully, A. (1992). Women's perceptions of cesarean and vaginal delivery: Another look. *Research in Nursing and Health, 15*, 439–446.

Freda, M. C., Anderson, H. F., Damus, K., & Merkatz, I.R. (1993). What pregnant women want to know: A comparison of client and provider perceptions. *Journal of Obstetric, Gynecologic, and Neonatal Nursing, 22*(3), 237–244.

Gottesman, M. M. (1992). Maternal adaptation during pregnancy among adult early, middle and late childbearers: Similarities and differences. *Maternal-Child Nursing Journal, 20*(2), 93–111.

Greydanus, D. E. & Railsback, L. D. (1985). Abortion in adolescence. *Seminars in Adolescent Medicine, 1*, 213–222.

Greydanus, D. E. (1983). Abortion in adolescence. In E. R. McAnamey (Ed.), *Premature adolescent pregnancy and parenthood*. New York: Grune and Stratton.

Harker, L., & Thorpe, K. (1992). "The last egg in the basket?" Elderly primiparity—a review of findings. *Birth, 19*(1), 23–29.

Harris, B. G., Sandelowski, M., & Holditch-Davis, D. (1991). Infertility.... and new interpretations of pregnancy loss. *Maternal Child Nursing, 16*, 217–220.

Harrison, A. O., Wilson, M. N., Pine, C. J., Chan, S. Q., & Buriel, B. (1990). Family ecologies of ethnic minority children. *Child Development, 61*, 347–362.

Henshaw, S. K., & Van Vort, J. (1989). Teenage abortion, birth and pregnancy statistics: An update. *Family Planning Perspectives, 21*(2), 85–88.

Hines, P. M., Garcia-Preto, N., McGoldrick, M., Almeida, R., & Weltman, S. (1992). Intergenerational relationships across cultures. *Families in Society: The Journal of Contemporary Human Services, 73*(6), 323–338.

Kammerman, S. B., and Kahn, A. J. (1988). *Mothers alone: Strategies for a time of change*. Dover, MA: Auburn House.

Kellner, K. R., Donnelly, W. H., & Gould, S. D. (1984). Parental behavior after perinatal death: Lack of predictive variables. *Obstetrics and Gynecology, 63*, 809.

Kennell, J. H., Slyter, H., & Klaus, M. H. (1970). The mourning response of parents to the death of a newborn infant. *New England Journal of Medicine, 283*(7), 344–349.

Kennell, J. H., & Trause, M. A. (1978). Helping parents cope with perinatal death. *Contemporary Obstetrics and Gynecology, 12*, 53.

Keye, W. (1994). Psychologic relationships. *Clinical Obstetrics and Gynecology, 37*(3), 671–680.

Khazoyan, C. M., & Anderson, N. (1994). Latinas' expectations for their partners during childbirth. *Maternal Child Nursing, 19*, 226–229.

Kirkley-Best, E., & Kellner, K. R. (1982). The forgotten grief: A review of the psychology of stillbirth. *American Journal of Orthopsychiatry, 52*(3), 420–427.

Klaus, M. H., & Kennell, J. H. (1982). *Parent-infant bonding* (2nd ed.). St. Louis: C.V. Mosby.

Kolker, A., & Burke, M. (1993). Grieving the wanted child: Ramifications of abortion after prenatal diagnoses of abnormality. *Health Care for Women International, 14*, 513–526.

Kubler-Ross, E. (1969). *On death and dying.* New York: Macmillan Publishing Company.

Lawson, L. V. (1990). Culturally sensitive support for grieving parents. *Maternal Child Nursing, 15*, 76–79.

Lewis, C. C. (1987). Minors competence to consent to abortion. *American Psychologist, 42*, 84–88.

Lewis, C. C. (1980). A comparison of minors' and adults' pregnancy decisions. *American Journal of Orthopsychiatry, 50*, 432–445.

Lindemann, E. (1944). Symptomatology and management of acute grief. *Journal of Psychiatry, 101*(3), 141–148.

Lowe, N. K. (1991). Maternal confidence in coping with labor. A self-efficacy concept. *Journal of Obstetric, Gynecologic, and Neonatal Nursing, 20*(6), 457–463.

Mackey, M. C., and Stepans, M. E. (1994). Women's evaluations of their labor and delivery nurses. *Journal of Obstetric, Gynecologic, and Neonatal Nursing, 23*(5), 413–419.

Major, B. N., Mueller, P., & Hildebrandt, K. (1985). Attributions, expectations, and coping with abortion. *Journal of Personalities and Social Psychology, 48*, 585–599.

Makosky, V. P. (1982). Sources of stress: Events or conditions? In D. Belle (Ed.), *Lives in stress: Women and depression.* Beverly Hills, CA: Sage.

Maloni, J. A., & Kasper, C. E. (1991). Physical and psychosocial effects of antepartum hospital bedrest: A review of the literature. *Image, 23*(3), 187–192.

May, K. A. (1993). Impact of maternal activity restriction for preterm labor on the expectant father. *Journal of Obstetric, Gynecologic, and Neonatal Nursing, 23*(3), 246–251.

McCain, G., & Deatrick, J. A. (1994). The experience of high-risk pregnancy. *Journal of Obstetric, Gynecologic, and Neonatal Nursing, 23*(5), 421–427.

Mechanek, R., Klein, E., & Kuppersmith, J. (1988). Single mothers by choice: A family alternative. In M. Braude (Ed.), *Women, power and therapy: Issues for Women.* New York: Haworth Press.

Mercer, E., & Ferketich, S. (1988). Stress and social support as predictors of anxiety and depression during pregnancy. *Advances in Nursing Science, 10*, 26–39.

Miles, M. S. (1985). Helping adults mourn the death of a child. *Issues in Comprehensive Pediatric Nursing, 8*, 219–241.

Miovech, S. M., Knapp, H., Borucki, L., Roncoli, M., Arnold, L., & Brooten, D. (1994). Major concerns of women after cesarean delivery. *Journal of Obstetric, Gynecologic, and Neonatal Nursing, 23*(1), 53–55.

Mueller, L. (1991). Second trimester termination of pregnancy: Nursing care. *Journal of Obstetric, Gynecologic, and Neonatal Nursing, 20*(4), 284–287.

Nath, P. S., Borkowski, J. G., Whitman, T. L., & Schellenbach, C. J. (1991). Understanding adolescent parenting: The dimensions and functions of social support. *Family Relations, 40*, 411–420.

Nichols, M. R. (1993). Paternal perspectives of the childbirth experience. *Maternal-Child Nursing Journal, 21*(3), 99–108.

Olson, M. R., & Haynes, J. A. (1993). Successful single parents. *Families in Society: The Journal of Contemporary Human Services, 74*(5), 259–266.

Olson, S. L., & Banyard, V. (1993). "Stop the world so I can get off for a while." Sources of daily stress in the lives of low-income single mothers of young children. *Family Relations, 42*, 50–56.

Pakizegi, B. (1990). Emerging family forms: Single mothers by choice—demographic and psychosocial variables. *Maternal-Child Nursing Journal, 19*(11), 1–19.

Parkes, C. M. (1972). *Bereavement: Studies of grief in adult life.* New York: International Universities Press.

Peppers, L. G., & Knapp, R. J. (1980). *Motherhood and mourning: Perinatal death.* New York: Praeger.

Pridham, K., Lytton, D., Chang, A., & Rutledge, D. (1991). Early postpartum transition: Progress in maternal identity and role attainment. *Research in Nursing and Health, 14*, 21–31.

Reece, S. M. (1993). Social support and the early maternal experience of primiparas over 35. *Maternal-Child Nursing Journal, 21*(3), 91–98.

Reed, K. S. (1992). The effects of gestational age and pregnancy planning status on obstetrical nurses' perceptions of giving emotional care to women experiencing miscarriage. *Image, 24*(2), 107–110.

Reichert, J. A., Baron, M., & Fawcett, J. (1993). Changes in attitudes toward cesarean birth. *Journal of Obstetric, Gynecologic, and Neonatal Nursing, 22*(2), 159–167.

Richardson, R. A., Barbour, N. B., & Bubenzer, D. L. (1991). Bittersweet connections: Informal social networks as sources of support and interference for adolescent mothers. *Family Relations, 40*, 430–434.

Rowe, J., Clyman, R., Green C., Mikkelsen, C., Haight, J., & Ataide, L. (1978). Follow-up of families who experience perinatal death. *Pediatrics, 62*(2), 166–170.

Rubin, R. (1975). Maternal tasks in pregnancy. *Journal of Advanced Nursing, 1*, 367–376.

Shrock, P. (1988). The basis of relaxation. In F. H. Nichols & S. S. Humenick (Eds.), *Childbirth education: Practice, research and theory.* Philadelphia: W. B. Saunders.

Stack, J., & Barnas, K. (1987). Stillbirth. *American Family Physician, 35*(2), 117–124.

Stafford, R. (1990). Recent trends in cesarean section use in California. *Western Journal of Medicine, 153*(5), 511–514.

Stainton, M. C. (1990). Parents' awareness of their unborn infant in the third trimester. *Birth, 17*(2), 92–96.

Stainton, M. C. (1994). Supporting family functioning in pregnancy. *Maternal Child Nursing, 19,* 24–28.

Stainton, M. C., McNeil, D., & Harvey, S. (1992). Maternal tasks of uncertain motherhood. *Maternal-Child Nursing Journal, 20*(2), 113–123.

Stenberg, L., and Blinn, L. (1993). Feelings about self and body during adolescent pregnancy. *Families in Society: The Journal of Contemporary Human Services, 74*(5), 282–289.

Stinson, K. M., Lasker, J. N., Tohmann, J., & Toedter, L. J. (1992). Parents' grief following pregnancy loss: A comparison of mothers and fathers. *Family Relations, 41,* 218–223.

Tilden, P. V. (1984). The relation of selected psychosocial variables to single status of adult women during pregnancy. *Nursing Research, 33,* 102–107.

Trad, P. V. (1993). Abortion and pregnant adolescents. *Families in Society: The Journal of Contemporary Human Services, 74*(7), 397–409.

U.S. Bureau of the Census. (1990). Household and family characteristics. *Current Population Reports*, Series p-20, No. 447. Washington, DC: U. S. Government Printing Office.

Van Riper, M., Pridham, K., & Ryff, C. (1992). Symbolic interactionism: A perspective for understanding parent-nurse interactions following the birth of a child with Downs' Syndrome. *Maternal-Child Nursing Journal, 20*(1), 21–39.

Wall, E. M. (1988). Assessing obstetric risk: A review of obstetric risk-scoring systems. *Journal of Family Practice, 27*(2), 153–163.

Wilcox, A. J., Weinberg, C. R., & O'Connor, J. F. (1988). Incidence of early loss in pregnancy. *New England Journal of Medicine, 319,* 189–194.

Williams, L. B., and Pratt, W. F. (1990). Wanted and unwanted childbearing in the United States: 1973-88. *National Center for Health Statistics. National Survey of Family Growth*, p.189.

Yoder, L. (1994). Comfort and consolation: A nursing perspective on parental bereavement. *Pediatric Nursing, 20*(5), 473–477.

Zayas, L. H., & Busch-Rossnagel, N. A. (1992). Pregnant Hispanic women: A mental health study. *Families in Society: The Journal of Contemporary Human Services, 73*(9), 515–521.

CHAPTER 27

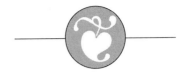

Psychosocial Adaptation of the Child, Adolescent, and Family With Physical Illness

Nell Baker

Knowledge of the normal development of socialization, judgment, and cognitive processes aids assessment of the psychosocial status of a child or adolescent. This chapter provides brief summaries of developmental tasks, play behaviors, and thoughts about physiological processes and death typical of various ages. Illness affects a child's development and the entire family system. Examples based on interviews with expert nurses describe behavioral interventions and effective tools to increase coping and adaptation by family members.

Clinical conditions covered, with assessment and intervention recommendations, include:

1. Congenital conditions and illnesses occurring in infancy
2. Acute major illness with anticipated recovery
3. Major chronic illness or condition
4. Terminal illness

Each section includes the following topics:

1. Effects and interventions with the child
2. Effects and interventions with parents
3. Effects and interventions with siblings
4. Case examples for various age groups

ILLNESS: A CHILD DEVELOPMENT PERSPECTIVE

A child is a developing person. At birth, a human being has no memories, pathways of thought for recall, or strength gained by successful performance. There is only genetic endowment. Personality, conscience, and judgment are developed as the child grows (Leckman, 1991). Ideally, the family will nourish, teach, love, and protect the child as he or

Patricia Barry: *Psychosocial Nursing:
Care of Physically Ill Patients and Their Families*, 3rd ed.
© 1996 Lippincott-Raven Publishers

she grows and learns—leading, guiding, and allowing individuation (Baker, 1994). Although the period of optimum parental influence usually is complete at the end of adolescence, adaptation and emotional growth take place throughout life (Erikson, 1963; Fawcett, 1993).

Physical illness is a stressor in the life of a child and family system. Whether the illness is congenital, acute with complete recovery expected, or the onset of a chronic disorder, it interrupts the process of development and the roles and interpersonal relationships of all family members. According to the nature of the disorder, symptoms may be continuous or episodic. Whether interventions take place in the home or hospital, family patterns are interrupted and treatment uses time and financial resources that the family may have chosen to use in some other way (Jackson & Vessey, 1992).

One responsibility of health care professionals is to strengthen the family's ability to impact favorably on the level of functioning the child is able to attain. This includes anticipating the stress associated with the illness and enhancing the family's ability to be cohesive and strong (Jackson & Vessey, 1992).

An appreciation of child development helps health care professionals assess the pediatric patient's ability to understand about body functioning, illness, and treatment expectations. Although each child is different, understanding of age-related capabilities helps to formulate explanations, evaluate responses, and design strategies to lessen anxieties related to disease and treatment (Leckman, 1991).

Comprehension increases as the child's ability to understand advances. Because a child appeared to understand an explanation given at an earlier time and developmental level, ongoing understanding is not guaranteed. Periodic evaluation of comprehension and psychosocial adjustment are necessary. For example, an adolescent whose disease was controlled well during childhood may be judged as noncompliant with health maintenance routines if the illness is exacerbated. However, assessment may indicate that, as parents relinquished control of treatment strategies to the young teen, rationales for treatment were not retaught. They assumed

that their child "just knew" the plethora of information they had acquired during years of parenthood.

ASSESSMENT

Because prevention or early intervention is preferable to treatment of established problems, ongoing psychosocial evaluation of development and adjustment are essential to producing competent individuals who function at the highest level possible. Evaluation of psychosocial functioning may be done by using standardized assessment instruments or by interviewing parents and child to determine if the illness is interfering with relationships with other family members, peers, or in performance at day care or school. Deviations from normal developmental expectations must be addressed by intervention strategies or by referral to mental health professionals to maintain optimal health (Sabbeth & Stein, 1990; Vessey & Caserza, 1992).

Successful assessment is based on the interviewer's ability to establish a trusting relationship. Empathy, observation, and open-ended questions lead to formulation of psychosocial diagnoses. The health care professional is the expert on assessment and interventions, but the parent is the expert on the child. Collaboration between them is based on mutual trust and respect. Urgency to gather information should never supersede the establishment of rapport. Whether in a quiet, private setting or in a busy, noisy environment, the successful interviewer uses space and proximity, eye-contact, tone, consideration, and careful attention to establish a therapeutic alliance (Vessey & Caserza, 1992). If parents believe that the health care provider is trying to help them solve their problems and enhance the quality of their lives, they work with more dedication to achieve their goals (Clunn, 1991).

DEVELOPMENTAL EXPECTATIONS

Thorough understanding of normal development, deviations from norms, and evaluative methods are essential for appropriate assessment and intervention. Below is a brief summary of developmental expectations and age-related thoughts on illness and death.

Infancy: 0–1 Years

If, during infancy, children consistently receive adequate nutrition, restful sleep, comfort, and nurturing touch, they develop trust and hope (Erikson, 1963). Without trust and hope, mistrust may contribute to depression and personality disorders later. A sense of self begins to develop as infants realize that the nurturer separates from them but returns to attend their needs. A further sense of self occurs as infants recognize the effects of actions they initiate (Clunn, 1991; Vessey & Caserza, 1992).

Without verbal skills to define their response to illness or pain, infants historically have been denied basic rights. They do experience and react however, and the reactions can be evaluated and treatment provided. (Acute Pain Management Guideline Panel, 1992). Although infants have no concepts to define death, they do react to loss (Ayoub, 1991).

Toddlerhood: 1–3 Years

As very young children begin to explore their environment, react with the joy of discovery, and express their needs verbally, they become more autonomous (Erikson, 1963). If nurturing continues, limits are set consistently, and movement is impeded only for safety, the child learns self-control without loss of self-esteem. Senses of dignity and justice emerge and conscience begins to develop (Ayoub, 1991).

Play with other children is parallel. There is awareness of others and imitation, but little interaction. Toddlers learn to relate emotionally to parents, siblings, and other people, but the key socializing agents are the parents (Clunn, 1993).

Shame and self-doubt occur if the developing will of a toddler is sharply challenged. Good/bad and right/wrong are associated with the consequences of actions. Words are understood literally and without discrimination for shades of meaning. While toddlers may use single-word utterances to represent whole sentences, they are developing an understanding of more complex forms of speech.

Abstract thoughts either are not understood or are translated into known concepts. Talking to the young child with long sentences and too many words clutters and obscures meaning.

The young child is likely to assume that illness emanates from himself or herself, that sickness and pain are punishments for misdeeds or bad thoughts. This is called "immanent justice" (Lewis, 1994). Tandem with this belief is "omnipotence," the child's belief that he or she has "all power" over what happens. These irrational cognitive processes are referred to as "magical thinking." Unless corrected, these interpretations lead to feelings of guilt or shame for causing illness (Schonfeld, 1991).

Death is likely to be perceived only in relation to loss. It is viewed as temporary and reversible. While not perceiving the seriousness of their illness, young children may be disturbed by parents' emotions and attribute the cause to themselves (Ayoub, 1991).

Preschooler: 4–6 Years

Imagination and initiative characterize the preschool age (Erikson, 1963). The physical world is explored with all senses. The child learns to be loving, relaxed, energetic, and task-oriented. Speech increases in complexity, and thought is concrete and tangible. At this age, children interpret objects and events in terms of their relationship or use to themselves. Because they are developing conscience and an inner sense of warning or threat, preschoolers are no longer guided only by others.

Children begin to play together but are unaware of perspectives other than their own. If the child retains a sense of initiative without impinging on the rights of others, the lasting outcome is a sense of direction and purpose (Clunn, 1993).

Preschoolers still believe that illness is a result of their thoughts or actions. This may cause additional worry unless it is countered with accurate information within the child's ability to comprehend. Preschoolers can understand causality based on a single external symptom or an illness within their experience such as a cold (Yoos, 1987).

Death and life may seem interchangeable to preschoolers, who have no basis for concepts such as "forever." Irrational fears may be stimulated by euphemisms adults use for death (Ayoub, 1991; Wheeler & Pike, 1993).

Middle Childhood: 7–10 Years

During school age, industry, productivity, and perseverance lead to task completion and a sense of competence (Erikson, 1963). Feelings of inadequacy and inferiority may occur if performance expectations are too high. Teachers and peers gain importance. School-agers learn physical and cognitive skills and how to organize facts and solve problems in a concrete fashion, reason inductively, consider points of view other than their own, respect authority, follow rules, and maintain social order (Modlin & Adams, 1993). Group games and sports are fun.

At this age children can understand that illness is caused by germs, but have little understanding of physiological processes. Although they can be taught the symptoms and treatment routines for chronic conditions, they may not report symptoms reliably because they fear retribution for causing the symptoms themselves. Attitudes about death are greatly influenced by adults, especially parents, but school-aged children are able to conceptualize death as inevitable, universal, and irreversible (Ayoub, 1991).

Early Adolescence: 11–13 Years

Early adolescence has hallmarks of middle childhood and adolescence, with reverberation between the two. A need to be nurtured vies with a need for independence. Idealism vies with doubt. Morality and values develop, and conscience is refined. Concern about physical changes may cause confusion about self-image. There is emphasis on friendship with one particular person, usually of the same sex. Peers assume greater importance and, if confidence is weak, overidentification with groups or gangs may result (Clunn, 1991).

Logical solutions to problems can be attained. Normally, an early adolescent has the cognitive ability to understand physiology, causality of illness, and treatment regimens. However, compliance with regimens may be difficult because of the desire to conform with peers. Early adolescents may blame themselves for illnesses over which they have no control or ignore treatments vital to health maintenance, e.g., "If I ignore it, it might go away" (Hogarth, 1991).

Adolescence: 14–18 Years

As the ability to think abstractly develops, older adolescents reconsider their disorders, health maintenance needs, and abstract concepts such as death and afterlife. In developing formal operational thought, they listen to each other and a few respected adults, and begin to formulate their own opinions (Kempe & Rawlins, 1993). If adolescent development is successful, young people grow in confidence, hone aptitudes, discover opportunities, and move toward economic independence and civic competence. Illness may be considered an inconvenience but tolerated as an element of one's identity. Selecting and preparing for an occupation may be of more concern than illness or death. Feelings of invulnerability and vitality are typical (Erikson, 1963; Wheeler & Pike, 1993).

Parents

Well-functioning parents are the single most important psychological resource for a sick child (Spirito & Fritz, 1993). Their dignity and position in the family is strengthened by giving them information in a way that can be understood and assimilated, and appraising them of professional opinions and plans (Jellinek et al., 1991). Like patients, parents' safety, physiological, emotional, and cognitive needs must be maintained for them to function as leaders of their families (Danielson, Hamel-Bissell, & Winstead-Fry, 1993).

Language is necessary for communication. Consent and treatment must be based on accurately translated information if parents do not understand English or are hearing impaired. The burden of translating should never be placed on a child, especially the patient. A child's attempt to translate unfamiliar words referring to physiological concepts which are not fully understood potentially leads to misinformation for the parent. More importantly, roles within the family are skewed when the parent is dependent on the child for information to make important decisions (Porter & Blackwell, 1991).

Beliefs and self-care traditions of other cultures must be considered. Ethnic groups, from Native Americans to recently immigrated Southeast Asians, often have strong practices and beliefs used traditionally to maintain health. Incorporating an understanding of cultural practices increases the hope of successful outcomes (Porter & Blackwell, 1991; Rairdan & Higgs, 1992; Siantz, 1994). See Chapter 5 for a full discussion of the influence of cultural practices.

Emotions impede communication with parents when their child is ill. Despite the parent's age, intellect, educational level, coping style, cultural assets, or support systems, there will be fear and anxiety. There may be actual or imagined guilt or shame that the illness was not prevented. Fears of inadequacy may compound emotions such as disappointment, grief, chronic sorrow, financial worry, and fatigue. Maladaptive coping may be seen in the form of demanding or irritable behaviors, hypervigilance, overprotectiveness, enmeshment with the ill child, or ingratiating and attention-seeking behaviors (Baker, 1994; Groves, 1978; Jellinek et al., 1991).

Screening for home care should include an assessment of parental coping skills and assistance provided to decrease anxiety. Unaddressed parental apprehension may lead to parents' thinking of the child as "vulnerable" and may cause overprotectiveness, sleep or eating problems, separation anxiety, or an inability to set limits. Efforts should be made to avoid the designation of vulnerability because it interferes with the age-appropriate activities essential to growth and development (Thomasgard & Metz, 1995; Boyce, 1992).

Siblings

If a sister or brother becomes ill, siblings may feel responsible for the illness, imagining that negative thoughts caused it. When parents' attention is directed to the ill child, the sibling may resent the loss of the parents' time. If death occurs, siblings may assume responsibility for the death and the family's grief. Inappropriate behaviors such as joking, giggling, irritability, or regression to earlier developmental levels may signal that loss and irrational guilt are too tremendous to acknowledge (Wheeler & Pike, 1993).

To prevent the pain of unwarranted guilt, siblings should be reassured that the illness is not their fault and that their parents continue to love them. Information about the sibling's disorder will help the well children avoid irrational feelings of guilt, shame, or stigmatization (Gallo et al., 1991).

PREVENTION STRATEGIES

Therapeutic communication and anticipatory guidance are key elements in prevention. Adversity at any age is linked to stress-induced alterations in immune and neuroendocrine function. Negative psychological and physical effects of stress may be lessened by supporting adaptive coping methods (Thomasgard & Metz, 1995; Irwin & Hauger, 1991).

CONGENITAL CONDITIONS AND ILLNESSES OCCURRING IN INFANCY

About 5% of babies are born with major malformations obvious at birth or detected in early childhood. Treatment of these conditions accounts for most of the hospitalizations of children. Approximately 9% of perinatal deaths are due to malformations (Behrman et al., 1992).

EFFECTS AND INTERVENTIONS WITH THE CHILD

Children who are born with anomalies accept the world as defined by the reality of their capabilities. Their concern about illness is recognized as it interferes with their comfort and attachment to their parents. Pain and other peoples' reactions to their limitations may cause them to develop emotional reactions (McCubbin & McCubbin, 1993; Vessey & Caserza, 1992).

Congenital problems and illnesses are often accompanied by pain or painful procedures. The management of pain has traditionally been ignored in the care of children

(Schechter, Berde, & Yaster, 1993). When pain is suspected or when procedures are known to be painful, healthcare providers should analyze their observations of the child's responses and provide analgesia and comfort measures based on the analysis. Untreated pain establishes physiological responses which enhance subsequent pain and cause negative attitudes and emotions associated with medical procedures (Tesler, 1994).

Pain has other consequences. It disrupts attachment between infant and parent; feeding; and adaptation to the environment. "From the infant's perspective, pain from lifesaving care may be indistinguishable from the pain of child abuse" (Gardner, 1994, p. 89).

EFFECTS AND INTERVENTIONS WITH PARENTS

When anomalies are associated with conditions that affect cognitive or physical development, parents may be characterized as victims of the chronic condition because of the worry, sorrow, and issues related to long-term effects of the handicap on their child's life (Austin, 1993).

When an infant's disorder, such as cystic fibrosis, is not correctable, DeWet and Cywes (1985) found that parents are likely to be critical of the healthcare professionals, citing negative factors such as bluntness of the teller who had no hope to offer, delays in receiving the diagnosis, and lack of adequate information. Obviously, such perceptions hinder the establishment of rapport and productive working relationships.

Interventions with families who cope well with congenital conditions are founded on good communication, avoiding factors which inhibit collaboration of parents and healthcare providers.

EFFECTS AND INTERVENTIONS WITH SIBLINGS

Parents are encouraged to discuss disorders in their newborn with their other children. Brothers and sisters infer problems from their parents' behavior. If problems are not discussed

and explained congruent with the children's cognitive level, they interpret the problem as secret and, perhaps, shameful. If the sibling has experienced jealousy or resentment because of the disproportionate amount of time the parents spend with the new baby, magical thinking and the irrational feeling of omnipotence may cause emotions such as guilt.

Unfounded emotions may become intolerable without supportive, nonthreatening words to help dispel the discomfort. Congenital conditions impact siblings. However, the siblings' behavior, social competence, and adjustment can be maintained despite the requirements of another family member, if their emotional needs are recognized and addressed (Gallo et al., 1991).

CASE EXAMPLE: INFANT WITH LOW BIRTH WEIGHT

Sally Adams, M.S., R.N., C.P.N.P., has a primary practice with infants of low birth weight in Dallas County, Texas. She describes how she establishes rapport with families to help normalize the life of children with special needs. Conditions such as respiratory difficulties, neurological conditions, or intestinal problems are associated with birth weight under 1500 g, and require strength and help from the extended family system.

I recognize that, although parents hesitate to express their disappointment, they may experience grief that they do not have the child of their dreams. They need to talk about their feelings of loss without guilt. I reassure them and do not judge them. I talk with them at least twice before the baby is discharged from the hospital to help them develop familiarity with me and, hopefully, to trust me. Their anxiety about taking home a tiny baby with special needs is usually so great that they may not hear and assimilate what I say at first. I can only help them to clarify reality and alter misconceptions if they trust me enough to tell me their fears.

I invite the baby's siblings, grandparents, aunts, and uncles to attend clinic or send their questions and observations by the parents for discussion. I pay attention to their opinions to encourage their participation and unify the support the parents will need. I suggest they think of the baby's growth based on a "start time" that is the actual birth date plus the length of time it was premature. This avoids the child being considered "slow" when compared with other children whose age is calculated from the end of a full-term pregnancy.

As the baby's primary care provider, I explain my availability and use events as they occur to help the parents solve problems and assess outcomes of alternative actions. Gradually, trust advances. In time, parents begin to think of me as someone who helps prevent problems by regular well-baby checks-ups, immunizations, and information. ❧

When confronted with anomalies requiring surgical correction, DeWet and Cywes (1985) report that parents' most acute fear is of losing the child. Positive factors in acceptance of the situation are a sympathetic attitude and hope for successful outcomes instilled by professionals who describe the problems and corrective procedures.

CASE EXAMPLE: INFANT WITH CONGENITAL HEART DEFECT

Paula Dimmitt, M.S., R.N., is in advanced nursing practice. An experienced Clinical Nurse Specialist in pediatric cardiology at Children's Medical Center of Dallas, she talks to parents about the hope which may be realized through corrective interventions with congenital heart defects. Because she talks to parents before the baby develops personality, she tries to shape their thinking with information and anticipatory guidance before the child is labeled "disabled."

I liken cardiac defects to birth marks: they are often repairable. I want the family to see this child is a person in their lives, neither an object to be pitied and indulged, nor ignored and neglected. I want them to maintain hope for the future, so I mention events like birthday parties when the baby is 3 or 4.

Some children with heart defects may not have as much energy as their sisters or brothers. I encourage the parents to allow the child to set limits for his own physical activities even if his color is blue—it's OK. The child will stop when he needs to.

I don't want the family to think of this child as "sick." They become overprotective and he ends up dependent and afraid. That leads to poor self-esteem and confidence and we'll end up with a "cardiac cripple" or a dare-devil who does crazy things to prove himself later on.

I briefly discuss with the parents their value system regarding discipline. If they have not yet developed a discipline style, I teach them about positive motivation, logical consequences, and time outs. I emphasize that consistency is important for all the children in their family.

Since 50% of children with Down syndrome have heart defects, I often talk to parents who must adjust to special learning needs in addition to physical defects. I say, "Susie may be slower," not, "She is retarded." I want them to know that she can be potty trained. It just might be when she is 4 or 5—not the same age as her cousin or neighbor. She can learn to add. It just might take longer. I don't want them to think of this child's situation as sad but challenging. She can become a productive member of society.

Some cardiac defects are accompanied by other anomalies which can be repaired. I want the parents to have the will, strength, and stamina to adjust to the demands of home care and multiple hospital stays. Maintaining hope is important. It is stressful to make frequent transitions from home with full responsibility for care, to hospital where others do most of the treatments, and back home with new duties.

Early in our relationship, parents frequently wonder if they were guilty of causing the birth defects. I assure them that heart defects occur before parents know that new life is forming. I redirect them from finding cause or placing blame, to planning for the future.

How do I talk to the child about his special needs as he gets older? To start with, the child and his sibs are in the room when I talk with the parents. I use words within their understanding and encourage them to ask me questions. The only time I talk with parents alone is if I am describing specific surgical procedures. Parents need details about physiological functions that have no meaning to young children but might frighten them.

When I prepare children for their heart surgery, I use similes. I know preschoolers are concrete thinkers and understand only what they have experienced. For example, a heart might be visualized like a valentine, not a pump with valves, veins, and arteries. To a 6- or 7-year-old, I speak about patching a hole "like Mommy patches a hole in your pants." With a teenager, I am aware that body image and being like other teens is important, so I emphasize positive outcomes in terms that are congruent with those needs.

Children and adolescents have less anxiety and are more cooperative after surgery if they have been introduced to the daily hospital routines in a matter-of-fact fashion. I teach children how to prevent pulmonary complications by deep breathing and help their parents to coach them. They are encouraged to ask for pain medicine as they need it after surgery. The only children I have seen have trouble after surgery are adolescents who shut out all information by saying, "I don't want to know. Don't tell me a thing about it!" 🎔

ACUTE MAJOR ILLNESS WITH ANTICIPATED RECOVERY

Trauma and physical disorders are classified as acute major illnesses if they have sudden onset and require nursing interventions at home or in the hospital, and if recovery is achieved within 3 months. Pain, unexpected onset of symptoms, unusual procedures and equipment, complex explanations, strangers, strange environments, and interrupted routines cause anxiety in children of any age. Anxiety intensifies pain and decreases a child's ability to cope adaptively. Thus, pain and anxiety become cyclic, difficult to interrupt, and cause difficulty in recovery, rehabilitation, and the attainment of developmental expectations. Treatment is most effective when psychological interventions are used in conjunction with medical methods of pain management (McGrath & Unruh, 1993).

EFFECTS AND INTERVENTIONS WITH THE CHILD

Geist (1979) wrote that a false belief in a child's resilience and emotional buoyancy delays judicious psychological intervention, often causing maladaptive psychological side effects that interfere with the child's life more than the physical disorder itself. Preventing psychosocial side effects includes helping a child minimize fear, maintain relationships with family and friends, and reenter school successfully after the acute phase of the illness. If regression occurs during an acute illness, previous developmental attainments will be resumed after recovery if emotional needs are successfully attended.

Infants need the presence of their parents or consistent surrogates, and daily routines as near normal as possible, to prevent emotional concomitants to their illnesses. Preschoolers through adolescents need developmentally appropriate explanations of physical processes, assuming little or no prior knowledge or understanding. The use of anatomical dolls aids understanding. Information should be given in small amounts with frequent reviews and reiteration. Encouraging children to explain the information to their family or other health care professionals helps integrate the knowledge they have just acquired.

Tours of special procedure rooms, surgical suites, and intensive care areas provide opportunities to explain treatments, answer questions, and give reassurance. Medical play with realistic equipment offers opportunities to explore emotions related to treatment modalities in a developmentally appropriate way (Francis, 1995).

Parents are often more successful in distracting children from painful procedures than are professionals, and if prepared and encouraged, normalize situations that might be intimidating. The child and parents can decide together in advance how to divert attention during an anxiety-provoking procedure. They may consider using a particular toy, book, videotape, story or poem to recite, relaxation/visualization exercise, computer game, or therapeutic touch (McGrath & Unruh, 1993; Ross & Ross, 1988). They may select different strategies for different days or procedures. Techniques learned with the support of professionals are useful later when parents must perform procedures at home (Bossert et al., 1990).

EFFECTS AND INTERVENTIONS WITH PARENTS

Helping parents cope with the demands of their child's illness plays an important role in the overall management of care. Timely information, support, and encouragement empowers parents in their roles. Daily meetings with team members to discuss the parent's views, concerns, the child's status, and care plans maintain a collaborative rapport. In the management of complex acute illnesses, care conferences provide an opportunity to coordinate social service, pastoral care, child life, and consultants from various specialty services with family and pediatric teams. If a team member prepares parents and supports their participation in care conferences, he or she allays anxiety and links them with the treatment team (Baker, 1994; Jellinek, et al., 1991).

EFFECTS AND INTERVENTIONS WITH SIBLINGS

For siblings, reassurance by the parents of their continued love is essential. If children have been associated with hospitalizations only when older family members have gone there for terminal care, they may harbor unfounded fears for the sister or brother. It is important for siblings to call and visit the hospitalized child; send and receive photographs or video-

tapes, notes, and drawings; and receive assurance that the hospitalized child will return home. Siblings need preparation for what they will see in the patient's room because a debilitated sibling and treatment apparatus can be frightening. Before the sick child comes home, siblings should be coached about the appearance and activities to expect during recovery (Landreth, 1991).

BEHAVIORAL AND PSYCHIATRIC INTERVENTIONS

Despite interventions to prevent psychological reactions, some children do not respond in a predictable manner. The following examples will describe interventions initiated by psychiatry consultation-liaison services when children and families had difficulty recuperating from acute illness (Lewis, 1994).

CASE EXAMPLE: CHILD AGED 0–1 YEAR

Chucky, a 10-month-old boy, and his family had vomiting and diarrhea. For the rest of the family it was an acute illness, relieved within a week. Chucky was referred to pediatric gastroenterologists when his unremitting vomiting and diarrhea caused significant weight loss. Diagnostic procedures did not identify a physiological cause for symptoms. The Psychiatry Clinical Nurse Specialist assessed his eating/feeding behaviors and formulated plans.

Chucky's developmental milestones and play behaviors were appropriate. He was the third child of caring and attentive parents. However, he was the first child for whom Dad was the primary care provider. Dad worked all night and slept in the hospital room most of the day as he did at home, leaving Chucky awake but quiet in the darkened room much of the time. When Dad awoke and fed his son, Chucky refused or vomited. Mom worked days and slept at night. During Chucky's hospitalization, she visited daily with his sister, aged 7, and 5-year-old brother. Both siblings were healthy and involved in school, church, and community activities. Each time Chucky vomited, Mom and his siblings looked at him with concern, cleaned his face, and murmured sympathetic remarks like, "Poor baby. What can we do?"

Chucky had neither aversion to food in his mouth nor difficulty swallowing. He ate a variety of food when fed by the nurse. When Dad fed him, he held Chucky in one arm, putting the spoon to Chucky's lips for him to suck the food into his mouth. Pureed fruit was all that was worth the effort. Dad gave the bottle in the position used for feeding an infant. When burped, Chucky vomited most of the fruit and milk.

A log was started to show the time, amount, and circumstance when Chucky ate and vomited. He vomited approximately 60 times a day in amounts that varied from an estimated 5 to 120 ml, and in all circumstances except when he slept. Eating occurred at irregular intervals due to Dad's sleep patterns.

Recommendations for change began with wiping Chucky's face when he vomited with no special comment. Other changes involved his schedule. To normalize Chucky's day, a special playroom program was developed to provide age-appropriate activities and social interactions for Chucky while his Dad slept. The parents agreed to provide for these activities at a day care center after discharge.

Because Dad worked at night, he needed a period of uninterrupted sleep each day. He and a staff nurse decided which meal the nurse would feed in order to maintain regular meal times for Chucky. The nurse put Chucky in a high chair and made eye contact as she fed him a combination of cereal and fruit, allowed him to feed himself or play with finger foods, and put milk in a "tippy cup" to let him experiment. He sat upright and held his own bottle after his meal. Dad sometimes observed this procedure and commented on the differences he saw. The nurse informally taught techniques for feeding a 10-month-old. Dad admitted that he had not thought to add cereal to the fruit Chucky liked. With the addition of cereal to his diet, Chucky's diarrhea ceased.

The Psychiatry Clinical Nurse Specialist had dinner with the family in Chucky's room to demonstrate how "time out" can be used to extinguish unwanted behavior. Chucky ate in his high chair at the table with them and was included in the conversation. If he vomited, his chair was pushed back with a soft but firm, "time out." He was observed peripherally for

safety but was not addressed directly during this time. As soon as the vomiting or spitting ceased, his chair was pulled back toward the table, his face was cleaned without comment, he was told, "Time in," and included in the social interactions. His siblings were assured that he would know that they still loved him if they talked and smiled when he was in "time in."

After these techniques were successful in the hospital, they were continued at home. At the follow-up visit, Chucky's mother brought the log which indicated only six episodes of "spitting up" which she characterized as "drool."

Analysis: Inadvertently, Chucky's needs for play and social recognition were not being met because of conflicting needs of other family members. A behavior, learned during an acute illness, continued because it helped him meet his needs, illustrating how people adapt conditions to fulfill needs. At the age of 10 months, Chucky made no conscious decision to vomit in order to be noticed by his parents, but he was gratified by their response when it occurred. Techniques of time out and time in (Christophersen, 1988) and rewarding the desired behaviors (Kazdin, 1991) helped to extinguish an unwanted, learned behavior (Vitulano & Tebes, 1991).

Outcome: Developmental, physical, and emotional needs were met and parental skills were increased.

CASE EXAMPLE: CHILD AGED 1–3 YEARS

Three-year-old Patti was in the hospital for IV antibiotic therapy. Her discharge was delayed because she refused to take oral medications. The usually effective techniques used by experienced pediatric nurses, her dad's cajoling, and her mom's admonitions did not get Patti to take the medicine. The treatment team was frustrated because a 3-year-old was delaying discharge. The insurance provider denied hospitalization and the family's rural community had no home care agency support.

When the insurance case manager was informed about a behavioral program to increase Patti's compliance and that the parents were learning how to use the strategy at home, he allowed additional hospital time. He suspected that oral medication would have prevented the hospitalization for IV therapy and that future hospitalization might be avoided if the parents learned to help Patti comply with oral medications.

A developmentally appropriate reward system was discussed with Patti and her dad. Her dad helped Patti make a wall mural. He drew trees and she colored sky and sun. Patti was intrigued by earning butterfly and flower stickers for her picture by taking medications. She took her pills, and clapped for herself each time she enhanced her wall mural (see Box 27-1).

Analysis: A preschooler did not comprehend the rationale for taking oral medication but did appreciate the attention caused by the struggle. A desired behavior was developed by helping her to approach her task in a playful way (Landreth, 1991) and by providing positive gratification (Werry & Wollersheim, 1989).

Outcomes:

1. Adaptive behavior became more rewarding than oppositional behavior.
2. Parents acquired a new skill. ❦

CASE EXAMPLE:
CHILD AGED 4–7 YEARS

Seven-year-old Ramon was afraid of taking pills because he choked each time he tried. His mom spoke little English. She was embarrassed by Ramon's fear and bewildered by his behavior. He could not be discharged without oral medications. Because Ramon was conversant in both English and Spanish, he frequently interpreted for his mom, attempting to translate physical concepts about which he had little understanding. Assessment showed a tense and anxious child.

BOX 27-1	Principles of a Behavioral Reward System
	• Clear communication about the behavior expected • Consistent reward with something valued by and in short supply for the patient, controlled and immediately attainable by the parent

To relieve Ramon from translating, an adult translator was obtained when discussion about medical and nursing interventions was necessary. In addition, Ramon learned muscle relaxation exercises and guided imagery. When asked to visualize something pleasant that opened wide, he described how his mom opens her arms when she welcomes him home from school. When this was translated for his mom, she demonstrated with her arms and added a big smile. He learned to relax throat muscles and swallowed pills successfully.

Analysis: Reestablishing roles and generational boundaries (Fawcett, 1993) and strengthening parental function decreased the child's anxiety (Givler, 1991). Visualizing and relaxing selected muscles increased the child's feeling of control (Titlebaum, 1988).

Outcome: Roles were resumed, dignity maintained, and treatment progressed to home care. ❦

CASE EXAMPLE:
CHILD AGED 7–10 YEARS

Ellie, a bright-eyed, cooperative child, was terrified by the idea of dental procedures. Many cavities had developed due to her aversion. Use of a general anesthetic was precluded due to a physical disorder. The dentist said restorative procedures could be delayed long enough to desensitize her fear.

Assessment indicated no trauma associated with her mouth which might have caused Ellie's dread of oral procedures. Neither she nor her mother knew the genesis of her panic. Ellie agreed, however, to try to control it.

In four sessions, Ellie learned muscle relaxation/imagery techniques. Concurrently, she developed a list of happy thoughts and a hierarchy of fears. She grasped the idea of "shuttling" her mind between happy and feared content areas. Ellie's mother was in the room with her each time she practiced these skills and was encouraged to praise the positive use of her bright mind and the courage it takes to control fears.

Ellie was coached to maintain relaxation as she ventured progressively into the treatment area, the dental chair, and, finally, a "rehearsal" with dentist and assistant gowning, gloving, and explaining the procedure. When restoration began, she signaled when her fear became uncomfortable. She was coached to regain her relaxed state, and said when she was ready to continue the procedure. Ellie's mom held her hand throughout this and two subsequent dental procedures.

Analysis: Anxiety and relaxation cannot coexist (Wolpe, 1973; Titlebaum, 1988). In vivo, systematic desensitization decreased anxiety and a new coping method was learned (Spirito & Fritz, 1993).

Outcome: Emotional comfort was restored and irrational fear was removed as a barrier to treatment. ❧

CASE EXAMPLE: EARLY ADOLESCENT AGED 11–13 YEARS

Molly, an 11-year-old girl, was in the pediatric intensive care unit (PICU) with multisystem failure caused by "cat scratch" disease. She required ventilatory support, peritoneal dialysis, and hyperalimentation. Pain management for pancreatitis was impeded by her parents' fear that she might become addicted. Complete recovery was possible if all systems were managed effectively during the acute and rehabilitation phases.

Visits from numerous pediatric specialty teams bewildered and frightened Molly and her parents. Molly's nightly bath stimulated her, sleep was difficult, and procedures caused frequent interruptions. Tracheostomy made communication difficult. Getting out of bed was frightening. She refused to do respiratory and physical therapy exercises. Her parents were overwhelmed by their emotions of anxiety, irrational guilt, and anger. Psychological concomitants were more debilitating than the disease because Molly's physiological disorders were managed expertly.

Molly wanted to sleep all day. When awake, she gestured with silent demand to the area of her cubicle where medication was prepared. In agitation, she pounded her arms and legs against the siderails if a sedative was not administered immediately. To avoid bruising, mechanical restraints were considered. Psychiatry was consulted because of her behavior.

Clearly, a care conference was in order. Responsibilities of the multidisciplinary care providers were discussed, and parental needs and roles were defined. Pain consultants assured the parents that analgesics for physiologically caused pain could be managed without adverse consequences.

When pain control measures were defined and Molly realized that she could be more comfortable, she stopped wanting to sleep all of the time. When a reward system for periods of time without tantrums was explained to her, she wrote, "I didn't know it mattered." With clear communication about the importance of her behavior, she controlled it.

Baths are not usually given in the morning in PICU because of medical and nursing rounds. However, because the evening bath was stimulating to Molly, the evening nurse taught Mom to give the bath without disturbing tubes and dressings so Molly could bathe in the morning. Dad was taught to lift Molly, and, because she trusted him, getting out of bed was less frightening. When the parents invested their energy in familiar parental activities, they were less afflicted by their fear and unrealistic feelings of guilt.

Molly's wish to sleep without interruption led to "clumping" or deferring nursing activities at night. With sleep and mobility improved, Molly concentrated on educational activities introduced by the hospital teacher and play activities provided by the Child Life Specialist. Her life became more predictable. Her appetite and elimination improved with the increased activity, and she was weaned from hyperalimentation. As oral intake increased, kidney output increased and peritoneal dialysis was discontinued. Molly was soon transferred from the PICU.

Molly's siblings visited her often. Because specially constructed dolls had been used to demonstrate procedures and explain physiological functions to her, she was familiar with the equipment. As her condition and endurance improved, she asked to use the dolls when she played with her younger sister and brother, helping them to understand some of her bandages and "boo-boos" without fear. The family left the hospital with emotions intact.

Analysis: Care conferences helped to clarify overwhelmingly complex clinical issues and address the family's emotional needs as well as physical and safety needs of the patient. Concrete suggestions helped the family become partners in Molly's care (Fritz & Spirito, 1993).

Outcome: An 11-year-old returned to family and school activities without emotional sequela after an acute illness (Geist, 1979). ❦

CASE EXAMPLE: ADOLESCENT AGED 14–17 YEARS

Pete, a 16-year-old, was referred far from his home community for diagnosis of an illness with acute onset. He became increasingly noncompliant with medications and irritable about his mother's hovering in his room. When the nurse asked Pete what was really bothering him, he said lack of privacy and missing his friends bothered him more than being sick. In short, he said, his mother was "making him crazy!" His mom explained that she stayed in the room all the time because she feared missing the doctor when he came to discuss Pete's condition.

Plans were made with Pete and his mom so both of them would have their needs met: Mom could leave the room and Pete would have her paged when the doctor came to discuss plans or test results; and Pete contracted with his mom to earn phone calls to friends by taking his medications as scheduled.

Analysis: Good communication about needs and what can be done to meet them helped the adolescent control his actions. Positive rewards were negotiated appropriate to adolescent developmental level (Mast, Schoppe, & Hogarth, 1991).

Outcome: Family members clarified their respective needs and maintained intergenerational boundaries. ❦

MAJOR CHRONIC ILLNESS OR CONDITION

Chronic illnesses are disorders with symptoms lasting for more than 3 months, or requiring hospitalization or extensive health services for more than 1 month in a 12-month period. Ap-

proximately 1 to 2 million children in the United States have diseases of such physiologic severity as to interfere with the child's usual daily activities (Perrin & Shonkoff, 1992).

EFFECTS AND INTERVENTIONS WITH THE CHILD

Although a child has been functioning well and developing normally, coping is affected when a condition is diagnosed which limits or changes established habits. Regression is likely to occur as the child and family attempt to adjust to new stressors. Children vary in their response to the onset of a chronic disorder as they vary in response to other major risk factors like divorce and abuse (Mrazek, 1991). Emotional concomitants of chronic illness may include anxiety, disappointment, grief due to lost functions, guilt, anger, or sorrow. Resilience, the ability to bounce back, is increased by social support and healthy self-esteem (Francis, 1995).

Important strategies for helping children to cope include providing information within a child's cognitive ability, and helping parents decide how to talk with children about illness. Early recognition of maladaptive coping, and psychological intervention, are more likely to occur with preplanned, integrated, biopsychosocial care (Sabbeth & Stein, 1990). Other potentially helpful strategies for decreasing anxiety associated with illness and treatment include relaxation exercises, choices about distraction techniques, cognitive strategies like imagery and calming self-talk, hospital play and rehearsal, and opportunities for discussion. Decisional control, when possible, helps a child's sense of efficacy. Self-esteem is increased by each successful event and positive appraisal from others.

A developmental approach to normalizing life despite a chronic disorder emphasizes the same factors that are important for all children. With adaptations to their particular capabilities, children should meet the same behavioral expectations their parents have for other children in the family: participation in new experiences, interaction with healthy peers, and regular school attendance (Clunn, 1991). Sawin and Marshall (1992) demonstrated that competency can be achieved by adolescents with chronic disabilities. Key factors in achieving competency in adolescents include opportunities for making decisions, interacting with friends, and making contributions to family functioning in a meaningful way.

EFFECTS AND INTERVENTIONS WITH PARENTS

Management of a child's chronic illness requires daily adjustment to accommodate the child's special needs (Deatrick & Knafl, 1990). While adjustment increases stress on the family system, some families respond to the challenge with resilience (Cadman, Rosenbaum, & Boyle, 1991).

Children and adolescents with diabetes comply with their medication regimes and function better if their parents provide guidance and control with warmth and concern (McKelvey et al., 1993; Lawler et al., 1990). The family's ability to respond to the relentless, daily demands of diabetes management dictates the quality of the child's and family's life (McCarthy & Gallo, 1992).

Parents' increased confidence in their ability to manage their child's asthma, as well as earlier intervention by health care providers, was achieved by educational interventions with parents from varied sociodemographic populations (Moe et al., 1992). With the mind-set that parents, as well as the ill child, are patients, health care professionals provide information, psychosocial support, and encouragement that lead to competent families despite the presence of a chronic disorder.

Psychosocial assessment of children and adolescents with chronic illness includes evaluation of strengths and stressors on the family system, competency or deficit in family coping skills, evaluation for genetic predisposition, and psychological testing. Children in multiproblem families are at risk for poor developmental, psychological, and educational outcomes. Poor outcomes are associated with parents' problems such as psychiatric disorder and disturbed emotional development, substance abuse, chronic illness, or impaired intellectual functioning (Adnopoz, Grigsby, & Nagler, 1991). Assessment of these factors leads to

multidisciplinary planning to achieve optimal outcomes for the child.

EFFECTS AND INTERVENTIONS WITH SIBLINGS

Some sisters and brothers of children with chronic illnesses experience more behavior problems than other children. However, in other families, siblings show positive effects, such as increased cooperation, self-esteem, empathy, and cognitive mastery (Fawcett, 1993).

BEHAVIORAL AND PSYCHIATRIC INTERVENTIONS

CASE EXAMPLE: CHILD AGED 1–6

Dodi was 4 years old when she had a craniectomy with gross total resection of a brain tumor. After surgical recovery, the relief and joy felt by her parents and brothers turned to frustration as they began coping with her day-to-day behaviors. Their style of parenting by guiding, coaching, and allowing progressive autonomy had been effective previously. Now Dodi seemed anxious and bewildered. They asked for guidance because of her oppositional behavior.

Psychological testing compared to presurgical evaluation revealed that Dodi's intellectual functioning was significantly diminished. This information helped the parents adapt their style and expectations. Parenting strategies, beginning with simple, direct communication (talking with fewer words), helped Dodi understand the meaning. Immediate rewards and brief "time outs" helped to shape the troublesome behaviors. Dodi's oppositionality decreased as she was able to process her parents' messages.

Analysis: Psychological testing provided information to help parents adjust to the needs of a child who was changed by treatment of a life-threatening condition (Graham, 1991; Williams, Pleak & Hanesian, 1991).

Outcome: The family adapted to the special needs and increased their ability to guide and protect the child. The child's anxiety decreased and her compliance increased when she understood her parents' expectations. ❦

CASE EXAMPLE: CHILD AGED 7–10

Keith, an 8-year-old boy, was 2 weeks post–liver transplant. He had no postsurgical complications. There were no signs of rejection and full recovery seemed imminent when Keith had a marked change in behavior. He began refusing all medications, screaming and throwing things, and avoiding eye contact and all attempts to reason or encourage him. Except for his tantrums, he was withdrawn. This was a change from the quiet, chronically debilitated, and dependent boy he had been before the transplant, and the cooperation and compliance he had shown immediately following surgery. His mother was frustrated and afraid because she knew the importance of medication to successful rehabilitation. She said, "I don't know what to do. I feel like spanking him."

Talking with Keith, the Psychiatry Clinical Nurse Specialist (CNS) thought he seemed disappointed. Keith had done everything everyone asked of him. He had been cooperative, believing and trusting the adults who told him he'd be OK when he got a new liver. At the age of 8, he heard "OK" to mean feeling well, playing, going places, and doing schoolwork. He had not understood that feeling well was contingent on compliance with a rigid routine.

When Keith felt well enough to go to the playroom, he was frequently interrupted. Twelve times a day he took medications, up to nine different kinds at a time. Eight times a day he had eyedrops, ointment on his skin, or medicine added to his IV. There were frequent blood draws and respiratory treatments. He was powerless to do anything about it, so he controlled the only things he could: what he put into his mouth, and his behavior.

The CNS asked Keith if he would like a program he could manage that had rewards he could earn and a poster to show everyone how well he was doing. He liked the idea. His favorite color was blue so the poster was blue and Keith helped to make it. He agreed to earn points based on time increments: 1 point for taking all medicines within 15 minutes at each medication time, 2 points for taking them within 10 minutes, and 3 points for finishing within 5 minutes.

Keith's job was to remind the nurse to time him and tell him how many points he earned. He used the points to buy special time with the nurse. She agreed to spend 20 minutes a day with him in an activity of his choice. (She preferred to spend the time for positive reward rather than coping with his tantrums.) The 20 minutes with the nurse provided his mom with some time alone. Also, his mother learned a strategy to use at home.

Analysis: An 8-year-old's concrete thinking and ability to process information about complex physiological functioning was recognized. He was given developmentally appropriate tasks and decisional control over specific activities.

Outcome: The program was so successful that Keith's transplant team thought it was "magic." The poster provided such positive recognition that it was converted to a "praise chart" to continue the tangible positive support after the unwanted behaviors were extinguished. ❦

CASE EXAMPLE: EARLY ADOLESCENT AGED 11–13

Maxine, a 13-year-old, had glomerulonephritis from birth. Her transplanted kidney had been rejected and she had sustained a stroke which left her unable to read or understand many spoken words. She disliked her short stature caused by renal disease and her appearance which was affected by the medications that failed to prevent rejection. She was depressed, isolative, and had no appetite. She and her parents still grieved the loss of Maxine's twin who died from complications of a renal transplant 18 months previously. Sorrow pervaded this family.

Maxine left her darkened room only for medical procedures. Her nutritional status was maintained by gastric feedings. Her mom embarrassed her and annoyed the health care team with her complaints and recriminations each evening during her hurried visits. Her dad disappointed her and angered her mom by avoiding hospital visits.

520   PART V—Psychosocial Interventions for Specific Age Groups and Clinical Settings

Antidepressant medications helped to lighten Maxine's mood. Maxine agreed to participate in a day treatment program in a psychiatry therapeutic milieu. There she was recognized for her smile, empathy, and support for other children with physical disabilities. Because family participation was an expectation of the program, her parents learned about activities they could share as a family, how to hold and touch Maxine so she could feel their warmth and compassion without words. Their avoidance and verbally offensive defenses were used less.

Analysis: Sorrow and grief affected the parents' ability to support their child throughout a chronic illness.

Outcome: Resilience was restored to a family by increasing their coping mechanisms in the face of almost unbearable stress (Francis, 1995).

CASE EXAMPLE: ADOLESCENT AGED 14–17

Chanta, a 17-year-old, was hospitalized for sickle cell pain so frequently, and for such long periods, in her senior year of high school that graduation was in jeopardy. Opioids and nonpharmacological methods of pain management failed to bring the resilience expected when pain is relieved. Symptoms seemed greater than the degree of pathology. Chanta had planned her suicide and was implementing the plans when psychiatric intervention was initiated.

Family therapy revealed that Chanta assumed responsibility for her mother, who needed financial assistance and nurturing for a chronic physical disorder. Although not an illicit drug user herself, Chanta had become a drug dealer to obtain money for her family. Anxiety and depression resulted from the incongruence in her ethics and exigency. Social services helped obtain legal financial support.

Analysis: Adult responsibilities incongruent with adolescent development resulted in the use of maladaptive coping mechanisms. Psychological factors impacted on physical well being (Lewis, 1994).

Outcome: When psychosocial issues were attended and the adolescent was relieved of responsibility for her family's well-being, her

pain crises abated. She completed high school successfully despite her chronic physical disorder.

When information and support are provided by trusted professionals in a timely manner, parents are more able to control their emotional reactions in frightening situations which may threaten their family members. With anxiety allayed, parents are more able to guide their children responsibly and to normalize their family's activities despite congenital, acute, or chronic illness. Competent coping averts potentially life-long maladaptation in patients and family members.

TERMINAL ILLNESS

Children's understanding of and reaction to death is individual. Thier reaction is affected by age and developmental level, personality, and coping style. The openness of the family and professionals to discussing facts related to the child's circumstances helps the child reconcile knowledge with beliefs and move through the emotional stages associated with dying: denial, anger, bargaining, depression, and acceptance (Kubler-Ross, 1969).

EFFECTS AND INTERVENTIONS WITH THE CHILD

Decisions about what information is given to children regarding their condition must be made by the parents. Health care professionals should help parents with techniques for therapeutic dialogue to keep the child and siblings in the information loop in developmentally appropriate ways.

If the child is anxious, the anxiety usually is more about fear of pain and loneliness than about death itself. One of the most difficult but valuable services that can be performed by trusted adults is to reassure the child and demonstrate that he or she is not and will not be alone (Clunn, 1991; Wheeler & Pike, 1993).

A question like, "Some kids want to know if they are not getting better; would you want to know?" lets the child indicate what he or she is ready to discuss. Denial is a defense against anxiety and should be respected if the child asks not to discuss his or her condition. Providing facts that a child does not want to hear precludes meaningful conversation. Conversely, withholding information to protect emotions leads to disbelief and hinders trust.

Hope can be interjected as the child is appraised of treatment, rationale, and expected results. If the adult asks for clarification of unclear remarks or draws or plays with the child, conversation may progress into thoughts the child has found difficult to express (Lewis, Lewis, & Schonfeld, 1991).

When death is imminent, friends and extended families sometimes avoid contact with the child and family for fear of saying something that may worsen the situation. They should be assured that simply sitting close is a valuable intervention. Seeing familiar faces helps a dying child remain calm and relaxed.

Favorite music and comfort measures such as mouth care, gentle backrubs or hand massage, cool sponge baths, and loose clothing may be soothing. Only foods that the child likes and that are easy to eat should be offered. Feeding should be slow and in small amounts several times a day (Whaley & Wong, 1991).

If questions are necessary, they should be answerable with "yes" or "no." Gentle talk, familiar topics, and the voice of a family member is reassuring. Conversations that may be troubling should take place outside the child's hearing even if the child appears to be asleep.

EFFECTS AND INTERVENTIONS WITH PARENTS AND SIBLINGS

Parents and siblings experience the same emotional stages as the child with the terminal illness, although the stages may not be concurrent or sequential (Kubler-Ross, 1969). Parents and siblings may not remain for discrete periods of time at any particular stage. They may repeat or skip stages (Parkman, 1992). If one parent is using the defense of denial while the other is angry, and the siblings at home are sad, the sick child's needs may not be met. Often, the health care professional's most difficult action is to help the parents find the strength to be honest with themselves, their sick child, and their other children.

Sometimes, asking the brother or sister if they want to say goodbye helps them realize that death is imminent. Preparing them to say goodbye should include information about how their sibling may appear, an explanation about equipment and sounds that they may see and hear, and coaching about what they may say and do (Parkman, 1992).

The response to death relates to the past experiences of each family member. Support in promoting the process of the family's bereavement may take the form of listening as parents relive events of the child's life, observing rage without feeling threatened or fearful, hearing wails of intense grief, or seeing the blank face of numbness. The lives of the family members will never be the same. Parents are losing their dreams concerning their family. Their concentration may be poor and questions may have to be answered repeatedly. Siblings may fear they have caused the death and their parents' grief. They need reassurance that they are not guilty at all (Parkman, 1992).

CASE EXAMPLE: THE DYING CHILD OR ADOLESCENT

Jody Slyter, M.S., R.N., is a Pediatric Nurse Practitioner in the Center for Cancer and Blood Disorders at Children's Medical Center of Dallas. She often provides emotional support to children and their families in the terminal phase of illness, including support at the time of death.

Helping a family to prepare for the inevitable death of their child, I assure them that I have never seen a child die in fear. Their concerns are about being alone or hurting. We can assure them that neither of those things will happen.

Over time, I help parents define what needs to be done to allow the sick child to die. I ask them to anticipate regrets beginning, "If only I had ...," "I wish I had let him or her ...." If they allow their fears to preclude their saying or doing certain activities, the consequence will be regret that opportunities were lost. Sometimes, the regret is having lost irretrievable time with the remaining children.

To protect siblings from pain, parents sometimes hinder what needs to be completed for a peaceful death. Children sometimes need to say goodbye. The dying child may want to give a treasured teddy bear, assure the care of a pet, or help reassign their bedroom.

Listening to Caroline, a 7-year-old who was dying, her parents and I realized that the words we heard had meaning. Caroline described spinning a straw. Sometimes it pointed toward a person dressed in white, sometimes in black. Quietly, we asked who the various people were. As Caroline named the people, the parents realized that the people in white had all visited recently to say goodbye. The people in black were the younger siblings and cousins who were being protected from her imminent death. Caroline needed to say or send special goodbyes to these children, too. What might have been interpreted as meaningless delirium described what Caroline needed to complete in order to attain a peaceful death.

Sometimes children feel that they must protect their parents from grief. Parents may need prompting to say, "I'll be sad" or "I'll miss you so much," not "I can't live without you" or "I don't know what I'll do without you."

Jason was a 14-year-old adopted son of older parents who chose all-out treatment despite a poor prognosis. They exhorted their son to continue the fight. He told me he didn't want to fight anymore but he feared that his dad would not survive his death. The weekend that death seemed inevitable, Jason's father refused to leave the room. Jason lingered. Only when his father left on Monday morning did Jason stop breathing. It was as though he protected his father to his last breath.

I cry with parents sometimes because what is happening is sad. Parents sometimes are afraid to cry in front of the child who is dying.

Brad was 10. He knew that he had relapsed and that chemotherapy prolonged the dying process but would not prevent it. His mom was stoic. She never cried in front of him and didn't smile much either. She told me that she thought it would hurt Brad to see her cry. I asked her what he thought was happening when she left the room and came back with a red nose. She let me help her talk with him about how she would miss him and they cried together. Then he talked about some things she could do when she didn't have to be at the hospital so much. She told me that it was like he gave her permission to go on living.

I go to funerals of patients, and encourage other professionals to attend services if they are so inclined. Parents have told me that it makes them happy to think their child was special to the people who worked with them.

Often, I send a card much later or call to see how things are going. Parents tell me that it feels strange when friends avoid talking about their child and they miss hearing the name.

Lacey died when she was 4 months old. Her mom wondered if people think she forgot she had a child by that name and, by mentioning it, they will cause new grief. She said, "I lost my precious baby. How can anything they say be worse than that? I like to remember her and hear that they enjoyed being with her too." I wondered with her what Lacey's voice would have been like if she had learned to talk, what her favorite toys would have been. We laughed together about the happy way she squealed when her mom walked into the room. She would have been a delightful little girl. ❧

CONCLUSION

Despite physical disorders, handicaps, or terminal illness, children have the capacity for love, the need to learn, and the ability to grow and adapt. Families may need assistance to find the resilience required to accommodate special needs. The role of health care professionals is to help parents adapt in order for them to lead and guide their family, and allow their children to individuate.

BIBLIOGRAPHY

Acute Pain Management Guideline Panel. (1992). *Acute pain management: Operative or medical procedures and trauma. Clinical practice guideline.* AHCPR Pub. No. 92-0032. Rockville, MD: Agency for Health Care Policy and Research, Public Health Service, U.S. Department of Health and Human Services.

Adnopoz, J., Grigsby, R. K., & Nagler, S. F. (1991). Multiproblem families and high-risk children and adolescents: Causes and management. In M. Lewis (Ed.), *Child and adolescent psychiatry: A comprehensive textbook.* Baltimore: Williams and Wilkins.

Austin, J. K. (1993). Families with chronically ill children. In C. S. Fawcett (Ed.), *Family psychiatric nursing.* St. Louis: Mosby-Year Book.

Ayoub, C. (1991). Emotional consequences of chronic physical illness. In P. Clunn (Ed.), *Child psychiatric nursing.* St. Louis: Mosby-Year Book.

Baker, N. A. (1994). Avoiding collisions with challenging families. *The American Journal of Maternal/Child Nursing, 19*(2), 97–101.

Behrman, R. E., Kliegman, R. M., Nelson, W. E., & Vaughan, V. C., III. (1992). *Nelson textbook of pediatrics* (14th ed.). Philadelphia: W. B. Saunders.

Bossert, E., Holaday, B., Harkins, A., & Turner-Henson, A. (1990). Strategies of normalization used by parents of chronically ill school age children. *Journal of Child Psychiatric Nursing, 3*(2), 57–61.

Boyce, W. T. (1992). The vulnerable child: New evidence, new approaches. In L. A. Barness, D. C. DeVivo, M. M. Kaback, G. Morrow, III, F. A. Oski, & A. M. Rudolph (Eds.), *Advances in pediatrics.* St. Louis: Mosby-Year Book.

Cadman, D., Rosenbaum, P., & Boyle, M. (1991). Children with chronic illness: Family and parent demographic characteristics and psychosocial adjustment. *Pediatrics, 87,* 884–889.

Christophersen, E. R. (1988). *Little people.* Kansas City, MO: Westport.

Clunn, P. (1991). *Child psychiatric nursing.* St. Louis: Mosby-Year Book.

Clunn, P. A. (1993). The child. In R. P. Rawlins, S. R. Williams, & C. K. Beck (Eds.). *Mental health-psychiatric nursing: A holistic life-cycle approach* (3rd ed.). St. Louis: Mosby-Year Book.

Danielson, C. B., Hamel-Bissell, B., & Winstead-Fry, P. (1993). *Families, health and illness: Perspectives on coping and intervention.* St. Louis: Mosby.

Deatrick, J. A., & Knafl, K. A. (1990). Management behaviors: Day-to-day adjustment to childhood chronic conditions. *Journal of Pediatric Nursing, 5*(1), 15–22.

DeWet, B., & Cywes, S. (1985a). The birth of a child with a congenital anomaly. Part I: Some difficulties experienced by parents in the maternity home. *South African Medical Journal, 67,* 292–296.

DeWet, B., & Cywes, S. (1985b). The birth of a child with a congenital anomaly. Part III: Response of parents to the diagnosis. *South African Medical Journal, 67,* 370–373.

Erikson, E. H. (1963). *Childhood and society.* New York: Norton.

Fawcett, C. S. (1993). *Family psychiatric nursing.* St. Louis: Mosby.

Francis, S. (1995). Disability and chronic illness. In B. S. Johnson (Ed.), *Child, adolescent and family psychiatric nursing.* Philadelphia: J. B. Lippincott.

Fritz, G. K., & Spirito, A. (1993). The process of consultation on a pediatric unit. In G. K. Fritz, R. E. Mattison, B. Nurcombe, & A. Spirito (Eds.), *Child and adolescent mental health consultation in hospitals, schools, and courts.* Washington, DC: American Psychiatric Press, Inc.

Gallo, A. M., Breitmayer, B. J., Knafl, K. A., & Zoeller, L. H. (1991). Stigma in childhood chronic illness: A well sibling perspective. *Pediatric Nursing, 17*(1), 21–25.

Gardner, S. L. (1994). Pain and pain relief in the neonate. *American Journal of Maternal/Child Nursing, 19*(2), 85–90.

Geist, R. A. (1979). Onset of chronic illness in children and adolescents: Psychotherapeutic and consultative intervention. *American Journal of Orthopsychiatry, 49*(1), 4–23.

Givler, T. L. (1991). Working therapeutically with parents of Hispanic and American Indian children and adolescents in the hospital. In R. L. Hendren & I. N. Berlin (Eds.), *Psychiatric inpatient care of children and adolescents: A multicultural approach.* New York: John Wiley and Sons.

Graham, P. J. (1991). Psychiatric aspects of pediatric disorders. In M. Lewis (Ed.), *Child and adolescent psychiatry: A comprehensive textbook.* Baltimore: Williams and Wilkins.

Groves, J. E. (1978). Taking care of the hateful patient. *New England Journal of Medicine, 298*(16), 883–887.

Hogarth, C. R. (1991). *Adolescent psychiatric nursing.* St. Louis: Mosby-Year Book.

Irwin, M., & Hauger, M. D. (1991). Developmental aspects of psychoneuroimmunology. In M. Lewis (Ed.), *Child and adolescent psychiatry: A comprehensive textbook.* Baltimore: William and Wilkins.

Jackson, P. L., & Vessey, J. A. (1992). *Primary care of the child with a chronic condition.* St. Louis: Mosby-Year Book.

Jellinek, M. S., Beresin, E. V., Herzog, D. B., & Sherry, S. N. (1991). Coping with the truly difficult parent. *Contemporary Pediatrics, 8,* 19–49.

Kazdin, A. E. (1991). Learning theory and behavioral approaches. In M. Lewis (Ed.), *Child and adolescent psychiatry: A comprehensive textbook.* Baltimore: Williams and Wilkins.

Kempe, A. R., & Rawlins, R. P. (1993). The adolescent. In R. P. Rawlins, S. R. Williams, & C. K. Beck (Eds.), *Mental health-psychiatric nursing: A holistic life-cycle approach* (3rd ed.). St. Louis: Mosby-Year Book.

Kubler-Ross, E. (1969). *On death and dying.* New York: Macmillan.

Landreth, G. L. (1991). *Play therapy: The art of the relationship.* Muncie: Accelerated Development.

Lawler, M. K., Volk, R., Vivian, N., & Menger, M. R. (1990). Individual and family factors impacting diabetic control in the adolescent: A preliminary study. *American Journal of Maternal/Child Nursing, 19*(4), 331–345.

Leckman, J. F. (1991). Genes and developmental neurobiology. In M. Lewis (Ed.), *Child and adolescent psychiatry:*

A comprehensive textbook. Baltimore: Williams and Wilkins.

Lewis, M. (1994). Consultation process in child and adolescent psychiatric consultation-liaison in pediatrics. *Child and Adolescent Psychiatric Clinics of North America, 3*(3), 439–448.

Lewis, M., Lewis, D. O., & Schonfeld, D. J. (1991). Dying and death in childhood and adolescence. In M. Lewis (Ed.), *Child and adolescent psychiatry: A comprehensive textbook*. Baltimore: Williams and Wilkins.

Mast, L. A., Schoppe, L. R., & Hogarth, C. R. (1991). Development of the healthy adolescent and family. In C. R. Hogarth (Ed.), *Adolescent psychiatric nursing*. St. Louis: Mosby Year Book.

McCarthy, S. M., & Gallo, A. M. (1992). A case illustration of family management style. *Journal of Pediatric Nursing, 7*(6), 395–402.

McCubbin, M. A., & McCubbin, H. I. (1993). Families coping with illness: The resiliency model of family stress, adjustment, and adaptation. In C. B. Danielson, B. Hamel-Bissell, & P. Winstead-Fry (Eds.), *Families, health and illness perspectives on coping and intervention*. St. Louis: Mosby.

McGrath, P. J., & Unruh, A. M. (1993). Psychological treatment of pain in children and adolescents. In N. L. Schechter, C. B. Berde, & M. Yaster (Eds.), *Pain in infants, children, and adolescents*. Baltimore: Williams and Wilkins.

McKelvey, J., Waller, D. A., North, A. J., Marks, J. F., Schreiner, B., Travis, L. B., & Murphy, J. N., III. (1993). Reliability and validity of the diabetes family behavior scale (DFBS). *Diabetes Educator, 19*(2), 125–132.

Modlin, T. J., & Adams, A. (1993). In R. P. Rawlins, S. R. Williams, & C. K. Beck (Eds.), *Mental health-psychiatric nursing: A holistic life-cycle approach* (3rd ed.). St. Louis: Mosby-Year Book.

Moe, E. L., Eisenberg, J. D., Vollmer, W. M., Wall, M. A., Stevens, V. J., & Hollis, J. F. (1992). Implementation of "open airways" as an educational intervention for children with asthma in an HMO. *Journal of Pediatric Health Care, 6*(5), 251–255.

Mrazek, D. A. (1991). Chronic pediatric illness and multiple hospitalizations. In M. Lewis (Ed.), *Child and adolescent psychiatry: A comprehensive textbook*. Baltimore: Williams and Wilkins.

Parkman, S. E. (1992). Helping families say good-bye. *American Journal of Maternal/Child Nursing, 17*(1), 14–17.

Perrin, J. M., & Shonkoff, J. P. (1992). Children with special health needs: An overview. In R. E. Behrman, R. M. Kliegman, W. E. Nelson, & V. C. Vaughan, III (Eds.), *Nelson textbook of pediatrics* (14th ed.). Philadelphia: W. B. Saunders.

Porter, N., & Blackwell, S. (1991). Working with resistance in families: A cross-cultural perspective. In D. O. Hendren & I. N. Berlin (Eds.), *Psychiatric inpatient care of children and adolescents: A multicultural approach*. New York: John Wiley and Sons.

Rairdan, B., & Higgs, Z. R. (1992). When your patient is a Hmong refugee. *American Journal of Nursing, 92*(3), 52–55.

Ross, D. M., & Ross, S. A. (1988). *Childhood pain: Current issues, research, and management*. Baltimore: Urban and Schwarzenberg.

Sabbeth, B., & Stein, R. E. K. (1990). Mental health referral: A weak link in comprehensive care of children with chronic physical illness. *Developmental and Behavioral Pediatrics, 11*(2), 73–78.

Sawin, K. J., & Marshall, J. (1992). Developmental competence in adolescents with an acquired disability. *Rehabilitation Nursing, 1*(1)41–50.

Schechter, N. L., Berde, C. B, & Yaster, M. (1993). *Pain in infants, children, and adolescents*. Baltimore: Williams and Wilkins.

Schonfeld, D. J. (1991). The child's cognitive understanding of illness. In M. Lewis (Ed.), *Child and adolescent psychiatry: A comprehensive textbook*. Baltimore: William and Wilkins.

Siantz, M. L. (1994). Child and family minority research: How are we doing? *Journal of Child and Adolescent Psychiatric Nursing, 6*(4), 6–9.

Spirito, A., & Fritz, G. K. (1993). Psychological interventions for pediatric patients. In G. K. Fritz, R. E. Mattison, B. Nurcombe, & A. Spirito (Eds.), *Child and adolescent mental health consultation in hospitals, schools, and courts*. Washington, DC: American Psychiatric Press, Inc.

Tesler, M. D. (1994). Children's pain: Part I. *Nurseweek, 1*(1), 5–6.

Thomasgard, M. and Metz, W. P. (1995). The vulnerable child syndrome revisited. *Developmental and behavioral pediatrics, 16* (1), 47–53.

Titlebaum, H. (1988). Relaxation. In R. Zahourek (Ed.), *Relaxation and imagery: Tools for therapeutic communication and intervention*. Philadelphia: W. B. Saunders.

Vessey, J. A., & Caserza, C. L. (1992). Chronic conditions and child development. In P. L. Jackson & J. A. Vessey (Eds.), *Primary care of the child with a chronic condition*. St. Louis: Mosby-Year Book.

Vitulano, L. A., & Tebes, J. K. (1991). Child and adolescent behavior therapy. In M. Lewis (Ed.), *Child and adolescent psychiatry: A comprehensive textbook*. Baltimore: Williams and Wilkins.

Werry, J. S., & Wollersheim, J. P. (1989). Behavior therapy with children and adolescents: A twenty-year overview. *Journal of American Academy of Child and Adolescent Psychiatry, 28*(1), 1–18.

Wheeler, S. R., & Pike, M. M. (1993). Families' responses to the loss of a child. In C. S. Fawcett (Ed.), *Family psychiatric nursing*. St. Louis: Mosby.

Williams, D. T., Pleak, R. R., & Hanesian, H. (1991). Neurological disorders. In M. Lewis (Ed.), *Child and adolescent psychiatry: A comprehensive textbook*. Baltimore: Williams and Wilkins.

Wolpe, J. (1973). *The practice of behavior therapy* (2nd ed.). New York: Pergamon.

Yoos, L. (1987). Chronic childhood illnesses: Developmental issues. *Pediatric Nursing, 13*(1), 25–28.

CHAPTER 28

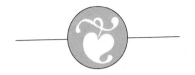

Psychosocial Assessment and Intervention with the Home Care Patient and Family

Marcia Miller
Janet Duffey

Psychosocial home care nursing is rapidly developing into a subspecialty of consultation-liaison psychiatric nursing. Beginning in 1979, when Medicare wrote the reimbursement guidelines for psychiatric nursing in home health, researchers began looking at the relevance of providing psychosocial nursing services in the home. An early review of the literature addressed issues such as using nontraditional treatment teams to deliver psychiatric services in the home (Soreff, 1983), and the role of the clinical nurse specialist in psychiatric home care (Klebanoff & Casler, 1986). Later articles discuss the application of theory to psychiatric home care (Duffey, Miller, & Parlocha, 1993; Lesseig, 1987; Miller & Duffey, 1993).

This chapter will focus on psychosocial assessment and intervention with the home care patient and family. Knowledge of systems theory, crisis theory, self-care theory, adult learning theory, social/ecological theories, milieu therapy, and the various brief psychotherapies

establishes a foundation for helping nurses assist patients with complex psychosocial needs and issues at home.

A MAJOR SHIFT FROM ACUTE TO HOME HEALTH CARE

In her article "Health Care in the Year 2000 and Beyond," Sandra Hellman (1991) cites some significant statistics relevant to the future reshaping of health care. As the baby boom generation ages, the number of elders in America will peak around the year 2010, when one-third of adults 65 and older will have at least one of their parents living. Major changes in ethnic mix will occur. Hispanic and Asian

Patricia Barry: *Psychosocial Nursing:*
Care of Physically Ill Patients and Their Families, 3rd ed.
© 1996 Lippincott–Raven Publishers

American communities will play a much larger role in American society. The average age of the American population is expected to increase from 28 to 38.

How does this affect disease incidence? Hellman continues, "The presence of senile dementia has multiplied ten times since the turn of the century" (p. 69). Acquired immune deficiency syndrome (AIDS) had been a previously unknown phenomenon in the health care world. Baby boomers are reaching midlife and are requiring more medical care as they age.

At a recent meeting of the National Association of Home Care (1993), the need for providing long-term home care for patients was seen as crucial based on the following factors:

1. The increased reliance on high-technology modalities for care.
2. More low birth weight children are surviving and growing to adulthood.
3. Terminally ill children are living longer.
4. Earlier detection of chronic illness.

THE IMPACT OF MEDICARE AND MEDICAID

Despite statistics that indicate we need more options for health care, the economic reality is that the funding of many health care programs is currently in jeopardy. Medicare reimbursement rates are decreasing. Federal Medicaid programs under state regulation continue to reimburse inconsistently for various psychosocial-related conditions. Increasing attention is being paid to managed care, health maintenance organizations, and preferred provider organizations as one means of providing cost containment and quality management.

Hospitals and health care providers are under increasing pressure from reimbursement sources to offer services that promote appropriate use of the continuum of care, with less emphasis on hospitalization as the place people receive health care. The *continuum of care* concept promotes cost-effective care from hospital to home (Lutz, 1993). One expanding part of this continuum is home health care.

Traditionally, home health care has been seen as a postdischarge resource for hospitalized patients. Since Medicare has been the primary payer for home care services, most home care agencies and programs have been designed to meet its standards (Health Care Financing Administration, 1989).

1. First, the person must be enrolled as a Medicare recipient.
2. The home health agency has an agreement with Medicare to participate in the Medicare program.
3. The services are reasonable and necessary, based upon documentation.
4. The plan of treatment is ordered by a physician and reviewed by the physician for a period of 2 months.
5. The patient is confined to home, or requires considerable and taxing effort to leave home.
6. The visits take place in the patient's residence.
7. The patient requires skilled nursing care.

The home health care industry is growing rapidly. Rather than exclusively operating as a post–hospital discharge resource, it is now being seen by many payers as a preventive measure to offset costlier forms of health care (Knollmueller, 1992). Curiously, the "birth" of home health care nursing as a discipline also stressed primary prevention rather than tertiary rehabilitation.

PREVENTIVE CARE: AN HISTORICAL PERSPECTIVE

Home care as a health care service began in the United States at the turn of the century. In New York, the Metropolitan Life Insurance Company was the largest insurer for the working class in 1908. At the time, one-fifth of all Metropolitan's death claims were attributed to an outbreak of tuberculosis. As part of a then-nationwide health care reform movement, Metropolitan's chief executive officers decided to launch a preventive tuberculosis health program, instructing their sales agents to begin to collect health care-related data on policyholders and to institute preventive instruction.

Unfortunately for Metropolitan, but fortunately for the future of public health and home care nursing, the sales agents balked at carrying out the plan themselves. Lillian Wald, director of the Henry Street Settlement House, knew of their plans. She felt public health nurses could do the data collection and teaching. On June 9, 1909, Ada Beazley, a Henry Street nurse, made the first visit to a Metropolitan policyholder. Thus, the Visiting Nurse Service of New York began. Soon, insurance companies across the country began using fledgling visiting nurse services to provide health promotion and disease prevention.

Clearly, a preventive focus was and still is a potentially profitable policy for most payer sources. While the focus of Medicare-driven home care has been on post–acute treatment modalities, it appears we are going back to a more preventive model (Hamilton, 1992).

DIAGNOSTIC AND RELATED GROUPS

A second reason for the growth of home health care is the advent of the use of diagnostic and related groups (DRGs) as standards for reimbursement for hospitals. Inpatient stays became shorter, and patients came home quicker and sicker (Naylor, 1990). In an effort to prevent costly rehospitalization, it was realized that support from home health care services could reduce relapse and recidivism. The literature reveals that this belief is, indeed, true (Cummings & Weaver, 1991; Kellogg et al., 1991). Over the past 5 years, the length of stay for acute care hospitalizations has dropped, while the number of visits for many large home care agencies has increased (Lutz, 1993).

In response to the need for more specialized services, agencies have developed various clinical programs. Once providing only medical-surgical care, many home care agencies have expanded to include the following specialty programs: hospice, infusion therapy, pediatrics, perinatal, respiratory, cardiovascular, geriatrics, and psychiatric home care services.

WHAT IS HOME CARE NURSING?

The Department of Health and Human Services Work Group defines home health care as:

That component of a continuum of comprehensive health care whereby health services are provided to individuals and families in their places of residence for the purpose of promot-

ing, maintaining or restoring health, or of maximizing the level of independence, while minimizing the effects of disability and illness, including terminal illness. Services appropriate to the needs of the individual patient and family are planned, coordinated and made available by providers organized for the delivery of home care through the use of employed staff, contractual arrangements or a combination of the two patterns. [Warhola, 1980, p. 806]

There are three major forms of reimbursement for home health services. The first type of reimbursement is private pay. Home health nursing is not to be confused with private duty nursing because, in general, home health services are provided on a time-limited, intermittent basis (such as three times per week for a number of weeks for an hour-long visit each time) regardless of payor source. Private duty nursing implies shift work or 24 hour attendant care in the home, which is paid for privately.

A second type of reimbursement for home care is Medicare. Agencies must follow Medicare guidelines to receive reimbursement. These guidelines are fairly detailed and define parameters for reimbursable services. For example, home care nurses cannot visit patients and perform skilled care in acute care settings that have registered nurses in place. However, home care agencies can see patients in settings other than the home and bill Medicare for those visits. Residential care facilities, board-and-care homes, and independent senior living facilities are some examples of settings outside the traditional home where patients receive care.

A third kind of reimbursement is developing in the era of managed care, with utilization of services regulated by the various managed care companies. Authorization for these services is usually carefully monitored by a case manager from the insurance company. While the widespread management of home health expenses and care delivery is new, it remains to be seen how this impacts clinical outcomes, patient satisfaction, and the financial stability of home health agencies.

THE MULTIDISCIPLINARY TEAM IN HOME CARE

The importance of the multidisciplinary team in home care cannot be overemphasized. Coordination of the home care team members is crucial for successful outcomes, for the team and patient alike. Moreover, interdisciplinary communication and documentation is required of Medicare-certified agencies. This process assures continuity of care and enhances the delivery of quality care.

The following is a description of the roles and responsibilities of the various members of the multidisciplinary team.

NURSING

A registered nurse is ultimately responsible for case management and coordination of the patient's care. The case manager is responsible for completing all the admission paperwork, identifying other necessary disciplines if not ordered at time of referral, and completing ongoing documentation to comply with legal and reimbursement requirements.

Case management in the home care setting follows the traditional nursing process. A case manager performs a comprehensive assessment of the patient's biopsychosocial and environmental status in order to assess the ability to function. An appropriate nursing diagnosis is formulated based on the data obtained. Next, the case manager develops a plan of care or plan of treatment which is shared with the patient, caregivers, and physician. Once feedback is obtained on the plan of treatment, it can be implemented. The plan of treatment includes such information as the patient's diagnosis, current medications, functional limitations, visit pattern, frequency, clinical findings, nursing orders, and goals.

The patient is part of the multidisciplinary treatment team. The case manager involves patients as active participants in their care as much as possible. Patient advocacy is emphasized at all times. During multidisciplinary treatment planning meetings, the case manager coordinates the care from all the other disciplines involved in the case.

Once the plan of treatment is implemented, the case manager (in most cases) makes the majority of the home visits, is responsible for discharge and recertification documentation, and assures that all interventions promote maximum independence and are carried out in a timely way.

A home care patient's condition can change frequently. The case manager must update the care plan, revising visit patterns and the direction of interventions. Typically, home care patients require more frequent visiting during the first few weeks on service and less frequent visits as the case is nearing closure. Ongoing communication with all parties involved is crucial for successful case management.

REHABILITATION

Rehabilitation is defined as the restoration of an individual's capability to achieve the optimal ability to function, both physically and cognitively. The home care rehabilitation team includes occupational, physical, and speech therapists who specialize in various aspects of rehabilitation. Each discipline completes a functional assessment and develops (with the physician) a plan of treatment congruent with the goals set jointly by the patient and/or caregiver and the therapist.

OCCUPATIONAL THERAPY

The focus of occupational therapy (OT) is to assist the patient in relearning the tasks of daily living or activities of daily living (ADLs). Basic self-care activities begin with toileting, bathing, dressing, and eating. As patients achieve independence in self-care, the scope of OT may broaden to include community and avocational activities. The occupational therapist uses interventions such as safety instruction, home modification, muscle strengthening, coordination, positioning, and cognitive/perceptual teaching to prepare a patient for optimum functioning.

PHYSICAL THERAPY

The focus of physical therapy (PT) is improving muscular strength, range of motion, and functional mobility. Treatment is based on the patient's physical limitations. Principles of neuro–re-education, gait training, in-home exercise programs, prosthetic instruction, the use of ultrasound, and the application of hot and cold packs are used to restore functioning. The use of assistive devices for ambulation and the prevention of falls at home and in the community is another important service of PT.

SPEECH THERAPY

Speech therapy (ST) concentrates on communication, as well as dysphagia and other swallowing problems. The speech pathologist evaluates and treats the following areas: expressive and receptive language difficulties, retention of information, reading and writing, and oral motor functions related to speech and swallowing. Among the goals of home ST are to restore functional communication and oral nutrition and to teach patients and caregivers techniques and strategies to compensate for limitations and to promote functioning.

SOCIAL WORK

Social work in home health care is a varied and multidimensional role which encompasses many functions. It utilizes a broad range of knowledge, synthesizing concepts from biological, psychological, and social development theories; interpreting cognitive and emotional processes; and determining their effects on physical illness and disability. The importance of the home milieu represents the key to effective intervention aimed at maximizing resources available to patients.

Social work in home care is task-focused, requiring interventions specifically linked to the patient's current medical necessity. There are two key issues addressed by medical social work services: functional loss necessitating lifestyle changes, and lack of support systems to meet care needs. The potential social and psychological stressors experienced by home care patients include loss, change, compromise, uncertainty, depression, anxiety, fear, anger, regression, and dependency. While these issues are addressed by both the social worker (MSW) and the psychosocial nurse, the interventions of the nurse and the MSW are distinct and complementary.

The MSW psychosocial evaluation of home care patients and families focuses on the patient's social, psychological, cultural, environmental, and financial situations. This information is then used in treatment planning and interventions. Special attention is paid to the patient's ability to live at home, home safety, and the availability of options for change or environmental manipulation. Neglect, abuse, lack of support, and suicide risk must also be closely assessed. Home care social workers must be aware of the mandatory reporting laws and regulations determining use of emergency services. Careful clinical assessment skills are critical.

Any new diagnosis resulting in functional loss, altered body image, terminal illness, and other responses to illness are areas in which counseling can achieve a positive impact. Other areas include depression, anxiety, poor coping, patient/family conflict, poor adjustment, poor compliance, poor motivation, and unresolved grief or loss.

Other MSW interventions include providing the patient and family with information about types of community resources available and how to connect with identified resources. Assessment of the patient's capacity to use community resources is essential. Can patients perform household chores and personal care? Do patients need respite care, adult day health, transportation, and referral to support groups?

Facilitating access to community resources includes providing assistance to ensure that the patients connect with services. Advocacy is an important role. Planning for care for after-discharge from home care necessitates ongoing follow-up and communication.

Team care planning and collaboration are mandated by most reimbursement sources. The MSW role in the interdisciplinary conference is to share specialized knowledge with other members of the home care team regarding psychosocial issues, for the purpose of incorporating comprehensive care into the total care plan.

In summary, MSW interventions must follow reimbursement guidelines by establishing the link between the services provided and the medical situation. The home environment provides a valuable framework in which to assess and intervene effectively.

HOME HEALTH AIDES

Home health aides provide personal care services, perform simple treatments as ordered by the case manager, and provide "light" homemaking services. Under Medicare, home health aides must provide some level of hands-on personal care, usually providing assistance with bathing and dressing. A *treatment* is defined, for example, as routine vital-sign documentation and weight documentation. Simple meal preparation may include making a sandwich or a light meal. Aides are also well-trained in skin care, transfers, care of the bedbound patient, and assistance with ambulation.

Care must be taken that home health aides are not required to do tasks that some would consider within the role of a housekeeper. Care and cleanliness of the sickroom is a priority for home health aides. However, they cannot be expected to clear the corners of cobwebs or clean the entire house in one visit.

Home health aides may be requested on the original referral or may be added by the case manager once the initial visit has been made. Regardless, it is the case manager who writes the specific orders for the home health aide. For example, orders for the bedbound depressed patient differ widely from the patient who is depressed but is relatively ambulatory.

As part of the multidisciplinary treatment team, home health aides are regularly supervised by the case manager in the patient's home. This supervision of the home health aide is a licensing requirement. As with other home care services, visits must be classified as intermittent, under the Medicare program. Consequently, home health aide visits are usually less than 2 hours in length.

Skilled home health aides can provide valuable observations about the patient's condition and report them to the case manager. At times, the home health aides see patients more frequently than does the case manager, and are attuned to subtle changes in the patient's behavior and condition. Home health aides also provide a level of social support to home care patients. In many cases, home health aides are an important factor in preventing psychological decompensation. The following is an example of how home health aides can achieve this.

CASE EXAMPLE

Bonnie is a 45-year-old woman with multiple sclerosis and major depressive disorder. She is only partially ambulatory and has extremes of mood lability. She takes multiple medications, including monthly B_{12} injections for a diagnosis of pernicious anemia. Prior to home care intervention, Bonnie had been hospitalized for depression and suicide attempts at least twice yearly for the past 5 years. Her physician decided to try home care following a recent hospitalization, despite Bonnie's objection.

The psychosocial nurse opening the case noted Bonnie's hopelessness and resistance to intervention. Bonnie was convinced her depression would never resolve, particularly in light of her worsening multiple sclerosis. Complicating matters was the fact that Bonnie herself was a nurse who had recently gone on medical disability. The home care nurse recognized the potential for transference/countertransference issues for both parties.

Following initial assessment, the nurse decided to order a PT and OT evaluation, an MSW, and a home health aide to provide personal care. Soon the home situation and Bonnie's physical condition stabilized, but her emotional lability persisted.

The home health aide was ordered three times per week. In contrast to the nurse case manager's difficult relationship with Bonnie during their weekly visits, soon Bonnie became quite fond of the home health aide. It appeared that consistent, early morning visits with the home health aide for personal care created a bond that was conducive to recovery.

As this bond developed, the home health aide began to detect subtle changes in Bonnie that the RN case manager was unable to discern. Specifically, Bonnie began to show signs of withdrawal and isolation, a precursor behavior that in the past had resulted in hospitalization when there was no psychosocial intervention.

The home health aide reported these changes in Bonnie's behavior during weekly multidisciplinary team conferences. Other observations about Bonnie's behavior were shared by the other members of the treatment team. A plan was devised whereby the nurse and the social worker would make a joint visit to Bonnie's home to discussed the noted behavior change.

With discussion, Bonnie admitted she was having suicidal thoughts again and had even started to develop a plan. The attending physician was contacted. The RN case manager visit frequency was increased to three times per week. Changes were made in Bonnie's medication because it was believed that some of her medications were contributing to her depression. Within 2 weeks, Bonnie had improved significantly. Clearly, the observations by the home health aide were essential in providing an optimal level of care for Bonnie and keeping her out of the hospital. ❧

A THEORETICAL FRAMEWORK FOR PSYCHIATRIC HOME CARE

Psychosocial assessment and intervention can incorporate a variety of ideas and theories that give the clinician a unique way of looking at problems and developing tools for intervention. These include crisis intervention, Orem's self-care model, and behavioral/cognitive therapies. This "blend" of ideas is described by Duffey, Miller, and Parlocha (1993) as being beneficial to a wide variety of psychosocial and medical problems as well.

CRISIS INTERVENTION THEORY

Crisis, in the purest sense, is defined as "psychological disequilibrium in a person that for him constitutes an important problem which he can for the time being neither escape nor solve with his customary problem-solving resources" (Caplan, 1974). Home care patients frequently face situations in which their previous coping mechanisms are inadequate, resulting in a crisis.

There are three commonly experienced types of crises: maturational, situational, and adventitious. A *maturational* crisis usually occurs at definable developmental stages throughout life, including adolescence, marriage, or

retirement from a career. A *situational* crisis results when the individual feels upset by external events. A few common examples seen in home care patients are worsening of health status, death of family members, or relocation to a new community. *Adventitious* crises are the least likely to be experienced in the home care population. These are events that affect society as a whole, such as earthquakes, floods, and wars.

While many individuals look forward to old age as being a peaceful and tranquil time, this seems to be less true than one would hope. The elderly seem more crisis-prone due to physical limitations related to the aging process, in combination with a lessened ability to deal with stressful events (Lang et al., 1990). These events include maturational and situational crises associated with retirement, decrease in income, role changes, and loss of physical and/or mental health, as well as death of family and friends.

Crisis resolution, then, becomes a common challenge for the elderly receiving home care services (see Figure 28-1). Crisis intervention, as described by Aguilera (1990), has the objective of "dealing immediately and vigorously with the patient's acute reactions to overwhelming situations" (p. 7). The role of home care services is to assist in the resolution of crisis with an awareness of the various types of crises and their impact on an individual's physical and mental health status. Therefore, the primary goal of crisis intervention is the restoration of functional equilibrium as soon as possible. Crisis intervention is a type of short-term, cost-effective therapy focusing on solving current problems quickly. Crisis assessment in home care begins with assessing the balancing factors that help patients to resolve crisis.

Crisis intervention starts by examining the stressful event that exceeds the individual's usual coping mechanisms. After identifying the precipitating event, the nurse assesses the patient's perception of it. Factors such as dependency needs, family dynamics, and psychological defense mechanisms will influence the patient's perception. It is critical that the home care nurse draw out the patient's perspective. For example, a nurse may expect a newly diagnosed, insulin-dependent diabetic

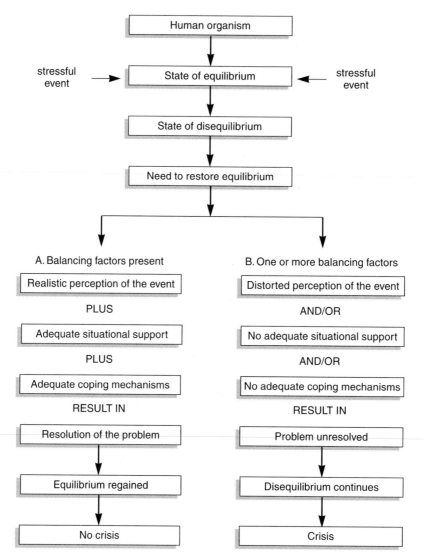

FIGURE 28–1. Crisis model. (Aguilera, D. [1994]. *Crisis Intervention: Theory and methodology.* 7th ed. St. Louis: CV Mosby, p. 32.)

to focus on dietary limitations, but the patient's perception might be that he or she is near death.

Situational supports are another balancing factor to assess in the crisis situation. The home care nurse is in a truly unique position to assess the home environment and the quality and quantity of socially supportive relationships. This assessment might include the social relationships within the home as well as the physical quality of the home. For example, are

family members able and willing to provide emotional and physical support to each other while weathering the crisis?

To assess coping mechanisms, it is useful to ask questions such as:

1. How have you handled past crises?
2. What are some of the positive and negative ways you relieve stress?

Homebound patients are very likely to overuse maladaptive coping behaviors, such as obsessive, negative thinking or withdrawal, which can make the crisis worsen. The identification of positive coping mechanisms readily available in the home is a critical part of the treatment plan.

By applying concepts from crisis intervention theory and assessing the patient's balancing factors, the nurse can gain a more accurate view of both the subjective and objective picture of the patient's crisis experience. If any of the balancing factors is absent or weakened, the next step is to look at the impact of these on a patient's functional abilities.

OREM'S SELF-CARE NURSING THEORY

Orem's self-care nursing theory focuses on three related theories: self-care, self-care deficit, and the theory of nursing systems. *Self-care,* according to Orem (1991), is defined as an adult's continuous contribution to his or her own continued existence, health, and well-being. Additionally, it is the practice of activities that individuals initiate on their own behalf in maintaining life, health, and well-being.

Typically, home health nurses complete an initial nursing data base which focuses on the various bodily systems. Orem's self-care requisites provide guidance on how we respond to each negative and positive finding. These self-care requisites are especially important as the patient and family members are active caregivers rather than passive recipients of care.

The assessment of self-care requisites in the home helps to focus both on behaviors and on resolution of functional limitations. These requisites include the maintenance of intake of air, water, food, fluid; adequate elimination, activity, and rest; solitude and social interaction; prevention of hazards; and promotion of normalcy. Each of these requisites addresses different areas of functioning. For example, *maintenance of sufficient intake of air* refers to the ability to breathe normally, without distress. Assessment of *intake of water and food* determines the adequacy of intake in supporting normal physiological processes. *Elimination* pertains to regular elimination patterns and their associated hygienic practices.

In an article that applies Orem's concepts to home health care nursing, Duffey, Miller, and Parlocha (1993) state "the next three requisites, namely activity and rest, solitude and social interaction, and prevention of hazards, are particularly appropriate for home care practice and are more observable in the home compared with the hospital" (p. 25). Assessment of the requisite to *maintain a balance between activity and rest* includes assessing the normalcy of sleep, wake, and rest cycles. *Solitude and social interaction* concerns the maintenance of bonds of affection, love, and friendship, as well as controlling impulses to use and abuse others.

Prevention of hazards to human life, functioning, and well being is especially useful and important in the home situation. This requisite includes response to predictable and unforeseen hazardous situations, as well as their impact on individual functioning. It is particularly important that the home care nurse assess both the patient and his or her environment for hazards.

The *promotion of normalcy* focuses on the attainment of optimal health and functioning within the context of the individual's existence according to his or her genetic makeup, character, and abilities. This global concept is negatively impacted by an inadequacy of other self-care requisites. In summary, Orem's self-care theory helps pinpoint precise areas for intervention.

BEHAVIORAL THERAPY

Home care patients often display a complex myriad of behaviors as a response to their acute medical illnesses. Behavioral approaches are useful in unraveling the complexities of these situations. Specifically, they ask, "What is causing this person to behave in this way right now and what can we do right now to change that behavior?" (Wilson, 1989, p. 257).

The focus of this type of therapy is to provide appropriate learning experiences where the patient develops new coping skills and communication styles and techniques, and learns how to discontinue maladaptive habits and self-defeating behaviors. To accomplish this, the nurse focuses on what the patient can do dynamically to change the situation. Unlike reflective stances observed in more traditional psychotherapies, the nurse may freely give advice or information. This fits very well with the time-limited nature of home care services as well as being easy to document in a clear, readable fashion for other clinicians and insurance reviewers.

CASE EXAMPLE

Mr. Smith is a 67-year-old man with chronic obstructive pulmonary disease (COPD) and a secondary depression. The initial physical assessment showed that he is noticeably short of breath at rest, has lungs with scattered rhonchi, and coughs frequently with a moderate amount of white sputum. Predictably, his endurance is poor and ambulation is slowed. Now he only walks within his home. His sleep pattern is quite disrupted; he sleeps both day and night. He complains of constipation and decreased appetite.

A mental status examination showed that Mr. Smith is alert and oriented, demonstrates depressed mood and poor concentration, but denies suicidal thoughts. However, he did express vague sentiments that the best part of this life was over, and felt overwhelmed by the chronic nature of his pulmonary illness. He also related that two of his close friends had died within the past month.

Crisis Assessment. Mr. Smith's perception of the events leading to his current state of distress is that his friends are gone and his COPD has once again become acute. This is a fairly realistic perception of the events. Next, we look at his situational supports. Unfortunately, with the loss of his two friends, he is left with diminished social contacts, although a neighbor calls him each day and a daughter who lives 60 miles away visits occasionally on weekends. His fairly isolated existence means that he has an inadequacy of social supports. His coping abilities have also been lessening along with his endurance. Specifically, he is no longer able to engage in meaningful hobbies such as gardening, reading, and hiking, which were his main mechanisms of relieving stress and maintaining a positive self-image in the past.

Through the use of crisis assessment, we have identified that, while Mr. Smith has a realistic perception of the events affecting him, his situational supports and coping mechanisms are not adequate to resolve his problems. Mr. Smith is an extreme state of crisis that is impacting on his functional abilities. To identify these functional limitations, we move on to assessment using Orem's Self-Care Requisites, outlined in Table 28-1. ❦

COMMON HOME CARE PROBLEMS

DEPRESSION

As noted in Chapter 18, depression is one of the most frequently observed psychiatric disorders in the United States. Between 1980-1985, the National Institute of Mental Health (NIMH) conducted a large epidemiological survey of adults seeking treatment for mental health-related problems. Data concluded that of U.S. adults seeking treatment in one year, 79.1% were diagnosed with major depression. The survey looked at those patients seeking treatment in both mental health settings and general medical clinics.

With the onset of serious emotional or medical illness, it is easy to envision a complex and frustrating situation taxing one's ability to cope. In addition, many illnesses, as part of their disease process and the medications used in their treatment, increase the incidence of depression. This is of interest as we look at who becomes depressed and why. With a "healthy" mix of both situational and biopsychosocial perspectives, the symptoms of depression often can be resolved in medically compromised individuals.

Depression has long been underrecognized and undertreated, especially in the medically ill and elderly populations. Within both groups, 25% to 50% of major depressive illnesses go undiagnosed and untreated (Esser & Lacey, 1989). According to Thobaben (1990), "If left untreated, the patient's self-care capacities may be further diminished; self-destructive behavior may result in further incapacity or death" (p. 33).

TABLE 28–1
Self-Care Assessment

The table below describes self-care requisites and Mr. Smith's corresponding condition.

Condition	Requisite
Lungs with scattered rhonchi; shortness of breath at rest; cough moist; thick, white sputum	Sufficient intake of air
Intake is adequate, no evidence of dehydration	Sufficient intake of water
Appetite poor, weight loss of 10 lb over the past month	Sufficient intake of food
Constipation, intermittent use of laxatives	Appropriate elimination and associated hygienic process
Poor tolerance of activity, sleep pattern disrupted	Balance between activity and rest
Very isolated, does not initiate social contact, circle of friends recently decreased.	Balance between solitude and social interaction
High risk for recurrent respiratory infection. Mild-moderate risk for self-harm due to vague suicidal ideation	Prevention of hazards
Not functioning within previous physiological or emotional norms	Overall normal functioning of individual

In the general population of the United States, 300,000 people attempt suicide annually, and 1 out of 10 of these attempts is successful (Kruse & Jones, 1990). The suicide rate for the elderly is especially important to home care service providers as the majority of their patients are elderly. While the overall population demonstrated a suicide rate of 12.8 per 100,000, the rate in the elderly population was 21.6 per 100,000. This means that elders comprise about 69% of all reported suicides in our country annually.

While these statistics only include reported suicides, it is quite possible that many others go undocumented. In addition, there is a wide spectrum of suicidal behaviors ranging from active to passive means. Active forms include guns, hanging, or jumping from a high place. Passive means of suicide, more difficult to detect, include medication noncompliance, not eating, or failure to carry out other vital self-care requirements.

Home health agencies and providers need clear standards for safe practice when a patient is at risk for self-harm or suicide. To facilitate this, a written policy and/or protocol for use by agency staff can assure a consistent and reliable response to an identified suicide risk. Discussion of this topic is quite anxiety-producing for medical and psychiatric staff alike. The ultimate result, however, is a heightened ability to deal more comfortably with a situation laden with legal and moral implications.

As part of the initial nursing assessment process, it is important to assess for suicidal ideation in all patients suspected of being depressed. This is important because not all suicidal patients have a primary diagnosis of depression or overtly present as being in danger of harming themselves. Some individuals openly express suicidal thoughts and intent to act out in a lethal manner, while others give only subtle behavioral indications such as neglecting grooming, giving away prized possessions, or making reference to "being gone." Once it is established that a patient has the intent of harming himself or herself, he or she should be asked questions directly, including:

1. Are you thinking of suicide?
2. Do you think about ending your life?

3. Do you feel that you would be better off dead?

Asking these questions will not precipitate suicidal thoughts but instead will confirm the presence of suicidal ideation.

The level of risk is also important. This is determined by the presence of a plan, availability of a chosen method, and its level of lethality. High-risk methods frequently seen in the home include guns, high-potency narcotics, drowning, and electrocution. Other less lethal methods of suicide include wrist-cutting, drug overdoses, and carbon monoxide inhalation. Regardless of the means or plan, all suicide threats must be taken seriously. One such tool, an "Intervention Decision Tree," was developed by Kruse (1990).

CASE EXAMPLE

Mr. Roberts is a 70-year-old man with severe arthritis. He has been making vague references to the nurse that he will not be needing her services much longer. When she asked why, he indicated that he thought he wouldn't be alive much longer. Further probing revealed that he planned to take an overdose of his pain medication since his life was filled with excruciating pain. The nurse determined that he was at moderate risk for suicide. This was based on determining that the method for suicide was of low lethality, the patient had available social supports, and the patient was able to contract not to harm himself. This allowed the medical team to attain optimal pain control. 🍎

DEMENTIA

Individuals with various types of dementing illnesses are being kept in the home with the assistance of the home care team, rather than automatically being placed in a skilled nursing facility. This presents many challenges for the patient, family, caregivers, and home health providers. The primary function of the multidisciplinary team (MDT) is supportive in nature.

One of the critical issues for designing appropriate care for the demented patient in the home is to assure that diagnostic studies have been completed to determine the cause of mental impairment. Some of the reversible and treatable causes of such impairment include profound depression, paranoid disorders, toxic deliriums, infectious diseases, and severe nutritional deficiencies. Once these have been ruled out and the type of dementia determined, anticipatory guidance and successful management techniques can be applied. The clinical interventions will differ only slightly for the diagnoses of Alzheimer's disease, vascular dementias, dementias due to other medical conditions, or acute delirium.

Assessment of the demented patient should be completed with the input and assistance of caregivers, with careful attention to the general health status, presenting behaviors, medications, and potential and actual safety hazards. This data is crucial for the development of a meaningful care plan. It contributes to successful implementation of an in-home treatment plan that will make it feasible for the patient to remain in the home rather than being placed in a more restrictive environment.

The careful, thoughtful analysis of disturbing behaviors can be accomplished by the use of the "ABC approach." This method explores the *Antecedent, Behavior,* and *Consequences* of behavior problems, in order to understand and manage them. The "ABC" approach advocates documentation of behaviors preceding the problematic behavior, the actual inappropriate behavior, and events occurring immediately after. This approach is helpful in identifying precipitating events, target behaviors, and interventions to modify behavior patterns (Alessi, 1991).

Applicable nursing diagnoses for individuals with dementia include:

Self-care deficit related to decreased mental alertness

Potential for injury related to restlessness and agitation

Ineffective family coping due to sleep disturbance

Alteration in thought processes related to delusional thinking

Potential for injury related to lack of awareness of environmental hazards

ANXIETY

Anxiety occurs as both a reaction to the stress of illness and an actual psychiatric condition (DSM-IV, 1994). Anxious patients are not able to concentrate, process, or retain information necessary to manage their illness in the home care setting. They typically visit emergency rooms and seek outside medical care while not in an actual medical crisis. The following case vignette demonstrates such an example.

CASE EXAMPLE

Mr. Lark is a 65-year-old man living alone. He is well known to the local hospital emergency unit and makes frequent calls to 911. He averages four visits to the emergency room by ambulance per month. Further evaluation of his physical and mental status revealed an underlying anxiety disorder with a high degree of somatization. ❦

Nursing diagnoses that can apply to this and other anxious patients would be:

Ineffective coping related to recent retirement (role change)

Ineffective coping related to physical changes

Anxiety related to perceived change in health status

Anxiety related to perceived lack of recognition from others

Anxiety related to cognitive impairment

Management of anxiety in the home care setting differs from management in the hospital only in that home care interventions are more self-directed and more preventative in nature.

ASSESSMENT OF AVAILABLE RESOURCES

The home care team provides skilled and intermittent care with a focus on strengthening resources in the home. Comprehensive treatment also includes identifying other mental health providers in the community. Some factors to consider when referring to additional resources are whether the patient can afford the resource and is willing to utilize other community mental health professionals and supportive community groups.

Traditional mental health care community resources include a wide variety of specialties, with different clinical focuses. Some of these resources include private psychiatrists, psychologists, psychiatric home care, partial hospitalization, group and individual counseling, community mental health clinics, geriatric outreach services, county-based social services, and private case management services. The clinical emphasis of these services and the patient's financial obligation are factors that impact on the availability of these services. For example, psychiatrists, psychologists, and counselors may facilitate support groups with a specific clinical issue in mind and be paid for partially, completely, or not at all by an insurance carrier.

Insurance reimbursement for various mental health services varies according to the overall benefit plan. A major determining factor is whether or not these benefits are "carved out" into a separate category and therefore subject to limitations as to the number of outpatient visits and inpatient days, or total annual lifetime dollar amounts. Careful review of insurance policies is advised. Skillful negotiation with insurance companies is, unfortunately, becoming part of the determination of who receives care and where it is received.

The spectrum of supportive psychosocial services does not end with the medical community. Various social groups within the community provide varied and useful services. These may include self-help groups such as Alcoholics Anonymous, Narcotics Anonymous, Alanon, and peer-led grief support groups. The richness of the community can be expressed in various service-related groups providing for the needs of individuals on a voluntary sliding scale. Some examples are meals on wheels, services for the blind, and even house repairs for low-income seniors. The home health care team, interacting with various members of the community, is in an ideal position to discover the "hidden," less-readily identified sources of informal support services that exist outside the medical community.

HOME ASSESSMENT OF RESPONSES TO ILLNESS

THE HOME AS A SYSTEM AND AS A THERAPEUTIC MILIEU

The initial nursing assessment of individuals and families in the home requires a working knowledge of the principles of general systems theory (von Bertalanffy, 1968). As in the hospital, the home care setting is a complex, interrelated system with both overt and covert feedback loops of communication. As part of a systems assessment, through the collection of objective and subjective data, it is important to consider the relationships and behaviors of the patient, caregivers, family members, and the overall environment as factors contributing to the patient's condition. While not always therapeutic, the home is the milieu where the patient will be treated.

According to Garritson (1992) the therapeutic environment (at least in the hospital) must promote safety and group well-being. The home care setting is no exception. The central task in home care is to balance the home environment with the patient's needs.

Patusky (1989), in an excellent chapter on psychiatric home care, discusses the role of the home milieu on psychosocial home care nursing assessment and intervention: "Assessment of living conditions and potential hazards goes hand in hand with an evaluation of the patient's ability to perform activities of daily living and exist in an independent setting without self-harm" (p. 651). If the home is not therapeutic, the patient's recovery will be slowed considerably.

A simple visual scan of the home environment can yield a wealth of data. The nurse must prioritize what part of the environment needs to be assessed first. Safety hazard assessment should occur routinely upon admission to home care and should be part of the nurse admission data base. What constitutes safety hazard assessment? The two major types of hazards experienced by most home care patients are falls and burns. Therefore, causative factors contributing to falls and burns must be noted. Loose rugs, frayed outlets, space heaters, and appliance malfunctioning must be corrected immediately to make the home environment less hazardous.

Changes in Nurse–Patient Dynamics

Part of assessing the home milieu is recognizing the differences in the nurse–patient relationship that can occur as a result of the nurse visiting in the patient's environment (Patusky, 1989). In the home, the patient is more in control than in other settings. The patient has so much control, in fact, that a nursing visit can be refused or the outcome sabotaged.

The dynamics of the home setting can change the formalities of the nurse–patient relationship. In the home, the nurse is frequently treated like a guest or a family member by the patient. The nurse can lose objectivity about the patient or become overinvolved. Transference and countertransference issues may emerge, which can hinder successful outcomes. Patusky likens the home care nurse's role to that of the old community family physician who makes house calls and is seen more as a family member than as an outsider.

Home care nurses must be aware of this change in the nurse–patient relationship. Bowers (1992) conducted a study in England of 12 community psychiatric nurses. Some psychiatric home care nurses felt that being in the patient's home exerted a kind of pressure towards an informal, friendship-based relationship; accordingly, they tried to distance themselves from patients. For example, some nurses refused an offered cup of tea. Others felt that the home setting was more conducive to chatty conversation than to therapy and psychoeducation.

Bowers concluded that only in matters seen by both participants as clearly medico-psychiatric will the nurse become more assertive. In other words, when psychiatric home care nurses could also perform medically oriented tasks, they were more comfortable with the "rules" of the relationship. Psychosocial home care nurses must be able to address the patient's medical concerns because, frequently, functional limitations express themselves medically. In addressing medical concerns, however, the role of the nurse as therapist may become blurred.

Cultural Factors

In the home as in other settings, it is extremely important to consider a patient's cultural background when assessing the patient. The home care nurse is in a unique position to view how culture impacts on the meaning of illness and health, influences compliance with the treatment regime, and defines the nurse–patient relationship.

For example, a home care nurse observed that one of her patients was noncompliant with the treatment regime. Despite teaching the essentials of a low-sodium diet, the patient continued to eat fatty foods and foods with a high sodium content. The nurse consulted with the psychiatric clinical nurse specialist (PCNS) on staff. Perhaps the patient had an underlying dementia and was forgetting the instruction. Or was the patient depressed? One thing was certain: the patient's blood pressure was dangerously high.

The PCNS made a visit and began talking with the patient. There was no evidence of overt depressive symptoms. A cognitive screening exam was essentially negative, ruling out depression and dementia as causes for noncompliance. The patient was very apologetic to the CNS about his blood pressure but refused to use salt substitute or minimize his sodium intake. He felt the home care nurses were making unreasonable demands on him.

After a lengthy discussion, the PCNS realized the patient's culture was the reason for his noncompliance. He had grown up in the Deep South where (in traditional Southern cooking) bacon or ham is used as a seasoning. Asking him to give up salt would, according to the patient, significantly interfere with his quality of life. He would rather risk the complications of high blood pressure than give up his high-salt diet!

The PCNS reported this factor to the patient's doctor and discussed findings with the treatment team. Unlike the hospital setting where a low-salt diet would be prepared for this patient, in the home he had more control over his own food preparation. The home care team realized that they had to develop a plan that would best meet the patient's cultural needs. The patient agreed that he would lower his salt intake somewhat if the physician could readjust his medication. That being done, the patient's blood pressure stabilized and his case was able to be closed.

Culture can also impact the dynamics of the nurse–patient relationship, as Bowers' study (1992) has already demonstrated. In many cultures (East Indian, for example), offering food to the nurse during the visit is a sign of hospitality and it should not be refused. Home care nurses must be sensitive to the diverse cultures seen in home health care.

Psychosocial Assessment With a Focus on the Elderly

Psychosocial assessment in home care must recognize those psychosocial considerations germane to the elderly (over 65) patient, the largest users of home care services. When assessing the elderly, it is important to understand and appreciate the following:

1. The strong feelings the elderly may have about "opening up" for fear of being labeled "psychiatric." Older patients are more uncomfortable talking about feelings than younger patients.
2. The role of informal as well as formal sources of social support (both past and present) impacting on the elder.
3. The potential influence of multiple losses experienced by this generation.
4. Communication problems occurring in the interview. This can be due to sensory impairments affecting the elderly, or time constraints within the interview process. The elderly typically take longer to interview.
5. The importance of a holistic assessment, one that is biological, psychological, sociological, spiritual, cognitive, and behavioral.

Some researchers cite four major categories of stressors common to the elderly (Wagnild, Hoffman, & Grupp, 1991):

1. Early hospital discharge
2. Condition at discharge
3. Home environment
4. Inadequate, inappropriate, or inaccessible resources

These potential stressors are expected to increase as hospitalization drops in priority as a treatment alternative site.

A final consideration when assessing the elderly, and often overlooked in the hospital, is the richness of past life experiences. Often nurses forget that their elderly patient is an individual with a past, and in most instances a colorful one at that. Home care nurses, because of their presence in the home, are more able to appreciate the contributions of one's past to one's present. Yet even well-seasoned home care nurses can forget the value that life experience brings to individuals.

CASE EXAMPLE

A psychiatric home care nurse was performing a psychosocial assessment on one of her elderly patients. As part of the assessment a cognitive screening tool, the Mini-Mental State Exam, was administered. Much to the nurse's surprise, she discovered the patient was severely cognitively impaired in all areas except serial-7s. Only when she discovered the patient had been formerly employed as a math teacher did she realize the reason for the discrepancy in her findings. ❧

Another example of the importance of considering a patient's life experience is illustrated in a recent article on the effect of music on decreasing agitation in the elderly. The authors recommend incorporating a music preference question into an admission interview. While the sample size was limited to five people, the study concluded that listening to music of their choice had a calming effect on some patients (Gerdner & Swanson, 1993).

Lastly, the nurse must consider not only the patient's own personal traits, culture, and feelings, but also the interpersonal dynamics that can occur. Love (1992) writes of the specific countertransference responses that can occur when working with the elderly. It is helpful for nurses to be aware of their own:

Feelings surrounding death and aging
Relationship issues with their own parents and grandparents
Beliefs that the elderly cannot change their ways
Beliefs that the elderly individual will die soon

Such beliefs can decrease a nurse's motivation to design an intervention plan. As home care nursing increases in prevalence, and the benefits are recognized more and more by patients and providers, the age range of home care patients will become more diverse. Regardless, the elderly will continue to predominate as the age group most commonly served by home care services.

THE IMPORTANCE OF FUNCTIONAL ASSESSMENT AND DOCUMENTATION

Home care reaches a segment of the population that may have otherwise been unable to seek outside medical care due to the presence of multiple functional limitations. A functional assessment of the patient is crucial. Nurse researchers have found that functional assessment improves the quality of patient care (Krach & Yang, 1992).

As stated above, reimbursement for home care services depends on the payor's ability to understand and interpret documentation to determine suitability for payment. Assessing the patient from a functional standpoint paints a visible picture of the patient's condition and helps guide the nurse in developing clear and concrete interventions. It also helps reviewers to understand that the nurse is providing a useful and, therefore, reimbursable service.

Home care psychosocial nursing, by its very nature, must focus on ongoing psychotherapeutic assessment and intervention. Principles of therapeutic communication, psychodynamic interpretations of the individual and family systems, and transference/countertransference issues must be addressed constantly. So, too, issues pertaining to the experience of illness also apply. According to Barry (1989), the various issues around illness are trust, self-esteem, body image, shame, control, loss, guilt, and intimacy. The well-informed psychosocial home care nurse will constantly keep these issues in mind when dealing with home care patients.

Reviewers of home care documentation are rarely trained in understanding the language of psychosocial nursing. Translating psychosocial concepts into functional limitations is the key to successful assessment, intervention, and documentation of provided home care services. Successful home care documentation focuses largely on functioning rather than on feelings alone.

MAINTAINING A SYSTEMS FOCUS

When considering individual and family responses to illness, it is important to remember that a family is a system within the larger home care system. The family is known as an open system with three important components.

Wholeness stresses the interactive nature of the family system. Patients must be assessed and interventions undertaken within the context of the existing family system. *Relationship* examines *what* is happening within the family system versus *why* something is happening. This focus on the "here and now" also complements the third component of the family system, *equifinality*, which assumes there is a problem with the current interaction in the family system that must be addressed. The concepts of wholeness, relationship, and equifinality can help the psychiatric home care nurse maintain a systems focus when dealing with a patient's problem (Foley, 1989).

In home care, the dynamics of the family impact more on assessment, intervention, and outcome than in any other setting. Frequently, family members serve as caregivers and are the primary "clients" within the family system, particularly when the patient is incapable of retaining instructions or benefitting from interventions. Often, just the mere presence of the nurse in the home introduces a "third party" (even when there are multiple caregivers) that can soften the tense family dynamics resulting from the impact of the illness.

The nuclear or extended family may not be identified by the patient as the real family. Many home care patients hire an outside attendant to be the primary caregiver. A typical scenario is the patient who lives with grown children who work; an unskilled attendant has been hired to care for the patient during the day. In this case, the attendant would be labeled the primary caregiver and contact person. The nurse may only rarely communicate with the grown children about the patient.

Another common scenario are those patients living in various assisted-living settings.

These settings may include small, licensed board-and-care homes, residential care facilities, or senior housing complexes. In these cases, the board-and-care home worker may be considered the patient's family and the primary caregiver or contact person. These patients are often particularly challenging cases. They may have few outside social contacts and are being managed by a conservator. The conservator, an individual legally designated to attend to financial matters or make decisions on behalf of an individual deemed mentally incompetent, may be a family member who is close to the patient, or an unconnected individual who is the local money manager for the patient, while the actual family lives at a distance.

PSYCHOSOCIAL NURSING INTERVENTIONS

Psychosocial nursing interventions for home care patients are based on principles of behavioral therapy, cognitive therapy, self-care theory, and crisis intervention as discussed earlier. Specific patient-related interventions are also based on the patient's diagnosis and presenting functional limitations. The following are some of the common general interventions used in psychiatric home care.

PSYCHOEDUCATION

Based on our experience and consistent with nursing's biopsychosocial approach to patient care, we believe a psychoeducational focus promotes successful outcomes. Current ideas are shifting away from the idea that the brain and the mind are two separate entities (McEnany, 1992).

In home care, patients are taught that their psychiatric illness is probably due to a biochemical change in the brain. By using this approach, the potential for optimal control and compliance is enhanced. There is less tendency for blame and the development of underlying feelings of guilt. Patients often refer to their medications as vitamins and liken their illness to vitamin deficiencies.

Patients also need to be taught the nature of their psychiatric illness or their emotional distress. Patients are often relieved to hear that vegetative signs are symptoms of depression, not laziness or lack of imagination. Patients in an acute crisis appreciate being taught about the nature of crisis resolution, i.e., that a crisis is, by nature, time-limited in its effect of producing stress.

A significant piece of psychoeducation is medication teaching. In home care, medication teaching and the development of a stable and consistent medication regime is crucial for optimum recovery. Medication teaching includes providing written instructions for patients about their medications and providing an in-home system which will achieve the best chance for compliance. Home care nurses often use items found around the house to help patients remember their medication schedule. Egg cartons are frequently used when over-the-counter medication reminder boxes are unavailable or too expensive.

REESTABLISHING
SELF-CARE ACTIVITIES

All psychosocial home care patients come to home care with some functional limitation that interferes with their ability to achieve their self-care requisites. Nursing interventions are behavioral and cognitively designed. The nurse may ask the patient to keep an activity diary and checklist, which can assist in structuring the patient's day. For example, the patient may be asked to socialize with at least one person during the week. It is expected that the patient will attempt to dress in street clothes, if possible, during the visit. Regaining self-care skills promotes self-esteem and normalcy.

BEHAVIORAL MANAGEMENT

In cases where problem behaviors are occurring, psychosocial home care nurses give patients, caregivers, and families concrete suggestions as to how to effect behavior change. Often, developing a behavioral program for a patient will introduce enough structure to encourage behavior control. For example, schizophrenic patients who respond to auditory hallucinations by yelling in public need to be taught that yelling in public is inappropriate. In a similar case, simple instruction on washing clothes may be helpful. For elderly demented patients in particular, caregivers and families need to be sure that the diagnosis of dementia is accurate, and that sundowning is an expected behavior. Simple sleep hygiene principles are emphasized.

ASSISTING WITH PROBLEM SOLVING

Patients who are coping poorly are frequently unable to prioritize or mobilize enough resources to solve problems. Simple problem prioritization can minimize anxiety so that the problems can be solved. "Pro" and "con" lists can help patients who are having difficulty making a decision about their situation.

IDENTIFYING POSITIVE
PAST COPING BEHAVIORS

The home care patient's reaction to crisis can cause him or her to feel unbalanced; accordingly, the patient may be unable to use prior coping skills to offset distress. The identification of positive, past coping behaviors can assist the patient in being able to resume them. Examples of these behaviors include simple activities such as knitting or reading the newspaper.

INDICATIONS FOR REFERRAL
TO MENTAL HEALTH SERVICES

While realizing that there is a full spectrum of mental health which can be complicated by many factors, there is common agreement about when a referral to mental health services is indicated. These include overt and covert symptoms that indicate a certain level of distress and impaired functioning. In some situations, symptoms may be identified easily as those of an acute mental illness, or they may be subtle as in failure to thrive, noncompliance, or other evidence of the inability to carry out self-care activities.

As the specialization of home care programs increases, it is important to utilize psychiatric nurse specialists when a patient experiences both physical and emotional distress. Referral for consultation, evaluation and treatment by a psychiatric nurse can be a critical part of the treatment plan, even if the primary diagnosis is medical in nature. Audits of existing home care medical records have consistently demonstrated significant emotional distress in approximately 20% of medical patients. If patients belonging to this group do not receive psychiatric care, they have an increased chance of further physical or mental complications and delayed recovery.

Some physical indications for closer assessment include malnutrition, dehydration, unexplained failure to thrive, and noncompliance with the in-home treatment plan. Psychiatric problems are more easily recognized. They include anxiety, depression, suicidal ideation, sleep disorders, delusions, hallucinations, dementias, and inappropriate behaviors. Patients whose medication profiles include antidepressant, antipsychotic, or antianxiety agents or mood stabilizers are also appropriate for consultation services.

CONCLUSION

Home care is a rapidly growing sector of health care charged with the task of caring for an increasingly acute and diverse population. This task includes increasing attention to mental health issues which previously have been underrecognized and therefore untreated. Psychosocial home care nursing is relatively new, but is gaining respect and credibility among providers, payers, and patients alike.

As part of the home care treatment team, the psychosocial nurse provides a unique service which is complementary to the entire MDT. By the application of relevant theories such as crisis intervention, Orem's self-care model, and behavioral and cognitive theory in the home setting, there is a greater potential for successful treatment outcomes for individuals experiencing noncompliance, depression, dementia, and anxiety. This benefit is not limited to the identified "client," but includes the caregiver, facility, and community as a whole.

ACKNOWLEDGEMENTS

The authors wish to thank Margaret M. Elms, B.S., O.T.R., Manager of Rehabilitation Services, and Mary Ellyn Abeliuk, L.C.S.W., B.C.D., Social Work Coordinator at the Visiting Nurse Association and Hospice of Northern California, for their contributions to this chapter.

BIBLIOGRAPHY

Aguilera, D. C. (1990). *Crisis intervention: Theory and methodology*. St. Louis: C. V. Mosby.

Alessi, C. (1991). Managing the behavioral problems of dementia in the home. *Clinics in Geriatric Medicine*, 7(4), 787–801.

Beyea, S., & Matzo, M. (1989). Assessing elders using the functional health pattern assessment model. *Nurse Educator, 24*(5), 32–37.

Bowers, L. (1992). Ethnomethodology II: A study of the community psychiatric nurse in the patient's home. *International Journal of Nursing Studies, 29*(1), 69–79.

Caplan, G. (1974). *Principles of preventative psychiatry*. New York: Basic Books.

Cummings, J., & Weaver, F. (1991). Cost effectiveness of home care. *Geriatric Home Care, 7*(4), 865–874.

Diagnostic and statistical manual of mental disorders. (1987). Washington, DC: American Psychiatric Press.

Diagnostic and statistical manual of mental disorders (4th ed.). (1994). Washington, DC: American Psychiatric Press.

Duffey., J., Miller, M., & Parlocha, P. (1993). Psychiatric home care: A framework for assessment and intervention. *Home Healthcare Nurse, 11*(2), 22–28.

Esser, A. D., & Lacey, S. D. (1989). *Mental illness: A home-care guide*. New York: Wiley.

Foley, V. D. (1989). Family Therapy. In Corsini, R. J. & Wedding, D. *Current Psychotherapies*. Itasca, Il: F. E. Peacock.

Garritson, S. H. (1992). Milieu therapy. In H. S. Wilson, & C. R. Kneisl (Eds.), *Psychiatric nursing*. Addison-Wesley.

Gerdner, L., & Swanson, E. (1993). Effects of individualized music on confused and agitated elderly patients. *Archives of Psychiatric Nursing, 7*(5), 284–291.

Hamilton, D. (1992). Research and reform—community nursing and the Framingham tuberculosis project, 1914–1923. *Nursing Research, 41*(2), 8–13.

Healthcare Financing Administration. (1989). *Medicare home health agency manual*. HFCA publication No. II, revision 222. Retrieval title P11R222. Washington, DC: U. S. Department of Health and Human Services.

Hellman, S. (1991). Health care in year 2000 and beyond. *Future Research Quarterly*, Spring, 67–81.

Kellogg, F., Brickner, P., Conley, L., & Conroy, M. (1991). Controlling hospital readmission of elderly persons living at home: A risk factor analysis. *Home Health Care Services Quarterly, 12*(2), 5–16.

Klebanoff, N., & Casler, B. (1986). The psychosocial clinical nurse specialist: An untapped resource for home care. *Home Healthcare Nurse, 4*, 36–40.

Knollmueller, R. (1992). Prevention and home care, not strange bedfellows. *Caring* (9), December, 4–11.

Krach, P., & Yang, J. (1992). Functional status of older persons with chronic mental illness living in a home setting. *Archives of Psychiatric Nursing*, 6(2), 90–97.

Kruse, E., & Jones, G. (1990). Development of a comprehensive suicide protocol in a home health care and social service agency. *Journal of Home Health Practice*, 3(2), 47–56.

Lang, M., Kraegel, J., Rantz, M., & Kreji, J. (1990). *Quality of health care for older people in America*. Kansas City, MO: American Nurses Association.

Lesseig, D. (1987). Homecare for psych problems. *American Journal of Nursing*, 87(10), 16–19.

Love, C. (1992). Applying the nursing process with the elderly. In H. S. Wilson & C. R. Kneisl (Eds.), *Psychiatric nursing*. Redwood City: Addison-Wesley.

Lutz, S. (1993). Hospitals continue move into home care. *Modern Healthcare*, January 25, 28–31.

McEnany, G. (1992). Biological therapies. In H. S. Wilson & C. R. Kneisl (Eds.), *Psychiatric nursing*. Addison-Wesley.

Miller, M., & Duffey, J. (1992). *Psychiatric home care program development manual*. Unpublished manuscript.

Miller, M., & Duffey, J. (1993). Planning and program development for psychiatric home care. *Journal of Nursing Administration*, 23(11), 35–41.

National Advisory Mental Health Council. (1993). Health care reform for Americans with severe mental illness: Report of the National Advisory Mental Health Council. *American Journal of Psychiatry*, 150(10), 1447–1465.

National Association of Home Care. (1993). Toward meaningful reform. *Caring*, 10(3), 4–10.

Naylor, M. Comprehensive discharge planning for hospitalized elderly: A pilot study. *Nursing Research*, 39(3), 156–160.

Orem, D. (1990). *Nursing: Concepts of practice*. St. Louis: C. V. Mosby.

Patusky, K. (1989). Psychiatric home care. In L. M. Birckhead (Ed.), *Psychiatric nursing*. Philadelphia: J. B. Lippincott.

Soreff, S. (1983). New directions and added dimensions in home psychiatric treatment. *American Journal of Psychiatry*, 9, 1213–1216.

Thobaben, M. (1990). Depression in the medically ill homebound patient. *Journal of Home Health Care Practice*, 2(3), 33-38.

Von Bertalanfy, L. (1968). *General systems theory*. New York: George Braziller.

Wagnild, G., & Grupp, K. (1991). Major stressors among elderly home care clients. *Home Healthcare Nurse*, 9(4), 15–21.

Wagnild, G., Hoffman, A, & Grupp, K. (1991). Theoretical perspectives of stress and coping among elderly home care clients. *Home Health Care Services Quarterly*, 12(1), 137–156.

Warhola, C. (1980). *Planning for home health services: A resource handbook*. Publication HRA 80-1401. Washington, DC: Public Health Service, Department of Health and Human Services.

Wilson, G. (1989). Behavior therapy. In R. Corsini & D. Wedding (Eds.), *Current Psychotherapies*. Itasca, Il: Peacock Publishers.

Zimmer, J., Groth-Juncher, A., & McCusker, J. (1985). A randomized controlled study of a home health care team. *American Journal of Public Health*, 75(2), 134–140.

CHAPTER 29

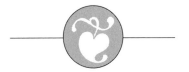

Emotional Support of the Older Adult and Family

Jane Neese
Anita Thompson-Heisterman
Miriam Hirsch

During the 20th century, the number of older Americans or those aged 65 and over has increased significantly. According to the United States Bureau of the Census, the number of older Americans has increased from 3.1 million in 1900 to 31.8 million in 1990. This demographic phenomenon, according to most projections, will continue throughout the 21st century (Schneider & Rowe, 1990). By the year 2030, it is estimated that there will be approximately 66 million older persons, more than twice the 1990 figure (American Association of Retired Persons, 1992).

The trend to manage the nation's health care needs for all ages in ambulatory settings has resulted in a larger percentage of older adults in acute care settings. Early discharge from acute care facilities and the inability of most families to afford long-term care necessitates that our society be prepared to address the needs of this growing segment of the population.

The health care system and many existing social programs for the elderly have become strained financially, causing many programs to be eliminated to reduce costs. The problem involves, however, more than a shortfall in revenue. Many older adults experience difficulties and disadvantages which are the direct results of widely held myths, misperceptions, and overgeneralizations about the aging process. In order to address the needs of older adults, to validate their involvements, to share a meaningful relationship with them, and to learn from their wisdom, one must recognize that few generalizations are valid.

DEFINITION OF AGING

Aging can be defined as the movement of the organism toward death over a course of time (Whitbourne, 1985), but the process of aging does not affect all organisms in the same way. There seems to be no normal curve of aging that applies to everyone (Chopra, 1993) and tremendous individual differences contribute

Patricia Barry: *Psychosocial Nursing:*
Care of Physically Ill Patients and Their Families, 3rd ed.
© 1996 Lippincott–Raven Publishers

to this. Some people escape certain symptoms, while others are afflicted with these symptoms long before old age (Chopra, 1993).

Becoming "old" is a unique individual experience that is not based on chronological age. When a 97-year-old woman was asked when she perceived herself to be "old," she replied, "I really did not feel old until I was in my mid-80s." When she was 82 years old, this woman had been maintaining an acre yard by mowing the grass and raking leaves. Therefore, applying age-related changes universally and as an inevitable outcome has proven to be difficult. Because of this, many researchers tend to be somewhat reluctant to define what is meant by aging. The individual differences in how age affects people has led researchers to formulate multidimensional explanations. Thus, when "normal aging" is mentioned, serious questions arise. Therefore, the term "successful aging," rather than normal aging, will be used in this chapter.

DISPELLING THE MYTHS OF AGING

Myth 1: Being old is synonymous with being sick.

One of the most damaging myths about old age is that age causes one to be sick. Physical changes do occur, but disease is not necessarily inevitable. A major component of many age-associated declines can be explained in terms of lifestyle, habits, diet, and an array of psychosocial factors extrinsic to the aging process (Butler, Lewis, & Sunderland, 1991). It is suggested that how our bodies age, in terms of critical life signs and cellular processes (Chopra, 1993), is strongly influenced by the lifestyles one adopts.

Research shows that what were once considered normal developmental changes with advancing age are really changes resulting from disuse and disease (Small, 1994). For example, presbycusis (age-related hearing loss) is considered "normal," but do loud noises hasten the process? Teenagers who listen to loud music will likely experience hearing loss well before they reach old age. Smoking, having a high-fat diet, and not getting enough exercise are all detrimental to the body. Noting

how these risk factors change with age and over time may be useful in distinguishing between those who age well and those who do not (Forbes & Hirdes, 1993). The fact is that most "young-old" people, those age 65 to 75, are in good health and recent studies indicate that two-thirds of the population over 75 years is also healthy (Averyt, Furst, & Daulton-Hummel, 1987).

Myth 2: Most older people are senile.

The development of an irreversible dementia such as Alzheimer's disease is not a normal part of the aging process. As many as 85% of older people are mentally alert and healthy. Approximately 5% of older adults, however, do suffer from severe memory impairment and 10% have symptoms of moderate impairment caused by dementia disorders, primarily Alzheimer's disease. Alzheimer's disease is estimated to be the cause of 50% to 60% of the cases of senile dementia. The chances of developing a dementing illness are shown to increase with advancing age. It is estimated, however, that one out of every four people diagnosed as having dementia is misdiagnosed (Friedan, 1993).

Myth 3: Most older people need to be taken care of and live in nursing homes.

Most older people live where they always have—at home in their communities. Ninety-five percent of those over age 65 remain in the community rather than in an institution (U.S. Bureau of the Census, 1990). Only 5% of older people live in long-term care facilities at any given time, and 25% will require a brief stay at some point of their life (Averyt, Furst, & Daulton-Hummel, 1987). Most older adults want to live independently and to remain at home because this insures their ability to maintain control over their lives. Most elders dread the thought of becoming a burden on their children and relatives, and "intimacy at a distance" is preferred (Averyt, Furst, & Daulton-Hummel, 1987).

Getting accurate information to dispel the myths of aging involves understanding the theories of adult development, as summarized in Table 29-1.

Although each of these somewhat static behavioral theories does make important points, none has proven to be valid in explaining the complexities of older adult development. Therefore, integrative theories, which emphasize biopsychosocial determinants of older adult development, are becoming more viable options. This synthesis of philosophy requires not only methodological sophistication and resources, but also investigators who are receptive to collaboration with multiple disciplines (Birren & Schaie, 1990).

SUCCESSFUL AGING

The best method to obtain information on what successful aging is and what older people need is to ask them. Those who have lived to experience old age are survivors and have experiences and knowledge that younger people can learn and benefit from.

One prevailing characteristic in those who appear to be aging successfully is a positive self-image that develops out of an awareness and acceptance of one's own aging, and a recognition of aging as a unique stage of life with limitations and developmental possibilities. As Dr. Bessie Delany (Delany, Delany, & Hearth, 1993), aged 102, says in *Having Our Say*, "If you asked me the secret to longevity, I would tell you that you have to work at taking care of your health. But a lot of it is attitude. I'm alive out of sheer determination, honey!" Older sister Sadie, aged 104, adds, "Life is short and it's up to you to make it sweet."

Although these sisters have experienced many losses in life, they still have a sense of purpose and accept the challenges and limitations of their age. Their sense of purpose in life and their determination is based on their desire for control over their lives and their struggle to maintain their independence and sense of competence. Some older people, however, are not as fortunate. They may become incapable with the passage of time; others always were incapable. But others only become incapable because they imagine themselves to be so, and society reinforces this view (Comfort, 1990).

ROLES OF OLDER ADULTS

Sociogenic aging refers to the roles which society imposes on people as a certain chronological age is reached (Comfort, 1990). These roles have a strong effect on one's self-esteem. The roles that people play can be a personal choice or they can be imposed. As Bessie and Sadie Delany said, remaining productive has kept them alive. Therefore, one of the secrets to longevity and successful aging is to make life

---

Table 29-1
Theories of Older Adult Development

Theory	Description
Disengagement theory (Cumming & Henry, 1961)	Proposes that older adults voluntarily withdraw from society to protect themselves from failure and rejection due to diminished capabilities. Society also withdraws from the older adult to make room for the younger, more capable members.
Activity theory (Havighurst & Albrecht, 1953)	Proposes that as one ages, loss of roles is a naturally occurring phenomenon, usually as a result of illness or disability; however, older adults will find replacement roles for those that were abandoned.
Exchange theory (Atchley, 1988)	Proposes that older adult behavior can be explained by the reciprocity of relationships and situations.

purposeful. This varies tremendously from person to person.

INTERPERSONAL RELATIONSHIPS

Interpersonal relationships are essential to one's existence because they arise out of a need for engagement with others. Needs for psychological support and stimulation are met when one interacts with others. An attraction to those with similar beliefs, values, and personalities is usually the foundation for these relationships. The characteristics of having mutual trust and feeling comfortable with another are powerful determinants in the formulation of friendship (Schultz & Ewen, 1988).

Friendship

Levels of friendship vary from casual to loving. *Loving* implies that someone or something is deserving of one's involvement and engagement and gives a person a reason for living. Because personality has been shown to remain relatively stable throughout the lifespan, the number of friends and the degree of that involvement also tends to remain stable. As one ages, the tendency to focus on those most meaningful relationships increases.

Sexual Intimacy

The intimate relationship, in addition to providing for the needs for social interaction and sharing, also serves as a means for sexual expression. Sexuality, for most people, is very important and is usually a lifelong interest and need. Many older people still want and have sexual intercourse. The need for sexual stimulation, closeness, sensuality, and being valued as a man or woman (Comfort, 1990) does not decrease with age per se, but can decline because of illness or attitude.

Older adults are not asexual and do not seek social isolation and deprivation. Older men in general do experience more difficulties in the act of sexual intercourse than do older females. Most of these difficulties, however, are due to performance anxiety rather than actual physical health problems (Com-

fort, 1990). A significant drop in sexual activity for any length of time also contributes to problems in performance. Diseases and side effects to medication may be responsible for some of the difficulties but the need for intimacy is still important. Careful assessment of the nature of the sexual dysfunction is critical no matter what the age of the patient. One must realize that older adults still have the capacity for and a "normal" interest in maintaining sexual relations.

ROLES IN THE FAMILY

One of the most basic social institutions is the family. Close family relationships often arise out of basic needs for intimacy, love, trust, and a sense of belonging. Interdependence among family members enables us to better satisfy our needs.

Like its members, the family too, has a life cycle. This cycle often begins with the marriage of two people who eventually become parents. The cycle ultimately changes with the death of or separation from a spouse. The life cycles of most families continue as the children establish their own family life cycles (Atchley, 1988). Each member has a variety of roles within the family which may include being son or daughter, sister or brother, wife or husband, grandmother or grandfather. Feelings of equality, self-disclosure, similarity, acceptance, agreement, trust, and cooperation among members keep the relationships strong.

ROLE OF WORK

Getting an education and eventually a competitive job are often seen as something that younger members of the family can accomplish more effectively than older ones. Technological advances such as those brought about in the computer age may cause older adults to feel left behind. Today there is more emphasis on observation and learning outside the family than in earlier times, when young people learned, traditionally, by watching their elders. Thus, the skills of some older people may no longer be viewed as valuable or as proficient. This is evident when older people are forced to retire at a certain age. Their ability to perform the work is not as much an issue as is the misperception that age causes an inflexibility and an inability to learn.

A young adult strives towards financial independence and wishes to start his or her own family. Becoming financially secure requires that one have a career, a profession, or a skill. But financial independence is not the exclusive need of the young. Older adults can continue to be, and many are, valuable contributors in our workforce. Many have chosen to remain vital and interested in life after retirement. They do so by continuing to grow, develop, and learn from experiencing new situations. Some volunteer efforts that contribute significantly to the overall well-being of others.

Our modern, industrialized society requires its members to be highly productive and competitive in a fast-paced environment. The emphasis on productivity, often defined in terms of financial gain, may foster the belief that making money is equivalent to being useful and valued. The shift from a rural, agrarian society in which family survival depended on the interdependence of its members, to an urban, industrialized society where interdependence is less important, has changed the structure of the American family. This shift has contributed also to some of the changes in the position of older adults within our society.

THE CHALLENGE OF PHYSICAL ILLNESS TO THE OLDER ADULT

For most elderly, the interpretation of losses, whether the loss is physical health or the death of a loved one, depends upon the individual's sense of self. Young health professionals, who have yet to experience the challenges of age, have difficulty comprehending the life of an older adult with physical conditions that may impair an active sex life and other activities.

In the following discussion of the meaning of chronic illness and terminal illness to older adults, the focus is on how the sense of self has been preserved or eroded. In the older adult, age-associated losses such as having a disabil-

ity, death of a spouse or close friends, and retirement, tend to corrode the sense of self (Tobin, 1991). For most people, personality or the core sense of self remains stable throughout life (Mezey, Rauekhorst, & Stokes, 1993).

Developmental Tasks of Aging

The individual is a product of all the developmental processes which have occurred over a lifetime. Although there is continuity of personality development and a stable sense of self-identity over time, this does not imply personality rigidity as one ages. The last stage of life may present unique opportunities for growth, since individuals are capable of change at any point in the life span (Bornstein, 1992).

The potential for successful resolution of developmental tasks depends in part on the range, flexibility, and appropriateness of coping styles. Older adults are more likely than their younger counterparts to have employed a wide range of coping responses. Elders who have successfully negotiated earlier stages of development enter old age with an armamentarium of coping mechanisms available to them.

The primary developmental task of older adulthood, according to Erikson (1963), is to achieve ego integrity instead of ego despair. This task is further delineated by Peck (Bornstein, 1992) into ego disintegration vs. work-role preoccupation, body transcendence vs. body preoccupation, and ego transcendence vs. ego preoccupation. These tasks refer to the ability to maintain a sense of selfhood apart from losses of work role and failing health, and the ability to make meaning out of one's life (ego transcendence).

Those who have successfully negotiated earlier developmental tasks will be equipped to deal with these final challenges. Both the ill elder and the unaffected spouse struggle with this developmental stage while coping with the challenges of caregiving demands and often chronic debilitating illness.

We do not become old suddenly. Aging occurs at a slow pace, allowing most individuals to cope with the various physical changes of the aging process as well as to integrate these changes into their perception of self. Even though each elder may maintain his or her sense of self in a unique way, most elders share similar processes in maintaining their sense of self. Among the elderly, especially the oldest-old, there is "an interchangeability of the past and present" (Tobin, 1991). Thus, the evidence of the past and present mold to support the self concept, in comparison to young adults, who define themselves through their current life events and relationships.

ISSUES OF IDENTITY

When elders describe themselves, they vacillate between present and past examples of themselves. If both the present and past fail, elders will use distortion and what they wish could be, to preserve their sense of self (Tobin, 1991). When warranted, elders preserve the self by a selective screening of reality and by accepting previously unwelcome characteristics.

During old age, the sense of self is the sum of experiences over a long life. Through this blurring of past and present, coupled with distortion, identity endures and remains stable. As Tobin (1991) proposes, "The task of the very old is to maintain a consistency of self when confronted with losses, which occurs within the awareness of having lived a life and with the acceptance of death, is achieved by a purposeful simplification of identity which reaffirms the self" (p. 9). Preservation of the concept of the self is a primary human motivation (Tobin, 1991).

A common complaint among young adults is that elders dwell in the past. In order to maintain their identity, elders use the past as self-validation because they may lack interpersonal relationships and roles through the death of others, or through age-associated losses such as retirement or the end of child-rearing. For some elders, there is a lack of cognitive ability to maintain interactions in the present. In addition, present interactions and abilities may not be congruent with how the older adult perceives himself or herself (Tobin, 1991).

CASE EXAMPLE

Ms. A continued to live alone in her old home that did not have central heat. She received homebound meals from a commu-

nity agency, and a nearby neighbor supplied her with firewood. Even though she had a severe heart condition, Ms. A continued to live in her crumbling home, walk up a flight of stairs to her bed, and carry her firewood from her front porch. When her clinical nurse specialist expressed concern about her heart condition with regard to climbing the stairs and carrying in the wood, Ms. A replied that she could use "the exercise" since she had been "so lazy" in keeping the rest of the house clean. She rationalized that "after all I have been sitting around all day."

In her past, Ms. A had worked hard on her family farm, maintaining a garden for the family's food and raising ten children and twenty grandchildren. For Ms. A, maintaining her sense of self meant preserving her independence by living in her home, sleeping in her bed, and contributing to taking care of herself by carrying the firewood in from the porch. The clinical nurse specialist did not intervene in this situation, but left Ms. A to continue maintaining her sense of independence in her own meaningful way. 🍎

THE MEANING OF CHRONIC ILLNESS

The likelihood of developing a chronic illness during the aging process is high. According to Eliopulos (1993), nearly one-half of the elderly suffer from arthritis, more than one-third have hypertension, nearly one-third have a hearing impairment, and more than one-fourth have a heart condition. Therefore, for many elderly, integrating the presence of a chronic illness into the sense of self is one of their developmental tasks.

How well an older adult can accomplish this process will affect the individual's concept of illness. For most elders, the development of chronic illness is an insidious process that does not occur suddenly, but slowly evolves. Thus, accommodating the limitations of the chronic illness is a daily occurrence. Since the process is slow, most elders learn to function with chronic illness and adapt their life accordingly. Coping with chronic physical illness will be discussed in a later section of this chapter.

THE MEANING OF TERMINAL ILLNESS

For most people, being told that you have a terminal illness means death is not far. Older adults who are attending to Erikson's developmental task of integrity versus despair are dealing with accepting death (Erikson, 1963). In examining the meaning of terminal illness among older adults, one must examine how they interpret and accept death.

Rappaport et al. (1993) found that the more successful an elder was in developing a life purpose, the less concern there was about death. On the other hand, the elder who was less successful in his or her search for meaning had considerably more death anxiety. Those elders who had a purpose for living viewed the future as a new perspective on life that offered more meaning. In other words, the individual with this perspective was a planner who looked to tomorrow to discover a new meaning for life and was not fixated on past anxieties (Rappaport et al., 1993).

According to Fry (1990), most elders are not concerned with death per se, but with the process of dying. Apprehensions about dying are focused on several factors: physical pain and sensory loss during the dying process; risk to personal safety around the time of death; suffering indignity and ingratitude at the time of death; dying alone without the support of a significant relationship; being permanently forgotten after death; and the uncertainty of life after death (Fry, 1990).

ADAPTATION TO PHYSICAL ILLNESS

An elder's adaptation to physical illness can be examined through the coping strategies he or she employs in the process of adaptation. Coping strategies may vary in method but have a similar outcome. An elder who becomes aggressive or rather assertive, evading the "normalcy" of developmental passivity, may be better able to cope than one who is passive (Tobin, 1991).

CASE EXAMPLE

Ms. B was a difficult, 83-year-old woman who suffered from chronic substance abuse, obesity, hypertension, and cardiac dis-

ease. She continued to maintain that she was "too mean to die." At every available moment, she fought staff regarding hospital routines, medication regimes, and dietary restrictions. She characterized her younger life as someone who had to "fight for whatever I got." In later life, she continued the same strategy.

Ms. C was the antithesis of Ms. B; she was known to staff as a compliant, never complaining, and "very sweet" lady who kept to herself. Unlike Ms. B, Ms. C did not have a history of substance abuse, but had hypertension, obesity, and congestive heart failure.

Ms. C became withdrawn and died shortly after she was moved to a nursing home, whereas Ms. B continued to control the staff when she was transferred to the nursing home. Ms. B was able to mobilize her anger positively by not blaming herself for unavoidable events or losses which may lead to depression. Her aggression also gave her energy to cope with the stress of physical illness and ventilate her rage, and reduced her sense of helplessness.

Spirituality enhances elders' adaptation to chronic illness. Seven out of ten elders believe in an afterlife that denotes reunions with deceased loved ones (Reed, 1991). These reunions are optimistically anticipated (Tobin, 1991). In a study by Reed (1991), the seriousness of an illness or the number of diagnosed illnesses correlated positively to spiritual involvement among elderly subjects. As the number of illnesses increased, so did the level of spiritual involvement, even though organized religious practices diminished (e.g., attending church or synagogue and social functions). Therefore, religious beliefs and practices influence the elder's adaptation to physical illness (Reed, 1991).

An additional technique, *magical coping*, is used to denote the self-enhancing illusion that the self has control of forces external to itself. In other words, elders who utilize magical coping with physical illness maintain the illusion that they have control over the disease. Even though this coping strategy is contrary to what is generally believed to be "good mental health," Taylor (1989) argues that positive mental health may be characterized not by accurate appraisals of reality, but by self-enhancing illusions. Magical coping may be closely linked with the individual's need to remain in control, and thus preserve the self.

SPOUSE OR SIGNIFICANT CAREGIVER RESPONSES

Caregivers of elders who suffer from disabling physical illnesses are plagued by many emotions. The caregiver role increases role overload and impacts the caregiver physically, emotionally, socially, and financially.

Contrary to popular belief, caregiver burden is perceived less when physical care needs are present than when there is psychological or cognitive impairment (Baillie, Norbeck, & Barnes, 1988). According to Baillie et al. (1988), caregivers are more at risk for psychological distress and/or depression when the elder is mentally impaired, the caregiving time has been continuous over a prolonged period of time, and the caregiver has few social supports.

Caring for cognitively impaired elders usually entails an extended period when the caregiver slowly loses sources of social support that were previously obtained though work, hobbies, or volunteer work. Robinson (1990) found that caregivers who had more affection, affirmation, and aid from their social network had higher self-esteem. Those caregivers who reported lower self-esteem had lost important relationships during the previous year. Therefore, social support networks tend to bolster the caregiver during the stressful period of caregiving (Robinson, 1990).

RESPITE CARE

A method of reducing caregiver stress, extending the caregiver's ability to provide assistance, and supporting the continuation of caregiving is by providing respite services. Respite services can be provided in the home or in an agency, depending upon the resources of the caregiver.

Methods of providing respite vary in many ways, including the duration of respite care rendered (i.e., hours or days); the time when care is delivered (day or night); location of respite services (in-home, day care center, nurs-

ing home, or other residential setting); the schedule of respite services (planned versus crisis intervention); and the aim of the service (custodial care or active rehabilitation [Brodaty & Gresham, 1992]). In Virginia, for example, most nursing homes provide respite services based on a daily monetary rate. Voluntary as well as fee-for-service respite care can be obtained. Having respite care available helps free up time for the caregiver to spend on household chores, running errands, part-time employment, and social activities.

Berry et al. (1991) found that caregivers reported positive physical and mental health as well as an improvement in the quality of their caregiving relationship when they were able to use respite services. Those caregivers using in-home respite services were able to reduce their time spent on caregiving, while caregivers who used out-of-home respite services reportedly spent the same amount of time in caregiving activities (Berry, Zarit, & Rabatin, 1991). From subjective reports, most caregivers praise the efforts of respite care and perceive a decrease in burden.

What effects do respite services have on the patient? Little research has been done to examine whether respite services have positive or deleterious effects on patients. Hirsch and colleagues (1993) found that short-term admission to nursing homes for the purpose of providing respite care for caregivers had brief negative effects on veterans with advanced dementia. Those with advanced dementia declined in self-care and behavior two days postdischarge from nursing home-provided respite services; however, within two weeks, they had resumed their prerespite status. The effect of respite care on patients remains unclear, but can be fertile ground for research.

Nursing Intervention

For nurses, understanding the barriers to respite care may help assist the caregiver in making a decision to use services. Two major barriers to using services are the caregiver's lack of knowledge about available respite services, and guilt about using them.

The first barrier is easily resolved by furnishing the caregiver with information regarding the different types of respite services available, finding out their cost, and discussing the caregiver's needs. Some caregivers mistakenly "save" respite services for emergencies such as caregiver hospitalization or time of crisis; this defeats the use of respite services as prophylaxis to prevent physical or emotional exhaustion. In such cases, caregivers need to be educated on how to use services (Brodaty & Gresham, 1992). The second barrier is more difficult to overcome. The nurse must be nonjudgmental but helpful in assisting the caregiver to explore the pros and cons of accessing respite services.

EFFECTS OF ILLNESS IN THE OLDER ADULT ON THE FAMILY

The illness of an elder family member can have a profound effect on the entire family, especially if the illness is chronic and requires caregiving on the part of other family members. Contrary to a popular notion, families do not rely on others to provide care for their elders. At considerable financial and emotional expense, most of the caregiving is done at home by family members, one-quarter of whom are themselves over age 65 (Harper, 1992).

Increased longevity of elders coupled with shorter hospital stays due to Medicare reimbursement policies has resulted in elders living longer with chronic illness and being discharged from hospitals after acute episodes of illness "quicker and sicker" than ever before. Community long-term care is the norm, not the exception, a trend that will only increase as the number of older adults increase into the next century. The American Association of Retired Persons (1990) predicts that by the year 2030, the proportion of persons age 65 and over may climb to 21.8%, compared to 12.6% in 1990.

POTENTIAL FOR FAMILY CONFLICT

The situational tasks of caregiving required are complex and challenging. Caregiving requires a wide array of skills and knowledge for which there often is no formal or experiential preparation. In general, families assume the caregiving role without a full understanding of what is involved or of the consequences of the long-term caregiving role.

In addition to providing nursing, counseling, transportation, cooking, and home maintenance chores, families also are expected to be their own advocate and case manager, discovering and negotiating the community services available for assistance. Often these community resources are inadequate, nonexistent, or disorganized, presenting a confusing array of diffuse services. Caregivers may become frustrated in attempting to negotiate a multiagency, multisystem service and health care delivery system. Accurate information on benefits and services is often difficult to obtain.

Role Conflicts

Role conflicts are inherent in families with an ill older adult. According to Temple and Fawdry (1992), roles are the expected and actual behaviors associated with one's position in a social system. Roles are learned by observing others in the role. *Role stress* occurs when role obligations are vague, irritating, and/or impossible to meet. *Role strain* occurs when a person experiences a subjective state of distress. *Role conflict* refers to a situation where existing role expectations are contradictory or mutually exclusive. With the addition of another role, the role of caregiver adds to already existing roles, resulting in role overload.

The caregiving experience is fraught with potential for role stress, strain, overload, and conflict. For example, when one member of a couple becomes ill, the healthy spouse may have to assume roles and responsibilities for which he or she was never prepared. A wife may have to learn how to handle the finances while a husband may need to assume more responsibility for the maintenance of the home or the family relationships.

The "Sandwich Generation"

Conflicting demands of generations may pose severe dilemmas and conflicts for the adult child caregiver. The generation of adults in midlife is often named the *sandwich generation* to describe their position between the younger and older generations, each requiring care and assistance. Caregiving tasks most frequently fall onto adult daughters who must find a way to balance competing and colliding roles of wife, mother, daughter, and employee, among others.

Parent care is composed of a complex collection of tasks and activities that change as the frailty and dependency of members shifts (Green, 1991). Role reversal between parents and their adult children is often painful for both since the parent needs to rely on the child for many of the functions he or she was once able to perform independently, and the child witnesses the decline of a beloved parent.

Frequently, psychological and situational tasks reactivate buried and unresolved conflicts between family members. These conflicts can occur between spouses, parents, children, and siblings. Consider the adult daughter who never felt appreciated and now is struggling to care for a demanding parent, or the wife who was in an abusive relationship with an alcoholic husband and now must care for him as his cognition declines due to his substance abuse. Sibling relationships also can be adversely affected by the demands of caring for an aging parent. The sibling geographically and/or emotionally closest to the parent frequently assumes the caretaker role. Such roles may have been assigned covertly early in life.

Women's Work?

Often daughters feel they are the ones expected to carry out the tasks of caregiving, although this expectation was never explicitly discussed. Some daughters experience a great deal of resentment towards the brother who is perceived to be the "favorite" child although he contributes little to their parents' care.

Societal expectations do place caregiving tasks under the heading of woman's work. Conflicts, while painful, do present an opportunity to improve relationships between family members. While 40% of siblings in a study by Strawbridge and Wallhagen (1991) reported a negative impact on the sibling relationship precipitated by parent care, 60% reported that

they had become closer and had a more satisfying relationship due to the experience.

DYSPHORIC RESPONSES TO PHYSICAL ILLNESS

Many, often-unanticipated, feelings may be generated by the illness of an older family member. Family members may fear the loss of the ill elder. Anticipatory grief can be productive, leading to a resolution of feelings regarding death for the afflicted elder and others, or can disintegrate into a sense of helplessness and fatalism. Feelings of sadness or dysphoria are typical.

Clinical depression with resulting loss of function may occur as a result of ineffective coping with grief and loss. A sense of hopelessness may lead to suicidal feelings. Suicide is a serious problem among the aged. While the elderly comprise 12% of this nation's population, they account for 25% of the nation's suicides (Lazarus, 1988).

A sense of one's own mortality, accompanied by feelings of helplessness and fear, may be elicited by an elder's illness. Fear may generate anger that this illness occurred to a loved family member. Anger may be acknowledged openly and expressed, or displaced onto others. Sometimes anger is handled behaviorally through acting out against authority or self-destructive measures.

Guilt is an emotional state frequently generated by the illness of a loved one. Guilt may be related to conscious concern over past conflicts, behaviors, or omissions, or may be unconscious and acted out in other relationships. Family members may see the illness as punishment for real or imagined "sins."

Anger and frustration about the situation of coping with the illness or being in charge of the care of an older adult may occur. Resentment regarding the lack of involvement of other family members is often experienced. A sense of loneliness, isolation, and despair may occur in the caregiver or the patient while coping with the illness. Feeling overwhelmed due to taking on roles and responsibilities for which one has no experience or training is typical.

The potential range of feelings and conflicts is multifaceted and may lead to opportunities for growth and a richer, more intimate relationship with other family members, or to ineffective coping responses. People may engage in fight–flight or approach–avoidance responses, with resultant indecision, displacement of feelings onto auxiliary caregivers (the professionals are not doing enough), self-neglect, overcompensation, and other responses.

Bornstein (1992) describes three patterns of nonproductive response to stress. These include compliant/helpless, aggressive, and moving-away behaviors, which eliminate external sources of assistance. For instance, a child or adolescent may act out feelings, using behavioral responses to express fear or anger about a grandparent's illness. These behaviors may push the parents further away at a time when the child needs more support and structure. Flexibility and a range of coping mechanisms are the keys to handling feelings, as well as to psychological and often physical health.

EMOTIONAL CRISIS AS A RESPONSE TO PHYSICAL ILLNESS

As one ages, the chances of developing an illness that may lead to a disability increase. Not only have advances in medical technology prolonged life in those with terminal illnesses, they also have increased the life span among the aging population. As people live longer, however, they are more vulnerable to acquiring chronic health problems (Lamm, Dungan, & Hiromoto, 1991). According to the American Association of Retired Persons (1990), most older people have at least one chronic condition and many have several; thus, the risk for needing assistance at some time usually increases with age.

The impact of these disabilities on older adults and their families is unique in several ways and has profound effects on personality and social environment (Lane & Hobfoll, 1992). Because most older people do not live in institutions but rather in their communities, a major channel for assistance is often provided through the family (Birren & Schaie, 1990). Emotional crises which often develop as a response to physical illness involve not only the older patient, but also the entire family system.

EMOTIONAL CRISIS OF THE OLDER ADULT PATIENT

Physical health strongly influences what people are capable of achieving. Often, choices of profession, occupation, hobbies, and other roles within society are based on one's ability to perform adequately. For many, these roles define who we are and make up the foundation of our self-concepts.

The effects of illness or disability force an individual to reevaluate or abandon previous roles, if the severity of the illness or disability decreases the individual's ability to perform those roles. Because of restricted roles and the development of new roles, such as the "sick role," feelings of inadequacy may arise. Feelings of inadequacy lower self-esteem and require that the individual readjust former roles based on current ability and available resources. Depending on the severity of the illness or disability, an increased dependency on others may be required. For older adults, this may be especially difficult because they have been independent for most of their lives, as well as having been the care providers for others (Atchley, 1988).

As contemporary research in health psychology suggests, chronic illness increases stress, which increases the need for social support (Lane & Hobfoll, 1992). These changes can lead to emotional crises. Older adults may also experience difficulty adapting to the losses associated with disability due to the death of spouses and friends. Retirement naturally eliminates several sources of support (Oxman & Berkman, 1990). The negative effects of widowhood, more commonly experienced by older people, are well documented. Although not well-understood, older widowed men have a higher rate of mortality than do older widowed women. The loss of friends through death or relocation can also influence coping.

Increasing disability may require housing alternatives as the social support network decreases. Income may also be reduced in later life because of retirement. Disability may require that the older person spend more money on services that he or she, or the spouse, once provided by him or herself or spouse (Atchley, 1988). Therefore, reliance on other family members may be necessary.

EMOTIONAL CRISIS OF THE FAMILY

For most older adults, the designated caregiver is usually a family member. The family is one of the most basic social institutions, for the members are usually interdependent on one another. The family unit is a system where change has repercussions for all members.

Health-related dependency can be viewed as a crisis that threatens the organization of the family system and the roles which each member plays within it. The effects of the illness "radiate" throughout all those who are interlinked to the member with disabilities. The situations within the family become more tangled as the crisis escalates (Birren & Schaie, 1990). This interlinking of the lives of family members is referred to as the "life-event web" (Pruchno et al., 1984).

Illness of a family member may cause disruption in many areas within the family system. The family's organization, emotional and interpersonal relationships, and energy that was directed towards personal growth and development change as a result of the physical disability of one member (Stuifbergen, 1990). The resulting change creates role tension and emotional distress and ultimately influences the system's organization and functioning. The changing demographics of the American family also have an impact.

Birren and Schaie (1990) have identified four types of macrosocial change experienced by families. It is important to recognize these in order to understand the organizational changes that occur and why caregiving has become such a visible social issue (Table 29-2).

Although the family system may experience many stresses resulting from the failing health of its member, positive outcomes from the crises may also emerge. Under stress, the family may experience a reemergence of old conflicts, a heightened motivation to resolve past issues, and an increase in the ability to communicate. As a result, the cohesiveness of the family unit or the relationships between individual members may strengthen (Jarvik & Small, 1990), and a sense of mastery may develop (Lane & Hobfoll, 1992). The affected member may feel that he or she was able to meet some of the needs of the supporter or caregiver (Lane & Hobfoll, 1992), thus enhancing self-esteem.

The stress that arises when a family member becomes chronically ill requires long-term lifestyle change. Nursing intervention should emphasize effective coping through problem-solving, improved communication and information, and control in assisting the family unit. It is important to understand that stress associated with caregiving is often normative because most families have functioned successfully until the crisis developed. Therefore, the perspectives of the patients and families and their reciprocal interactions around the experiences of illness should be the primary concern in the design of caring interventions (Donnelly, 1993).

ASSESSMENT OF THE GERIATRIC PATIENT

Assessment is the systematic review and evaluation of patient, family, and environment, and is the core and foundation of psychogeriatric nursing practice. Assessment is the initial step in the development of a comprehensive plan of care, implementing that plan, and evaluating its effectiveness. Assessment is continuous and is used throughout the nursing process cycle of observation, understanding, intervention, and evaluation.

Psychogeriatric nursing assessment requires a broad and complex knowledge base on the part of the nurse. Nurses must understand how the aging process unfolds, as this serves as a baseline for comparison and for determining what is normal and what is not. Nurses must understand the myriad psychiatric, behavioral, psychological, and social problems that can be found in the elderly, and merge this understanding with their nursing knowledge. Nurses must know how physical health, mental health, and environmental and social problems all interact to

Table 29-2
Macrosocial Changes Affecting Families

Macrosocial Changes	Results
Increase in life expectancy	More middle aged people with parents and grandparents
Decline in fertility and birthrate	Smaller families and fewer children to assist family members in times of crisis
Increase in vertical or "bean pole" structure of family	Increase in longevity of family members
Increase in the number of generations alive at the same time	The middle or sandwich generation cares for both the younger and older generations

Source: Birren & Schaie, 1990

complicate the picture of the older patient, caregiver, and family in need (Thompson-Heisterman, Smullen, & Abraham, 1992).

In the elderly, physical and mental health interact closely. Many physical illnesses may have psychiatric manifestations, often before physical signs and symptoms of illness are apparent (Lipowski, 1989). Psychological problems may occur due to physical illness or functional deficits. Drug reactions and interactions, drug toxicities, or other adverse reactions can present themselves physically or psychiatrically. When social problems such as poverty or living in isolation are added, it is apparent that psychogeriatric problems may be the result of complex interactions of biological, psychological, and social factors.

Creating a Therapeutic Environment

The creation of a therapeutic environment in which to conduct the interview of the elderly patient is the first step in the assessment process. Attention to the interview environment is critical (see Table 29-3 for the elements of a therapeutic environment).

Cultural and educational background, as well as the expectation of illness as a normal concomitant of aging, cause many elderly people to underreport symptoms (Kane, Ouslander, & Abrass, 1989). The stigma attached to mental illness further contributes to the underreporting of symptoms, as do denial and fear of illness and disability. In addition to

these psychosocial factors, the elderly may have altered physiological responses, such as decreased sensation, which further predispose them to underreport symptoms. To assure a comprehensive assessment, a systematic approach is recommended to reduce the likelihood of underreporting or nonobservation (Thompson-Heisterman, Smullen, & Abraham, 1992).

While some elderly patients underreport symptoms, others overreport somatic complaints. Due to the value systems of this generation of elderly, it is much more acceptable to have a physical illness than an emotional or psychological problem. The interaction of psyche and soma is well documented, yet many elderly find it difficult to discuss stressful life events, preferring instead to focus on very personal somatic concerns. A careful and thorough assessment, along with the use of effective communication skills, will elicit data critical to the plan of care.

The *Psychogeriatric Nursing Assessment Protocol* (Abraham et al., 1990) was developed by a multidisciplinary team. Nursing assessment focuses on the interaction of physical, psychological, cognitive, behavioral, and social stressors, and recognizes resources and strengths as they affect the functioning, health status, and quality of life of elderly individuals and their families. The Protocol is a comprehensive guide to structure and direct nursing assessment of geriatric patients with psychiatric or neurobehavioral problems (see Table 29-4)

Table 29-3
Establishing a Therapeutic Environment

Intervention	Rationale
A relaxed, quiet setting free from distractions	Assists patient in concentrating on questions
Establish rapport	Speak in conversational tone, make "small-talk," reassure the patient the interview is important and a step in developing a plan of care, and enjoy the process of the interview
Have good lighting, free of glare	Enhances performance on visual cues and decreases distortions and misperceptions of nonverbal communication
Schedule appointments for late morning or early afternoon	Older adults need more time to perform their ADLs
Keep interview at a reasonable length	Avoids fatiguing the older adult
Be prepared for disabilities	Make sure that the room can accommodate a wheelchair or walker; speak louder and deeper if the elder is hearing-impaired; have larger print and good lighting for the visually-impaired; allow some time for responses—older adults are slower to respond

Source: Thompson-Heisterman et al., 1992

Assessing Caregivers and Family

There are several compelling reasons to include caregivers and family in the psychogeriatric assessment process. Contrary to conventional wisdom, it is known that most care of the elderly in the United States is done by family members. Interviewing family members, including the primary caregiver, enables nurses to view the patient in the context of the larger family system. The family can offer information which the cognitively impaired patient may not be able to provide. Often, the family or caregiver may provide information which the patient is embarrassed to provide.

Interviewing the family and patient together gives information about family dynamics and communication patterns, while interviewing them separately often provides information which they do not wish to share with each other for various reasons. Further, interviewing the caregiver and family builds support for the family in the caregiving role, which often can make the difference between the patient's premature institutionalization or continuing residence in the home (Thompson-Heisterman, Smullen, & Abraham, 1992).

Often, it is the family, not the identified patient, that requires intervention. The impact of caring for an elderly person on the caregiver's health and well-being is well known. A careful assessment of the family can often result in interventions which not only support the identified patient in the home, but serve a preventive function for all family members involved.

Caregiver and family assessment should include a description of the family configuration, the dynamics, the perceived burden of caregiving, coping mechanisms, and strengths. Finally, psychogeriatric nursing assessment needs to be sensitive to the cultural, ethnic, and racial backgrounds of patient and family, specifically attitudes, dialects, and health practices. The nurse must consider behaviors within their cultural context. What may seem like pathology to one culture is merely eccentric behavior to another (Thompson-Heisterman, Smullen, & Abraham, 1992).

Assessment of elderly patients is one of the most challenging aspects of psychiatric mental health nursing. Physical, psychological, and socioeconomic factors interact in complex ways to influence the health and functional status of the elderly. Therefore, comprehensive eval-

Table 29-4
Parameters of the Geriatric Assessment

Assessment Domain	Assessment Strategy
Functional Status	Physical ADLs; instrumental ADLs
Mental Status	Mental status exam; sleep/wake cycle; mood; speech; general appearance; description of typical day; history of any sudden behavior changes; suicidal ideations
Behavioral Status	Dress; hallucinations/delusions; wandering; sundowning; cooperativeness/resistance; aggressive or sexual behavior; repetitive behaviors; screaming/loud outburst; catastrophic reactions
Nutritional Status	Use open-ended question to assess daily intake including food and fluids
Medications	Prescriptive and "over-the-counter" medications; "brown bag" method— have the patient bring *all* the medications he or she uses; alcohol and drug use history
Sensory Assessment	Vision and hearing problems; mobility
Home Environment	Daily patterns; interactions among residents; safety of kitchen, bathrooms, and inside and outside areas

Source: Abraham et al., 1990

uation requires assessment of each of these domains. Though nurses view all individuals holistically and from a biopsychosocial perspective, assessment of elderly patients is especially complex but equally rewarding, using all the clinician's skills.

CRISIS INTERVENTION

The first step in any crisis is to identify the precipitants and obtain a thorough assessment. The nurse can then use the assessment to plan effective interventions. Acute anxiety often accompanies the news that a patient has an illness that may necessitate painful and invasive treatments and/or may cause serious adjustments to ability to function, self-image, and finances, among other areas. Interventions that decrease severe anxiety are critical because no learning or healing can occur when anxiety levels are too high.

Alzheimer's Disease

The diagnosis of probable Alzheimer's disease can create a crisis with acute anxiety for both patient and family. The assault to ego integrity by a disease that attacks the very essence of personhood, the ability to think and reason, is tremendous. The fear of losing one's mind that accompanies this diagnosis is often overwhelming when the diagnosis is made early enough in the disease process so that the patient can comprehend its meaning and repercussions. The disintegration of ego causes severe anxiety. Often, the patient has suspected that something is wrong and has made efforts to hide the declining cognitive impairment. In addition, great anxiety is engendered by the fear of becoming dependent on one's spouse, or especially one's children. A sense of hopelessness often accompanies this diagnosis, as people feel little can be done to ameliorate the progressive decline of the disease process.

Anxiety in the family of a patient with probable Alzheimer's disease is also acute, with concomitant feelings of being overwhelmed. Very often the demands of caregiving have already been great, with attempts to understand and manage disruptive behavior, compensate for declining memory, and cope with the myriad feelings generated by the situation. With the diagnosis comes confirmation of the worst case scenario and the prospect of more months and years of progressive disability and decline and increased caregiving tasks.

The nurse can intervene by offering hope, information, and resources once the meaning of the illness to patient and family have been explored. The family can be educated that the disruptive aspects of Alzheimer's disease are often caused by hallucinations, physiological conditions about which the patient is unable to communicate (for instance, a urinary tract infection or pain), or environmental precipitant (i.e., the care aide's tone of voice). These factors cause agitation which can be ameliorated through the use of a low-dose neuroleptic for hallucinations, attention to physiological states and needs, and attention to environmental precipitants.

Catastrophic reactions that are precipitated by misinterpretation of the environment can be particularly frightening to the patient as well as the caregiver. Discovering the precipitating event is the key to intervening. For example, taking a shower can trigger a catastrophic reaction, where the patient believes he or she is outside being subjected to a thunderstorm. In case of catastrophic reactions, the best course of action is to stop whatever is triggering the reaction and try at a later time. Resources such as support groups, respite care, home care, and written material should be offered to patient and family. Ongoing support from a concerned person outside the family is helpful to caregivers.

Financial and guardianship planning information is useful to provide to the family and patient. Interventions used by others coping with problematic behavior should be offered, with a caveat to family members that they are the true "experts" on their particular situation, as they are the people dealing with the crisis of dementia day-to-day. Although each situation is unique, much material and support is available to provide guidance and ameliorate the anxiety that accompanies the diagnosis.

COMMON EMOTIONAL RESPONSES TO PHYSICAL ILLNESS

ACUTE CARE SETTING

In the acute care setting, the overriding initial response of patient and family most likely to be expressed is fear and anxiety, because the pa-

tient would not be in acute care unless an acute physiological crisis existed. Fear may generate anger, which is sometimes displaced onto caregivers in the acute care setting. The family or patient may complain that the staff is not doing enough. Conversely, fear may create passivity and helplessness, with resulting reluctance to offend the professional staff lest retaliation occur.

In the older adult, the expectations of the staff in an acute care facility and the complexity of treatment modalities only tends to heighten the anxiety the individual is experiencing. Dysphoria related to actual or potential losses of function or role performance caused by the illness can occur in the patient and the family. Adult children may feel sadness due to the loss of a former relationship with a parent; this includes seeing the strong, independent parent decline. Stoic responses to pain and illness are not atypical. Cognitive attempts to achieve mastery and control of the illness and/or the environment can be assisted by teaching the family about the technological equipment in the acute care setting.

HOME CARE SETTING

The home care setting presents additional emotional responses in both patient and caregiver. Illness treated in the home care setting is usually chronic. It is characterized by progressive deterioration and decline accompanied by periodic, chronic, unremitting caregiving responsibilities. These responsibilities can create frustration, anger, and anxiety over being unable to handle the complex tasks, feelings, and responsibilities. It can also create resignation, with related feelings of helplessness and hopelessness.

Responses ranging along a continuum from sadness, dysphoria, and clinical depression with vegetative symptoms, to suicidal ideation can occur, especially in the affected adult. The caregiver more typically manages to cope overtly, with underlying emotional and physical costs. The effects of caregiving demands can be experienced through stress-related illness. Stress leads to a compromised immune system that can lead to illnesses such as arthritis. Other stress-related disorders include hypertension and gastrointestinal disorders (Kiecolt-Glaser, 1992). Poor self-care results in undetected and untreated illness as well as poor health habits. Poor nutrition along with lack of exercise, sleep, and diversion result in further compromised health for caregivers.

While the focus has been on the negative aspects of illness, disease also provides an opportunity for the patient and family to incorporate the experience into their spiritual belief system and to find meaning in the suffering and adversity. A spiritual belief system can have a profound effect on life and health. Those elders who feel that life has meaning are more likely to be resilient and make successful adjustments to life's losses and disappointments (Wagnild & Young, 1990).

NURSING INTERVENTION FOR CHRONIC INEFFECTIVE COPING

According to Barry (1989), the degree of emotional distress that occurs as a result of inadequate ego defenses depends on the patient's normal personality style and coping ability, his or her perception of the illness and the degree of threat it poses, and the availability and strength of a support system. Crises, whether developmental or situational, provide an opportunity for growth as successful resolution enhances future coping potential. The nurse's role nurse is to build on the strengths and compensate for the disabilities of patients and families.

INTERVENTIONS WITH THE PATIENT

Crisis Intervention

In the acute care setting, psychosocial nursing interventions are often based on crisis intervention principles. A crisis is a turning point; crisis intervention is a short-term therapy approach that focuses on solving immediate problems in a person's life in order to reestablish emotional equilibrium. The goal of crisis intervention is to restore the person to a precrisis level of functioning or to promote growth to a higher level of functioning through successful resolution of the crisis. In order to help the patient achieve resolution and restoration, the nurse promotes a realistic perception of the event, mobilizes social and situational support systems, and strengthens and supports individual and family coping mechanisms. Van Auken (1991) found decreased anxiety in those elders who were prepared for a move to a long-term care facility using anticipatory guidance, along with other crisis intervention techniques.

Acute crisis situations can and do occur in community psychosocial nursing. The following case study illustrates this fact.

CASE EXAMPLES

Mr. B, an 81-year-old, white, widowed male living on his family farm with his 27-year-old son, was referred to the psychiatric clinical nurse specialist after being evaluated by a nurse practitioner for physiological concerns. Upon assessment the nurse practitioner noted that Mr. B was very dysphoric and she requested a consultation from the clinical nurse specialist to evaluate Mr. B for depression.

Upon evaluation by the clinical nurse specialist, Mr. B appeared severely depressed with neurovegetative signs. His appetite was decreased, with a 15-pound weight loss over the previous year. He had sleep disturbance with initial, middle, and delayed insomnia, anhedonia, and anergy. Mr. B was dysphoric, frequently tearful throughout the interview, and had suicidal ideation with a partial plan, means, and method. He had considered shooting himself and, since his son hunted, the home contained several rifles and shotguns.

The clinical nurse specialist contracted with Mr. B not to hurt himself and asked the son to remove the guns from the home. Consultation was obtained from a geriatric psychiatrist who made a home visit with the nurse to evaluate Mr. B for antidepressant medication. Consultation was provided to Mr. B's family practice physician who would prescribe the antidepressant. Mr. B was started on Zoloft, which, along with psychosocial interventions by the nurse, made a significant difference in his mood. He continues to be monitored for medication side effects and mood changes. ❧

Be Alert to Medication Effect

Polypharmacotherapy can precipitate an acute crisis and is a tremendous problem among the elderly. It has been estimated that 9 million adverse drug reactions occur in older adults each year, and that more than 30% of all hospital admissions in the elderly are precipitated by untoward drug interactions or reactions. Though the elderly represent 13% of the population, they use 30% to 40% of the more than 1.5 million prescriptions written yearly (Harper, 1992). Drug reactions and toxicities can occur rapidly, given the changing pharmacodynamics and pharmacokinetics of aging. Francis (1992) notes that the most common cause of delirium in elders is medication-related.

Many physical illnesses have psychiatric manifestations, often before physical signs and symptoms are apparent. The following situation encountered by a community mental health nurse illustrates the acute and chronic effects of medication on psychological and physiological conditions.

CASE EXAMPLE

Ms. C was an 80-year-old, white female who lived with her 83-year-old husband in a remote, rural area. She was referred by her primary physician at the regional community health clinic to the mental health outreach nurse for assistance in evaluation of her symptoms, to determine if she had dementia or depression, or a combination of both.

Ms. C had several chronic medical problems including COPD, osteoarthritis and rheumatoid arthritis with severe crippling of the fingers of her left hand, macular degeneration, hypertension, and bilateral mastectomies 5 years prior to referral. Her medication included Tri-ampterene/HCTZ 75/50 mg 1/2 qd; Premarin 0.3 mg 1 qd times 25 days, then 7 off; Theophylline 300 mg 1 bid; Sulindec 200 mg 1 bid after meals; Lorazepam 1 mg 1/2 bid prn; and Ventolin Inhaler 34 gm prn.

Upon evaluation by the clinical nurse specialist, Ms. C related that she had become very confused after arriving home from a visit to her son's home in Louisiana. Upon return, she was unable to remember details of her trip and was unable to perform ADLs. During the trip to Louisiana, Ms. C had visited the grave of her daughter, who had died 6 years previously. The couple strongly considered a relocation to Louisiana and had even looked at a home.

Ms. C became tearful when discussing her daughter's death. Additionally, Ms. C was very short of breath and since her return was unable to perform simple tasks without becoming anoxic and anxious. She was having difficulty sleeping at night, needing to sit in her recliner to breathe and sleep. Ms. C reported poor appetite, with significant weight loss of 15 pounds in the previous 3 months. She denied suicidal ideation and described her mood as more "jittery" and anxious than dysphoric. Ms. C scored very well on the mini–mental status exam, revealing no cognitive impairment.

Evaluation of this case indicated that Ms. C had suffered from a delirium episode shortly after her return from Louisiana and that she had no current indication of significant cognitive difficulties. These findings were shared with her primary physician, who revealed that Ms. C had likely had a drug-induced delirium during her return home from Louisiana due to a theophylline level three times normal. All of her workup for dementia including thyroids, B_{12}, and serum thyroid studies were within normal limits. A CT scan revealed "diffuse cerebral atrophy and periventricular white matter disease." These findings had been shared with Ms. C and her family, who felt that it must mean she had Alzhheimer's disease and that they needed to "prepare for the worst."

The geriatrician was consulted, and stated that these findings did not necessarily mean dementia in a patient of this age. The patient and family continued to need reassurance that she did not have Alzheimer's disease. The differential diagnosis after sorting through the findings was more indicative of a depression related to unresolved losses and current attempts to adjust to chronic disability. Two weeks following the initial assessment, Ms. C was started on oxygen after a visit to her primary physician. Some of her transient memory loss was undoubtedly related to hypoxia. She was subsequently able to perform more of her own ADLs, which had improved her mood, though she still had many losses to resolve. Counseling was instituted by the nurse to assist Ms. C in resolving her losses. ❦

A Case Management Approach to Chronic Illness

Nursing interventions in the home care setting are most frequently centered on relieving the effects of chronic illness. The nurse is more likely to enjoy a longitudinal relationship with the patient; accordingly, principles and interventions central to case management and home care nursing apply. Case management has as many definitions as there are practitioners. Case managment is formulated, defined, and practiced based on how the nurse is grounded professionally and theoretically and the setting in which he or she practices.

Clinical Case Management

Kanter (1989) developed a model of clinical case management which combines well with long-term care nursing practice. Clinical case management is concerned with all aspects of a patient's physical, social, and biochemical environment. The patient is assessed within the context of his or her environment. The goals of clinical case management are to facilitate the patient's physical survival, personal growth, community participation, and recovery from or adaptation to chronic illness (Kanter, 1989). Principles of clinical case management include continuity of care, knowledge of insurance benefits, titration of support and structure, use of the case management relationship, flexibility, and facilitating patient resourcefulness.

The use of the case management (or the nurse-patient) relationship is critical to care. It enables the nurse case manager to assess, plan, intervene, and evaluate treatment strategies most effectively. A comprehensive understanding of a patient often requires repeated personal contact, observation, reports from significant others, and a thorough review of prior functioning and treatment. The relationship may be the critical variable in preventing further decline. Without a trusting relationship, interventions will be unsuccessful. For example, a patient may be willing to take a specific medication or treatment based on his or her trust of the nurse case manager.

Applying Case Managment Principles

The principle of continuity of care reflects an appreciation of the patient's need for support and treatment over an extended period of time. Titration of support and structure enables the nurse to provide interventions at the appropriate level. For example, high levels of support may be needed posthospitalization, but may be limiting or intrusive if carried beyond the acute need. The goal of intervention is to support patient and family strengths and to compensate for disability. The principle of flexibility is important in order to be able to respond to a patient's changing functional needs over time. Interventions can then be tailored to the patient. The final principle of case management is the facilitation of patient resourcefulness. The nurse case manager assists the patient in learning how to negotiate his or her environment and manage the illness.

The assessment of the patient's financial and health care benefits is extremely important since most elders live on modest, fixed incomes. Most elders are eligible for and receive Medicare benefits. The burden of paying the additional 20% of health care costs, including medication, can quickly reduce their monthly income. The benefit packages of those elders who have retired on pensions may have included continued health care that covers the 20% costs that Medicare does not pay. For most elders, however, this additional health care coverage is nonexistent. As a case manager, the nurse assists the patient in locating alternative resources, such as state-supported health care (i.e., Medicaid), to assist in defraying health care expenses.

Stages of Nursing Case Management

The stages of nursing case management are identical to the nursing process. A complete assessment of the patient in the context of his or her environment forms the basis of care and intervention (Thompson-Heisterman, Smullen, & Abraham, 1992). A comprehensive understanding of a patient requires repeated personal contact, observation, reports from significant others, and a thorough review of prior functioning and treatment. Planning for care is done with the patient, formulating measurable goals so that interventions can be evaluated for effectiveness. Kanter (1989) addresses the need for case managers to be aware of the conflicting needs and unconscious motives of patients in order to formulate useful plans. Unless the conflicts are realized and made explicit, interventions and plans can often fail.

Interventions made by the case manager on behalf of patients are extensive, encompassing both the patient and his or her environment. These include linking the patient with community resources, consulting with families and other caregivers, maintaining and expanding social networks, collaboration with physicians and other care providers, and advocacy. Patient-centered interventions include intermittent, individual psychotherapy; instruction in independent living skills; and patient education. Crisis intervention is both patient- and environment-centered (Kanter, 1989).

Specific interventions in caring for elders in the community are elaborated by Snustad, Thompson-Heisterman, Neese, and Abraham (1993). Individual psychotherapy can be employed within the context of the case management relationship. The following clinical vignette illustrates this point.

CASE EXAMPLE

Ms. W is a 77-year-old, white, married female who was referred to the outreach nurse following a hospitalization for a left hip fracture. While hospitalized, Ms. W related that she was experiencing some of the same symptoms as did her son, who died of intestinal cancer the year before. Ms. W was experiencing difficulty swallowing, anorexia, and weight loss with no apparent physical cause.

Prior to his death, Ms. W had provided total care for her son and she had always been close to him. She never expressed nor resolved her grief regarding his death, though she was able to recognize the expression of her grief through the development of symptoms similar to his.

Brief expressive therapy was provided to Ms. W in her home by the clinical nurse specialist, with the focus on Ms. W's resolution of her grief regarding the loss of her son. Ms. W was able to make use of this intervention. During the 12-week therapy all of her symptoms abated and she gained back nearly all of the 18 pounds she had lost during the year after her son died. ❧

Encouraging Reminiscence

Elders can often benefit from reminiscing, both individually and in a reminiscence group. This technique is also referred to as life-review work. It facilitates completion of the final developmental task of adulthood by helping elders to resolve involutional grief and accept losses. Reminiscence allows the elder to relive positive accomplishments, define his or her identity, and give meaning to his or her life (Moore, 1992). Reminiscence, like brief therapy, can be useful to expiate guilt, exorcise problematic childhood identifications, resolve intrapsychic conflicts, reconcile family relationships, and transmit knowledge to those who follow (Moore, 1992).

Referral to Community Resources

A key component of community mental health nursing is the relationship that clinicians maintain with other community providers and agencies. To remain functionally independent, elders often require a wide range of coordinated services. If the nurse has contacts within community agencies, referral can be facilitated. Referrals to agencies on aging, which in many areas provide a wide range of services, are important. These services include home-bound meals, home safety assessments and equipment, socialization through senior nutrition sites, and friendly visitors. Linkages with social services for evaluation of entitlements, care aide assistance, fuel assistance, and transportation are useful.

Referrals may be instituted to hospice programs when indicated, as well as to the public health department, home health agencies, and outreach programs providing physical assessment and screening. Mental health referrals may be made to the local community mental health clinic and to support groups such as the Alzheimer's Disease and Related Disorders support group. Housing service referrals for repairs are useful for impaired and/or impoverished elderly no longer able to maintain their homes. The following case study illustrates some of the range of community services needed by elders and families.

CASE EXAMPLE

Ms. W was an 86-year-old, widowed, African-American female who lived with her 64-year-old daughter, EW. Ms. W had been severely demented for several years due to a stroke. Her daughter, EW, had been providing the care of her mother during those years. The caregiving, although very important to EW's self-concept, resulted in an admission to the behavioral medicine unit of a local hospital for major depression with psychotic features. During this time the mother was admitted to the hospital also, since there was no other available caregiver. Referrals were made to an outreach nurse to provide caregiver support posthospitalization.

After evaluation by the nurse, several referrals were made to various community services. Social services provided a care aide 3 days a week to assist EW in caring for her mother. The community mental health nurse facilitated EW's follow-up at the local mental health center by arranging a referral and helping to arrange transportation. Since she did not have a physician, a referral was made for the mother to the geriatric clinic.

The mental health nurse also referred the family for homebound meals, including liquid supplement, because the 86-year-old mother was unable to eat well due to the condition of her teeth. Her daughter was unable to obtain groceries regularly due to the lack of available transportation. She also feared leaving her mother even when the care aide was present. On a few occasions, the mental health nurse delivered the homebound meals. This was necessitated because the area agency for aging did not have a driver for the area of the county in which the family lived, and the home was nearly inaccessible due to its location on the side of a mountain.

During the summer, the mental health nurse contacted social services regarding obtaining a fan for the family; the home had no air conditioning and was uncomfortably warm. The nurse gave EW information about caring for her demented mother. The consulting psychiatrist made a home visit to evaluate Ms. W for low-dose haloperidol (Haldol) to help manage the hallucinations that precipitated her agitated behavior. ❧

INTERVENTIONS WITH CAREGIVERS

In the acute care setting, crisis intervention strategies are as appropriate for families and caregivers as they are for individual patients. The nursing principles are to strengthen the family coping mechanisms, mobilize additional supports, and help the family realistically appraise the acute care situation. Barry (1989) discusses the importance of assessing family coping mechanisms to determine if they are helping to resolve the crisis or contributing to it. Family dynamics may undermine the patient's coping ability. In such situations, the nurse needs to intervene and refer the family to a social worker, counselor, pastor, or other resource if he or she is not able to provide counseling to them.

Long-term Effects of Caregiving

Long-term care of elders at home is more common, complex, and long-lasting than ever before due to the increased longevity of elders and decreased acute hospital stays. Gaynor (1990) studied the long-term effects on caregivers of caring for a medically disabled patient and found that the negative effects of caregiving on the caregiver's health were greater if the task was prolonged. Caretakers who provided care for more than 2 years had more physician visits and more ill health than did cohorts who did not provide prolonged care. The younger women in the sample experienced more of a sense of psychological distress (burden), while those over age 55 suffered more somatic effects.

Citing an earlier study she conducted, Gaynor (1990) discovered that one-third of admissions to a hospital respite program were for reasons directly related to caregivers' health. High levels of hypertension and heart disease were common among this sample of female caregivers. Gaynor states that, while caregiving may be viewed as an obligation or a choice, it may be detrimental to the physical and emotional health of the caregiver. When assessing a geriatric patient, the nurse also assesses the caregiver's health and sense of burden, social supports, and knowledge of resources (Gaynor, 1990; Thompson-Heisterman, Smullen, & Abraham, 1992).

Caregiver Support and Intervention

Both individual and group counseling and support of caregivers are efficacious, although a study by Knight, Lutzky, and Macofsky-Urban (1993) revealed that individual psychosocial interventions to caregivers, along with respite support, was more effective than group intervention. Green (1991) describes a group intervention with adult daughters of aging mothers or parents in which the goals of intervention are to:

1. Normalize the experience
2. Give a historical context to the relationship
3. Come to terms with the caregiver's own aging
4. Obtain assistance
5. Separate the caregiver's own issues from those of the parents'
6. Become aware of choices
7. Gain knowledge of community resources

Caregiver education is an important intervention, as the caregiver is often the only factor between the elder and institutionalization. Caregivers need to be provided with information related to normal aging, management of the chronic illness, specific techniques for managing troublesome behaviors if the patient is cognitively impaired, and negotiating the health and social service care maze. This information is a small part of the vast amount of knowledge caregivers need to have in order to function most effectively. In addition to education and psychosocial support, modified family counseling or therapy may be indicated. The following case study illustrates this concept.

CASE EXAMPLE

Mr. G is a 77-year-old, African American, married male with a 10-year history of Parkinson's disease. He was referred to the outreach nurse following a hospitalization for delirium related to his antiparkinsonian medication and depression.

Mr. G and his wife had long-standing marital discord exacerbated by Mr. G's increasing dependence on her secondary to his Parkinson's disease. Mrs. G states that Mr. G has always questioned her marital fidelity and has been mistrustful of her, though she has given him no cause to do so. At times, since Mr. G has had Parkinson's disease and been on Sinemet, he has become delusional, accusing her of adultery and becoming pregnant by another man.

Though traditional couples therapy is not possible due to Mr. G's mental status, the clinical nurse specialist meets with the couple regularly in order to allow them to discuss openly their concerns regarding one another in a forum that can allow possible resolution of specific issues. Mrs. G has been able to discuss her embarrassment about his sharing his concerns with others outside the family and he has been able to share his anger about her using his money for household expenses. This counseling intervention has provided an outlet for the couple that helps diffuse the anger between them and enables Mr. G to receive the care he needs.

CONCLUSION

Working with the geriatric patient is both challenging and rewarding. The challenge comes from confronting one's personal stereotypes of aging and developing an eclectic perspective towards the aging process that does not discount the wisdom and growth potential of the geriatric patient. In caring for the older adult, the nurse must understand the normal process of aging and how the aging process impacts on the individual, physically and psychologically, in order for the nurse to be able to interpret symptoms of pathology.

This chapter has focused primarily on the normal aspects of aging and their consequences on the patient and the family. The rewarding aspect of caring for the elderly unfolds as the nurse discovers through the patient the wisdom and acceptance of the patient's life.

As with other individuals, assessment and interventions with the geriatric patient should always include the designated caregiver and/or family. Caring for an aging parent can be stressful for adult children who are balancing employment, children, social responsibilities, and spousal relationships.

BIBLIOGRAPHY

Abraham, I. L., Fox, J. M., Harrington, D. P., Snustad, D. G., Steiner, D. A., Abraham, L. H., & Brashear, H. R. (1990). A psychogeriatric nursing assessment protocol for use in multidisciplinary practice. *Archives of Psychiatric Nursing, 4*, 242–259.

American Association of Retired Persons. (1990). *A profile of older Americans*. Washington, DC: American Association of Retired Persons.

American Association of Retired Persons. (1992). *A profile of older Americans*. Washington, DC: American Association of Retired Persons.

Arpin, K., Fitch, M., Browne, G. B., & Corey, P. (1990). Prevalence and correlates of family dysfunction and poor adjustment to chronic illness in specialty clinics. *Journal of Clinical Epidemiology, 43*(4), 373–383.

Atchley, R. C. (1988). *Social forces and aging*. Belmont, CA: Wadsworth Publishing Co.

Averyt, A. C., Furst, S., & Daulton-Hummel, D. (1987). *Successful aging: A source book for older people and their families*. New York: Ballantine Books.

Baillie, V., Norbeck, J. S., & Barnes, L. A. (1988). Stress, social support, and psychological distress of family caregivers of the elderly. *Nursing Research, 37*(4), 217–222.

Barry, P. D. (1989). *Psychosocial nursing: Assessment and intervention* (2nd ed.). Philadelphia: J. B. Lippincott.

Berry, G. L., Zarit, S. H., & Rabatin, V. X. (1991). Caregiver activity on respite and nonrespite days: A comparison of two service approaches. *The Gerontologist, 31*(6), 830–835.

Birren, J. E., & Schaie, K. W. (1990). *Handbook of the psychology of aging* (3rd ed.). San Diego, CA: Academic Press, Inc.

Bornstein, R. (1992). Psychosocial development of the older adult. In C. S. Shuster & S. S. Ashburn (Eds.), *The process of human development: A holistic life span approach* (3rd ed.). Philadelphia: J. B. Lippincott.

Brodaty, M., & Gresham, M. (1992). Prescribing residential respite care for dementia: Effects, side-effects, indications, and dosage. *International Journal of Geriatric Psychiatry, 7*(5), 357–362.

Butler, R. N., Lewis, M., & Sunderland, T. (1991). *Aging and mental health: Positive psychosocial and biomedical approaches* (4th ed.). New York: Macmillan Publishing Company.

Chopra, D. (1993). *Ageless body, timeless mind: The quantum alternative to growing old*. New York: Harmony Books.

Comfort, A. (1990). *Say yes to old age: Developing a positive attitude towards aging*. New York: Mitchell Beazley Publishers.

Cumming, E., & Henry, W. E. (1961). *Growing old: The process of disengagement*. New York: Basic Books.

Delany, S. L., Delany, A. E., & Hearth, A. H. (1993). *Having our say: The Delany sisters' first 100 years*. New York: Kodansha America, Inc.

Donnelly, G. F. (1993). Chronicity: Concept and reality. *Holistic Nursing Practice, 8*(1), 1–7.

Eliopulos, C. (1993). *Gerontological nursing* (3rd ed.). Philadelphia: J. B. Lippincott.

Erikson, E. H. (1963). *Childhood and society*. New York: W. W. Norton.

Forbes, W. F., & Hirdes, J. P. (1993). The relationship between aging and disease: Geriatric ideology and myths of senility. *Journal of the American Geriatrics Society, 41*(11), 1267–1273.

Francis, J. (1992). Delirium in older patients. *Journal of American Geriatrics Society, 40*(3), 829–838.

Friedan, B. (1993). *The fountain of age*. New York: Simon & Schuster.

Fry, P. S. (1990). A factor analytic investigation of homebound elderly individual's concerns about death and dying, and their coping responses. *Journal of Clinical Psychology, 46*(6), 737–748.

Gaynor, S. E. (1990). The long haul: The effects of home care on caregivers. *Image, 22*(4), 208–212.

Green, C. P. (1991). Midlife daughters and their aging parents. *Journal of Gerontological Nursing, 18*(3), 35–39.

Harper, M. S. (1992). Home and community based services for the elderly. In K. C. Buckwalter (Ed.), *Geriatric mental health nursing: Current and future challenges*. Thorofare, NJ: Slack.

Havighurst, R., & Albrecht, R. (1953). *Older people*. New York: Longmans Green.

Hirsch, C. H., Davies, H. D., Boatwright, F., & Ochango, G. (1993). Effect of a nursing-home respite admission on veterans with advanced dementia. *Gerontologist, 33*(4), 523–528.

Jarvik, L., & Small, G. (1990). *Parentcare: A compassionate, commonsense guide for children and their aging parents*. New York: Crown Publishers.

Kane, R. L., Ouslander, J. G., & Abrass, J. B. (1989). *Essentials of Clinical Geriatrics* (2nd ed.). New York: McGraw-Hill.

Kanter, J. (1989). Clinical case management: Definition, principles, components. *Hospital and Community Psychiatry, 40*(4), 361–367.

Kiecolt-Glaser, J. K. (1992). Psychoneuroimmunology: Can psychological interventions modulate immunity? *Journal of Consulting Psychology, 60*(4), 569-575.

Knight, B. G., Lutzky, M. A., & Macofsky-Urban, F. (1993). A meta-analytic review of interventions for caregiver distress: Recommendations for future research. *Gerontologist, 33*(2), 240–248.

Lamm, B., Dungan, J. M., & Hiromoto, B. (1991). Long-term lifestyle management. *Clinical Nurse Specialist, 5*(4), 182–188.

Lane, C., & Hobfoll, S. E. (1992). How loss affects anger and alienates potential supporters. *Journal of Consulting and Clinical Psychology, 60*(6), 935–942.

Lazarus, L. (1988). *Essentials of geriatric psychiatry*. New York: Springer.

Lipowski, Z. B. (1989). Delirium in the elderly patient. *New England Journal of Medicine, 320*, 578–582.

Mezey, M. D., Rauekhorst, L. H., & Stokes, S. A. (1993). *Health assessment of the older individual* (2nd ed.). New York: Springer Publishing Company.

Moore, B. G. (1992). Reminiscing therapy: A clinical nurse specialist intervention. *Clinical Nurse Specialist, 6*(3), 170–173.

Oxman, T. E., & Berkman, L. F. (1990). Assessment of social relationships in elderly patients. *International Journal of Psychiatry in Medicine, 20*(1), 65–84.

Pruchno, R. A., Blow, S. C., & Smyer, M. A. (1984). Life events and interdependent lives. *Human Development, 27*(2), 31-41.

Rappaport, H., Fossler, R. J., Bross, L. S., & Gilden, D. (1993). Future time, death anxiety, and life purpose among older adults. *Death Studies, 17*(4), 369–379.

Reed, P. G. (1991). Spirituality and mental health in older adults: Extant knowledge for nursing. *Family and Community Health, 14*(2), 14–25.

Robinson, K. (1990). The relationships between social skills, social support, self-esteem and burden in adult caregivers. *Journal of Advanced Nursing, 15*(7), 788–795.

Schneider, E. L., & Rowe, J. W. (1990). *Handbook of the biology of aging* (3rd ed.). San Diego, CA: Academic Press, Inc.

Schultz, R., & Ewen, R. B. (1988). *Adult development and aging: Myths and emerging realities.* New York: Macmillan Publishing Co.

Small, N. R. (1994). Importance of self-care among the elderly. *Geriatric Care, 26*(2), 8–9.

Snustad, D., Thompson-Heisterman, A. A., Neese, J. B., & Abraham, I. L. (1993). Mental health outreach to rural elderly: Service delivery to a forgotten risk group. *Clinical Gerontologist, 14*(1), 95–111.

Strawbridge, W. J., & Wallhagen, M. I. (1991). Impact of family conflict on adult child caregivers. *Gerontologist, 31*(6), 770–777.

Stuifbergen, A. K. (1990). Patterns of functioning in families with a chronically ill parent: An exploratory study. *Research in Nursing and Health, 13*(1), 35–44.

Taylor, S. E. (1989). *Positive illusions: Creative self-deceptions and the healthy mind.* New York: Basic Books.

Temple, A., & Fawdry, K. (1992). Kings theory of goal attainment: Resolving filial caregiver role strain. *Journal of Gerontological Nursing, 18*(3), 11–15.

Thompson-Heisterman, A. A., Smullen, D. E., & Abraham, I. L. (1992). Psychogeriatric nursing assessment. In K. C. Buckwalter (Ed.), *Geriatric mental health nursing: Current and future challenges.* Thorofare, NJ: Slack.

Tobin, S. S. (1991). *Personhood in advanced old age: Implications for practice.* New York: Springer Publishing Company.

Trice, L. B. (1990). Meaningful life experience to the elderly. *Image, 22*(4), 248–251.

U. S. Bureau of the Census. (1990). *The need for personal assistance with everyday activities: Recipients and caregivers.* Current Population Report Series No. 19. Washington, DC: U. S. Government Printing Office.

Van Auken, E. (1991). Crisis intervention. Elders awaiting placement in an acute care facility. *Journal of Gerontological Nursing, 17*(11), 30–33.

Wagnild, G., & Young, H. M. (1990). Resilience among older women. *Image, 22*(4), 252–255.

Whitbourne, S. K. (1985). *The aging body: Physiological changes and psychological consequences.* New York: Springer-Verlag.

PART VI

APPLYING
PSYCHOSOCIAL
NURSING
PRINCIPLES TO
NURSES' SELF-CARE

The final chapter in this book is for nurses themselves. There is stress in caring for chronically or critically ill human beings who are reacting to some of the most frightening experiences they will ever know. The need for constant precision in dealing with patients and medications, the pressures of administrative responsibilities and changing policies, and sheer physical exhaustion also lead to stress for nurses.

Nurses are expected to focus constantly upon the needs of others in their work. They may forget that their own needs can be provided for, and that there are ways to deal with the everyday and exceptional stresses of nursing. This chapter is written for nurses everywhere in the hope that it will provide for them some of the care they so readily give to others.

CHAPTER 30

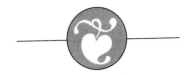

Coping With Stress in Nursing Practice

Ann Robinette

Stress is a difficult, complex topic. Stress impinges on many aspects of professional nursing, some more widely reported than others. Among the least discussed stressors in nursing are the "suffering" aspects defined by Benner & Wrubel (1989). These are the stressful parts of caregiving that have no obvious solutions or quick fixes. The complexity of "suffering," our own and that of others, can make us feel more helpless and inadequate than any other stressor.

As described in Chapter 6, *stress* is the response to an external or internal demand or stressor. A stress response can be manifested physiologically or psychologically. Stressors are a necessary and important part of life; they challenge us to do our best, to perform optimally. For example, before taking an exam, stress can create an energetic, hyperalert state, a positive stress response which can motivate and stimulate. Stress can, however, be harmful.

Hans Selye's (1978) classic work on stress, and the more recent work of Lazarus and Folkman (1984), both are helpful models in understanding how stressors affect us and what factors can help to mitigate them. Concrete examples of application of these theories will be presented later in this chapter under the discussion of specific stress management strategies.

THE STRESSORS OF NURSING PRACTICE

Lewis and Levy (1982) describe the "caregiving" experience as "filled with complex expectations, along with identified and unidentified stresses, disappointments, and gratifications" (p.158). Focusing on *caregiving* is the key to understanding the stresses of nursing practice. "Caring is a basic way of being in the world—caring sets up what counts as stressful and what coping options are available" (Benner & Wrubel, 1989, p. xi). Most of the stress management literature today, based on modern technological self-understanding, does not accurately portray stress and coping in health and illness or in nursing practice. Health, illness, and caregiving stressors can be complex and multidimensional.

SOURCES OF STRESS

In her classic work, Marshall (1980) presents one of the clearest pictures of stresses among

Patricia Barry: *Psychosocial Nursing:
Care of Physically Ill Patients and Their Families*, 3rd ed.
© 1996 Lippincott–Raven Publishers

nurses. She outlines sources of stress and their effects on the nurse: the environment; uncertainty and responsibility within the job; the heavy responsibility of the role; the relationship with patients and their families; the relationship with physicians; nursing's low status; immediate working relationships with colleagues; the need to fulfill others' expectations and those of the organization; and conflicts between work and personal life. Marshall's major concern is the personal cost to the nurse of providing both medical services and emotional comfort and support to patients, pitted against the nurse's own need for nourishment.

Distinct Features of Nursing Stress

Marshall (1980, p. 20) notes three "distinct features that set nursing apart as a special case in the stress literature." The first involves "primary task aspects," the core requirements of the nursing role. Nurses must be cognitively and emotionally aware of the condition of their patients.

Lazarus (1966) believes that the critical psychological process that defines stress is the perception of threat. The nursing professional can experience stress as a result of perceiving that his or her ability to heal is on "trial" while caring for a patient (Marshall, 1980, p. 20). Menzies (1970) found that nurses' main coping technique for managing stressful stimuli was avoidance, causing repression of emotions and leading to secondary stressful effects. Consequently, both the primary task and the means to manage it become stressful to nurses (Marshall, 1980).

The second distinct feature of nursing stress is the fact that nursing is highly visible work that produces unequivocal success or failure. The third feature is the expectation that nurses should *not* be or act stressed, for their co-workers' and patients' sake, as well as their own.

From this evidence, Marshall (1980) concludes, "The nurses' role is therefore implicitly and chiefly one of handling stress. The nurse is a focus for the stress of the patient, relatives, and doctors as well as her own" (p. 21). All of these stresses can erode the nurse's spirit.

PERSONALITY CHARACTERISTICS OF NURSES

There are personality characteristics of nurses that not only make them "good" nurses, but also contribute to their stress. Any strength becomes a liability if overused or if used too unconsciously.

Perfectionism and Commitment

Some of these characteristics include perfectionism and an extremely strong sense of dedication and commitment. For example, a nurse who has already worked a 48-hour week with her critically ill, neutropenic patients agrees to work a double shift because there is "nobody else available." In this situation, a strong sense of dedication and commitment becomes a liability.

Too often, nursing professionals do not say "no" or set limits on what they will do because of fear of the reaction of others. Will my head nurse get mad at me? Will "they" not like me? Will "they" say I am remiss in my duty? Will "they" think less of me? An overdeveloped sense of responsibility may create unrealistic goals and self-expectations wherein the person takes responsibility for actions beyond the self.

Self-Denial

When a child grows up in an environment where expectations are focused on meeting another's needs (usually a mother's and/or father's), rather than learning to be in touch with, identify, and then meet his or her own needs, this individual can become an expert in meeting others' needs. There is much about this dynamic that works well for nursing practice. However, this dynamic becomes negative when nurses focus on others' needs and neglect their own needs. Many nurses feel guilty or "selfish" for taking time for themselves—to eat lunch, take a break, or focus on meeting personal or spiritual needs, such as reading a book alone or exploring a special interest. Some have learned self-denial so well that there is no awareness of personal wants or needs.

Linda Arnold (1990) says, "Most nurses never went to 'want school.'" There are lots of needy people out there and nurses are "dying to take care of them" (Snow & Willard, 1989). Ignoring or denying personal needs sends them underground where they emerge at the most inopportune time, usually unconsciously and to the detriment of the individual. Nurses cannot be everyone's filling station when their own tanks are empty. Personal needs must be acknowledged and met to ensure that the filling station has fuel when it is needed.

A Need for Control

Many in nursing have a high need for control. This is a valuable trait when administering high-dose chemotherapy or extremely toxic antibiotics, or when monitoring that patient on the ventilator. It is not a useful trait, however, when applied to the newly admitted patient who is a successful lawyer frightened by the unfamiliar environment and her impending surgery, and who communicates this fear by refusing to do things on the "hospital's schedule." The nurse, who needs to be in control, is likely to get into a power struggle with this patient, causing the nurse stress.

Some of the nurse's stress from this struggle is avoidable. A nurse caring for such a patient must recognize that it is the patient who needs to be in control. In order to be therapeutic for the patient, the nurse should resist being lured into such a power struggle. In addition, the nurse should resist taking on the burden of feeling responsible for everybody and everything, and accept responsibility only for personal actions. Narrowing this range of responsibility contributes to a more consistent sense of personal competence.

PERSONAL AND PROFESSIONAL BOUNDARIES

While caring is an essential ingredient of healing, overidentification with patients and their families can compromise judgment. When working with the medically ill, the limits between professional and personal boundaries can become blurred, allowing personal feelings and behaviors to override professional ones.

Physically caring for people, regardless of setting, is a very intimate experience which engenders many warm, close feelings in both the patient and the caregiver. Many of us do this work to get exactly that kind of gratification, connection, and meaning. It becomes problematic when the caregiver doesn't have "a life" in addition to nursing work; nursing becomes the caregiver's "life." The dynamic of putting others first comes into play here. Table 30-1 illustrates the differences between personal and professional relationships.

Struggling with professional/personal relationship conflicts does not eliminate the associated stress. It does provide awareness that there are guidelines for appropriate behavior which, if followed, will reduce the nurse's stress.

There are two crucial points to keep in mind:

1. Be conscious of your personal feelings for a patient and/or the family and monitor how those feelings are affecting your patient care.
2. Place the patient's needs first in the work setting.

In psychotherapy, the goal is to help people *get* better, not to make them *feel* better. The same is true for nursing. The key is to avoid being seduced by both the nurse's and the patient's wish to have the patient feel better in the moment.

CARING FOR DIFFERENT PATIENT POPULATIONS

Caregivers face different stresses from different illnesses, different patient populations, and the care required by different groups.

In a research study about oncology caregivers, Herschbach (1992) hypothesized that oncology nurses and doctors had more stress than their nononcology colleagues. Analysis of his research data revealed that oncology caregivers do not have *more* stress; rather, they experience stress from a different cause than that of cardiac, intensive care, and surgical caregivers. Institutional factors, lack of staff, and inadequate supplies were the causes of stress for the cardiac, intensive care, and surgical care-

Table 30-1
Personal vs. Professional Intimacy

Aspect of Intimacy	Personal Intimacy	Professional Intimacy
Goal	Closeness itself	Healing
Relationship	Symmetrical (give and take)	Complementary (teacher to pupil)
Range	Unlimited	Circumscribed (serve client according to role)
Duration	Unlimited	Circumscribed (until set time)
Behavior	Spontaneous	Disciplined (do right thing whether we want to or not)
Contract	None	Customary (signed agreement, understand services rendered)
Sex	Yes	No
Confidentiality	Loose	Tight
Legal Accountability	No	Yes

From Racy, J., in Friedman, N. & Huls, J. (1991). Intimacy: The cornerstone of caring. *American Journal of Hospice and Palliative Care, 8*(2), 31–5, 44. Used with permission.

givers studied. In the oncology settings, emotional involvement and self-doubt caused stress.

Similarly, bone marrow transplant (BMT) nurses who work in laminar air flow (LAF) cope with the tremendous dependency of patients in LAF, in addition to the isolation that LAF imposes. All of this intensifies the already "absurdly stressful" context of the BMT treatment regime.

It is a common phenomenon that those who care for members of discriminated-against and disenfranchised groups take on the characteristics and feelings of those for whom they care (Benner & Wrubel, 1989). This translates into a major source of stress for those caregivers.

For example, the psychiatric emergency services staff of a large metropolitan hospital daily treats the most severely mentally ill and the most destitute and impoverished of all psychiatric patients. Because this hospital is chronically short-staffed as well, staff members are constantly asked to take on more responsibility with constantly dwindling resources. Even though they deliver excellent care under the circumstances, the staff members are often angry at the system, suspicious of authority, and, frequently, bleak about the future. These feelings are also characteristic of their patient population.

PRACTICE SETTINGS

Another major source of stressors for the nurse professional is the changing practice arena. As the economic pressure on health care has increased, many patients whose acuity made them appropriate for ICUs are now cared for on medical-surgical units. Those patients who were previously on floors in the general hospital now receive their care from home health care providers. These changes have placed new care demands on the nurses in these areas and, consequently, created new tensions. It is well documented that hospital nurses are having to care for "sicker patients quicker."

Stressors of Home Care Nursing

A review of relevant literature indicates that the caregiving experience of home health care nurses includes these specifics:

- Complex and extensive paperwork on which reimbursement depends (Harris, 1988: Monica, 1988; Morrissey-Ross, 1988)
- High expectations of productivity, with reimbursement based on a per visit basis (Harris, 1988)

- A sicker population of patients including more elderly, more chronically ill, and more terminally ill (Harris, 1988)

The sicker population exposes these caregivers more frequently to suffering which may not be alleviated (Benner & Wrubel, 1989). Handy (1988) and Volk (1988) note that high-technology home care requires the competence to deliver such complex nursing care and provokes anxiety about delivering such care in the home setting, increasing stress.

The home care setting lacks the structured, external boundaries typical of traditional health care (i.e., the hospital or outpatient setting), thereby denying the caregiver a certain sense of security associated with that structure. The patient and family, rather than the health care providers, define and control the environment. Resources usually available to the caregiver are missing. The home care environment demands that the caregivers use their own internal boundaries to define the situation, or be overwhelmed by it (Hillman, 1986).

The unique setting and the autonomy of home care nursing practice contributes to these nurses' isolation from other professional caregivers (Hillman, 1986). These issues easily lead to feelings of overinvolvement with patients and their families, of being too responsible for too much, and a feeling that patients and families are too dependent on the caregiver (Benner & Wrubel, 1989). In addition, the caregiver is exposed to urban dangers: increased poverty, filth, homelessness, violence, and drug use. These factors not only make delivery of urban home care risky, but create added stress.

STRESS RESPONSES

Stress in nursing practice can be manifested in physical, emotional, or intellectual responses, as detailed in Table 30-2. Each individual's response to stress is unique. Some responses may be learned, others may be neurobiologically based.

For example, the nurse who blames herself when a situation becomes chaotic and out-of-control may do so because she watched her mother accept blame when situations became chaotic at home. The nurse also may have inherited her father's sensitive GI tract, and may experience diarrhea and stomach cramps when stressed. This nurse might learn to manage her stress response by recognizing her personal stress signals and accepting them as cues to initiate a stress reduction regime.

STRESS MANAGEMENT STRATEGIES

Benner & Wrubel (1989) draw on the work of Lazarus and his colleagues to offer this definition of stress: "Stress is defined as the disruption of meanings, understanding, and smooth function so that harm, loss, or challenge is experienced, and sorrow, interpretation, or new skill acquisition is required" (p. 59). They further state that "coping is not an antidote to stress," but rather what one does with the disruption (p. 62).

The goals of stress management strategies include eliminating those stresses that can be eliminated; mastering the stress that cannot be eliminated; or developing techniques for recognition and modification of our own stress responses.

Stress vs. Suffering

Before stress management strategies can be effectively implemented, it is important to distinguish between stress and suffering. When asked to free associate to the word *stress,* typical responses might include lack of time, not enough staff, not getting the requested time off, too many conflicting demands, too much to do, not enough or the lack of the right equipment, and lack of direction from above. Free associations to the word *suffering* might include pain; untimely deaths (e.g., those of children or young adults); causing pain with medical/nursing treatments; birth defects; homelessness; addictions/substance abuse; AIDS; downsizing.

Associations to the word *stress* are about loss of control, poor management, overload, a sense of time urgency—bureaucratic-type stressors. On the other hand, free associations to the word *suffering* often are concerned with meaningful losses and things which pose a threat to significance (Benner & Wrubel, 1989).

Table 30-2
Effects of Stress

Physical	Emotional	Intellectual
• constant state of fatigue • sleep disturbance • change in food, alcohol, drug, and/or cigarette intake • changes in physical appearance • repetitive accidents • change in sexual behavior • exacerbation of physical illness • muscular pain (e.g., neck and lower back)	• angry outbursts • irritability • feelings of worthlessness, helplessness • depression • isolation from others • self-criticism • feelings of guilt • inability to identify and express feelings • difficulty forming and maintaining intimate relationships • martyrdom • numbing feelings through addictions • cynical and negative feelings towards patients, families, and co-workers • whining	• forgetfulness • preoccupation • mathematical and grammatical errors • lack of concentration • lack of attention to details • denial • assuming responsibility for the behavior and feelings of others • indecisiveness • difficulty setting limits • lying when telling the truth would be easier • past, rather than future, orientation • diminished productivity • impaired problem solving • resistance to change • change to abstract and analytical thinking • feelings of powerlessness • breakdown in effective communication • strict adherence to rules rather than considering the uniqueness of others • objectifying patients (e.g., "the new leukemic") • pessimism • uncooperativeness • tardiness or absenteeism

Cunningham, M. (1992). Professional issues in cancer care. In J. Clark & R. McGee (Eds.). *Core curriculum of oncology nursing*. Philadelphia: W. B. Saunders.

The Limits of Problem Solving

It is important to distinguish between stress and suffering because the strategies needed to cope with the stress associations are different from the strategies needed to cope with suffering. Using the same coping strategies to manage both issues denies these differences.

Strategies appropriate for the stress associations are frequently problem-solving oriented. The popularized view of stress is of a modern-day folk disease which excludes normal meaningful losses and in which scientific findings are enmeshed in popular self-understanding and interpretation of illness (Benner & Wrubel, 1989). This is *not* to negate the value of problem solving for certain situations and issues. However, problem solving is a limited strategy and is not productive when applied to issues identified as causing suffering.

The use of problem solving to address the causes of suffering may be too simplistic.

When problem-solving techniques are used to manage suffering, anguish levels about these issues do not lessen. Stress levels may even *increase,* causing further distress. Diminished spirits and feelings of failure provide additional stress.

Solutions to manage the stress of human suffering include strategies such as engagement and involvement, increased control, and distance—strategies that promote discovering meaning in the midst of pain, suffering, loss, growth, and change. It may mean enduring while maintaining one's concerns and meanings (Benner & Wrubel, 1989).

CASE EXAMPLE

In the 1989 Loma Prieta earthquake, the Marina district in San Francisco was badly damaged. A number of men and women who lived there either died tragically or suffered devastating losses.

In one family, the husband had just kissed his 43-year-old wife and 5-month-old son goodbye and was biking to a nearby store when the earthquake began. His wife was coming down the stairs of their two-story house when the first rolls of that 7.1 (on the Richter scale) earthquake were felt. She was unable to keep her balance, fell forward and the baby flew out of her arms. The wife's shoulder was dislocated, but more tragically, her young son was killed by the fall. The wife was admitted to a nearby private teaching hospital.

All of the immediate participants were severely traumatized—the wife by her own injuries and the loss of her baby. She felt extremely guilty for the baby's death and blamed herself for not being able to hold on to him tighter and protect him from harm. All efforts to dissuade her from this point of view were futile. Although clearly stunned by the loss of his child, her husband also felt guilty that he had escaped injury.

Interestingly enough, the surgical nurses were stressed by caring for this family. They felt guilty as well. They, too, had lived through the same earthquake, but had not suffered the same level of physical or emotional losses. They wondered why nothing bad had happened to them, why these bad things had happened to their patient and her family, and how to make sense of it all.

In working with this nursing staff, the goal was to help them recognize that there were no easy answers to these questions. What *was* helpful was sharing their concerns with one another, recognizing they were not alone in their feelings, and hearing how others made sense of the events. This was accomplished through a support group on the unit. ❧

SPECIFIC STRATEGIES

Social Support

The concept of social support is addressed in a model by Norbeck (1988). Dr. Norbeck cautions that the model is "over-simplified, but shows that stress is related to health outcomes and that social support buffers the effect of stress on health. Social support also has direct effects on stress and on health outcomes" (p. 86). There is disagreement among researchers regarding the exact components of social support.

For purposes of this discussion, Cobb's (1976) classic definition of social support will be used: "information leading the subject to believe that he is cared for and loved, esteemed and a member of a network of mutual obligations" (p. 300). In addition, those identified categories of behaviors that are theorized to be supportive (Barrera & Ainlay, 1983) are used:

Material aid—providing tangible materials in the form of money and other physical objects

Behavioral assistance—sharing of tasks

Intimate interaction—traditional, nondirective counseling behavior such as listening and expressing esteem, caring, and understanding

Guidance—offering advice, information, or instruction

Feedback—providing individuals with input about their behavior, thoughts, or feelings

Positive social interaction—engaging in social interactions for fun and relaxation

One coping strategy effective in managing the stress of human suffering, as illustrated in the case example above, is the use of social support in a group context. Pearlin and Aneshensel (1986) distinguish four functions of coping and social supports:

1. Prevention of the stressful situation through the acquisition of the "wisdom" that the group imparts to the members, both in the ability to anticipate problems and, once recognized, to adopt avoidance strategies.
2. Alteration of the stressful situation through exercising instrumental versus expressive support (i.e., the giving of material help, assistance, or information).
3. Changing the meaning of a stressful situation through the interaction in a group. Shared ways of defining situations, which are natural byproducts in groups, help an individual change the way he or she assesses a particular event. The group legitimizes and reinforces the perception as threatening, or helps reshape it as ordinary, trivial, ignorable. Also, groups mediate the stress process by helping the individual maintain a positive self-concept in the face of hardship (Pearlin et al., 1981). "The support group helps the individual maintain self-esteem and a sense of mastery by interpreting the stressful situation as one that does not reflect negatively on these prized elements of self. This is a crucial defense against stress" (p. 423).
4. Management of the symptoms of stress so they do not overwhelm the individual. Using the Lazarus and Folkman model (1984), this is emotion-focused coping rather than problem-focused coping. Validating the individual's response to stress is one way that social support mitigates the symptoms. In the support group, the individual can do things to relieve tension.

ADMINISTRATIVE AND ORGANIZATIONAL INTERVENTIONS

Administrative interventions that can be implemented to manage nursing stress include adequate staffing and reasonable work loads; adequate supplies and functioning equipment; minimal noise and crowding in the environment; rotating assignments for difficult cases; providing a less stressful "get-away" place for staff; regular staff meetings to deal with organizational matters; well-defined administrative policies; good orientation for new staff; inservice education; opportunities for professional growth; recognition of skilled performance; variation in assignments to prevent boredom; special benefits such as privileges, pay, or vacation; and the planning of social activities (Caldwell & Weiner, 1981; Marshall, 1980; Norbeck, 1985). The above interventions are examples of all three categories of stress management strategies: elimination, mastering, and modifying responses.

A STRESS-REDUCING PROCESS FOR THE INDIVIDUAL

The first step in a stress-reducing process is to believe that we have the right to take care of ourselves, and that doing so is not bad or selfish. From this belief comes a commitment to self-care.

Conducting a Self-Assessment

Once this commitment to self-care is a reality for the individual, a self-assessment must be made. What are our needs? Motivations? Goals? Who and what make up our support system? How do we respond to stress? Do we show physical symptoms? What are they? How do we react emotionally? How is our intellect affected? What is our communication style? Are we passive, aggressive, assertive? Or, like most people, do we use a combination of all three, depending on the situation? How does our communication style work for us? What about our time management skills? Always behind? Or are we driven by so many deadlines that it's hard to tell? How do we manage conflict? And lastly, what are the sources of our stress?

Part of the assessment process involves reflection on the possible answers to these questions. From this appraisal, we can begin to develop a stress-reduction care plan.

Developing a Self-Care Plan

The first step to effective self-care is to take excellent physical care of ourselves. We need to eat well-balanced meals, get a moderate amount of exercise, and get enough sleep, all on a consistent basis. This is the foundation which helps us manage the stressors in our lives. The other crucial piece is to "follow your bliss" as Joseph Campbell (1988) says. We must do what we love; no amount of stress reduction techniques can make up for the stress of doing what we hate.

There are other self-care strategies and approaches for stress management to consider. It is important to have as many choices and resources as possible to help cope with stress. If a carpenter only has one tool—a hammer—he can only hammer a nail. If he has a whole toolbox full of tools, he can build a house. We all need to have "full toolboxes," allowing us to be more successful in building our own customized stress-reduction homes.

What are some activities that we might include in this self-care plan? Increased physical activity; engaging more in social activity; becoming open to emotionally intimate relationships in our personal life; establishing realistic goals and expectations; identifying and working to eliminate irrational beliefs; seeking professional counseling; practicing relaxation techniques; maintaining a personal journal to record and analyze feelings and thoughts; taking responsibility when appropriate; delegating when appropriate; acquiring new skills through education, such as time management, dealing with difficult people, and conflict resolution techniques.

Administrative Options

In addition, there are options that administrators can implement to help staff deal with stress. Nurses themselves can advocate in the work setting for stress-reducing options such as support groups; balanced nurse-patient ratios that support quality patient care; employee benefit packages that provide for vacations, mental health days, and reimbursement for professional counseling; recognition and financial incentives that reward quality performance; the establishment of an ethics committee; participatory decision making; and increased multidisciplinary collaboration.

THE IDEAL VS. THE REALITY VIEW

In their book, *The Primacy of Caring* (1989), Benner and Wrubel talk about a technique to manage the stress of a situation that cannot be eliminated. If used enough, the technique can become an attitude, a way to approach the world, and a way to deal with stress. This technique is based on the ideal vs. the reality view.

The *ideal view* is based on standards and ideals which can be important for goal setting, providing us with guidance. A person searches for ideal, preconceived choices and views a situation only in relation to prespecified standards. Consequently, behavior, actions, and outcomes almost never measure up, because no one and nothing is ideal or perfect. Instead, behaviors, actions, and outcomes show up as deficient. In actuality, clinging to the ideal view may present obstacles, clouding recognition of the real possibilities in a situation.

In the *reality view,* a person looks for possibilities inherent in a specific situation, allowing him or her to view the situation as a field of possibilities and constraints. Shifting perspectives opens up new avenues for action; it's a more flexible strategy. This view decreases the sense of disappointment and powerlessness. Looking for the possible (rather than the *im*possible) is a good antidote for reality shock. The reality view involves asking questions that open up a world of possibility: What can be done now, in the meantime (before the ideal can be realized)? Is there another way to achieve the same end (other than the ideal)? Is the end in sight (the ideal) the most worthy?

We break out of the "less than ideal" deadlock by asking ourselves these questions and truly heeding the answers. The other key to having the reality view become an attitude and not merely a technique is this: We have to recognize the results as *achievements,* not compromises. Most people "settle" for the reality view, but still feel cheated and on some level inadequate for doing so. The "reality" is far from that. This case example illustrates the point.

CASE EXAMPLE

Ms. W, a psychiatric nurse with nearly 20 years experience, found herself in need of a short-term, flexible hours, staff position during her graduate school experience. She took "the worst job in my whole career" on a geroneuropsych unit in a 100-year-old, major metropolitan county hospital. The unit was the most run-down and neglected in the whole hospital, probably reflecting the status of its patients (remember the earlier point about this?). The majority of the staff were medical-surgical nursing staff, not psychiatric. The patients were poor and mostly without resources. Since it was a short-term job, Ms. W decided she could live with it.

One night, she was assigned to the unit's most refractory and stumping patient, Mr. G. He was a man in his early 60s who was admitted after becoming incontinent of stool on his wife's favorite Persian rug. He did not talk, had waxy facies, and could move only with assistance and then only to and from his wheelchair and the bed. He continued to be incontinent of stool and urine. Several complete work-ups revealed no physical cause for his behaviors and no psychiatric explanation why Mr. G acted as he did. Consequently, Mr. G was to be transferred the next day to a long-term care facility, since his wife could not meet his needs at home.

Ms. W decided to make his last evening on the unit a good one. It had been many years since she had been a staff nurse on an inpatient unit and she was determined to show she hadn't lost her "stuff." Her colleagues had a thorough care plan to manage Mr. G's incontinence. Ms. W introduced herself to Mr. G in his four-bed room, and explained how she as his nurse would be following the prescribed care plan to help him not be incontinent. Because Mr. G did not speak or respond nonverbally, Ms. W told him she assumed his assent to the plan.

Ms. W left. On her return, she helped Mr. G into his wheelchair to go into dinner. At that time she realized he had wet himself in the interim and she set about cleaning him up. Her

conversation with him swept away any possibility that this untoward event would happen again on her shift that night and she vowed silently not to get angry with him, even though she was disappointed that the "plan" hadn't worked so far. She was sure Mr. G didn't really sense how distressed she was.

The dining room in that cheerless place was on the unit, but at the far end of the hall. When she arrived with Mr. G, all other patients were already seated and eating. As she wheeled Mr. G into place, a voluminous yellow puddle appeared under his chair and spread out under the other tables. Ms. W was aghast. It was okay to inconvenience himself, but to ruin the others' dinner by this inappropriate action was unconscionable. You would have thought Ms. W had urinated on the floor herself.

She left him to eat dinner in his soggy trousers while she mopped the urine up from the floor. She was angry now, but highly conflicted; her anger didn't fit with the image she had of how she should feel toward a patient, particularly one as helpless as Mr. G. However, at the moment, she felt he was acting pretty passive-aggressive and she did not like it one bit.

After dinner, Ms. W brought Mr. G back to his room, determined even more to try to reinstate the care plan (the ideal view). As she helped him out of his wheelchair, the odor of feces assailed her. That was it! Not only was he still wet from his accident, Mr. G had now soiled himself as well. Ms. W lost it in front of Mr. G and two of his roommates: "I am so angry and frustrated with you! I know you can't like soiling yourself, but I don't know what else to do with you! I tried to follow the plan, but that hasn't worked. I feel so helpless."

At that point in her tirade, Ms. W noticed a lone tear rolling down Mr. G's face. She knew then she was the worst nurse that had ever practiced. She immediately began to apologize. "I am so sorry, Mr. G, I didn't mean to lose my temper and yell at you. I know you are *not* doing this on purpose; sometimes it just feels like you are. I am sorry I upset you. I am upset, too." And with that she cleaned him up and put him to bed, as they were both exhausted from the evening's encounters. However, as she put the side rail up, she hung the urinal, saying, "I'll just leave this right here in case you need it (that was part of the plan).

Don't worry if you wet yourself again, I'll be glad to clean you up. Good night." And she left to tend to her other patients.

About 45 minutes later, the light in Mr. G's 4-bed room went off. When Ms. W went to check, Mr. G's urinal was full of urine. Ms. W was astounded, asking "How did this happen?" Though another patient was in the room, Mr. G had no explanation either. Ms. W decided that since she was trying not to take responsibility for Mr. G. wetting himself, she probably shouldn't take credit for him not wetting himself. However, she was very pleased and told Mr. G so.

It was then that Mr. M (Mr. G's roommate) turned to Ms. W and said, "You are such a good nurse." "Me?!" Ms. W exclaimed, "Why do you say that, I feel like I'm a terrible nurse tonight." Mr. M said, "It's obvious you care about us and what happens to us." And that's when Ms. W understood that she didn't always have to do the *ideal* thing; what mattered was that she cared about her patients and tried to help them as best she could. In doing so, she conveyed her willingness to struggle with them about their difficult issues. They understood she wasn't perfect; neither were they. But they felt and sorely appreciated the caring her willingness conveyed. And in that place, with those people, that clearly was an accomplishment, not remotely a compromise. ❧

Viewing situations this way can release us from some of the most stressful aspects of our caregiving. It also serves as a challenge to see how creative we can be in the face of situations far less than ideal. It helps to recognize that "caring is a profound act of hope" (White, 1986). This is true for the professional nurse as well as for patients.

CONCLUSION

The stresses inherent in nursing practice are complex. It's no simple task to figure out coping strategies for all of these complex stressors. By recognizing the many causes for feeling stressed, each nursing professional can begin to recognize that the solution is a process.

There is no "one" or "right" way to cope with stress. Rather, managing stress is an ongo-

ing process, a lifelong endeavor, that changes and evolves as we do. By valuing and acquiring as many tools and strategies as we can, we will be able to tailor a plan to cope with any particular stressful situation. And, as we successfully deal with day-to-day stressors, our overall ability to cope with stress improves.

Dealing well with stress and taking good care of ourselves has a positive impact on our work. As we take better care of ourselves, the pleasure we get from our work is no longer obscured by all the suffering and less-than-ideal situations that we encounter. We continue to practice nursing because we get satisfaction from it. And we need to do all we can not to let this potential for enjoyment and fulfillment become lost to us through stress.

In her chapter on the "Psychological Problems of Staff and Their Management" in the *Handbook of Psychooncology* (1990), Marguerite Lederberg has some profound advice for nursing professionals. Although she is talking specifically about cancer care, the thoughts expressed are relevant to all aspects of nursing care.

> The features that make working with patients special can cut either way; they can make you feel stressed or make you feel valuable and worthwhile. For example, you can repress anger or you can feel strong enough to be generous. You can feel numb or you can feel capable of tolerating the human condition. You can flee from overemotional encounters or feel privileged to share extraordinary moments. You can feel guilty or you can feel a special gratitude and refined appreciation for life. You can feel intellectually overwhelmed or intellectually challenged. You can feel useless or proud of your unique personal contribution. You can feel alienated or anchored in a valuable human enterprise. [p. 639]

BIBLIOGRAPHY

Arnold, L. J. (1990). Codependency, part I: Origins, characteristics. *Association of Operating Room Nurses Journal, 51*(5), 1341–1348.

Barrera, M., & Ainlay, S. L. (1983). The structure of social support: A conceptual and empirical analysis. *Journal of Community Psychology, 11*(2), 133–143.

Benner, P., & Wrubel, J. (1989). *The primacy of caring.* Menlo Park, CA: Addison Wesley.

Caldwell, T., & Weiner, M. F. (1981). Stresses and coping in ICU nursing: I. A review. *General Hospital Psychiatry*, *3*(2), 119–127.

Campbell, J. (1988). Joseph Campbell and the power of myth (sound recordings). With Bill Moyers. Montauk, NY: Mystic Fire Video.

Cobb, S. (1976). Social support as a moderator of life stress. *Psychosomatic Medicine*, *38*(5), 300–314.

Cunningham, M. (1992). Professional issues in cancer care. In J. Clark & R. McGee, (Eds.), *Core curriculum for oncology nursing*. Philadelphia: W. B. Saunders.

Friedman, N. & Huls, J. (1991). Intimacy: The cornerstone of caring. *American Journal of Hospice and Palliative Care*, *8*(2), 31–5, 44.

Handy, C. M. (1988). Home care of patients with technically complex nursing needs: High technology home care. *Nursing Clinics of North America*, *23*(2), 450–459.

Harris, M. D. (1988). The changing scene in community health nursing. *Nursing Clinics of North America*, *23*(3), 559–568.

Herschbach, P. (1992). Work-related stress specific to physicians and nurses working with cancer patients. *Journal of Psychosocial Oncology*, *10*(2), 79–103.

Hillman, S. M. (1986). Assessing the patient in the home environment. In S. Stuart-Siddall (Ed.), *Home Health Care Nursing*. Rockville, MD: Aspen.

Lazarus, R. S. (1966). *Psychological stress and coping process*. New York: McGraw-Hill.

Lazarus, R. S, & Folkman, S. (1984). *Stress, appraisal and coping*. New York: Springer.

Lederberg, M. (1990). Psychological problems of staff and their management. In J. C. Holland & J. R. Rowland (Eds.), *Handbook of psychooncology*. Oxford: Oxford University Press.

Lewis, A., & Levy, J. (1982). *Psychiatric liaison nursing: The theory and clinical practice*. Reston, VA: Reston.

Marshall, J. (1980). Stress amongst nurses. In C. L. Cooper & J. Marshall (Eds.), *White collar and professional stress*. London: John Wiley & Sons.

Menzies, I. E. P. (1970). *The functioning of social systems as a defense against anxiety*. London: Tavistock Institute.

Monica, E. D. (1988). Documentation. In M. D. Harris (Ed.), *Home health administration*. Owings Mills, MD: National Health.

Morrissey-Ross, M. (1988). Documentation: If you haven't written it, you haven't done it. *Nursing Clinics of North America*, *23*(2), 484–490.

Norbeck, J. S. (1985). Perceived job stress, job satisfaction, and psychological symptoms in critical care nursing. *Research in Nursing & Health*, *8*(3), 253–259.

Norbeck, J. S. (1988). Social support. *Annual Review of Nursing Research*, *6*, 85–109.

Pearlin, L. I., & Aneshensel, C. S. (1986). Coping and social supports: Their function and applications. In L. H. Aiken & D. Mechanic (Eds.), *Applications of social science to clinical medicine and health policy*. New Brunswick: Rutgers University.

Pearlin, L. I., Lieberman, M. A., Menaghan, E. G., & Mullan, J. T. (1981). The stress process. *Journal of Health and Social Behavior*, *22*(4), 652–663.

Racy, J. (1991). Personal and professional intimacy: Drawing the line. In N. Friedman & J. Huls, Intimacy: The cornerstone of caring. *American Journal of Hospice and Palliative Care*, *8*(2), 31–5, 44.

Selye, H. (1978). *The stress of life*. New York: McGraw–Hill.

Snow, C., & Willard, D. (1989). *I'm dying to take care of you...nurses and codependence: Breaking the cycles*. Redmond, WA: Professional Counselor Books.

Volk, E. R. (1988). High-tech home care. In M. D. Harris (Ed.), *Home health administration*. Owings Mills, MD: National Health.

Index

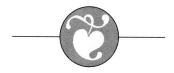

Page numbers followed by *f* indicate figures; those followed by *t* indicate tabular material; those followed by *b* indicate boxed material.

Hypomania, 188b
Hypothalamus, 9, 109, 115
Hypothyroidism, 201t
Hysterectomy, 353–357
Hysterical psychosis, 472
Hysterical traits, 276
ICU (intensive care unit) psychosis, 317
Id, 36–37
  defense mechanisms and, 51
Ideas, flight of, 189
Identification
  as defense mechanisms, 49
  of self, 168
Identity
  maternal, 479–480
  older adult and, 550
  in trauma, 469
Illness. *See also* Coping, stress and
  acute, 461–466. *See also* Acute
      illness
    child and, 512–516
  adaptation to, 460–461
    older adult and, 551–552
  Barry Holistic Systems Model and,
    153
  basic needs in, 273
  chronic, 360–372, 414–417,
    517–520. *See also* Chronic
    illness(es)
  coping risks of, 163–180
    body image and, 169–171
    control and, 171–173
    guilt and, 178–179
    intimacy and, 179–180
    loss and, 173–178
    self-esteem and, 167–169
    trust and, 165–166
  crisis intervention and, 293–294,
    297–298
  drive theory and, 34
  emic versus etic view of, 92
  emotional crisis response to,
    555–556
  ethnic explanatory models and,
    83–84
  explanatory model of, 91–92, 93b
  family and, 6–7, 10, 128–129
  family boundaries and, 137
  meaning of, 127
  older adult and, 546
    challenge for, 549–552
    effect on, 553–555
    emotional crisis and, 555–556
    spouse or significant caregiver
      response to, 552
  perception of, 128–129, 232f, 240,
    461

psychogenic, 51
psychosocial crisis and, 288, 289,
  297–298
psychosocial intervention and,
  301–321. *See also*
    Psychosocial intervention
psychosocial risks of, 11, 235f,
  244–246
stress and, 103–120, 294
terminal, 174, 176–177
Illness behavior, culture and, 82–87
Illusions, psychosocial nursing
  interventions and,
  319
Imagery
  anxiety and, 309–312
  chronically ill child and, 517
  conversational, 309–312
  guided, 379
  visual, 309
Imagery script, 310b–311b
imipramine (Tofranil), 214t
Immature defense mechanisms, 46t,
  47–48
Immature justice, of toddler, 507
Immune system, neurotransmitters
  and, 116, 118
Inadequate personality, 281–282
Independence-dependence, cancer
  and, 423
Inderal (indomethacin), 216t
indomethacin (Indocin), 216t
Industry, 43t
Ineffective coping, 45, 108, 163–164,
  223
  chronic in older adult
    intervention and, 561–563
  nursing diagnoses of
    in family members, 441–442
Infant
  acutely ill
    behavioral and psychiatric
      interventions and,
      513–514
    effects and interventions in, 512
  body image and, 169–170
  drive theory and, 34
  illness and, 507
  psychosocial stages of development
    and, 41–42
  self-esteem and, 167
  trust and, 165, 507
Infection
  cognitive mental disorders and,
    207–210
  depression and, 328b
Inferiority, 43t

Infertility, 340–343
  cancer and, 422
Informal contracts, nurse-patient,
  27
Information
  cancer patient and, 428–429
  crisis and, 287
  effective coping and, 462
  family need for, 466, 467b
  primiparous mother and, 480
  sibling of sick child and, 509
  withholding of, 443
Informed consent, cancer patient
  and, 427
Initiative versus guilt, 43t, 178
Instinct, 34, 45
Instrumental denial, 414
Instrumental support, effective
  coping and, 462
Integration, 61–62
  in trauma, 468
Intellect
  dementia and, 198, 199t
  development of, 39–40
  differentiation of self and, 133
Intellectualization
  caregivers of dying patients and,
    451, 452b
  controlled personality and, 275, 276
Intensive care psychosis, 317
Interactions
  cultural and effective health care,
    87–88
  psychosocial in home care,
    541–543
  social in coping, 462, 463b
Interferons, 420
Interleukins, 420
Internal locus of control, 172–173
Internal resources, 155, 156b
Interpersonal self, 168
Interpersonal styles, 273–281. *See
  also* Personality styles
  assessment interview and, 465–466
  assessment of, 247
  state versus traits and, 274
Interpreter
  guidelines to using, 90b
  roles of, 89–90
Interpreting, 26–27
Intervention
  Barry Holistic Systems Model and,
    154
  case management and, 564
  crisis, 288–292. *See also* Crisis
  interpersonal
    depression and, 328, 329, 331